Essentials of
Health and Wellness

Essentials of Health and Wellness

James Robinson III, EdD, FAAHE

Professor, Department of Social and Behavioral Health
School of Rural Public Health
Texas A&M University System Health Science Center

Deborah J. McCormick, PhD

Assistant Professor
Department of Health Promotion
Northern Arizona University

Technical Writer: **Lee Haroun**, EdD

San Diego, CA

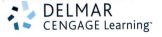
DELMAR
CENGAGE Learning™

Australia • Brazil • Japan • Korea • Mexico • Singapore • Spain • United Kingdom • United States

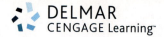

Essentials of Health and Wellness
James Robinson III, Deborah J. McCormick

Vice President, Health Care Business
Unit: William Brottmiller

Editorial Director: Cathy L. Esperti

Acquisitions Editor: Marah Bellegarde

Developmental Editor: Juliet Byington

Editorial Assistant: Erin Adams

Marketing Director: Jennifer McAvey

Marketing Coordinator: Kimberly Duffy

Art and Design Specialist: Jay Purcell

Production Coordinator: Jessica
McNavich

Production Assistant: Kate Kaufman

Project Editor: David Buddle

For product information and technology assistance, contact us at
Cengage Learning Customer & Sales Support, 1-800-354-9706

For permission to use material from this text or product,
submit all requests online at **www.cengage.com/permissions**
Further permissions questions can be emailed to
permissionrequest@cengage.com

Library of Congress Control Number: 2003027377
ISBN-13: 978-1-4018-1523-3
ISBN-10: 1-4018-1523-5

Delmar
Executive Woods
5 Maxwell Drive
Clifton Park, NY 12065
USA

Cengage Learning is a leading provider of customized learning solutions with office locations around the globe, including Singapore, the United Kingdom, Australia, Mexico, Brazil, and Japan. Locate your local office at **international.cengage.com/region**

Cengage Learning products are represented in Canada by Nelson Education, Ltd.

For your course and learning solutions, visit **delmar.cengage.com**

Visit our corporate website at **www.cengage.com**

Printed in the United States of America
4 5 6 7 11 10 09 08

Contents

unit **3**

PHYSICAL HEALTH 135

unit 4

MENTAL HEALTH   223

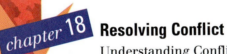

unit 5
SOCIAL HEALTH 295

Preface

Essentials of Health and Wellness is an approachable, inviting, straightforward text that provides high school students with the essential body of health information they can use to develop their health and wellness knowledge and skills. This may be the only health course many students will ever encounter, and the vital skills and behaviors covered will help students develop wellness behaviors now that they will carry into a healthy adulthood. It is also recognized that many school districts have very crowded schedules and are unable to include a full year of health education. The essentials nature of this text provides the student and the teacher with the core information that can easily be covered in a single academic semester but that can also be expanded to fill an entire school year. The many special features and activities included in the text make learning core health and wellness concepts engaging, interesting, and fun. Our goals were to provide a teacher-friendly text that motivates students to practice wellness for a lifetime and to provide a framework for the development of health literacy skills.

ORGANIZATION OF TEXT

The text is composed of 30 chapters that are organized into eight units. The first unit defines and describes health and then develops the wellness concept. The remaining units progress from personal, physical, and mental health issues presented in the early chapters to the more global health issues of family and community later in the text. The text is designed to provide numerous opportunities for student interaction and exercises intended to engage the student in developing a set of wellness skills. Many of these activities, as indicated by a special icon, give students the opportunity to do research, perform interviews, and write down personal information that they can save and refer to later. It is recommended that each student create a *Health Folio* to keep track of his or her personal health information. This can be something as simple as a file folder or as elaborate as a binder system and can be taken with the student after the course is finished so he or she can benefit from this resource on the path toward a healthy adulthood.

CHAPTER ORGANIZATION

Each unit contains a number of chapters related to the central theme of the unit. The teen stories that open each chapter feature a teen dealing with a real wellness issue. Each chapter contains a list of *Chapter Objectives* that can be used to ensure understanding of the noteworthy wellness elements in the chapter. In addition, each chapter opens with a list of *Key Terms* featured in the text along with a glossary entry in the margin for each key term. Early in each chapter is a *Personal Assessment* designed to measure student understanding of the chapter theme or to assess individual student behaviors associated with the chapter's wellness message. Interpretations of the answers to the Personal Assessments are included at the end of each chapter for student review. Special features, photographs, figures, and tables support and enhance key information in each chapter and help keep students engaged with the material. *Glossary Terms* are highlighted in the text and defined in the margins to facilitate comprehension. Each chapter also contains a section called *Building Your Wellness Plan* that empowers the student to take positive steps toward a healthier lifestyle. This unique feature ties key chapter topics with suggestions for healthy actions or wellness behaviors that can easily be incorporated into the student's life. Finally, each chapter concludes with *End-of-Chapter Activities* to reinforce learning. Students can complete short answer and discussion questions as well as test understanding of key vocabulary terms. In addition, there are *Weblinks* that provide dependable Web sites for further information on issues covered in the chapter. And each chapter provides *Application Activities* that connect wellness content to core instruction areas (language arts, mathematics, science, and social studies), allowing teachers to integrate core instruction into the health class.

Features

In addition to many tables and illustrations, each chapter contains a number of feature activities.

- *What's News?* This feature delivers late-breaking research and information on selected topics within each chapter.
- *Did You Know That . . . ?* Students are exposed to little-known facts that can reinforce chapter topics in an entertaining manner.
- *Teen Forum.* Students are presented with a topic that can be viewed from a number of viewpoints. The teen forum responses can be presented in class discussions or in written assignments that are retained in the Health Folio.
- *Take It on Home.* This feature presents wellness issues that teens can discuss with their families. The findings from these family discussions are written up by the student and included in the student Health Folio.

- *Real Teens.* Each chapter includes a story of a real teen who uses his or her health literacy skills to address important wellness topics.
- *Weblinks.* At the end of each chapter are links to Web sites that include more information on chapter topics.
- *Building Your Wellness Plan.* The wellness plan is a self-directed way of developing lifelong wellness skills. The student may find something new to add to the overall wellness plan as he or she goes through each chapter. To assist each student with the development of an overall plan, each chapter includes a wellness plan form to help develop wellness skills for that chapter.

EXTENSIVE TEACHING AND LEARNING PACKAGE

A number of ancillary materials accompany this text. These materials are designed to support student learning and provide the teacher with easy-to-implement activities intended to reinforce learning and skill development.

Teacher's Edition to Accompany Essentials of Health and Wellness

ISBN 1-4018-1524-3

Instructors will find material to support instruction in the *Teacher's Edition to Accompany Essentials of Health and Wellness*. For each chapter there is:

- An outline of chapter content for preparing lessons
- Suggested teaching activities
- Answers to all the end-of-chapter activities
- A chapter quiz and answer key
- A Wellness Plan worksheet to photocopy for student use

Essentials of Health and Wellness Online Companion

ISBN 1-4018-1527-8

Teachers can access a free Web site developed by Delmar Cengage Learning that specifically supports this text with numerous teaching materials, including:

- Lesson plans for each chapter
- Timely health updates
- Classroom activities and accompanying activity worksheets (including Spanish versions)
- PowerPoint presentations that can be used and adapted for lectures
- Teaching tips and tricks

- Sketches of pertinent health and wellness dilemmas students can read aloud, followed by questions to prompt thoughtful discussion
- Additional personal assessments for each chapter
- Material from the *Teacher's Edition* that can be downloaded and printed (in PDF format) for instructor and classroom use

Sexuality Supplement to Accompany Essentials of Health and Wellness

ISBN 1-4018-1525-1

For school districts that desire an expanded sexuality instruction unit, the *Sexuality Supplement* augments the existing content in the core text. In addition to the material in the core text, the *Sexuality Supplement* covers topics such as love and affection, sexual attraction, sexual orientation, sexually transmitted infections, and birth control.

Computerized Test Bank to Accompany Essentials of Health and Wellness

ISBN 1-4018-1526-X

For school districts and instructors who would like a database of over 1,100 questions and answers from which to build test and quizzes, there is the *Computerized Test Bank to Accompany Essentials of Health and Wellness*. For each chapter, as well as for the *Sexuality Supplement*, there are 35 to 40 questions—including true/false, matching, and multiple choice—that can be used as is or modified by teachers to meet their instructional needs.

ABOUT THE AUTHORS

James Robinson, III, EdD, FAAHE

James Robinson is currently professor in the Department of Social and Behavioral Health in the School of Rural Public Health at the Texas A&M University System Health Science Center. Dr. Robinson received his BS in health and physical education and his MEd in health education from West Chester University and his EdD in health education from the University of Northern Colorado. He taught health education for five of his 11 years as a faculty member in the Downingtown Area School District, Downingtown, Pennsylvania. After his doctoral studies, he held faculty appointments at California State University–Northridge, the University of Northern Colorado, and Texas A&M University. Dr. Robinson's health education consultations include school districts in California, Colorado, Texas and Wyoming, as well as the state health and education departments in Colorado and Texas. Dr. Robinson is author or co-author of more than 25 professional publications and has delivered more than 50 professional presentations to local, state, and national audiences. He is currently the co-editor of the *Journal of Drug Education.* Dr. Robinson has served on numerous committees and boards of the American Association for Health Education and the American School Health Association. The American Association for Health Education honored him with Fellow status in 1999 and with the Professional Service Award in 2003. In addition to his teaching, scholarly activity, and service, Dr. Robinson has generated approximately $2.5 million in grant support for his research and projects.

Deborah J. McCormick, PhD

Deborah McCormick is currently an assistant professor in the Department of Health Promotion in the College of Health Professions at Northern Arizona University in Flagstaff, Arizona. She received her BS in health and physical education from the University of Mary Hardin-Baylor, her MS in health and physical education from Baylor University, and her PhD in health education from Texas A&M University. Dr. McCormick has held faculty appointments at Lamar University, University of Texas at San Antonio, and Texas State University. She has delivered more than 50 professional presentations to local, state, and national audiences on topics related to health promotion.

Acknowledgments

A project of this magnitude is not brought to fruition without assistance from many individuals. The authors thank the following professionals who contributed to the development of this text:

Brian L. Clinton, BS, CHES, Health Content Consultant

Daphne Fulton, MPH, Health Content Consultant

Mary Katherine Sanchez, MPH, Health Content Consultant

Beth McNeill, MS, Assessment Consultant

The authors also wish to express their appreciation to those individuals who contributed to the book's production:

Lee Haroun, EdD, whose technical writing expertise added immensely to the completed manuscript

All the students and parents who served as photographic subjects and the organizations who provided photographic subjects

The many individuals who offered suggestions, comments, and professional insights on the first draft of this text. Their feedback was essential in producing a text that meets the needs of high school health educators. Their time and effort is greatly appreciated.

Dr. Robinson would also like to express his heartfelt gratitude to all those who provided personal support for the development of this manuscript:

Dr. Danny Jean Ballard, his wife, friend, and professional colleague, for her patience and willingness to support the project

Dr. Betty Dabney, School of Rural Public Health colleague, for her photographic expertise

Netti-Anne Robinson and James Robinson IV, his teenaged children, for their reviews and comments

Dr. Ciro V. Sumaya, Dean of the School of Rural Public Health, for his friendship and support during the writing of this text

The numerous teenagers in Bryan and College Station, Texas, who provided insightful comments on the text design

Dr. McCormick would like to extend her gratitude and appreciation to the following people for their personal and professional support:

Bradley Sutton, spouse and friend, for his patience and unselfishness during the writing of this text

Dr. Rhonda M. Johnson, Northern Arizona University colleague, for her encouragement both in beginning and completing this project

Family, friends, and professional colleagues for their direct and indirect support during the writing process

REVIEWERS

Amy Beard
Nutritionist
Little Rock, AR

Kathleen Bush, RN
Cedar Bush, UT

Rhonda Dunn, RN
Greenbrier High School
Evans, GA

Janet Gower, RN
Ygnacio Valley High School
Concord, CA

Geoffry Alan Haines
Crooms Academy of Information
Technology
Sanford, FL

Michelle Mancuso, MPH
Public Health Promotion and
Disease Prevention
San Francisco, CA

Dawn Marinich
Fox Lane High School
Carmel, NY

Elisa Elizabeth Huston McNeill
Texas A&M University
College Station, TX

Charlene Parharm
The Academy of Irving ISD
Hurst, TX

Fontina L. Rashid, PhD
Psychologist
Stockton, CA

Cynthia Snyder, Ed.S.
Crooms Academy of Information
Technology
Sanford, FL

Vicki Taylor, RN
Lake Chelan School District
Chelan, WA

How to Use Essentials of Health and Wellness

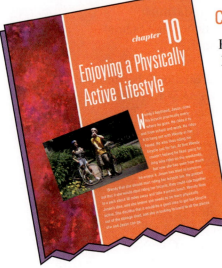

CHAPTER OPENER

Every chapter begins with a story about a teen faced with real-life health and wellness concerns. These stories give you an idea of what you will learn about in the chapter. They are also a place to see how other teens handle different situations and for you to think about what you might do if you were in their place.

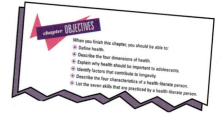

CHAPTER OBJECTIVES

Review this series of goals before you begin reading a chapter to help you focus your study. When you have completed the chapter, review these goals to see if you understand the key points.

KEY TERMS

These are the critical vocabulary words you will need to learn for each chapter. These terms are highlighted within the text, and definitions are included in the margins. You will also find these terms listed in the glossary section at the back of the book. Use this listing as part of your study.

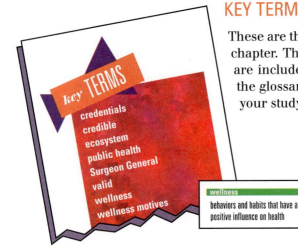

HEALTH FOLIO

Whenever you see this icon, there is a written activity that you can place in your Health Folio. Your Health Folio is a place where you can collect all your personal assessments, Take It on Home reports, Wellness Plans, and other activities. When you have completed your health class, this is a great resource you can refer to.

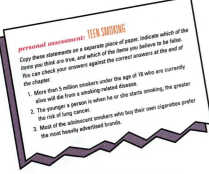

PERSONAL ASSESSMENT

Take the Personal Assessment at the beginning of each chapter. Write your answers on a separate piece of paper and check them against the feedback located at the end of the chapter. Some Personal Assessments give you insight into your personal health and wellness behaviors; others quiz you on what you already know about a topic. These are a fun way to learn more about yourself.

DID YOU KNOW THAT . . . ?

Check out these boxes for interesting facts and trivia. These are a great place to learn more about all kinds of health and wellness issues and will help you grasp the key concepts of each chapter.

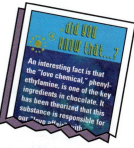

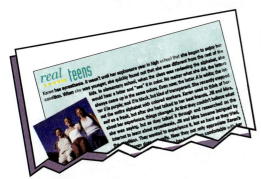

WHAT'S NEWS?

For current events in health, read the What's News? boxes. You'll find interesting information on new health-related research and hot topics. This is a good place to see how the information covered in the chapter has real-life applications.

TAKE IT ON HOME

These activities ask you to share what you are learning about health and wellness with your family and to ask them questions about their experiences. This is a chance for you to learn more about your family and to help keep them thinking about health and wellness. Take notes of your discussions with your family members and keep these in your Health Folio.

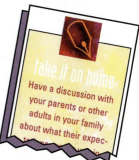

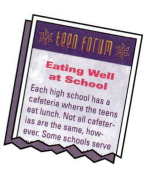

REAL TEENS

These stories are your chance to see how other teens deal with health and wellness challenges and dilemmas. Use this feature to better understand the information being presented and to think about what you might do if you were in that teen's shoes.

TEEN FORUM

Use the Teen Forums to spark critical thinking and classroom debate. Each Teen Forum presents an issue related to the information in the chapter and asks you for your opinion. You can think about the issue yourself, or you can discuss it with classmates, friends, or family members.

BUILDING YOUR WELLNESS PLAN

Health and wellness is more than something you learn about in books; it is a way of life. Your wellness plan is a list of actions you can take to develop positive health behaviors now that will follow you into adulthood. These boxes look at information you learned about in the chapter and offer suggestions for applying that information to your life.

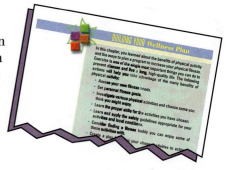

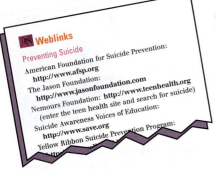

WEBLINKS

Use these dependable weblinks to find more detailed health and wellness information on the Internet.

SHORT-ANSWER AND DISCUSSION QUESTIONS

Use these questions to review what you know about the information in each chapter. Short-answer questions are looking for just a few words in the answers, whereas discussion questions are looking for more complete, thought-out explanations of your answer.

CHAPTER VOCABULARY

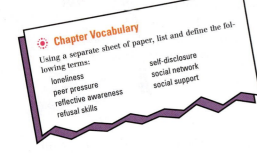

Test your understanding of key chapter terms by defining the chapter vocabulary on a separate piece of paper. You can check your definitions against the glossary at the back of the book.

APPLICATION ACTIVITIES

The information and behaviors you learn in your health class have many applications to science, math, language arts, and social studies. Use the application activities to learn about health and wellness while you practice the skills you've learned in your other classes, such as writing, math, research, and analysis.

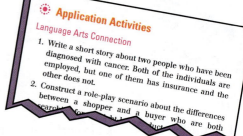

unit 1

Developing Health and Wellness Skills

Introduction

Who's responsible for your health? If you answered, "I am," congratulations! You have taken a giant step forward into adulthood. For much of your life, your health was probably in the hands of others: family members, doctors, nurses, or other adults. As an adult, you will be completely responsible for taking care of yourself. You may also have some responsibility for taking care of the health needs of your family members. You can prepare for those responsibilities by learning all you can about ways to prevent illness and injuries. The information and activities in this book and the things you will do in your classroom are designed to help you prepare for a healthy adulthood.

You will learn that threats to your health come in many forms. Some threats are biological, like bacteria and viruses; some are chemical, such as pesticides; others, like drug abuse, are social in nature. Recognizing these threats or risks is an important first step in maintaining your health. The purpose of this unit is to help you to learn more about health and the concept of wellness and to develop skills that will help you practice behaviors that keep you well.

chapter 1

Health for Adolescents

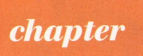

Corey often thinks about her future. As do many teens, she wonders what the coming years hold for her. She is happy that she is able to do well in school. She works very hard to learn and earn good grades. She is also happy that she is in good health. She appreciates the help and support she gets from her family to make good health decisions. Corey is sure that with her good health and the energy that comes with it, she will be able to achieve all the goals she has planned for her future.

chapter OBJECTIVES

When you finish this chapter, you should be able to:

- ☀ Define health.
- ☀ Describe the four dimensions of health.
- ☀ Explain why health should be important to adolescents.
- ☀ Identify factors that contribute to longevity.
- ☀ Describe the four characteristics of a health-literate person.
- ☀ List the seven skills that are practiced by a health-literate person.

key TERMS

chronic diseases
diabetes
genes
health literacy
homeostasis
infectious diseases
life expectancy
metabolic rate
optimal health
osteoporosis

Introduction

Before you begin reading this chapter, take a few moments and think about the kind of life you want for yourself, now and in the future. Chances are, you want to feel well and have plenty of energy for your daily activities and the things you like to do. The good news is that no other group of young people in history has had as much personal control over their own health as you do. What you are learning today can make the difference in how long and how well you will live.

The teen years can be both exciting and challenging. It is exciting that you are becoming more independent and enjoying more freedom than you did as a child. It is challenging because you have more responsibility and are learning the life skills you will need as an adult. Some of the most important of these skills are related to your health and well-being. This book and your health class will provide you with the information you need to make good decisions about your health. By taking advantage of these learning opportunities, you can better enjoy your teen years and lay the foundation for the future as a happy, healthy, productive adult.

personal assessment: HEALTH AND MY BEHAVIORS

Think about the things you are doing or not doing that can have an effect on your health. On a separate piece of paper, indicate for each of the following behaviors if it is true or not true for you. Feedback is at the end of the chapter.

1. I currently have all the immunizations I am supposed to have.
2. I do not smoke cigarettes.
3. I make an effort to eat fruit and vegetables every day.
4. I choose not to use drugs or alcohol.
5. I use a safety belt every time I ride in an automobile.
6. I am able to deal with stressful situations without anger or urgency.
7. I have someone I can talk to when I need help solving problems.
8. I can communicate well with members of my family.
9. I make decisions that are good for my health and act on them.

YOU AND YOUR HEALTH

Tremendous progress has been made in medical research and in the development of cures and treatments for diseases and injuries. We understand more about how the human body works—and does not work—than at any time in history. Until about 60 years ago, possibly within the lifetime of your grandparents, the major killers of humans were **infectious diseases**, over which people had little control. Until the discovery of vaccines and antibiotics, people had few ways to protect themselves from infection and disease. Without the variety of modern drugs and advanced surgical techniques commonly available today, people who were seriously ill or injured in the past had little chance of surviving. Look at Table 1-1 and examine the differences between the leading causes of death in 1900 and 2002. You will see that there are distinct differences among the top three causes of death.

Today, the three leading causes of death in the United States are not infectious diseases; they are heart disease, cancer, and stroke. All three of these leading causes of death are greatly influenced by how we live. You may think that these, and other serious diseases such as **diabetes** and **osteoporosis**, are for older people to worry about. But there is evidence that many of the habits you practice when you are young will determine the state of your health in later adulthood. Your eating habits and how much you exercise, for example, not only affect how fit and healthy you are now but also may affect how long you live and how well you live.

infectious diseases

diseases caused by organisms that can spread through water, food, air, or human contact

diabetes

disease in which the pancreas does not produce enough insulin, which is needed to properly use sugar for energy

osteoporosis

a condition in which the bones lose their density and strength

Table 1-1 Leading Causes of Death in the United States, 1900 and 2002

1900		2002	
Cause of Death	**Number of Deaths per 100,000 People**	**Cause of Death**	**Number of Deaths per 100,000 People**
Pneumonia and influenza	202	Heart disease	258
Tuberculosis	194	Cancer	201
Diarrhea, abdominal infections	143	Stroke	61
Heart disease	137		44
Senility, ill-defined death, or unknown	117	Accidents	36
Stroke	110	Diabetes	25
Kidney disease	89	Pneumonia and influenza	24
Accidents	72	Alzheimer's disease	18
Cancer	64	Kidney disease	13
Diphtheria	40	Blood infection	11

THE HEALTH CONTINUUM

Your health is constantly changing, varying from day to day and even from hour to hour. Sometimes changes come suddenly; you wake up one morning with a fever and a headache. At other times, changes are not quite as obvious. As a person ages, his or her body may develop conditions that lead to heart disease or cancer and the person may not feel any symptoms at all. Because a person can have an illness without feeling symptoms, as we get older, it is a good idea to get medical examinations that detect illnesses such as these.

The health continuum was developed to show changes in health. Figure 1-1 illustrates how health can range from **optimal health**, the highest level of health a person can possibly have, to life-threatening illness.

Your health does not usually remain at its optimal level for long periods at a time. If you are a typical teen, however, your level of health will often be close to the optimal end of the continuum. When physical health problems do develop, **homeostasis** is interrupted and the body

optimal health

the condition in which a person is the healthiest he or she can possibly be

homeostasis

the state of balance in which all the body's systems are working in harmony

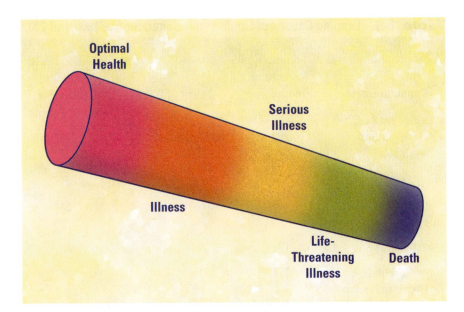

Figure 1-1
The health continuum

gets out of balance. Injuries, such as a strained muscle, and bodily reactions, such as a fever, disrupt homeostasis. When homeostasis is disrupted, the body works overtime to return to a balanced state. The more serious the illness or condition, the greater is the struggle for homeostasis. What do you think are the effects of a serious injury on the body's homeostasis?

WHAT DO WE MEAN BY "HEALTH"?

How would you define *health*? Is it the way you feel? Does it mean not being sick? Most people think of health as a physical condition, but it is much more than that. Health is a measure of how we feel physically, mentally, socially, and spiritually at any point in time. Are you surprised to see the words *mentally*, *socially*, and *spiritually* in a definition of health? The World Health Organization (WHO), an agency of the United Nations, expanded the definition of health in 1948, when it was created to work on international health issues. Members of the WHO believed that they should be concerned about the total quality of a person's life. Their definition of health states that it is "a state of complete physical, mental and social well-being and not merely the absence of disease or infirmity." It is now common to describe four dimensions of health, which all have an effect on the quality of our lives:

1. Physical health

2. Mental and emotional health

3. Social health

4. Spiritual health

Your Physical Health

Physical health refers to the condition of your body. For example, it includes the state of your muscles, organs, and bones. When your physical health is affected, you may experience signs or symptoms that include pain and discomfort. Common examples are stomach pain, headaches, painful joints, and a sore throat. Some teens have unhealthy physical conditions, such as leukemia or early HIV infection, but have no obvious symptoms. What are some symptoms that let you know you may have problems with your physical health? Can you think of other examples of illnesses or conditions that don't have symptoms?

Your Mental and Emotional Health

Mental and emotional health refers to the state of your mind and the ability to balance your emotions. It includes how you react to conditions around you. For example, a measure of mental health is how you respond to stress and the problems of daily life. A person who has poor mental health may respond to normal situations with unusual or inappropriate behavior.

People often fail to recognize the symptoms of poor mental and emotional health. They may be unaware that their behavior is unusual. Lack of self-awareness can be one of the signs of poor mental health. Many people don't spend much time thinking about their mental health until they have trouble dealing with daily life. Even then, it may take a friend or family member to encourage them to seek medical help.

Are you satisfied with your ability to handle stress? Would you feel comfortable seeking counseling or medical help if you had trouble coping with daily life? Would you encourage a friend or family member to seek help if it appeared to you that he or she was mentally or emotionally unhealthy? These are important things to consider as you enter adulthood and encounter new, perhaps stressful, experiences.

Your Social Health

Social health refers to the quality of the relationships you have with other people. It is a measure of how you get along with all types of people, from family and close friends to people you do not know well. The degree of tolerance and respect you have for others is part of social health. Your ability to develop and maintain friendships that add value to your life is another measure of your social health. Problems with social health can seem especially troublesome to teens because this is a period of life when having friends and being accepted by **peers** is very important.

did you know that...?

The music at rock concerts can get as loud as 110 decibels. This is the same level of intensity as a gunshot or jet engine. Do you think this noise level can damage a person's hearing? What might be the long-term effects of attending many rock concerts? Learning about conditions that can damage your body and making sensible choices on the basis of this information are part of accepting responsibility for your own health.

peers

people in your age group; those with whom you have something in common, such as level of education, musical interests, or religion

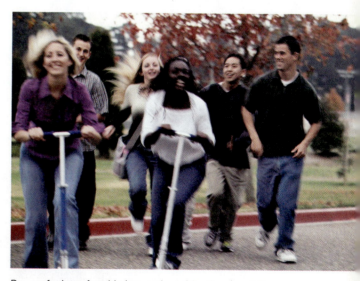

Do you feel comfortable interacting with other people? Do you have friends you feel you can trust? Do you think people can learn to be socially healthy?

Your Spiritual Health

Spiritual health refers to the values on which you base your life. It reflects the forces that have shaped your morals. Morals are the beliefs that guide your decisions about what is right and wrong. Stated another way, they are your standards of behavior.

Spiritual health does not necessarily refer to religious beliefs, although for many people it does. Spiritual health is that part of us that goes beyond the physical and mental and considers the meaning of life. Of all the dimensions of health, spiritual health is the most difficult to measure.

What are the factors in your life that contribute to your spiritual health? What might be a sign that you are having trouble with your spiritual health? These are good questions to ask yourself as you determine your overall personal health.

Your Total Picture of Health

When determining your overall state of health, evaluate all four dimensions. The dimensions may be on different levels as shown in Figure 1-2. For example, a person with good physical health but very poor social health would not be described as having a high level of overall health. Consider the case of Jim, a varsity football player. Jim is in great playing condition but has a short temper, often gets into fights, and has been in trouble with the law. Lately, he has been trying to develop his spiritual self to overcome his social and mental weaknesses. Although Jim is physically strong and fit, his social health and emotional health are weak. It is important to remember that health is more than if

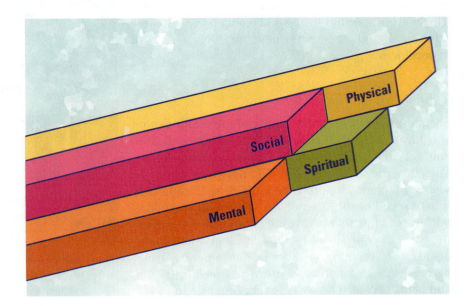

Figure 1-2
The dimensions of health

you feel good or bad in a physical sense. It will be in your best interest to be mindful of all four dimensions so that when you plan ways to achieve and maintain good health you can attend to all of your health dimensions.

How the Four Dimensions of Health Interact

Do you know anyone who has become physically ill from stress? We are learning that the four dimensions of our health are interconnected. Medical researchers are discovering more about how emotional stress can cause physical symptoms. Some activities, once considered to be only emotional or spiritual in nature, appear to have an influence on physical health. Meditation, which simply means clearing the mind of thoughts, is one example. Meditation has been shown to influence physical health by lowering the blood pressure. High blood pressure is a contributing factor to stroke and heart disease.

WHY SHOULD HEALTH BE IMPORTANT TO YOU?

An ancient proverb states, "He who has health has hope, and he who has hope has everything." Do you agree with this proverb? Many people believe that good health is more important than money or fame. In fact, good health increases your chances for achieving whatever it is you want in your life. Dealing with injuries and illnesses makes it difficult to participate fully in the activities you want to do. You can't perform well in a sport if you are injured or sick. It's difficult to do well in your classes if you are sick much of the time. Even hanging out with friends is not enjoyable if you do not feel well. Being healthy makes life more fun.

Good health also means having enough energy for study, work, and play. There are many demands on teens these days. Maybe you participate in sports or other school or community activities and have a job, in addition to your responsibilities at home. The more you do and want to do, the more important it is to have good health.

How would you rate your overall health? Do you feel well most of the time and have the energy you need? Are there any health dimensions you want to work on improving?

Good Health Starts Now

What you do now will influence your future health. Believe it! Good habits started now will have a cumulative effect because some of the things you do now will encourage you to develop other healthy practices as you grow older. Healthy behaviors help reduce the risks of getting diseases. This statement is especially true for **chronic diseases**. They are often caused by a lifetime of poor health choices that can cause serious problems later in life. In the same way, a lifetime of good choices can contribute to a healthy adulthood and old age.

chronic diseases

diseases that last for a long time with little change

An example of a good choice is choosing to eat well, maintaining a healthy weight now. Doing so will make it easier to keep a healthy weight when you are an adult. A healthy weight reduces your risk of developing heart disease and diabetes. An example of a poor choice is choosing to smoke. Almost all adults who die from lung cancer started smoking in their teens. The cumulative effects of years of tobacco exposure can lead to tragic results. The choice is now yours; good health behaviors now for good health later or bad health behaviors now for health risks as you get older. Do you have any habits you would like to change to increase your chances of being a healthy adult?

Your Life Expectancy

How would you like to live to be 100 years old? Living to that age was once considered rare, but more and more people are living for an entire century or even longer. The number of years that a person might live is called **life expectancy**. It is usually stated in terms of life expectancy at birth, but it can be determined at any age. The number of years given as one's life expectancy is the estimated years of life remaining. For example, a teen who has a life expectancy at age 16 of almost 62.5 years should live to be about 79 years old. A person who is 50 years old and has a life expectancy of about 26 years should live to be 76 years old.

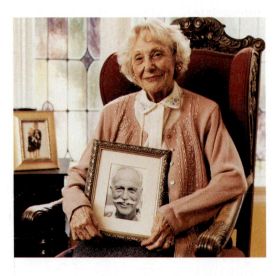

Life expectancies are determined by health scientists when they analyze the death certificates for every age. An interesting fact is that, at birth, females in the United States have a longer life expectancy than males. In fact, they can expect to live six years longer. Why do you think females have a longer life expectancy than males?

There is no single thing that helps a person live a long time. The length of time that a person lives is called **longevity**. Your longevity is influenced by several factors:

- Heredity
- Personal health behaviors
- Environment
- Economics

Heredity

You inherited traits, such as eye color, from your mother and father. Each parent contributed 50% of the traits that make up the unique person you are. Some traits, such as hair color, skin tone, and height, can be seen. Some traits, such as **metabolic rate**, cannot be seen. These biological traits were passed to you from the **genes** you received from your father and mother at the time you were conceived.

life expectancy

a measure of how long a person has left to live based on data related to current causes of death

longevity

the length of a person's life

metabolic rate

the rate at which your body uses food and oxygen to carry out various body processes

genes

the small units of hereditary material found inside the nucleus of a cell

Some of what you inherit has an influence on your health. For example, your metabolic rate has an impact on how easy it is for you to maintain your weight at a healthy level. Some health conditions, such as heart disease and diabetes, are more likely to occur in someone who has family members who had the disease than in someone whose family members did not have the disease.

Personal Health Behaviors

Your personal health behaviors and habits have more influence on how long and how well you will live than do heredity, environment, or economics. Many people rely on doctors and hospitals to keep them well, but evidence shows that since the 1960s the greatest contribution to increasing life expectancy in the United States is related to good health practices. Medicine cannot cure every illness and repair every injury. Your own actions have the most power in determining your level of health.

Environment

Some events that occur in your environment are beyond your control. For example, in places where there is war, disease, or natural disasters, people might not live as long as people in safer environments. Less dramatic examples of environmental factors that affect health include air pollution and toxic waste, which can cause health problems and shorten people's life expectancy.

Economics

People with higher levels of education and more financial resources tend to live longer than people with less education and fewer financial resources. When people cannot afford preventive care or medical attention when they first notice symptoms, they tend to wait until health problems become serious and are more difficult to successfully treat. Health insurance is one way to pay for health care, but it can be too expensive for many people. In fact, the Centers for Disease Control and Prevention (CDC) reported that in 2000 there were 45 states in which 10%–20% of the adults did not have adequate health insurance.

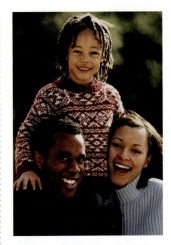

Your parents gave you genes that contribute to your health status and your appearance.

did you know that...?

In 1776, a person's life expectancy at birth was 23 years of age.

In 1900, a person's life expectancy at birth was about 48 years of age.

In 2001, a person's life expectancy at birth was about 77 years of age.

What do you think contributed to the increase?

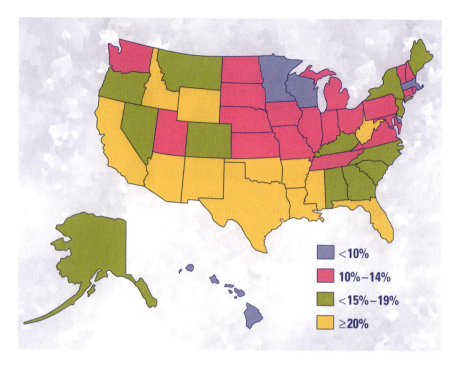

Figure 1-3
Adults (18–64 years old) with no health insurance, 2000

- ■ <10%
- ■ 10%–14%
- ■ <15%–19%
- ■ ≥20%

Living Well

Life quality is determined not only by how long you live but also by how well you live. Although some health conditions are to be expected with aging, you want to have optimal health as long as possible. As an older adult, you'll want to feel well and have the energy and ability to do the things you enjoy. But having good health is not something that will just happen. Part of becoming an adult is getting involved in making the right decisions and practicing the behaviors that lead to good

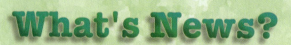

What's News?

School officials across the country are concerned about the weight students are carrying in their backpacks. Each year about 5,000 young people end up in emergency rooms for treatment of backpack-related injuries, according to the U.S. Consumer Product Safety Commission. Some schools have addressed the problem by setting a rotating schedule for homework assignments to lessen the load. In 2002, at least two states were attempting to pass laws that would limit the total weight of the textbooks in a student's backpack.

The American Society of Pediatrics recommends that students carry no more than 10%–20% of their body weight and that backpacks should typically weigh less than 15 pounds. If you carry a backpack, you may want to weigh it. If it is too heavy and you carry it on one shoulder, you increase the risk of injury or deformity. It is best to carry your backpack on both shoulders.

health. The first step is to recognize that there are things you can do now to help make your life both long and healthy. The information in this book and the activities you do in class will help you develop behaviors and habits that will increase your chances for a long, healthy, enjoyable life.

Financial Benefits

Good health can help you financially. People who practice good health habits tend to miss few days of work, to have a high level of energy throughout the workday, and to be productive. Individuals who take responsibility for their health also have lower health care expense than do people with poor health habits. In the United States, we spend more than $1 trillion each year on health care. This means that our average cost for each person is more than $5,000 per year.

If more people practiced good health habits, we would all save money. Healthy individuals use fewer medical services than do unhealthy persons. A reduction in the use of medical services would reduce the cost that insurance companies pay for services. In turn, insurance companies could charge less for health insurance. In this case, we would all win – more healthy people and fewer dollars spent.

In addition to enjoying financial benefits, when you practice good health habits you become a positive example for others, including family members and friends. Children often look up to and copy the behavior of teens. You might be surprised at how much influence you have on the people around you.

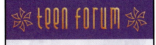

Paying for Health Care

People who practice poor health habits tend to be sick more often than people who do all they can to practice good health behaviors. Those who smoke cigarettes, for example, eventually need to use more health resources than nonsmokers. Some health professionals believe that individuals who practice poor health habits, such as smoking, should be required to pay more for their health care than do people, such as nonsmokers, with good health habits.

- Do you agree or disagree? Explain your response.

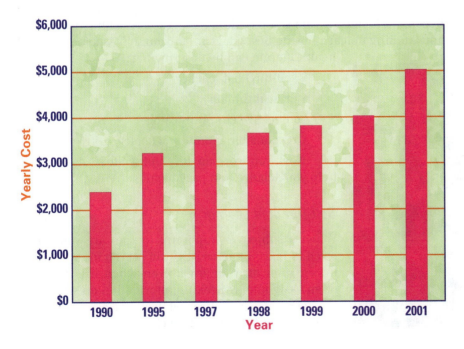

Figure 1-4
Costs of health care per person

DEVELOPING YOUR HEALTH LITERACY SKILLS

Do you know where to find reliable information about health topics? Can you take care of simple injuries, such as cuts or bruises? These are skills that demonstrate **health literacy**, the ability to obtain, interpret, understand, and apply basic health information and services. People who are health literate can properly use the information and services to advance their own health and the health of others. Here are more examples of health literacy skills:

- Interpreting a doctor's written instructions
- Correctly using a prescribed medication
- Understanding a hospital's billing statement
- Using library resources to design a nutrition program
- Recognizing the symptoms of common diseases
- Locating valid health information on the Internet
- Understanding basic health and medical terms
- Knowing when to consult a doctor

If you are health literate, you increase your chances for enjoying good health. It is estimated that 90 million adults in the United States have limited health literacy skills. This group had more visits to the doctor and required more hospitalization than did people with higher health literacy skills. This group's care resulted in $73 billion spent on health care.

The Health-Literate Person

Becoming health literate starts with believing that health is important and wanting to learn how to best take care of yourself. A person who is health literate can be described as:

- A self-directed learner
- A critical thinker
- An effective communicator
- A responsible member of society

Next, you work on developing life skills that will help you acquire and practice positive health habits.

Self-Directed Learner

When a subject is important to you, are you interested in learning more? Do you search for additional information on your own, even when it is not part of an assignment? Seeking information on your own is a sign of a self-directed learner, a person who doesn't limit learning to the classroom or to what he

health literacy

the ability to obtain, interpret, understand, and apply basic health information and services

Health literacy begins with you!

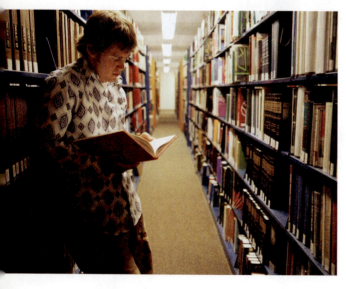

or she learns from family members. Classroom learning serves as a starting point for lifelong learning.

Because health affects the quality of your life now and in the future, health is much more than a subject to study in school. As a self-directed learner, you will seek additional information to help you make good health choices. Medical science is changing so rapidly that some of what you are learning now may be outdated in only a year or two. Scientists are continually learning more about how we function and are discovering new treatments and drugs. Think of your health class as a good foundation for future learning.

Critical Thinker

When you hear something presented as a fact, do you look for ways to make sure that the information is correct? Do you try to solve difficult problems by comparing several possible solutions before deciding what to do? Critical thinkers listen, observe, and read carefully to gather information. They check the credibility of their sources and learn to distinguish between **facts** and **opinions**.

Many popular health **fads** you hear about today, especially those that advertise easy cures for difficult problems, are not based on scientific evidence. It is important to apply critical-thinking skills to make choices that are helpful instead of useless or even harmful.

Effective Communicator

Can you express yourself to others so they understand what you mean? Do you listen attentively when others are speaking? Effective communicators give clear messages and listen carefully to incoming messages. They check their understanding by asking questions and using **feedback**. Feedback results in exchanges that are helpful to both you and others.

Giving accurate and complete information is an important health literacy skill. This does not mean you have to be a great speaker. It simply means that you take the time and make the effort to give accurate and complete health information to others in a form they can understand and use.

Responsible Member of Society

Do you participate in community activities such as food drives for the poor? Are you willing to volunteer for projects that make your community a safer place to live? Responsible members of society take an interest in the health and needs of others. They stay away from activities that threaten their own health or the health of others. Responsible people realize that their actions can make a positive difference in their community.

did you know that...?

The increase in life expectancy Americans now enjoy is the result of people's use of health information and health education to create improved health behaviors. Practicing healthy behaviors has done more for improving health than has the advancement of medical procedures.

fact

something that has actually occurred or has been proved to be true

opinion

a belief based on what seems to be true rather than on tested knowledge

fad

something that is very popular for a short period of time

feedback

a way to check if you understand what someone has said. A common method is to restate in your own words what you heard and to ask the speaker if this is what he or she meant

real teens

Carlos has been driving for about a year now. He likes driving and thinks he is a pretty good driver. Until recently he wasn't in the habit of wearing his seat belt. He knew that state law required every-one in the vehicle to wear their seat belts, but he figured this law didn't really apply to him because he was such a good driver. Why use a seat belt if he was never going to have an accident? He thought it was kind of cool to be a confident driver who didn't need to worry about stuff like that. Besides, Carlos had heard of people who had died in accidents because they were wearing seat belts and got trapped in burning cars, so seat belts didn't sound so safe after all.

One day Carlos read something in the newspaper that changed his mind. A girl at another high school was out with friends one night when their car was hit by someone who ran a stop sign. The girl was killed when she was thrown from the car. A police officer was quoted as saying the girl would probably have survived the accident if she had been wearing a seat belt. This story got Carlos to thinking that he needed to find out more about whether seat belts are really worth using. After all, no matter how good a driver Carlos is, he can't control people with bad driving skills or people who are careless or even under the influence of drugs or alcohol. Someone else could be at fault and cause an accident. Carlos had to do a report for his language arts class at school, so he decided to research the value of seat belts. He learned how to search the Web to find information and research reports from the National Highway Traffic Safety Administration. Carlos discovered that seat belts do save lives. The thing that really convinced him to wear his seat belt was a new advertising slogan: "When you are going to crash, how fast can you buckle up?" It took Carlos a few weeks to really get in the habit of buckling up, but now he won't drive without fastening his seat belt.

HEALTH LITERACY SKILLS

How would you rate yourself today on health literacy? This textbook and your health class provide you with many learning opportunities to become health literate and to make good health choices to fulfill your potential for a healthy, happy life. You will be challenged to develop your skills in seven areas:

1. Understanding health promotion and disease prevention
   - Knowing about the policies and programs organized by the government and private agencies to promote good health
   - Promoting and participating in the activities sponsored by those organizations

Examples: Participating in the Walk for Multiple Sclerosis to raise funds

Volunteering for community cleanup projects at public parks

2. Accessing valid health information and health-promoting products and services
   - Knowing where to gather reliable information
   - Investigating to see if the information is based on facts

   Examples: Researching and evaluating products that promise quick and easy weight loss

   Finding out where a friend can receive free medical care

3. Practicing health-enhancing behaviors
   - Learning about healthy behaviors
   - Making the behaviors lifelong habits

   Examples: Finding a sport or activity to enjoy at least three times a week

   Visiting the dentist regularly

4. Recognizing the influence of culture, media, technology, and other factors on health
   - Learning to examine ideas you have always taken for granted
   - Examining your beliefs in view of what you learn about health
   - Learning to resist pressures to engage in unsafe behaviors

   Examples: Deciding to eat fewer fast foods after studying the basics of nutrition

   Turning down someone's offer of a cigarette at a party

5. Using communication skills to promote health
   - Listening attentively to information about health topics
   - Orally explaining in a clear manner

   Examples: Describing health concerns to a physician

   Explaining a first aid technique to a friend

6. Setting goals and making decisions
   - Making plans to achieve optimal health
   - Designing and following health improvement programs for yourself
   - Gathering information and thinking about alternatives when making decisions

   Examples: Creating an exercise program you can stick with

   Deciding whether to get a job on the weekends or to spend the time studying and participating in outdoor activities

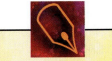

take it on home

Use the information from the health literacy section to make up a short questionnaire to measure health literacy. Ask each of your family members to take the questionnaire. Ask if they think more about their personal health now than they did when they were your age. Do they wish they had done anything differently? Are there habits they started as teenagers they have found difficult to change? Write a summary of their responses and compare the summary with your own health literacy skills.

advocate

to speak or write in support of something or someone

7. **Advocating** for personal, family, and community health
   • Being willing to state that health is important
   • Speaking out about health issues

   Examples: Explaining to a friend the dangers of use of illegal drugs

   Sharing with family members what you've learned in your health class about nutrition

BUILDING YOUR Wellness Plan

This chapter provided you with information about the different dimensions of health. You also learned that health is a condition that is measured at any point in time and is always changing. The remaining portion of this book and the work you do in your classroom will focus on a new concept: wellness. In the next chapter, you will learn about wellness and the first steps you can take toward developing a personal wellness plan. Your wellness plan will become a collection of ideas to be put into action as you practice wellness.

You may want to create a personal folder, file, or notebook to use as your Health Folio. The Health Folio will be a place to store copies of your personal assessments, chapter activities, and wellness plans. You may also include other papers and projects that are assigned by your teacher. This is a great way for you to keep track of your health!

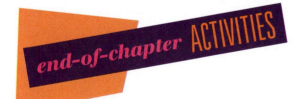

end-of-chapter ACTIVITIES

Weblink

Alliance for Aging Research:
  http://www.livingto100.com

Short-Answer Questions

1. Name the four dimensions of health.
2. List three reasons why health is important to teens and adults.
3. List four factors that would be described as environmental conditions that can affect health.
4. Name three things that can influence life expectancy.
5. List the characteristics of a health-literate person.

Discussion Questions

1. Develop a list of reasons why practicing good health behavior is important.

2. Explain the significance of the four dimensions of health.

3. Diagram and explain what is meant by the health continuum.

4. List and describe the characteristics of a health-literate person.

5. List and discuss the seven skills of a health-literate person.

Chapter Vocabulary

Using a separate sheet of paper, list and define the following terms:

chronic diseases	infectious diseases
diabetes	life expectancy
genes	metabolic rate
health literacy	optimal health
homeostasis	osteoporosis

Application Activities

Language Arts Connection

Imagine that you are 10 years older than you are now. You just heard from your local hospital that it wants to begin an experimental program designed to save the facility money and make health care less expensive for people who practice good health habits. Your task is to write a letter to the hospital listing and explaining the things you do to keep yourself healthy. Use the search you performed for health literacy and identify your health literacy skills in the letter.

Math Connection

Go to your school or community library. Use a computer, encyclopedia, or almanac to find tables on life expectancy. Explore various ways of determining life expectancy. Look for the life expectancies of people who are the following ages: newborn, 5 years, your age, 30 years, 50 years, and 70 years. If you add the corresponding life expectancies from the tables to these ages, are the total years the same for all the ages listed? Explain why you think they are or are not the same.

Social Studies Connection

Gather information about your own life expectancy. Conduct a search on the Web. You can visit the sites listed in this chapter or enter "life expectancy" into a search engine. Visit more than one site and look for information about the factors that affect your life expectancy. Write a summary of those factors. Include a section at the end of your paper that contains two health behavior goals you would like to add to your personal behaviors that could have a positive effect on your longevity.

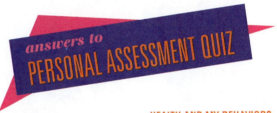

answers to PERSONAL ASSESSMENT QUIZ

personal assessment: HEALTH AND MY BEHAVIORS

It is hoped that you answered "true" to each of the personal assessment statements, but you may not have. You will see, as you progress through this book and your health course, that each of the behaviors listed can be good for your health.

chapter 2

The Wellness Lifestyle

Life is much more enjoyable when you have good health than when you are sick or injured. Being outdoors and having a good time with friends is a lot of fun. Brendon and Lisa like getting outside to visit beaches, parks, and other outdoor attractions. Whenever they get the chance, they gather up a few friends and go. Both Brendon and Lisa find outdoor activities to be much more fun than staying home watching television. They really enjoy the time outdoors together hiking, picnicking, and exploring new places. These teens may not realize it, but they have chosen activities that provide healthy benefits. They will be learning about wellness this year in school and will see how outdoor activities are related to wellness.

chapter OBJECTIVES

When you finish this chapter, you should be able to:

- Explain the relationship between health and wellness.
- Describe several wellness behaviors that protect and promote health.
- Explain the purpose of the nation's health objectives.
- List the Leading Health Indicators.
- Describe the various forms of wellness.
- Explain how to develop a personal wellness plan.
- List and describe criteria for evaluating the validity of health Web sites.

Introduction

In Chapter 1, you learned about the importance of health. You also learned that health refers to much more than just how you feel physically. Health is a measure of your physical, social, mental, and spiritual condition at any point in time.

If someone asked you right now, "How are you doing?" you would quickly do a mental check of yourself. Your answer could be, "Fine, except for my headache." Or perhaps, "Well, I'm upset that I didn't get the job I wanted." You may complete a quick assessment, think about all your health dimensions, and say, "I'm great!" Describing how you *are* takes into account all the dimensions of your life.

Reaching optimal health is a goal most people can agree is important. In this chapter, you will learn about practicing wellness to attain that goal. Your knowledge of wellness behaviors and how to apply them to your life can make the difference in the level of health you reach now and in the future.

key TERMS

credentials
credible
ecosystem
public health
Surgeon General
valid
wellness
wellness motives

personal assessment: MY HEALTH HABITS

Copy the questions listed below onto a sheet of paper and then answer each one with a yes or no. Keep the paper in your Health Folio to use later. Feedback is at the end of the chapter, but you can also read on to see how your answers can affect your future.

1. Do you avoid the use of tobacco?
2. Do you exercise regularly?
3. Do you believe you maintain a normal weight?
4. Do you restrict your eating between meals?
5. Do you eat breakfast every day?
6. Do you sleep at least eight hours each night?
7. Do you avoid the use of alcohol?

WELLNESS AND HEALTH

wellness

behaviors and habits that have a positive influence on health

Wellness is the process that gives you personal power over your health. Whereas health is a measure of how you feel at any point in time, **wellness** means practicing behaviors that have a positive effect on your health. The goal of wellness behaviors is to move you along the health continuum toward optimal health. You can see in Figure 2-1 that wellness develops with education and produces behaviors that result in good health.

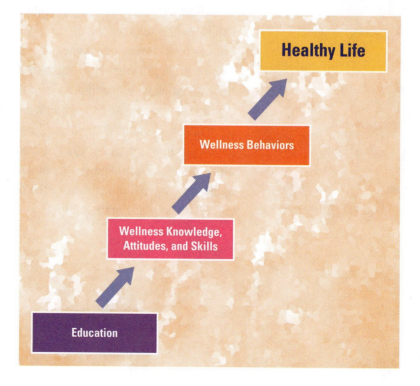

Figure 2-1
The relationship between learning and health

Wellness can be practiced by all people regardless of their health condition. For example, two young women are leaving a hospital at the same time after recovering from serious accidents. They both suffered spinal cord injuries, and neither is expected to walk again. One of the patients, Kathy, feels miserable about her injuries and refuses to see her friends. She spends her time feeling angry and sad. Marta, the other patient, has been grateful for visits from her friends and family. She looks forward to their continued support and hopes one day to participate in activities such as the Wheelchair Olympics. Both young women may be low on the physical health dimension, but Marta is practicing wellness behaviors and, as a result, is much healthier overall than Kathy. Can a person with a spinal cord injury obtain optimal health? Why or why not?

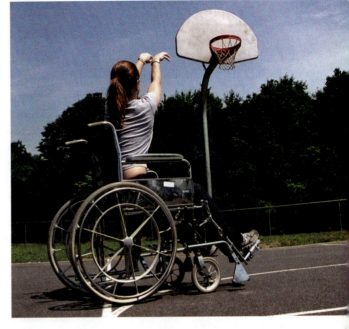

Wellness can be an exciting concept because it implies that you can exercise a lot of control over your life. You can express your independence as you make decisions about your health and create your own wellness lifestyle. Becoming interested in wellness provides you with opportunities to:

- Take responsibility for your health and how you feel
- Learn about wellness behaviors from this book and your health class
- Make decisions about your present and future health
- Protect yourself from harmful behaviors and conditions
- Reduce or delay the need for health care

WELLNESS BEHAVIORS

In the personal assessment at the beginning of the chapter, how many questions did you answer with a yes? Each question is related to a wellness behavior that research has shown to have a positive impact on health. In fact, medical research in the 1980s confirmed that personal health behaviors have a significant influence on longevity and quality of life. A research study of almost 30,000 people in California, conducted over a 12-year period, found that people who practiced the seven behaviors listed in the personal assessment enjoyed better health and had a longer life expectancy than people who did not practice the behaviors. Here are some interesting facts from the study:

- People who practiced six or seven of the behaviors lived longer than people who practiced fewer than six of the behaviors.
- Men who practiced none or only one or two of the behaviors were three times more likely to die prematurely than were men who practiced four or five of the behaviors.

did you know that...?

Sixty-five percent of all adult deaths are caused by heart disease, cancer, or stroke. Many of the behaviors that help prevent these conditions are formed during adolescence. Wellness practices you engage in now can make a difference in the years to come.

teen forum

Is Health Care a Right?

The United States has one of the finest health care systems in the world, yet not every person has access to this system. Some people cannot afford health care, and others live in rural areas, long distances from hospitals, doctors, and dentists. The increased cost of health care has caused some people to actively engage in disease prevention. Others believe that health care is a right and that everyone should be able to get medical treatment.

- What do you think? Should we be more responsible for maintaining our own health, or should we depend on hospitals to keep us well?

- Women who practiced none or only one or two of the behaviors were almost 3½ times more likely to die prematurely than were women who practiced four or five of the behaviors.

- People who did not eat breakfast had a 50% higher risk of premature death than did people who did eat breakfast.

We have also learned about specific connections between personal habits and whether a person gets heart disease or cancer. These two diseases account for almost two-thirds of American deaths each year. Knowing the connections between personal habits and these two diseases gives people some control over preventing them. Four behaviors related to those listed in the Personal Assessment can reduce the risk of both heart disease and cancer:

1. Follow good nutritional practices.
2. Stay away from all tobacco use.
3. Engage in regular physical activity.
4. Practice known prevention strategies, such as annual physical examinations and cancer screenings.

Take another look at your answers. Are you on the road to optimal health and longevity? Are there behaviors you'd like to develop and habits you want to change? As a teen, you have the time and the opportunities to develop wellness habits that can make a difference in your life. What you are studying in this class is good for much more than passing a test or getting a grade. The things you have the opportunity to learn are designed to help you understand what it is that you can do to stay healthy. Take advantage of this opportunity to learn wellness behaviors that can have a positive influence on your entire life.

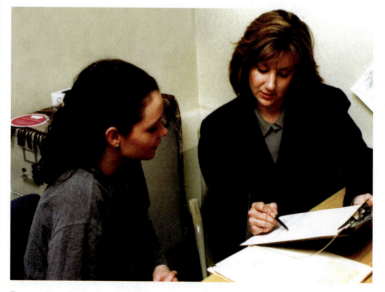

Researchers have found that practicing the seven behaviors listed in the personal assessment leads to better health and a longer life.

HEALTH PROMOTION

Health promotion is a combination of policies and activities designed to help people practice wellness and improve along the health continuum. Education and risk-reduction programs are conducted in communities, workplaces, and schools to help prevent or solve common health problems. For example, a hospital might offer nutrition information for pregnant women attending birthing classes. An example of risk reduction is a program that provides free infant restraint car seats to low-income parents. Health promotion is sponsored by both public and private organizations. Whether the programs are intended for small groups or the entire community, they stress the prevention of illness and injury and the promotion of wellness. Some employers realize that healthy employees are more productive than unhealthy ones, so they offer wellness-promoting activities such as exercise classes and stress-management workshops.

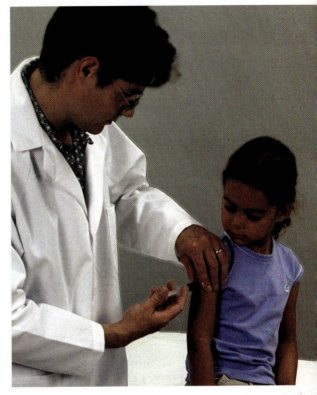

U.S. Health Objectives

The U.S. Public Health Service has taken an active role since 1979 in promoting wellness. Before then, our health care system focused mainly on medicine and its ability to cure illnesses. This meant that people went to the doctor or hospital *after* they got sick. In many cases, they received treatment too late to improve their health status or to save their lives. For example, by the time cigarette smokers felt the symptoms of lung cancer, it was usually too late to save their lives.

In 1979, an event occurred that changed the way the medical community and the public looked at health issues. That event was the release of the first *Surgeon General's Report on Health Promotion and Disease Prevention.* The **Surgeon General** is the highest medical official in the country, and the report focused on using the **public health** system to prevent disease instead of simply trying to cure it. This report identified five major goals aimed at improving the health and quality of life for all Americans and 225 specific objectives that would support the achievement of the goals.

In 1980, the report was revised, and a new list of goals was presented in *Promoting Health/Preventing Disease: Objectives for the Nation.* You can see from the title that the emphasis was on helping Americans achieve better health. The belief was that if businesses, communities, and individuals worked together to achieve the objectives, the need for medical care could be reduced.

Health officials evaluated the outcomes of *Objectives for the Nation* and concluded that the emphasis on prevention was working well. Meeting with health professionals and citizens at meetings held across

Surgeon General

highest-ranking medical officer in the United States

public health

sum of the federal, state, and local health agencies and organizations that work together to promote health and prevent disease for the community as a whole

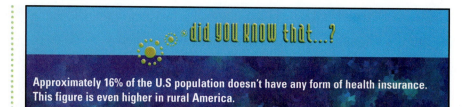

the nation, officials developed objectives for the 1990s. A report called *Healthy People 2000*, published in 1990, was the result. The very latest report is *Healthy People 2010*, and it is being used to guide the development of health programs and medical interventions for continuing the improvement of the nation's health to the year 2010.

As did the earlier reports, *Healthy People 2010* includes objectives that address the health of teens. In fact, 107 objectives were written specifically for teens. Of the 107 objectives for teens, 21 were identified as critical by the Adolescent Health Work Group. Figure 2-2 lists some examples of objectives the group considered to be critical.

Healthy People 2010 calls for even more personal responsibility and behaviors than did the previous reports. It also added a feature called "Leading Health Indicators." These are the 10 most important public health issues facing Americans at this time; they are listed in Table 2-1. Most of the indicators represent areas we as individuals can control by our choices and behavior. A major purpose of the indicators is to motivate people to accept responsibility for their health and get them to practice wellness behaviors.

As you are becoming interested in your health and start practicing wellness behaviors, you may want to join planned health promotion activities. In addition to helping you achieve a better life, you will be helping to meet the nation's health objectives.

Figure 2-2

Examples of *Healthy People 2010* critical health objectives for adolescents

- **Reduce deaths caused by motor vehicle crashes**

- **Reduce the suicide rate**

- **Reduce the proportion of children and adolescents who are overweight or obese**

- **Increase the proportion of adolescents who engage in vigorous physical activity that promotes cardiorespiratory fitness three or more days per week for 20 or more minutes per occasion**

- **Reduce tobacco use by adolescents**

Table 2-1   Leading Health Indicators Adapted from *Healthy People 2010*

Indicator	Reason for Including
1. Physical activity	There are numerous benefits from regular exercise, including a healthy body, reduced stress, and prevention of premature death. Yet only 75% of teens and 15% of adults exercise at least three times a week.
2. Overweight and obesity	Overweight and obesity are major contributors to many causes of preventable death and disability. More than 11% of all young people ages 6–19 are overweight or obese.
3. Tobacco use	This is currently the most preventable cause of disease and death in the United States. Almost 25% of adults are smokers, and in 1999, 35% of teens surveyed reported they had tried at least one cigarette in the past 30 days.
4. Substance abuse	Alcohol and illicit drug use are related to many of America's most serious problems, including violence, injury, and HIV infection. In 1995, the cost of dealing with drug abuse was estimated at $110 billion.
5. Responsible sexual behavior	Unintended pregnancy and sexually transmitted diseases, including HIV infections, can result from unprotected sexual behaviors. Abstinence is the only behavior that can completely prevent these conditions.
6. Mental health	Approximately 20% of the U.S. population is affected by mental illness each year. Depression is a real threat to both adults and teens.
7. Injury and violence	More than 400 Americans die each day from car crashes, murder, poisoning, drowning, and falls. These deaths are preventable.
8. Environmental quality	It is estimated that 25% of all preventable illnesses worldwide are related to environmental conditions. In the United States, it is believed that 50,000 premature deaths each year are related to poor air quality .
9. Immunization	Among the most important advances of the twentieth century, immunizations prevent numerous diseases, yet 28% of our nation's children are not immunized.
10. Access to health care	Not everyone has access to quality health care because some people lack financial resources and education. Approximately 20%, or more than 50 million people under the age of 65, have no health insurance.

take it on home

Prepare a list of the 10 Leading Health Indicators and take the list home to discuss with your family. Talk about the health practices and attitudes of the family members as they are related to each of the 10 health indicators. You can use the information to encourage family members to examine their wellness behaviors to see if there are some they might like to improve or reinforce. Remember, if the *Healthy People 2010* objectives are to be reached, we all need to do our part. Write a summary of your conversations and include it in your Health Folio.

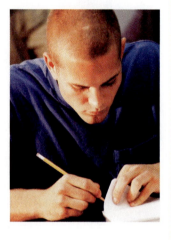

DEVELOPING A PERSONAL WELLNESS PLAN

It is one thing to know and appreciate the value of a wellness lifestyle; it is something else to put wellness into action. As you move toward adulthood, you will be given more and more responsibility for your health. It is up to you to determine what your wellness lifestyle will be. You need goals and a plan to get started. This section will help you set those goals and make that plan. Be sure to make your wellness plan fun. Practicing wellness behaviors is something you will do for your entire life; you should enjoy it!

Dimensions of Wellness

Wellness is a way of living. It involves making good decisions and performing behaviors that contribute to a high quality of life. It means doing those things that ensure not only your good health but the health of the people around you as well. Wellness is a complex process, and it extends beyond you as an individual. It includes your friends, family, and the environment. Just as there are several dimensions of health, there are several categories of wellness to address all aspects of health:

1. Personal wellness
2. Social wellness
3. Emotional wellness
4. Intellectual wellness
5. Environmental wellness
6. Cultural wellness
7. Spiritual wellness
8. Community wellness

Figure 2-3 illustrates how all the categories of wellness work together to influence your overall picture of personal wellness.

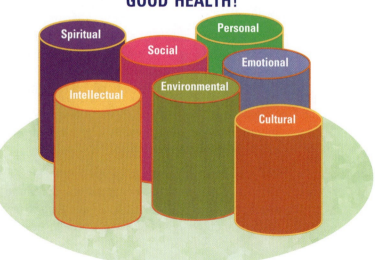

Figure 2-3
Wellness includes a number of components at different levels of intensity.

Although the importance of each component may differ from person to person, each component must be considered when you develop your personal wellness plan.

Personal Wellness

Personal wellness means accepting responsibility for using your health-related knowledge, skills, and opportunities to continually strive toward optimal health. It includes developing positive attitudes about yourself and about health. Personal wellness also means gathering the information necessary to make good health decisions. People practice personal wellness if they do things such as eating well, getting exercise, or staying well-groomed.

One way that Carrie practices personal wellness is to make careful and healthy food choices when she eats lunch at school and when she makes her own snacks at home. Jerry makes it a point to ride his bike at least five miles three days a week. There are many ways for you to practice personal wellness. What are some things you can do?

Social Wellness

Social wellness means learning to form positive relationships with other people. It is developing the interpersonal skills needed to interact effectively with others. Social wellness enables you to be comfortable with people at home, at school, and at work. Perhaps you can recognize social wellness characteristics in people around you.

Have you ever known someone like Frank or Sarah? Frank is a popular eleventh-grade student. Perhaps he is popular because he is a very sociable person. He is nice to everyone. People find him polite and note that he never has anything bad to say about anyone. Frank is socially well.

Sarah works at the ice cream shop on weekends. She sometimes finds some of the customers she waits on to be unlikable, but she makes a special effort to treat all her customers with respect. She is finding that this effort helps her be more accepting of people in general, even when she is not at work.

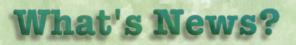

What's News?

A recent nationwide study of more than 68,000 people in the United States reported that 7 of 10 Americans do not exercise regularly. This is a surprising finding because of the proven benefits that come from regular exercise and the fact that lack of exercise contributes to approximately 300,000 deaths each year. Do you exercise every day? Do you exercise every week? Is exercise something you can include in your personal wellness plan?

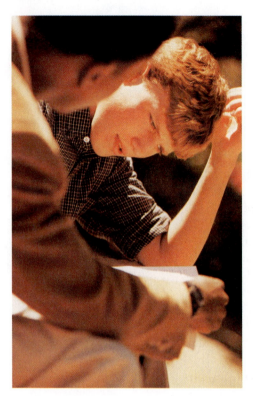

Emotional Wellness

Emotional wellness means developing high self-esteem, a strong self-image, and a positive attitude about life. An emotionally well person can effectively deal with the emotional and sometimes challenging situations that are part of everyday life. We all experience setbacks in life, such as performing poorly on a test, not getting the part-time job we applied for, or losing someone we love. It is natural to feel uncomfortable, even angry, when we face these kinds of difficulties. The feeling itself isn't unhealthy. What is unhealthy is to express our hurt or disappointment in unproductive, even damaging ways, such as losing our temper, yelling at someone, or turning to drugs for comfort and escape. The emotionally well person finds constructive ways to deal with life's problems. For example, Rashonda had a disagreement with her best friend this past weekend. She knew that even though she was angry with her friend, she did not want to lose the friendship. She decided to make a special effort to visit her friend and practice her assertive communication skills.

The emotionally well person also uses good communication skills to address problems. For example, Drew did not do well on his math test last week. He was very disappointed but knew it was not the end of the world. He put his wellness skills to work by talking with his teacher to find out what he could do to improve.

Intellectual Wellness

Intellectual wellness means enjoying learning and pursuing it beyond the classroom. It involves exploring new topics, learning new skills, and developing the ability to solve problems and to think critically. There are many ways to learn, such as reading, using the Internet, and talking with friends and family members about topics of interest. People who are intellectually well use a variety of methods to increase their knowledge and skills. Consider Maria. She loves to learn. She reads a lot, and instead of watching television she often uses her computer to learn new things. She not only finds it satisfying to uncover new information; she also finds that learning is fun. Do you use a computer to learn about new things that interest you?

Environmental Wellness

ecosystem

a complex collection of living things that share a specific environment

Environmental wellness means understanding and caring for the environment. As do all other organisms, we live in an **ecosystem**. We share our environment with other living things and depend on each other to use resources respectfully so we can keep the environment healthy.

Practicing environmental wellness involves looking for opportunities to protect the environment. For example, Danny learned about environmental issues in his tenth-grade science class. Since then, he has been very aware of the environment. He recognizes that he is only one person, but he has dedicated himself to developing a lifestyle that includes recycling and minimizing waste. He even taught his family how to make a compost pile. Danny knows that the things each person does will make a difference, and he recognizes the importance of setting an example for others.

Cultural Wellness

Cultural wellness is being aware of your own cultural background as well as understanding and appreciating the diversity and richness of other cultures. It involves interacting well with others, regardless of their gender, and accepting people of different races, backgrounds, abilities, ethnic backgrounds, and ages. Cultural wellness also means passing on the traditions of your family while blending them with the traditions of new family members.

Practicing cultural wellness is easy for Coleman. His family heritage is African American, and his family gets together every year for Kwanza, an African American festival held in late December. It is easy to do, too, because almost every one of his relatives lives in the state. Coleman's best friend, Ira, celebrates Hanukkah. Coleman and his friend get together each year and share the experiences of both holidays.

Spiritual Wellness

Spiritual wellness means looking within yourself and getting in touch with your spiritual self. This might mean reading a holy book, attending a religious service, practicing relaxation, or simply sitting in a quiet place to think about the world. Spiritual wellness may or may not include any particular religion or belief in a higher power. It does include setting aside quiet time for yourself to think about who you are

real teens

Shemikia is a junior in a Midwest high school. She loves her family, enjoys being with her friends, and is training for the high school swim team. Shemikia has developed her wellness skills and feels good about her high level of health. Recently, she has become interested in the environment. In her biology class, she learned about ecosystems and the interaction of living things in the environment. She realizes the importance of a healthy environment and knows that human beings have not always done a good job caring for it. She watches people tossing trash on the highways, putting grass clippings in plastic bags and sending them to the dump, and wasting water. She wants to do something to care for the environment but does not know where to start. Shemikia asks herself, "Whom can I talk to? Where can I find information? Can I make a difference by myself?" She decides that the best place to start is to talk with her biology teacher. She is also planning to perform a Web search to help her find some answers to her questions.

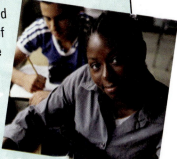

wellness motives

the sum of knowledge, beliefs, and values that contribute to forming reasons that encourage wellness behaviors

and what you stand for, to reflect on your life's purpose and goals, and to mentally explore possible solutions to important problems. Good places to seek quiet time include your home, a park, a beach, a forest, or a place of worship.

It is easy for Mike to be in touch with the spiritual part of his wellness lifestyle. His father is a minister, and Mike has been involved in church activities his whole life. His friend Jan is quite different. Jan's parents don't believe in organized religion, so Jan does not go to church. There are many occasions, however, when Jan and Mike talk about religion and what it brings to a person's life. Jan is very curious about Christianity and may go to church with Mike sometime. Mike, on the other hand, has gained a fresh perspective on his own beliefs by talking with Jan about ways her family practices spiritual wellness.

Community Wellness

Community wellness is engaging in activities that protect the health of the community. The health of a community depends on the individuals who live in it. Even if your community is very large, your individual behavior can have an impact. Your actions can set an example for others, either positive or negative.

Arnie and Sarah have been dating for a couple of months. One of the things they have in common is compassion for people who are less fortunate than they are. Each month, they volunteer to work at the homeless shelter downtown, serving meals and planning activities for the children of homeless families. They feel good about helping others and knowing that their actions can really make a difference in people's lives.

Realizing Your Personal Value

Wellness truly starts with you. As a teen, you have a lot of control over your personal habits. For example, you make choices about what you eat, how much you exercise, and whether you use substances proven to be harmful to your health.

A first step toward wellness is to develop a positive attitude about yourself and your well-being. This means forming positive attitudes such as:

- "I have value."
- "My health is important to me."
- "I am willing to take responsibility to practice wellness."
- "I want to live a long, healthy, satisfying life."

A positive attitude can help you motivate yourself to practice wellness behaviors. Having good **wellness motives** is important because some behaviors require self-discipline. Have you ever started an exercise program and then quit because it just seemed like too much trouble? At such times, there are some strategies you can use to keep yourself motivated:

- Keep the end result in mind. Concentrate on how good you will feel, how much energy you will have.
- Look for additional rewards. If you are exercising, for example, think about how you are protecting your heart, managing your weight, and reducing your stress.
- Challenge yourself to have fun. Look for healthy foods and recipes that taste good. Find a physical activity or sport you enjoy.
- Enjoy your success. Plan rewards as you achieve your wellness goals. Give yourself credit for sticking with a wellness program. Let yourself feel good about yourself and what you have accomplished.

Setting Wellness Goals

Goals are important because they give direction to your life. They provide you with a kind of compass to help you stay on course. If you think about it, everything around you is the result of someone's goals. Take the common lightbulb, for example. Developing a way to produce light was Thomas Edison's goal. He stayed with it even though he produced hundreds of bulbs that didn't work. Edison saw those "failures" as experiments and learned something from each one.

Goals keep you focused on solving problems. Here are some suggestions for setting good goals:

1. Your goals should be something you really want.
2. Be clear about exactly what you want.
3. Set a reasonable number of goals so that you will not get frustrated trying to achieve them all.
4. Make sure your goals are attainable.
5. State them in the positive rather than the negative. For example, "wanting to be smoke free" is better than "wanting to not smoke."
6. Write them out. The act of writing goals down helps reinforce them and increases the chance that you will achieve them.
7. Identify the barriers that may prevent you from reaching each goal. Then think about ways you can eliminate the barriers.
8. Identify the resources such as people, things, and money that can help you reach them.
9. Develop a plan for reaching each goal. Write out the plan.

Once you have planned and written out your goals, use the following strategies to increase your success rate:

- Keep your list of goals where you will see it often.
- Make a commitment with yourself to achieve your goals.
- Keep a mental picture of the goals and their outcomes.
- When faced with obstacles, use your resources.

- Repeat methods that *do* work.
- Do something to move toward your goals *every* day.
- Have someone close to you help you with your goals.
- Evaluate your progress regularly and reward yourself for your accomplishments.
- Be persistent. This is the main ingredient in achieving goals: *persistence.*

The Power of the Positive

Your wellness plan is likely to include some behaviors that you already do, but your plan may also include some behaviors you want to eliminate or change. Say you now spend a lot of time on the sofa watching television or in the house playing video games. You decide that exercise is to be part of your wellness plan. You will be more successful carrying out your plan if your goal is stated in terms of what you plan *to do*, rather than what you plan *not to do*. You will increase your chances of success if you say "I will exercise for at least 30 minutes at least four times a week" instead of "I will quit watching so much TV." Research tells us that people are more successful adopting new improved behaviors than they are at quitting bad behaviors. Replace the time you spend watching television with exercise and you will be substituting a new, positive behavior, rather than struggling to get rid of an old one.

ACQUIRING WELLNESS INFORMATION

You need accurate and meaningful information to make good wellness decisions. Finding many sources of information can be easy, but determining whether the information is **valid** is not so easy. And many of the facts about health seem to contradict each other or to change with every new study. How do you know what to believe? The best way is to determine whether the information is based on evidence or supported by scientifically accurate data. For example, many "wonder diets" have not been tested in a scientific manner. The diets are almost always advertised using the **testimony** of pleased customers. The diets are not based on valid research.

Family and Friends

Friends and family members are often good sources of information. But how do you know if the information they give you is accurate? The truth is, their intentions may be good, but what they tell you may be inaccurate. It is your task to validate the information you get from others. One good way to check validity is to find the same information in several sources. For example, if you hear something from a friend, read the

valid

based on evidence or supported by scientifically accurate data

testimony

a firsthand declaration of fact

> ### did YOU KNOW that...?
>
> Some health food companies publish their own newsletters and magazines. They use the publications to print articles explaining why health foods and products are needed for good health. If you read some of the articles in these publications, you will notice that the companies producing the magazine also advertise their own brand of the products the articles claim are needed.

same thing in your city's daily newspaper, and then locate the same information in a book, you have validated the original source. Finding out for yourself is important when it comes to health and wellness because poor information can result in wasted money or worse – on products and practices that are actually harmful to your health.

Printed Materials

You can read books, magazines, journals, and newspapers to gather information, but you need to be careful because not all printed material is accurate. Materials range from unbelievable and ridiculous articles, sometimes printed in tabloid newspapers sold at supermarket checkout stands, to reports of carefully conducted scientific studies, found in journals published by major universities or professional organizations. Here are some tips for determining the validity of written information:

- If a claim seems unbelievable, it almost certainly is. Follow your common sense.
- Locate more than one source and compare the information. If it is repeated in a number of reliable publications, the chances increase that it is true.
- Check the **credentials** of the authors. They should have the proper education and experience to know the subject.
- Determine the purpose of the writing. If it is to sell a product or to promote its own viewpoints, question the "facts" carefully.

The Internet

The Internet offers a wide variety of information. Using a good search engine, you can search almost any topic. Here are three of the most powerful search engines:

1. Google: **http://www.google.com**
2. Hotbot: **http://hotbot.lycos.com**
3. Ask Jeeves: **http://www.ask.com**

credentials

titles, education, or training that verify a person's intellectual or professional ability

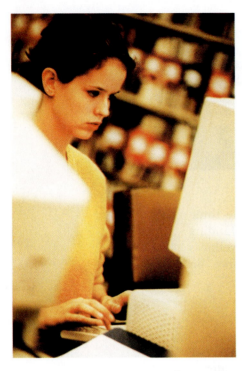

When you visit these Web sites, simply type in the topic you are researching and the search engine will supply you with Web sites that may contain information about the topic. If your topic has more than one word and you enter the words in the search window, the search engine will look for Web sites that have them, but not necessarily together or in the order you wanted. To obtain a more precise search, look for an "Advanced Search" button, and click to go inside. Enter your term as an "Exact Phrase," and the engine will search for the two terms together.

Once you have found a Web site that looks interesting, how do you know if the information is accurate? The following tips will help you evaluate health Web sites:

- Check the credentials of the person who put the information on the Web site. Medical and advanced graduate degrees, such as M.D. and Ph.D., are often indications that the person is knowledgeable. If there is no author listed, look for the sponsoring organization. Universities, health agencies such as the American Cancer Society, and federal and state health departments can be reliable sources of information.

- Determine the purpose of the Web site. Is it trying to sell you something? Be careful of Web sites that promise that your life will be better if you buy what they are selling. If the purpose is only to provide information, there is a greater chance the information is **credible** than if the purpose is to sell products.

- Look for same the information on other Web sites. See if they present the same facts.

- Check the date of the material. This should be stated on the Web site. Dates are especially important with health information because it changes frequently as new discoveries are made.

- Evaluate how the information is presented. Watch for sweeping generalizations, forcible language, personal testimonies, and claims without scientific references.

When using the Internet, remember that Web sites can come and go without notice. The most valid Web sites tend to be those that stay around. Explore the following Web sites to find good information about wellness:

- Accent Health: **http://www.accenthealth.com**
  This Web site is a product of CNN (Cable News Network) and has a search engine that gives you a wide range of medical information.

- Discovery Health: **http://health.discovery.com**
  This Web site is operated by the same company that produces the Discovery Channel on television, but this Web site contains only

credible

believable; reliable

health information. Click on "Health News" for recent news stories on health topics.

- Go Ask Alice! **http://www.goaskalice.com**
This is the health question-and-answer Internet service produced by Columbia University.

- Healthfinder: **http://www.healthfinder.gov**
This is a free guide to reliable consumer health and human services information. It was developed by the U.S. Department of Health and Human Services. In addition to covering a wide variety of health and wellness topics, it contains many links to other useful Web sites.

BUILDING YOUR Wellness Plan

A carefully developed wellness plan will help you easily meet the health and wellness goals you select for yourself. This chapter covers the components of wellness and offers information on setting personal goals. Thinking about your level of wellness now will help you decide what aspects of your wellness you would like to improve. Here are some things you may want to consider:

- Look at the eight components of wellness and identify one or two ways you are practicing wellness for each. Identify at least one way you can improve your wellness in each category.

- Think about your current attitude toward wellness. List at least three attitudes you might need to develop that will help you achieve your wellness goals.

- Use the suggestions for setting goals to set one wellness goal you can work toward this week. Try some of the strategies to increase your success rate to discover which suggestions work well for you.

- Visit the National Institutes of Health (NIH) Web site and read about *Healthy People 2010*. Choose one of the objectives and list personal wellness goals you would like to achieve that are related to that objective.

- Think about ways to increase your health literacy skills. Use the World Wide Web to obtain health information for yourself and your family. Practice evaluating the content of some health-related Web sites.

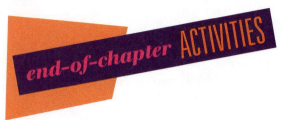

Weblinks

Consumer and Patient Health Information System: **http://caphis.mlanet.org** (click on "for health consumers")

Healthfinder—Quality of Information: **http://www.healthfinder.gov** (search for "website evaluation")

Healthy People 2010: **http://www.healthypeople.gov**

Short-Answer Questions

1. List three health behaviors that have been shown to contribute to longevity.
2. Name the two diseases that contribute to almost two-thirds of the deaths in the United States each year.
3. State the purpose of the nation's health objectives.
4. List three ways a person can practice spiritual wellness.
5. Name two good search engines on the World Wide Web.

Discussion Questions

1. Explain the relationship between health and wellness.
2. Explain the significance of *Healthy People 2010.*
3. List and describe several components of wellness.
4. Explain how you would advise someone to develop a wellness plan.
5. Describe three characteristics to look for when choosing sources of health and wellness information.

Chapter Vocabulary

Using a separate sheet of paper, list and define the following terms:

credentials	Surgeon General
credible	valid
ecosystem	wellness
public health	wellness motives

Application Activities

Language Arts Connection

Use the library or Internet to find information about the U.S. Surgeon General. Use your report-writing skills to prepare a report that includes the following:

1. What is the role of the Surgeon General?
2. Why does the Surgeon General wear a uniform?
3. Identify two individuals who have served as Surgeon General.
4. What qualifications are necessary to be the Surgeon General?
5. Who is the current Surgeon General?
6. What are the major health issues being addressed by the current Surgeon General?

Social Studies Connection

Use your Internet search skills to locate information about the health beliefs of people in other countries. Investigate both industrialized and less-developed countries. Try to determine the extent to which people in other countries practice wellness skills. Write a report that includes the following:

1. Are people more likely to practice wellness behaviors in industrialized or less-developed countries?
2. What are the differences in the health care systems in the countries you investigated?
3. List three health beliefs that people in these countries have that are different from yours.

Science Connection

Find three health Web sites other than the ones listed in this chapter. Use the tips given in the chapter to evaluate the Web sites. Write a report on each Web site, including the following:

1. Web site address
2. Web site title
3. Your evaluation of the Web site using the criteria presented in the chapter

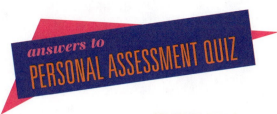

answers to
PERSONAL ASSESSMENT QUIZ

personal assessment: MY HEALTH HABITS

On the basis of research information:

1. Tobacco use, specifically cigarette smoking, is a major health risk. Each cigarette a person smokes will shorten his or her life by 14 minutes.

2. Regular exercise is health protective. Exercise can protect from heart disease, cancer, obesity, and diabetes and can help relieve stress.

3. Normal weight is health protective. Overweight contributes to diabetes, cancer, and heart disease. Severe underweight can be a sign of serious mental problems and can be life threatening.

4. People who eat between meals are not as healthy as people who do not. If you do eat between meals, eat only healthy snacks.

5. People who do not eat breakfast are ill more often than are those who do.

6. The healthiest people sleep between seven and eight hours each night.

7. Use of alcohol can lead to health problems, especially if it is used to excess. Alcohol also increases one's risk of auto accidents.

chapter 3

Problem Solving

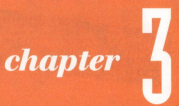

Netti is faced with a problem and has an important decision to make. She has worked and saved all the money she could to buy her own car. She only has enough money to get a used car, and she's worried that she may make the wrong choice and buy one that won't be reliable. Netti knows that buying a used car can be risky, and she doesn't really know much about how cars work or how to take care of them. Before Netti makes a final decision, she wants to analyze all possibilities. She will use her problem-solving skills to identify what she wants and needs in a car and to help her make a good decision.

chapter OBJECTIVES

When you finish this chapter, you should be able to:

- Explain the significance of health risks.
- Describe the purpose of the Youth Risk Behavior Surveillance System.
- Explain why problem solving is an important skill.
- List the skills associated with problem solving.
- Demonstrate how to develop a mind map.
- Explain each step in the problem-solving process.

key TERMS

brainstorming
deductive reasoning
inductive reasoning
mind mapping
morbidity
mortality
risk factors

Introduction

Human beings are unique in their ability to solve problems. We spend a lot of time each day solving problems. Some problems are fairly simple, such as finding a misplaced object, deciding how much time to devote to schoolwork, or choosing what food to eat for lunch. Other problems are much more complicated: choosing the right college, determining which car to buy, or trying to figure out how to manage a new relationship. Some of our problems are related to choices we have to make to protect our health. As a young adult, you will be developing an awareness of risks to your health. Knowing about these health risks is one thing; being able to take steps to control them is something else. In this chapter, you will receive information to help you sort through the complicated elements associated with health risks and make good decisions. Being able to problem-solve effectively is an important wellness skill.

Personal Assessment: YOUTH RISK BEHAVIOR

Here are some of the actual questions from the U.S. Centers for Disease Control and Prevention's 89-question Youth Risk Behavior Surveillance System survey. Answer each of these questions for yourself to see if you are engaged in or exposed to any high-risk behavior. You can review an interpretation of these items at the end of the chapter.

1. When you rode a bicycle during the past 12 months, how often did you wear a helmet?
   a. I did not ride a bicycle during the past 12 months.
   b. Never wore a helmet
   c. Rarely wore a helmet
   d. Sometimes wore a helmet
   e. Most of the time wore a helmet
   f. Always wore a helmet

2. How often do you wear a seat belt when riding in a car driven by someone else?
   a. Never
   b. Rarely
   c. Sometimes
   d. Most of the time
   e. Always

3. During the past 12 months, how many times has someone threatened or injured you with a weapon such as a gun, knife, or club on school property?
   a. 0 times
   b. 1 time
   c. 2 or 3 times
   d. 4 or 5 times
   e. 6 or 7 times
   f. 8 or 9 times
   g. 10 or 11 times
   h. 12 or more times

4. During the past 12 months, did you ever feel so sad or hopeless almost every day for two weeks or more in a row that you stopped doing some usual activities?
   a. Yes
   b. No

5. Have you ever tried cigarette smoking, even one or two puffs?
   a. Yes
   b. No

6. During your life, on how many days have you had at least one drink of alcohol?
   a. 0 days
   b. 1 or 2 days
   c. 3 to 9 days
   d. 10 to 19 days
   e. 20 to 39 days
   f. 40 to 99 days
   g. 100 or more days

7. How do you describe your weight?
   a. Very underweight
   b. Slightly underweight
   c. About the right weight
   d. Slightly overweight
   e. Very overweight

8. During the past 7 days, how many times did you eat fruit? (Do not count fruit juice.)
   a. I did not eat fruit during the past 7 days
   b. 1 to 3 times during the past 7 days
   c. 4 to 6 times during the past 7 days
   d. 1 time per day
   e. 2 times per day
   f. 3 times per day
   g. 4 or more times per day

9. On how many of the past 7 days did you exercise or participate in physical activity for at least 20 minutes that made you sweat and breathe hard, such as basketball, soccer, running, swimming laps, fast bicycling, fast dancing, or similar aerobic activities?
   a. 0 days
   b. 1 day
   c. 2 days
   d. 3 days
   e. 4 days
   f. 5 days
   g. 6 days
   h. 7 days

HEALTH RISKS

We are all exposed to circumstances and have engaged in behaviors that can contribute to disease, death, or injury. These conditions are known as **risk factors**, which means that exposure to them may result in a harmful outcome. Some risk factors are easier to identify than others. For example, driving while under the influence of alcohol is an obvious risk factor. Breathing secondhand cigarette smoke is not as obvious, but it is still a risk factor. Some risk factors are short term because they can result in immediate harm. An example is riding a bicycle without a helmet. Other risk factors do harm over a long period of time. Eating a high-fat diet for many years is an example of a long-term risk factor. What kinds of short- and long-term risk factors have you experienced?

There can also be compounding effects of risk exposure. This means that the more risk factors you are exposed to at one time, the greater the likelihood of a negative outcome. Take the skateboard example. Riding a skateboard without a helmet is one risk factor. Using the skateboard on a busy traffic area would be a second risk factor. Performing stunts that are dangerous would be an additional risk factor. Now imagine that the rider is also under the influence of alcohol or drugs. The possibility of an accident increases with each additional risk factor.

Threats to Your Health

The threats to your health as a teen are not likely to be from conditions such as heart disease or cancer. For young adults in your age group, there are four causes that contribute to almost 75% of all **mortality** and

---

risk factors

identifiable conditions or behaviors that increase one's risk of getting ill or injured

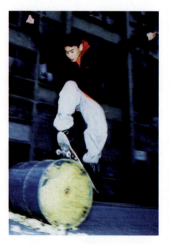

Performing stunts without the benefit of protective equipment increases one's risk of serious injury.

mortality

pertaining to the number of deaths in a given number of people

---

�֎ teen forum ֎

Robert's Wellness Decision

Robert and Ty decided to go swimming at a river not too far from their homes. This is their first time at this swimming spot, where a railroad bridge crosses the river. Ty suggests that they climb up to the bridge to make the 10-foot jump into the river. When they get on the bridge, Robert looks down at the dark water and has a flash of anxiety about jumping into the water. Ty says, "Let's go, man!" and springs off the bridge into the water below. As Ty is plunging to the water, Robert wonders what awaits Ty when he lands.

- Do you think there are risks associated with Ty's behavior?
- If you do, what might they be?
- If you were with Robert and Ty, would you have some concerns?
- Is there anything they could do to minimize their risk?
- Have you ever been in a similar situation?
- What did you do?

many instances of **morbidity**. You can see from Figure 3-1 that at least 78% of deaths among teens are not the result of diseases. Many of these deaths are caused by poor decision making and the practice of personal behaviors that are under the teen's control. Notice that many are the results of short-term risks.

In contrast, the leading causes of morbidity and mortality among adults are often the result of long-term risk factors. The causes of death among adults are shown in Figure 3-2. Research indicates that the risk factors associated with these diseases are tobacco use, poor eating habits, and physical inactivity. All these behaviors are also under our control. You can see that to a very great extent, we have opportunities throughout our lives to choose the behaviors that will decrease our chances of disease, death, and disability.

morbidity

pertaining to the amount of illness in a given number of people

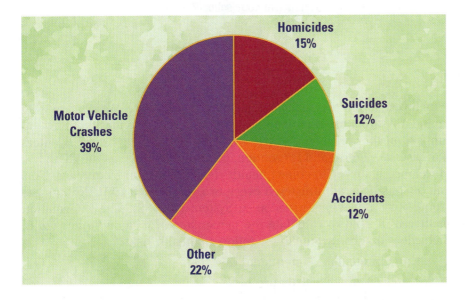

Figure 3-1
Major causes of death among teens 16–19 years old, 2000

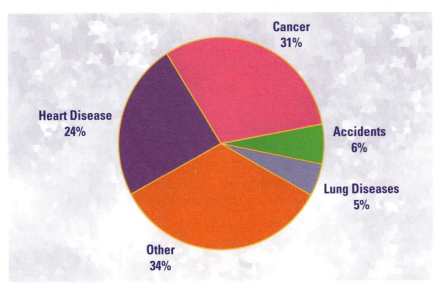

Figure 3-2
Major causes of death among adults 20–75 years old, 2000

What's News?

"Health and Human Services report shows teens making more responsible decisions." So stated a recent press release from the U.S. Department of Health and Human Services. The 2001 Youth Risk Behavior Surveillance System survey results indicated that, compared with the results of surveys in the 1990s, high school students in 2001 were:

• More likely to wear safety belts when riding in a car

• Less likely to ride with a person who had been drinking alcohol

• Less likely to seriously consider suicide

• Less likely to carry a weapon

• Less likely to smoke cigarettes on a regular basis

• Less likely to have had sexual intercourse

Do you think these trends are true for the students in your school?

Teen Risk Factors

The investigation of risk factors has become a science. We are now able to identify the most significant risk factors and behaviors that have an impact on the well-being of teens and young adults. The U.S. Centers for Disease Control and Prevention, commonly known as the CDC, has developed a survey to collect health risk information from teens. This survey has been administered every two years since 1991 through the Youth Risk Behavior Surveillance System (YRBSS). The information gathered is used to calculate the percentage of teens who engage in behaviors that contribute to the following health risks:

• Unintentional and intentional injuries
• Alcohol and other drug use
• Tobacco use
• Unintended pregnancy and sexually transmitted diseases (STDs)
• Unhealthy dietary behaviors
• Lack of physical activity

Risks You Can Control

You have personal control over many risk factors. These are risk factors that are related to your own behavior. Here are some examples of behaviors that involve personal choices:

• Wearing protective gear when skateboarding, biking, skiing, or doing other activities in which injury is possible
• Using a safety belt when riding in a car
• Choosing not to smoke cigarettes
• Avoiding excessive amounts of high-fat foods

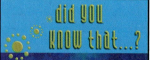

did you know that...?

At least one adolescent (12–19 years old) dies of an injury every hour of every day, or about 12,000 die each year. Injuries kill more adolescents than do all diseases combined.

Can you think of some other risk factors that are within your behavioral control?

Motivation and concern for your safety are important factors when you are addressing personal risk factors. If you value your well-being and you are committed to a wellness lifestyle, you can effectively deal with risk factors. By choosing to avoid risky situations and taking protective measures to ensure good health, you will be practicing **risk reduction** at the same time you are practicing wellness.

THINKING AS A WAY TO CONTROL RISKS

Developing and applying the wellness behaviors you learned about in Chapter 2 will require you to call on your brain power and thinking skills. Your brain is, without question, the most valuable 3 pounds in your body. The brain contains approximately 100 billion nerve cells. All these nerve cells work continuously to process calculations and to perform commands that control your very existence. Despite all the brain's power, most people use no more than 10% of their brain power. How much of your brain power do you think you use?

In Chapter 2, we talked about acquiring wellness information. Thinking is necessary to gather, compare, and evaluate this information so you can make healthy decisions. Applying what you learned from these processes can lead to healthy behaviors you can practice for a lifetime.

risk reduction

activities and behaviors intended to reduce the threat of a disease or to minimize the possibility of accidental injury or death

take it on home

Talk with your family members about your relatives. Draw a family tree that starts with your grandparents—the parents for *both* your mother and your father. Then include your other relatives:

- grandparents' brothers and sisters (great aunts and uncles)
- grandparents' children (your parents and your aunts and uncles)
- cousins

Talk with your relatives to find out who is living, who has died (and from what causes), and who is still living but has or has had a serious illness. Try to determine if there are any health conditions that may have a hereditary link (for example, several of the people on your mother's side had or have breast cancer). On the basis of the information you gather, what health condition do you think might be a risk for you? Keep a copy of the family tree and a summary of your findings in your Health Folio.

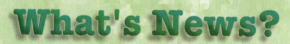

THE NEED FOR PROBLEM SOLVING

An important part of taking responsibility for your own health is developing the ability to solve problems. Our lives are filled with problems of all kinds. As hard as we may try to prevent them, problems arise. Some are minor, such as deciding which of two items to buy when you can afford only one. For example, if you have only $20, do you go see that movie you have been waiting for, or do you buy a CD you really want? Other problems are major, and your decisions can have a big impact on your life and on the people around you. One major problem you will be faced with is deciding whether to go to college or to find a full-time job after graduating from high school. Your ability to solve problems will help you make the right decisions for all the types of problems you will encounter.

Problem solving takes energy, and the more serious the problem, the more work it takes to find a satisfactory solution. But problem solving is a skill you can learn to do well by developing certain mental abilities and applying a five-step problem-solving process, described later in this chapter.

Critical Thinking

critical thinking

evaluating the worth, accuracy, or authenticity of issues and information, leading to a level of conclusion that can direct thoughts or actions

Critical thinking is not something only very intelligent people can do. In fact, it is a skill that can be learned by almost everyone. You have probably used critical thinking to solve math problems, organize a term paper, and judge the validity of health food claims. Although critical thinking has been defined in many ways, it generally means that a person can:

- Recognize problems: identify and understand their importance.

- Analyze: separate an idea into parts and examine in detail.

- Synthesize: put parts of ideas together in a meaningful way.

- Evaluate: judge or determine the worth or quality of something.

These skills require more than simply memorizing and recalling facts, as you do when taking most true-or-false and multiple-choice tests. Can you think of times when you have used critical thinking?

Reasoning

Thinking critically often requires the use of reasoning, which means drawing valid conclusions from facts or observations. There are two types of reasoning: deductive and inductive. **Deductive reasoning** begins with general statements and proceeds to a conclusion about something specific. It is based on known laws or rules about the nature of things. Two or more of these laws and rules, known as premises, are used to reach a conclusion. Here is an example of an argument using deductive reasoning:

Premise: All dogs have four legs.

Premise: Tipper is a dog.

Conclusion: Tipper has four legs.

Inductive reasoning is not based on laws and rules but is based on using your experience and observation. General conclusions are drawn from specific things that we know and see.

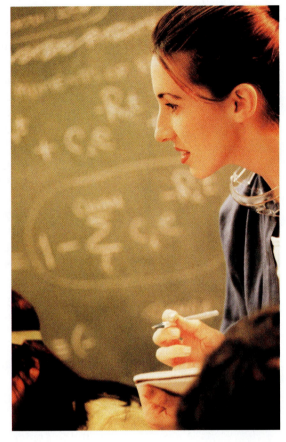

Creativity

Creativity plays an important role in critical thinking and problem solving because it enables us to see the world in a variety of ways. Not every problem has an easy solution, and many problems are quite complex. When faced with difficult or complex problems, we can use creativity to come up with new solutions and then apply critical thinking and reasoning skills to see if they might work.

deductive reasoning

reasoning that begins with the general and ends with the specific. Arguments are based on laws, rules, and established principles. Conclusions are based on two or more premises

inductive reasoning

reasoning that moves from the specific to the general; reasoning in which arguments are based on experience or observations rather than on laws or proven facts

did you know that...?

People can score high on creativity but low on critical thinking and reasoning. The following actual laws, created by politicians to protect the public, show why all these skills are needed.

- The Chico, California, City Council passed a ban on nuclear weapons, setting a $500 fine for anyone detonating one within city limits!
- Whaling is an illegal activity in Oklahoma!
- And how about *this* creative thinker? Police in Wichita, Kansas, arrested a 22-year-old man at an airport hotel after he tried to pass two $16 bills!

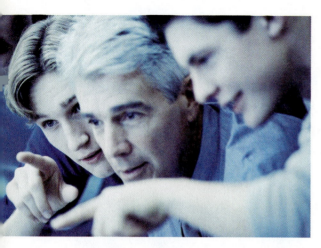

Some problems can be solved using known rules; others can be solved by creating new ideas.

Thinking creatively has often been described as "thinking outside the box." This means seeing the world in many different ways, considering new ideas, and having the courage to be inventive. It starts with mentally walking around a problem and seeing it from various angles. It continues with proposing solutions that are different from "what we've always done" and trying to come up with something new and original. It means using known ideas and things in new ways. For example, have you ever used a screwdriver as a doorstop? This is an example of using something in a new, perhaps unexpected, way.

Brain Teasers. Brain teasers are like gymnastics for the mind. They are little puzzles that give you a chance to test your mental skills in a fun way. Using your mental energies to work through the problems provides you with the opportunity to test your ability to problem-solve. There are similarities between finding solutions to brain teasers and finding solutions to more complex problems in your life. You recognize and define the problem and think it through to a solution. Problem solving is a skill, and as does any other skill, it improves with practice. Here is an example of a brain teaser:

> Daisy, Rose, and Lily each entered the county fair's flower competition. Coincidentally, the flowers they entered were a daisy, a rose, and a lily, but none of the girls entered her namesake flower. If Daisy did *not* enter a rose, which flower did each girl enter?

mind mapping

a technique that enables you to organize and illustrate your thoughts using both sides of your brain

Mind Mapping. **Mind mapping** is a technique that enables you to more freely use your brain. Our brains have two sides. We use the left side for logical, structured thinking and the right side for artistic, creative thinking. In classroom settings, we are more likely to use the left side. For example, we are often encouraged to think and write in outline form, moving systematically from one level to the next.

Mind mapping is a technique you can use to write down, organize, and illustrate your thoughts. A mind map represents a single major subject and consists of words, images, lines, and objects about the subject that are then connected to show relationships between them. You can color or illustrate mind maps any way you like. Essentially, a mind map has four major features:

1. A center image or circle that represents the major subject
2. Main themes that radiate off the center as branches
3. Minor themes that are linked to the main themes
4. No particular order required for adding themes

Figure 3-3 is an example of a mind map about camping. It provides a structure that could be used for preparing an oral report on camping. How might this technique be used to take class notes?

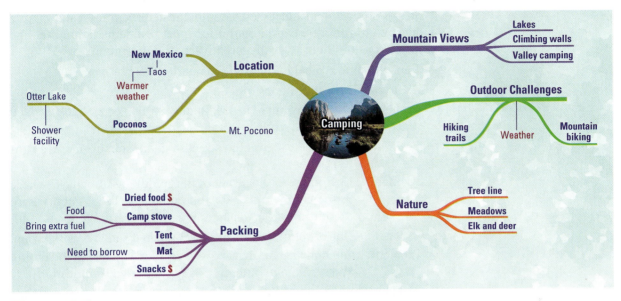

Figure 3-3 Sample mind map: camping

You can create mind maps by hand using colored markers, pens, and pencils. There are also software programs that make mind maps, but these can limit your personal creativity and artistic ideas. Regardless of which method you use, there are some standard guidelines:

1. Use a single sheet of paper in landscape format (longer from side to side than from top to bottom).

2. Begin by drawing an image and label for your subject in the center of the paper.

3. Draw branches from the main image to key words associated with the subject. Use images in place of the key words if you wish.

4. Add detail words and connect them to the key words with small wavy branches.

5. Continue to add key words and supporting details until you exhaust your thoughts about the subject. You can come back and add to your map later if you get more ideas.

Mind mapping is a useful skill for schoolwork, personal projects, and organizing your ideas when you are problem solving.

PROBLEM-SOLVING PROCESSES

The need to solve problems is part of everyday life. But many people never learn effective ways to handle problems. They fail to put all their skills to work to find a solution. Good problem solving also requires patience because complex problems take time, and a quick-fix mentality does not work. Some problems won't be solved on the first attempt, and others have more than one solution. Still others have underlying issues that need to be addressed. Despite these difficulties, solutions, or at least compromises, can be found for most problems if you take the time to work on them logically, creatively, and thoroughly.

Look at some typical daily problems in the life of a teen.

6:30 A.M.	The alarm goes off.
Problem:	Do you get out of bed right now, or do you go back to sleep for a little while?
7:55 A.M.	You need to cross the street to get to school. You are running late.
Problem:	Do you cross the street in the middle of the block, where traffic is moving, or do you go back to the corner, where there is a traffic signal?
2:00 P.M.	One of your teachers has just assigned you to a work group.
Problem:	You don't get along very well with two people in the group. Worse yet, one of them was named the group leader.

A teen faced with these problems may work through them without realizing problem-solving skills are being used. When Leslie's alarm goes off, she wants to hit the snooze button, but she has to take a makeup quiz for her biology class before school starts and she decides that sleeping a few more minutes is not worth hurting her quiz grade. Leslie made this decision without employing formal problem-solving techniques, but she did use her good problem-solving skills.

Other examples of problems that need your attention include deciding what foods to choose in the school cafeteria at lunch, how much time to spend on homework, and whether to get a cheap car now or wait until you save more money. The problems you face as a teen are more complex than those you faced as a child. Some of them may even affect your health, such as whether to smoke cigarettes or how to deal with people who mistreat you. People approach problems in many different ways. The teen years are a great time to learn and practice a formal problem-solving process to help you deal with increasingly difficult and sophisticated problems.

The typical problems in a teen's daily life, such as deciding whether to get out of bed and where to cross the street, are fairly simple and probably wouldn't require a formal problem-solving process. Deciding how to work with people with whom you do not get along, however, could be handled effectively using a structured process such as IDEAL, presented in the next section. It has been used by scientists and mathematicians for years and can be applied to any type of problem.

Using IDEAL to Solve Problems

acronym

a word that is formed from the first letter or letters of a series of words

The problem-solving process consists of five distinct steps. To help you remember these steps, use the term IDEAL. This is an **acronym**, which means a word that is formed from the first letter or letters of a series of words. In this case, IDEAL is an ideal reminder of the following steps:

1. **I**dentify the problem.
2. **D**escribe possible solutions.
3. **E**valuate each solution and reach a decision on which one to use.
4. **A**ct on the chosen solution.
5. **L**earn.

Identify the Problem

Identifying the problem is the logical first step. You might think that this is rather easy and obvious, but defining the true nature of a problem is not always that simple. Consider the sample problem about the group assignment from page 52. What do you think is the actual problem? If you say, "being put in a group with some people I don't really like," you are partially correct. But that is only a general description of the problem. Further, it is a generalization framed by emotions. This is a common but ineffective way of beginning to deal with a problem. It takes time and patience to uncover the real problem in many situations. In this example, the *real* problem will depend on the actual circumstances and the condition of your relationship with the two other people in the group. The real problem is not being forced to work with them but might be one of the following:

1. Can I work successfully with these people to learn something and get credit for the assignment?
2. Would I be better off being assigned to a different group?
3. What is it about these people that I don't like?

It is important to take the time to develop a clear picture of a problem as the first step in seeking a solution. A mind map can be a useful tool. As you map a problem, the following questions may help guide your thinking:

- What do I already know about this problem?
- Do I have all the information I need to understand this problem?
- Who can help me map out the problem?

If a problem seems too large and overwhelming, divide it into smaller subproblems. Once you have identified the subproblems, **prioritize** them: that is, rank them in order of importance. Begin with one or two subproblems you can address right away and work your way through the rest of them.

prioritize

rank items in order of importance

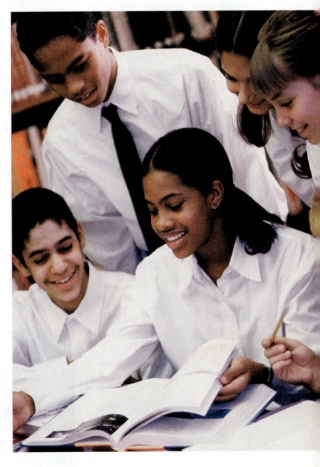

brainstorming

generating a list of possible solutions to a problem through free and creative thought

Describe Possible Solutions

Once you have clearly defined the problem, along with the issues that are related to it, you can begin to generate solutions. **Brainstorming** is a good way to discover possibilities. Brainstorming means listing all the solutions you can think of, even seemingly silly and impractical ones. You don't judge any of the solutions. The idea is to keep the list going until you have run out of ideas. You can invite friends and family members to join you in brainstorming. Involving other people sometimes works well because the interaction among people encourages them to think of more ideas than they would have if they were working alone. Just be sure everyone understands the most important rule of brainstorming: all ideas are acceptable during the generation phase. Judging ideas too early in the brainstorming session can stifle creativity. Evaluating the ideas for their usefulness comes after you have completed the list.

Evaluate Each Solution

Evaluate each solution on your list of brainstormed possibilities. You will need to decide on certain standards, or criteria, that solutions must meet to be acceptable. Here are a few questions that suggest commonly used criteria:

- Is the solution legal?
- Is the solution cost effective? Cost refers not only to money but also to the time needed to implement the solution.
- Is the solution creative? Sometimes people simply stick with their favorite ideas. They use them because they are familiar, instead of looking for new, more challenging, and possibly better solutions.
- Is the solution likely to solve the problem?

Deciding on the best alternative may require extensive research and consulting with friends, family members, or even experts such as a physician. The amount of time spent on this step corresponds to the complexity and seriousness of the problem.

Act on the Chosen Solution

Once you decide on the best alternative, you will need to act on it. You will be able to act on your choice with the confidence that you evaluated it among other alternatives.

teen forum

Power in Herbal Supplements

Several herbal remedies that are supposed to have a positive effect on mental wellness have received lots of attention the past few years. Two of these herbs, ginkgo biloba and ginseng, have been used by the Chinese for centuries to improve mental functions and energize the body. Research studies in the United States have not had consistent results. Some studies have shown that people using ginkgo biloba and ginseng demonstrated an increased ability to solve problems rapidly; other studies have not.

- Do you think that taking an herb can improve brain performance?
- How could you use your critical-thinking skills to answer that question?

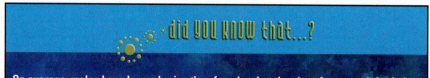

did you know that...?

On average, males have larger brains than females, but the size of a person's brain has nothing to do with intelligence. For example, the brain of the great physicist Albert Einstein weighed 1,230 grams. This is much less than the average brain weight of 1,400 grams.

Learn

Observe what happens when you put your selection to work. See if it is working. Is it doing what you expected it to do? Has it taken care of the problem? If not, you may have to go back and choose another alternative.

Decision Making

Decision making is an important part of problem solving and will play a very important role in your wellness lifestyle. At times, you may be tempted by the media or friends to take part in risky activities. Resisting these temptations and sticking with your wellness plan will require you to make some decisions. Some decisions will be pretty easy to make, such as deciding to eat an apple instead of a candy bar for a snack. Other decisions have a more serious impact on your health and well-being. An example would be deciding if you want to try smoking cigarettes.

As a teen, you are at an age when your decision-making powers will be tested far more they were before. You spend more time away from your family than you did as a child. And you now have life experiences and information you lacked when you were younger. As children grow and mature, they are generally given more opportunities to make decisions for themselves. Look at Figure 3-4 to see how, in a general sense, decision making shifts over time from parent centered to child centered. Consider the task of buying clothes. A parent would take an 8-year-old child shopping and would most likely decide which clothes to buy. The child might be allowed to choose the colors. Parents might also take a 14-year-old to buy clothes and specify the amount that can be spent. The teen, however, would be allowed to select the clothes.

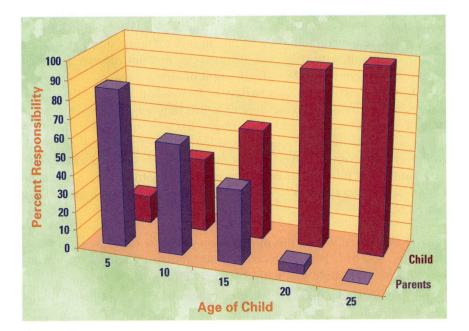

Figure 3-4
Responsibility for decisions

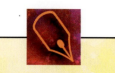

take it on home

Write up the steps in problem solving to take home. The next time a problem comes up in your family, share the steps and encourage everyone to get involved in a brainstorming session. Be sure to write down everyone's suggestions. Then facilitate a discussion of the possible solutions and choose one as a group. Implement the family's choice and conduct an evaluation to see how it worked out. Write up the experience and put it in your Health Folio. How is problem solving different when it is done in a group than when a person works alone?

By the time a child is 17, he or she is probably responsible for shopping, selecting, and perhaps even paying for the clothes. As children mature, parents entrust them with more and more opportunities to make decisions. This is probably true for you. The amount of freedom you have is likely to be related to how well you have made decisions in the past.

Using a Decision-Making Model

Choosing an alternative to put into action is a key problem-solving skill. Using a decision-making process will help you select the best alternative to solve your problem. A handy model for decision making is shown in Figure 3-5.

Step 1: List the Alternatives. The first step in decision making is to list alternative solutions from which to choose. This step may sound pretty basic, but many people fail to develop good problem-solving skills because they consider only one solution. Every problem has many possible solutions, and when people don't even consider them they lose the opportunity to apply decision-making skills. Sometimes it takes courage to think about different alternatives. Some may be painful or costly at the time but will be the best choice in the long run.

Step 2: Identify Advantages and Disadvantages. Once you have brainstormed a list of alternatives, you can go to the second step and examine each one to determine its advantages and disadvantages. You might want to write them down, especially if this is an important decision such as which college to attend. At this point, you want to keep the promising alternatives and reject the ones that are obviously unsuitable.

Step 3: Predict the Consequences. Step 3 is predicting the possible consequences of each alternative. This means asking, "What would happen if . . . ?" You may want to have a friend, family member, or other trusted person help you with this task. People who are not directly involved with the problem may offer a fresh point of view.

Consequences exist in a variety of forms. Some alternatives have psychological consequences, meaning you may experience emotional pain if you choose them. Or you might have to motivate yourself to adopt a new behavior. Some consequences are financially harmful; others are rewarding. Still others might require you to learn a new skill. The important thing is to consider each alternative and its possible consequences very carefully so you can determine what you are willing to accept.

Step 4: Prioritize. Using the information you now have, you can move on to step 4, which is to prioritize the alternatives. The following guiding questions can help you with this part of the process:

1. Which alternatives are *suitable* to address the problem? Some solutions may seem appealing, but if they do not take care of the

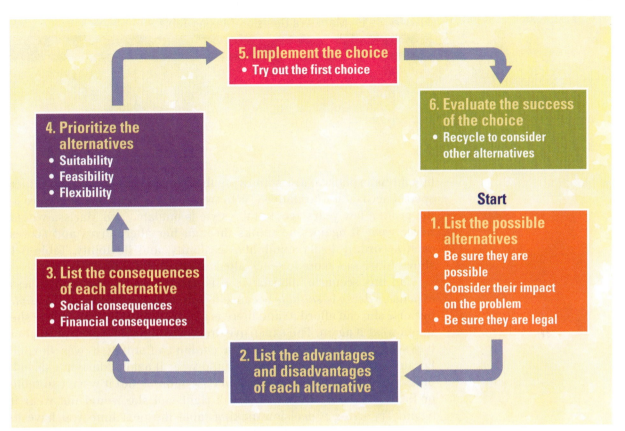

Figure 3-5 Decision-making model

problem, they are not suitable. Suitable also means that the alternative is **ethical**.

2. Which alternatives are *feasible*? Can you really implement the solution? Is the solution costly? What is the level of certainty that the alternative will work?

3. How *flexible* is the alternative? Is it compatible with other related situations or with circumstances that may arise later? Can the alternative be modified to apply to similar problems in the future?

Using a Decision Table. To help with your decision making, you can create a decision table. This is a convenient way to compare your alternatives. Suppose you have narrowed the possible alternatives for a problem down to three. Use the table to judge your alternatives according to the amount of suitability, feasibility, and flexibility by assigning each a score from 0 to 2. For example, imagine that Marissa is trying to decide what she will wear to the prom and she has three alternatives. Alternative A is to buy the dress that she loves; it is the most expensive dress she has seen and she really doesn't have the money for it, but she would probably wear it for other special occasions. Alternative B is to

ethical

conforming to moral standards

Table 3-1   Marissa's Decision-Making Table

Alternative	Suitability	Feasibility	Flexibility	Total
A	2	0	2	4
B	2	2	1	5
C	1	2	1	4

buy a less expensive dress knowing that she might wear it for another special occasion. Alternative C is to wear a dress that her sister wore to the prom a few years ago, but the style is outdated and Marissa would never wear it again. She thinks through her alternatives and scores each according to its suitability, feasibility, and flexibility. Table 3-1 shows Marissa's score for each alternative.

In this scenario, alternative B is Marissa's best choice. The less expensive dress is *suitable* because it will meet her needs; it is *feasible* because she can afford it; and there is a degree of *flexibility* because she might wear it again. The expensive dress was suitable for the prom, but it wasn't feasible because Marisa couldn't afford it; it was flexible because she knew she probably would wear it again. Marissa's sister's dress was feasible because it would cost nothing, but it wasn't suitable or flexible because the style wasn't right and she would not wear it again. Try using a decision-making table the next time you have to choose among several alternatives.

Step 5: Implement and Evaluate. The last step in the decision-making process involves steps 4 and 5 of IDEAL: Act on the chosen solution (implement it) and Learn (evaluate the alternative you have carried out). Did the solution work? You may have made the correct choice and that's great. But even if you have gone through all the steps in the process, your choice might not be the right one. In that case, you can make revisions, or you may have to start over and try something different.

A Few Helpful Hints

Decision making is a skill that can be learned, but it takes practice to do it well. Your teen years will present you with many opportunities to call on this skill. Here are a few more guidelines to consider:

- When the decision is very important, consider all possible solutions carefully. Don't just make a quick "I'll do this . . . " choice. The more important the decision, the more planning and care you should use in applying the decision-making process.

- If you avoid making a decision, you are making the decision not to act.

• You won't know if your decision is correct until you act on it. Only then can you evaluate the results.

Making Decisions on Your Own

What happens when you are not with your family? Friends become increasingly important during the teen years, and you probably spend a lot of time with yours. You are likely to encounter many situations in which you must make difficult decisions on your own. You may have already found yourself in these kinds of situations. Perhaps one of your friends offered you a cigarette, someone at a party offered you a beer, or an obviously intoxicated friend arrived to drive you to a movie. At times such as these, your health values are challenged. You find yourself having to decide whether to go along and place yourself in a high-risk situation or to follow your wellness plan, which calls for you to minimize obvious risks. You need an approach to decision making that will help you determine the best course of action. Being prepared will help you avoid being pressured to make poor decisions and having to live with the consequences of those poor decisions.

BUILDING YOUR Wellness Plan

One of the most important skills in your wellness plan is your ability to solve problems. You will have to make several key decisions to develop and follow a good plan. Before you can make these decisions, you must first identify any problems you might have with your current health habits. Then you can apply the problem-solving process to find solutions and develop wellness behaviors that will work for you. The information in this chapter will help you to:

• Understand the problem-solving skills you currently have and identify what additional knowledge or skills you need to improve your problem solving

• Learn to think critically and use reasoning skills to become a successful problem solver

• Practice identifying and describing your problems so that you can successfully solve them

• Solve problems by using any of the tools provided in the chapter, including mind mapping to clarify all the parts of a problem, the IDEAL model for problem solving, and the decision table to help with difficult decisions

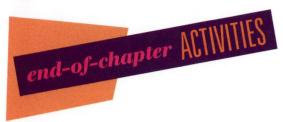

 Weblinks

Brain Teasers

Archived Brain Teasers: **http://www. louderthanabomb.com/brain_teaser_old.htm**

Butlerwebs.com: **http://www.butlerwebs.com/jokes/brainteasers.htm**

Psychtests.com: **http://www.psychtests.com/mindgames**

Health Risk Appraisal

Teen Net Health Promotion for Teens: **http://teennet.binghamton.edu/teensurv.htm**

You First: **http://www.youfirst.com**

Short-Answer Questions

1. Name one controllable and one uncontrollable risk factor.
2. State the technical medical term for measuring death in populations.
3. Name the leading cause of death among teens.
4. Name a type of reasoning based on known rules or policies.
5. What the acronym IDEAL stand for?

Discussion Questions

1. Describe the significance of the CDC's Youth Risk Behavior Surveillance Survey.
2. Why should people be aware of and concerned about risk factors?
3. Name and explain at least four risk factors that can affect your health.
4. What is the difference between inductive and deductive reasoning?
5. Describe the steps of the problem-solving model.

Chapter Vocabulary

Using a separate sheet of paper, list and define the following terms:

brainstorming	morbidity
deductive reasoning	mortality
inductive reasoning	risk factors
mind mapping	

Application Activities

Language Arts Connection

You can practice creativity and polish your writing skills with this exercise. It is called stream of consciousness writing. Choose a problem and set aside a specific amount of time to spend on your exercise. Try starting with three minutes. Begin writing and just let your thoughts flow while you write them down. Don't stop writing until your time is up. You may find that you have written a lot of nonsense, but that's okay. That is a sign that you are overriding the structural part of your brain. Set your paper aside for a while. Go back to it later and highlight the words and phrases that mean the most to you in the passage. Use the words and phrases to complete your final paper.

Social Studies Connection

Make a list of professional people who serve your community. Examples could include judges, doctors, firefighters, city commissioners. You may want to include the professional role you see yourself in some day. Select a few of the professional roles and write a paragraph for each one in which you describe how people in those roles might use problem-solving techniques.

Science Connection

The type of problem-solving process used by scientists is known as the scientific method. Some steps in the scientific method are similar to those in the problem-solving model:

1. Observe some aspect of the world around you.
2. Invent a tentative description, known as a *hypothesis*, that is a statement about your observation.
3. Make some *predictions* about the accuracy of your hypothesis.
4. Test those predictions by *experiments* or further observations, and modify or verify the hypothesis on the basis of your results.

Use library or Internet sources to create descriptions of the italicized terms. Prepare a report for your Health Folio explaining the scientific method and define the terms in your report. Explain how these terms apply to the steps in your problem-solving model.

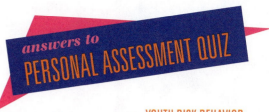

answers to **PERSONAL ASSESSMENT QUIZ**

personal assessment: YOUTH RISK BEHAVIOR

There are no correct answers to the questionnaire items, but some responses indicate higher levels of risk than others. You are taking healthy steps toward reducing risk factors mentioned in the questions if your answers were the following:

Item 1. f	Item 7. c
Items 3 and 6. a	Item 8. g
Item 2. e	Item 9. h
Items 4 and 5. b	

chapter 4

Communicating for Wellness

Carl and Jennifer have noticed that some kids at the high school have started smoking. Even some of their friends are now smokers, and their smoking bothers Carl and Jennifer a lot. The smoke irritates their eyes, and when they hang around a group of smokers, their clothes pick up the odor. Their friends sometimes encourage them to "be cool" and give smoking a try, but both Carl and Jennifer are sure this is something they don't want to do. They have strong feelings about smoking and have been able to say no every time someone offers them a cigarette. But even though they know they don't want to smoke, sometimes it is hard to say no to their friends. Carl and Jennifer have talked about how it feels when their friends don't listen to their reasons for not wanting to smoke. It gets frustrating, sometimes, but they are committed to wellness and plan on sticking up for their beliefs about saying no to smoking.

chapter OBJECTIVES

When you finish this chapter, you should be able to:

- Describe the components of the communication process.
- List and explain factors that can interfere with the communication process.
- Describe good listening skills.
- Compare the characteristics of different communication styles.
- Explain the importance of being assertive.

Introduction

Good communication is one of the keys to a healthy and satisfying life. Think about how much time you spend each day engaged in some form of communication. As a teen, you depend on your communication skills to accomplish many important tasks that will help you build a healthy and satisfying life:

- Acquiring information to develop adult life skills
- Building strong friendships
- Performing well in school
- Getting along with family members
- Dealing with difficult people
- Saying no to unhealthy suggestions

The quality of your communications affects all aspects of your wellness. In this chapter, you will learn about the communication process, different styles of communication, and ways you can become a better communicator.

key TERMS

active listening
body language
communicator
decode
empathy
encode
feedback
mirroring
paraphrase

personal assessment: YOUR COMMUNICATION STYLE

On a separate sheet of paper, write the numbers for each of the statements in the assessment. Then read each statement and write next to the number the letter of the response that most closely matches your behavior. The interpretation of your responses can be found at the end of the chapter.

1. When you go to a party where there are a lot of people, you are most likely to:
   a. Interact with a lot of different people.
   b. Talk one-on-one with people you know.
   c. Try to get some time to talk with people you think are important.
   d. Try to leave as soon as you can.

2. If you could be famous, which career do you think would fit you the best?
   a. Movie star
   b. Head of a company
   c. Inventor
   d. Humanitarian

3. If the phone rings, what are you most likely to do?
   a. Answer it immediately and talk for a while.
   b. Wait a few rings before you answer it.
   c. Answer it and finish the call as quickly as possible.
   d. Hope someone else will answer it.

4. Which of the following appeals to you most?
   a. Taking action on a calculated risk
   b. Creating good human relationships
   c. Discovering the secret in a complex mystery
   d. Going to an exciting social event

5. If you and a friend have an argument, your first reaction is to:
   a. Make sure the friend understands your position.
   b. Make sure the relationship doesn't get damaged.
   c. Avoid that person for a while.
   d. Find a compromise so you both get part of what you want from the situation.

EFFECTIVE COMMUNICATION

How many people have you communicated with today? Chances are you have had exchanges with a wide variety of people of different backgrounds, ages, and interests. Think about how you interacted with each person. Did you communicate in a different way with each one?

Most people take communication for granted. After all, almost everyone can speak, and talking is what communication is about, right? Actually, this is not true. Good communication involves a cluster of skills that not everyone has mastered. For example, do you ever feel that some people just don't listen to you? Good listening is an essential part of good communication. It's not difficult for most people to talk. But it can be a challenge to communicate effectively. The good news is that everyone can learn and develop excellent communication skills.

The assessment you completed at the beginning of the chapter revealed the type of communication style you favor. None of the styles are better or worse than the others. The style you demonstrate the most is reflective of your personality and how you respond to the world around you. Knowing what your style is may help you develop your communication style to its utmost.

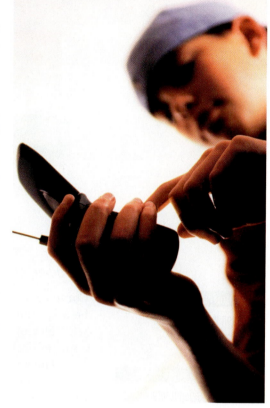

The Communication Process

Communication can be looked at as a process that consists of several steps. These steps can help us understand the nature of back-and-forth interaction as people take turns speaking and listening. Figure 4-1 is a diagram of the communication process. Each step is necessary for truly effective communication to take place. Can you think of people in your life who are great talkers but poor listeners? Do you consider your communications with them to be effective?

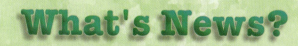

What's News?

Many teens like to use their cellular phones, but using a phone while driving an automobile is not safe. Current research indicates that young adults who use a cell phone while driving take longer to react to emergencies and are more likely to experience accidents than are people not using a cell phone. Some states have made it illegal to drive and talk on a handheld cell phone, and others are considering similar laws. Depending on where you live, talking on the phone while driving might be more than just dangerous, it might get you a ticket!

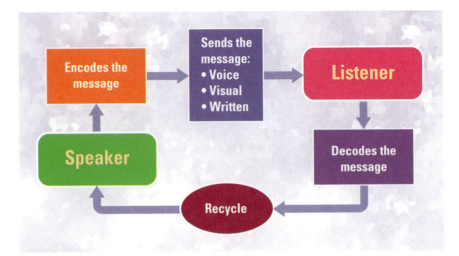

Figure 4-1
The communication process

Encoding and Sending Messages

communicator

a person who is transmitting information to another

encode

to develop a thought into a word or behavior pattern

Communication begins with the **communicator**. The communicator can be a speaker, a writer, or a performer. To simplify our discussion, we will refer to the communicator as the speaker. But the conditions that apply to oral communication apply to the other forms as well.

The speaker starts by determining the purpose of his or her communication. Then the message to be sent is developed and **encoded**. Encoding means that the speaker's thoughts associated with the message are converted into words and sentences or some other form that the listener (receiver) will understand. It is extremely important that the process start with a clear message because this forms the basis for the communication encounter.

Messages can be delivered in many ways. For example, they can be spoken and given in person, on a video, or over the phone. Or they can be written, as in a letter or e-mail. They can even be delivered visually as in the case of a photo, painting, or performance. An unusual but effective form of communication is pantomime. Have you ever seen a mime tell a story?

Decoding Messages

decode

to interpret a word or behavior pattern

Once the message has been delivered, the listener **decodes** (interprets) the message he or she has heard or seen. Sometimes this interpretation is not what the speaker had in mind. A number of things can influence how the receiver decodes a message:

- *Poor encoding.* The speaker has to present the message using words and terms that the receiver understands. Have you ever talked with someone who uses language that is way beyond your level of understanding?

- *Interference.* Sometimes messages are sent when there is noise in the background or conversation from people nearby. It is difficult to hear and concentrate on what is being said. The best communication takes place in a quiet environment.

- *Distraction.* Communication is difficult if there are distractions in the environment. Suppose two people need to have an important conversation, and they try to talk while watching television, while playing a video game, or while sitting at a sporting event. It is difficult to listen and understand if people don't give their full attention to the interaction.

- *Language.* If the people engaged in the conversation speak different languages or if they have very different vocabularies, communication can be hampered. The participants may spend so much time trying to figure out what the words mean that they lose the content of the messages.

Communication is a two-way interaction. The speaker and listener exchange roles throughout the conversation, taking turns sending and receiving messages. An important part of the exchange is **feedback**. This is a special kind of message used to confirm the listener's understanding of the original message. Using feedback to check meaning is what is meant by recycling in Figure 4-1. See Table 4-1 for examples of feedback. Can you think of other ways to check your understanding of the speaker's message?

feedback

special messages used to check understanding of the original message

Table 4-1 Did I Understand You?

Feedback Technique	What It Means	Examples
Paraphrasing	The listener restates the speaker's message in his or her own words.	• "So you're saying that you're having a lot of trouble understanding algebra?" • "Let me make sure I have this right. The assignment is to summarize Chapter 5, and it's due on Monday."
Reflecting	The listener repeats part of the message and asks the speaker to complete it.	• "You can't go to the concert on Saturday because _____." • "You want to buy a new CD player, but _____."
Clarifying	The listener asks questions about the speaker's meaning.	• "What do you mean when you say you think he's 'strange'?" • "You say I should join the club because it's fun. What kind of activities do they sponsor?"

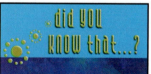

did you know that...?

Sign language is the fourth most used language in the United States. Many deaf and hearing-impaired individuals communicate with sign language. The most widely used form is American Sign Language (ASL). You can use ASL techniques to sign in two ways. One way is by learning the ASL alphabet and using finger spelling. The finger-spelling alphabet is shown in Figure 4-2.

Another type of sign language communicates entire concepts using the hands without the need to spell them out. For example, closing the index finger of your right hand and pivoting it on your right cheek communicates "apple."

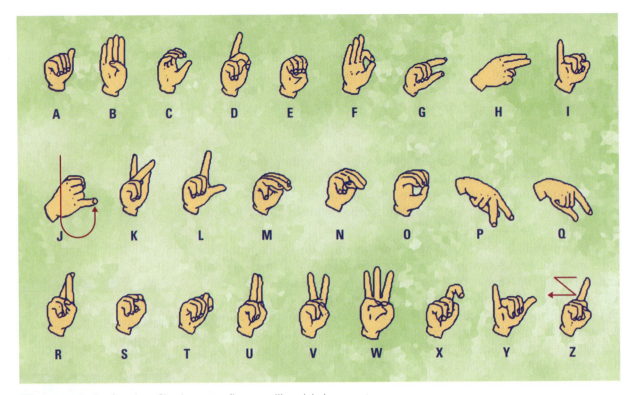

Figure 4-2 American Sign Language finger-spelling alphabet

Breakdown in Communication

Read each of the following examples after you have obtained a clear understanding of the communication process shown in Figure 4-1. Answer the questions at the end of each example to test your understanding of how to communicate effectively.

Ben and Carla

Ben and Carla have a problem. Carla expected to meet Ben at her house last night to study for an upcoming biology test. She is angry because he never showed up and never called her. Ben said he could not come because he went out with his family for his sister's birthday. He said he had told Carla when they discussed the study session that he would call her *if* he was free. His studying with her depended on which night his family was going to go to dinner with his sister. Given that Ben and Carla had their conversation at the very end of the lunch hour in the noisy cafeteria, there may have been miscommunication. What do you think caused the miscommunication? What could Ben and Carla have done to avoid the problem?

Netti and Brent

Netti and Brent have been going out with each other for about three months. Netti does not have strong feelings for Brent and wants to break up with him. She wants to be honest with Brent, though she knows it will be difficult to end the relationship without deeply hurting Brent. She spent the better part of the weekend going over what she plans to say when she is alone with Brent. What part of the communication model is Netti putting to use when she formulates her "good-bye" message?

Georgie

Georgie gave a speech in English class yesterday. It did not go as well as Georgie had planned. The grade was less than the A Georgie had expected. Although Georgie felt the presentation went well, the teacher's critique indicated that Georgie seemed to jump from one topic to another and used a lot of terms Georgie's classmates and the teacher did not understand. What communication problem did Georgie encounter that resulted in the lower grade?

NONVERBAL COMMUNICATION

We don't communicate only with words. In fact, more than half of our meaning is communicated through body language. **Body language** is the nonverbal part of communication expressed through facial expressions, gestures, movements, postures, and appearance. It is estimated that 60%–70% of our communication comes from body language. Communication research has found that if we notice a conflict between a person's words and body language, we tend to believe the body language. For example, if you are talking to someone who is leaning away from you with her arms crossed in front of her body, this posture may be a sign that she is not interested in what you have to say. On the other hand, a listener who is sitting up and leaning slightly toward you and making good eye contact is probably involved and interested in the conversation. What other types of body language have you noticed when you are talking with friends and family members?

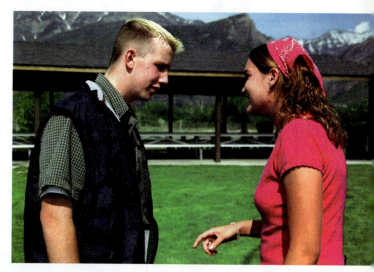

Without knowing the content of the conversation taking place, what do you observe about the body language?

LISTENING SKILLS

Communication is not just talking. Listening is just as important. In fact, you will spend about 45% of your communication time listening. Unfortunately, many people think that listening is the same as hearing

body language

the nonverbal part of communication expressed through facial expressions, gestures, movements, postures, and appearance

did you know that...?

There are approximately 100,000 words in the English language. The average individual uses between 30,000 and 60,000 of them. People who study speech estimate that we have about 750,000 nonverbal communication symbols.

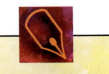

take it on home

Spend some time listening to and observing the interactions between males and females in your home or neighborhood. Take notes on how the people communicate with each other verbally and nonverbally. Can you identify traits that are different for males and females? Can you describe and explain behaviors that seem effective and those that seem less so? Record your observations in your Health Folio.

and don't do a very good job with it. The average person retains about 65%, or the majority, of what he or she hears for only a few minutes.

What do you think is the difference between hearing and listening? If you say that hearing takes little or no effort for the average person, you are correct. We hear sounds when they occur. Listening, on the other hand, means paying close attention and interpreting what we hear. It takes some effort to listen. And it takes a *lot* of effort to listen *well*.

Suppose you are in a park with a friend and his family. You spend the afternoon talking, picnicking, and playing ball. Your friend has talked about some problems he is having with his parents. You think you are paying attention, but your mind is also taking in the sounds of birds, kids laughing, and traffic on a nearby street. When you get home, you spend some time thinking about what your friend said and realize that you really are not sure how serious his problems are. You missed a lot of the details because, although you heard what he said, you weren't really listening. You plan to call him later and make an effort to learn more about his situation.

Listening, then, is not something you just do. It is a skill that can and should be learned. Listening carefully is an essential part of being a good communicator. It helps you decode messages and promotes good interpersonal relationships because it shows other people you care what they have to say.

Characteristics of a Good Listener

What do you think makes a good listener? Are there people you enjoy spending time with because they show an interest in what you have to say? Here are some of the characteristics of a good listener:

- Good listeners make an effort to empathize with the speaker. They maintain good eye contact and use appropriate nonverbal cues that indicate they are paying attention with interest.
- Good listeners listen for general ideas as well as for facts.

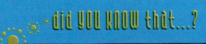

did you know that...?

First impressions are important! Research shows that when you first meet someone, you have approximately 20 seconds to make an impression. How can you make it a good one? Well, your appearance sends a nonverbal message about who you are, so if you want the impression to be favorable, it's a good idea to dress appropriately for the occasion and to be well groomed. Making eye contact with the person you meet, smiling, and showing interest tells a person that you are trustworthy and friendly. Good posture and a comfortable handshake will communicate self-confidence. All is not lost, however, if you fail to capitalize on the first impression. If you feel your first impression did not go well, use your problem-solving skills to correct the situation.

- Good listeners are patient with the speaker. They don't interrupt but wait for their turn to speak.

- Good listeners focus on what the speaker is saying instead of thinking about what *they* are going to say next. They listen to everything the speaker has to say before responding.

- Good listeners focus on the speaker, even if the information is not very interesting. They listen for something of value.

What other characteristics can you add?

Improving Your Listening Skills

How would you rate your own listening skills? Are you an **active listener**? This is someone who becomes completely engaged in the communication process and pays attention to the other person's verbal and nonverbal messages. Listening is one skill that everyone can improve. Here are some tips to show you how:

- Make it your goal to be a good listener. As it does in many other wellness skills, motivation plays a role in whether you become a good listener. The first step is really wanting to be a good listener.

- Stop talking and listen. Try to increase the amount of time you spend taking in and interpreting information.

- Ask questions to learn more or when you don't fully understand the speaker's message.

- Develop a set of nonverbal habits that indicate you are in tune with the speaker. These include good eye contact (with "smiling eyes" and not frowning) and body posture that is upright or leaning forward. You can show interest by leaning forward, silently nodding, or saying things such as, "I see" and "Tell me more." These actions tell the speaker you are listening and care what is being said.

active listening

paying attention and being completely engaged in the communication process

take it on home

Try an experiment when you go home today. Each time a family member speaks to you, stop what you are doing—whether you are eating, watching television, or playing video games—make eye contact with the person who is speaking to you, and *listen*. Don't do anything else while you are actively listening. Record in your Health Folio your observations and explain how it felt to do this exercise.

Mirroring Dialog	
Speaker	**Listener**
Hojoon, his eyes wide in excitement, says, "I can't believe it. I wanted to go for a bike ride. I went to the garage to get my bike, and it was gone!"	Frank makes good eye contact with Hojoon. He leans slightly forward with an expression of surprise on his face.
Hojoon's expression turns to sadness. "I worked almost the whole summer to raise the money for that bike."	Frank's surprised expression begins to change to one of worry.
Hojoon's expression turns to pleasant surprise. "Oh, I forgot! I told my sister she could borrow it first thing in the morning to go to swim practice. She's not home yet."	Frank mirrors his pleasant expression. "Man, that *is* a relief. I would have hated to see you go through the hassle of trying to get it back if it had been stolen."

Figure 4-3
Mirroring while actively listening shows empathy for the speaker.

mirroring

repeating, copying, or paraphrasing the speaker's communication style

empathy

sensitivity to and understanding of another person's emotions

paraphrase

to restate the speaker's message in your own words

Mirroring

Mirroring is a response pattern you can use to show **empathy** for the speaker. Ways of mirroring include copying the way the other person is sitting, **paraphrasing** some of his or her key points, and speaking at the same speed as him or her. In the example in Figure 4-3, Frank mirrors his friend, Hojoon.

Showing empathy lets others know that you care about them. It not only improves communication but also strengthens interpersonal relationships. Can you think of other ways to show empathy?

COMMUNICATION STYLES

Knowing how communication works is an important part of becoming a good communicator. You can enhance your communication skills if you understand that not everyone communicates in the same way. In fact, psychologists have identified many communication styles. Table 4-2 illustrates four major types.

Communication styles tend to reflect the speaker's personality type. *Passive* individuals tend to be meek. They lack self-esteem and fear that if they challenge another person, that person will become angry and dislike them. They communicate in a soft voice, avoid eye contact, and give the message that they will not present a challenge. For example, Simon has been waiting in line a long time at the record shop to get the latest record from his favorite group, and he has to hurry and catch the bus home. Then two kids come up and go to the counter ahead of him. One of the pair looks at Simon, but Simon just shrugs his

Table 4-2 Characteristics of Four Common Communication Styles

	Communication Styles			
	Passive	**Aggressive**	**Passive-Aggressive**	**Assertive**
Description	Communicator puts the rights of others before his or hers	Communicator puts personal rights above others' rights at all costs	Communicator avoids confrontation but attempts to get even through manipulation	Communicator presses for personal rights while respecting the rights of others
Consequences	Communicator loses, receiver wins	Communicator wins, all others lose	Communicator loses, others lose	Communicator wins, others win
Messages given	I'm sorry. I don't count.	You don't count. I am right.	I am right and I will teach you a lesson	I count. You count.
Behavior cues	No eye contact, insecure statements, head down	Glaring eye contact, hostile body language, loud voice, swearing	No immediate action, passive demeanor; the "lesson" will come later	Use of "I" statements, steady eye contact, easy manner

shoulders, looks away, and says nothing. His communication style on this occasion is passive. He is not communicating what his needs are.

Individuals who are *aggressive* are just the opposite. They feel a need to have their way at any cost. They are easily angered, tend to bully the people around them, and make it clear that it is their way—or else. Their communication style is loud and confrontational. If Simon had used an aggressive communication style in the example above, he would have yelled at the guys that butted ahead and would have said something like "Hey, jerk! I'm next. Go to the back of the line." Can you see why this type of communication does not work well? Can you imagine how the person he spoke to would have reacted if he also had an aggressive communication style?

Passive-aggressive people don't take responsibility for the events in their life. They tend to procrastinate and work inefficiently, then blame others for their lot in life. Their communication indirectly expresses their anger, but their intention can be to punish others. For example, they may fail to state clearly what they want from others, then put them down by lying about them to their friends. If Simon were passive-aggressive he would have handled the situation above by tossing the album on the counter, saying to the clerk, "Forget it, I've waited long enough," and kicking the door on the way out of the store.

Assertive individuals exhibit the healthiest communication style. They state clearly what they think, what they feel, and what their needs are. But they do it in a way that does not threaten or belittle the listener. An assertive Simon would have said, "Sorry, but I have been waiting for some time and need to catch the bus. Please let me get my album and go." He is also prepared to say "Thanks" if his request is met.

USING COMMUNICATION EFFECTIVELY

Understanding how communication works is one thing. Using communication to your best advantage is another. Let's examine some ways of using communication-related behaviors to enhance your well-being.

real teens

Carl has a friend named Brian who was badly burned when he was four years old. Brian's burns were so severe that his damaged skin did not grow with him. Over the years, he has had more than 80 surgeries to prevent his skin from restricting his growth, but he remains severely scarred. Many people in school find it difficult to talk with Brian. They seem to be uncomfortable being around him and have a hard time making eye contact. Carl is different. He and Brian have known each other for a long time. Carl knows that good communication includes making eye contact and being a good listener, so he makes a special effort to include these skills when he talks with Brian. These skills helped him solidify his friendship with Brian, but they have also made him a better communicator with his other friends.

Assertiveness

Assertiveness is an important life skill, but it is especially useful for teens. As a child, you tended to live with many rules: "Don't do this," "Don't do that," "You should be . . . ," and "You must . . . ." Many of these instructions came from your parents or other adults because they wanted to keep you safe and teach you the importance of rules. As a teen, you have more opportunities to choose your actions. Assertiveness skills will help you stand on your own and follow rules that make sense to maintain your safety and well-being. Here are some suggestions for those times when you meet challenges that require you to assert yourself:

- *Be true to yourself.* You have had many life experiences with family, friends, neighbors, teachers, and clergy. As a result of these experiences, you have developed a set of standards and values, a sense of right and wrong, that provides you with an ethical compass to guide your life. These standards are important tools that help you with your decision making. You know what is good and evil, you know what is honest and dishonest, you know what is good for your life and what is bad. Use these values to make wellness decisions you *know* are good for you.

- *Be courageous.* As a teen you will encounter challenges to your beliefs and wellness decisions. Standing up for yourself and defending your beliefs takes courage. It isn't always easy to act in a way that is different from the behavior of others in your group. It's easy to just agree and go along with others. Doing what you believe is right can be more challenging.

- *Plan ahead.* Think about how you will respond if faced with situations that call for you to follow your beliefs. Suppose a friend asks you to sneak into a concert without paying. You know sneaking in is wrong and don't want to do it. Do you have an idea of what you would say? Would you know how to respond to your friend assertively?

- *Keep the "we" in mind.* When faced with a difficult situation, you want to express yourself and state what you believe to be right. But you want to do it in such a way that the other person feels valued. One effective way is to use "I" statements. For example, saying "I would like to go home now" works better than "You are nuts for wanting to stay, and for wanting me to stay with you."

- *Be prepared to defend yourself.* You may be challenged when you make assertive statements about what you are and are not willing to do. People may call you "a wuss," "a loser," or some other term implying that you are not "cool." What would you do if you found yourself in this kind of situation? How would you reply?

- *Stand up for yourself.* When you are defending your actions, make firm eye contact with the person challenging you. If you look away, look down, or look apologetic, your reply will be perceived as weak. This perception will open the door for you to be challenged. Restate your position in a firm but nonthreatening voice. Don't give a response that leaves room for an argument, and don't state your reply in a way that sounds apologetic.

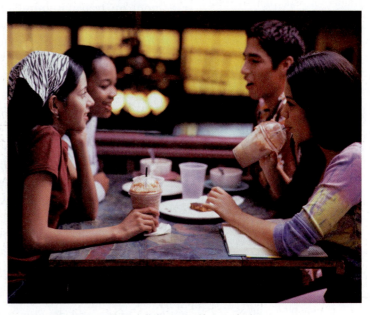

It takes courage to calmly explain yourself assertively.

Handling Aggressive Communication

Have you had experiences dealing with people who behave and communicate aggressively? Having to deal with aggressive people is not uncommon among teens. You may find this kind of person at school, at work, and even in your own family. In general, individuals who communicate aggressively do so because they lack the personality traits and skills to communicate any other way. In times of stress, their communication style becomes even more aggressive. There are some effective ways to deal with aggressive people:

- *Avoid them.* If you know people who are verbally aggressive, try to avoid them. If you do come into contact with them, keep the communication simple. Don't engage in discussions that can lead to conflict, especially if they are bullies.

- *Don't try to be more aggressive than they are.* One aggressive person challenging another can lead to an escalating conflict. Sometimes you have to call on all your assertive communication skills and self-discipline to stay calm. The more calmly you respond, the greater the likelihood that the other person's level of aggression will diminish.

- *Be polite.* This suggestion may sound out of place, but allowing the other person to speak without interruption tends to relieve the tension. Trying to interrupt and "correct" the speaker will only feed the aggressiveness.

- *Clarify what the argument is.* In a polite way, keep your opponent on track. Remind him or her what the argument is about. Don't let the discussion wander to other issues, especially those that become destructive personal attacks.

- *Avoid the use of "you" statements.* Statements attacking the other person, such as "You don't even understand what I'm saying. You are so stupid!" will only feed the fire of aggression.

- *Present logical arguments, not personal attacks.* When someone comes at you in an aggressive style, recognize that arguments involve ideas. Even if you are being personally attacked, do not return in kind. Use logic and reason to address the topic, and resist verbally attacking your opponent.

- *Know when to quit.* If the aggression continues to escalate, feel free to stop the communication. You can simply say, "I don't want to keep talking to you. I feel like our conversation isn't going anywhere."

Communication and Feelings

As you progress through your teen years, you will have many opportunities to apply and develop your communication skills. Many of your communication interactions will be motivated by feelings. In fact, feelings will probably play a major role in determining the nature of your interactions with others. Strong feelings are often involved when we communicate with people close to us, such as parents, friends, classmates, and teachers. These feelings can be very joyful, but sometimes we experience sadness, anger, frustration, and disappointment in our relationships. Maybe you disagree with your parents about going out with your friends instead of attending a family function. Or your feelings have changed for someone you have been dating for a few months. Or perhaps you have lost someone you cared for very much and need to talk about it.

There is nothing wrong with experiencing strong feelings. The challenge is knowing how to best communicate your feelings. It is best to be honest. First, be honest with yourself that the feelings exist. Don't try to stifle them or stuff them away. Expressing your feelings is healthy and contributes to your well-being. It also improves your relationships with others. No one likes to hear bad news, but it's better to know and deal with the truth than to have it hidden.

Honesty and dealing directly with other people takes courage. It is important to consider the feelings of the other person and to present issues in a way that is not hurtful and is as comforting as possible. Do you know anyone who is able to communicate kindly about difficult and emotional issues? What have you observed about that person's communication behaviors?

BUILDING YOUR Wellness Plan

Good communication skills are among your most important life skills. With attention and practice, your communication skills can become useful tools in your wellness plan. These skills can help you negotiate for the things you want in life and enhance your relationships with other people. The essential communication skills you should take from this chapter and add to your wellness plan include:

- Understanding the communication process, especially the significance of encoding and decoding information
- Using effective body language to enhance verbal communications
- Being an active listener
- Developing an assertive communication style
- Appreciating the diversity of communication styles
- The ability to respond appropriately to an aggressive communication style

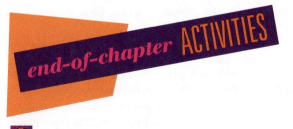

end-of-chapter ACTIVITIES

Weblinks

ASL signing: **http://commtechlab.msu.edu/sites/aslweb**

Effective communication: **http://kidshealth.org**
  (search for "talking to your doctor")

Finger-spelling alphabet (animated):
  http://www.where.com/scott.net/asl

Finger-spelling alphabet (scrambled):
  http://www.iwaynet.net/~ggwiz/boggle/scramfs.htm

☀ Short-Answer Questions

1. Why should teens be interested in developing good communication skills?
2. What is the importance of encoding in the communication process?
3. What is wrong with an aggressive communication style?
4. What behaviors would you use when listening actively?
5. List and describe things you can do to become a better listener.

☀ Discussion Questions

1. Diagram and explain the components of the communication process.
2. Discuss the characteristics of good listeners.
3. List and explain some characteristics of assertive communication.
4. How would you handle a discussion with someone who is communicating in an aggressive and threatening manner?
5. Why would a person use a mirroring technique when listening?

☀ Chapter Vocabulary

Using a separate sheet of paper, list and define the following terms:

active listening	decode	feedback
body language	empathy	mirroring
communicator	encode	paraphrase

☀ Application Activities

Language Arts Connection

Rent a movie you haven't seen. Instead of watching the whole movie right away, watch just enough to learn the names of the characters. Then fast-forward the movie to any scene in which two or more of the characters are in a conversation. Watch that scene with the sound turned off. Take notes during the scene and try to determine what the conversation is about by observing body language. Use your notes to write a script for the movie using the names of the characters. After you have completed your script, watch the scene with the sound turned on. Write a description of the scene and what was actually said. Report your observations.

Social Studies Connection

Imagine that you are a high school principal. You find that bullying and ridicule are taking place frequently at your school. Do some research on the Web to learn about the consequences of these behaviors for both the bully and the recipient. Develop a speech that you could give to a student assembly to discourage bullying behavior.

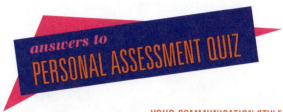

answers to
PERSONAL ASSESSMENT QUIZ

personal assessment: YOUR COMMUNICATION STYLE

Compare the answers you selected with the response table below. Collect the number of As you chose, the number of Ds, and so forth.

1. a. D	b. N	c. A	d. C
2. a. D	b. A	c. C	d. N
3. a. D	b. N	c. A	d. C
4. a. A	b. N	c. C	d. D
5. a. A	b. N	c. C	d. D

You probably will have one letter that appears more often than any of the others. That letter corresponds to the labels below, along with descriptions of the various types of communicators.

A = Asserter Fast-paced and direct. Asserters are hardworking, ambitious, leader-type people. They tend to be lawyers, politicians, or self-employed. Some famous asserters are Muhammad Ali, David Letterman, and Clint Eastwood.

D = Demonstrator People-oriented and enthusiastic. Demonstrators are idea people who like to be in the limelight. They tend to make good entertainers, social directors, and personnel managers. Some famous demonstrators are Robin Williams, Elvis Presley, Jim Carrey.

N = Narrator Slow-paced and indirect. Narrators are warm and friendly. They are likely to be nurses, counselors, or ministers. Some famous narrators are Bill Clinton, Florence Nightingale, Barbara Walters.

C = Contemplator Task-oriented and slow-paced. Contemplators are analytical thinkers. They are likely to be accountants, scientists, engineers, or bookkeepers. Some famous contemplators are Albert Einstein, Al Gore, Carl Sagan.

unit 2 | Personal Health

Introduction

During your teen years, you will find that health-related decisions are no longer the sole responsibility of the adults in your family. If you are like most teens, you have an interest in your appearance and personal grooming and want to take care of these things on your own. In this unit, you will learn about the chemical changes that take place in your body during your teen years and how they impact personal grooming. Many of these changes also affect the physical side of you, making you a reproductively capable adult.

This unit will also help you understand the mechanisms that make your senses work for you. Often we take our senses for granted, using them daily and trusting that they will function well the rest of our lives. It is hard to imagine that what we do or don't do to care for our senses will affect the quality of their performance as we age. Loud music and other noises, sunlight, and other environmental factors can reduce the quality of our senses through adulthood and into old age. In this unit, you will be able to develop the wellness skills you need to protect the quality of your senses for a lifetime.

chapter 5

Caring for Yourself

Brett is about to start his senior year in high school. But this year he will be surprising some people when he gets back to school. Until now, he didn't take a lot of pride in his appearance and was more interested in "dressing down." His old clothes were baggy and comfortable, and besides, he didn't believe that clothes made a person. He didn't bathe or wash his hair as often as he should have, so it wasn't surprising that people often shied away from him. Brett often told his friends and family that appearance was not as important as the person. Actually, there was some truth to what he said because he's a good kid—intelligent, kind, and considerate. His attitudes were challenged last spring when he learned in his social studies class that appearance does count. His teacher explained that psychological tests show that neat, well-groomed people are better liked than those who are messy. Brett thought a lot about this idea and decided he would "reinvent" himself for his senior year. Over the summer, he developed better grooming habits. He even changed his hairstyle and spent some of his summer earnings on new clothes. He's curious to see if he'll notice people acting differently toward him.

chapter OBJECTIVES

When you finish this chapter, you should be able to:

◉ Describe behaviors that contribute to healthy skin.

◉ Discuss how sun exposure causes skin damage.

◉ Explain how to prevent and treat acne sores.

◉ Describe the health risks associated with tattooing.

◉ Explain good hair care techniques.

◉ Explain how to properly care for the teeth and gums.

◉ Describe the practices that promote good sleep.

Introduction

key TERMS

actinic keratosis

circadian rhythms

dermis

epidermis

follicles

melanin

ozone layer

sebaceous glands

sebum

sun protection factor

Your parents were responsible for your personal care when you were a child. As a teen, that responsibility is shifting to you. At the same time, your changing body presents new challenges for grooming and personal hygiene. Appearance is very important to most teens, and, as you will learn, how you look is very much influenced by your wellness habits.

As a young adult, you will make a number of health decisions as you care for yourself. What are the best ways to take care of your skin, hair, and teeth? What kinds of grooming products should you use? What are some of the consequences of popular practices such as tanning and tattooing and piercing? Knowing the facts will help you make good decisions about these and other habits that affect your health. As a teen, you want to be liked and accepted by your peers. At the same time, you want to safeguard your current and future health. This chapter will give you information about habits you can incorporate into your wellness plan that will have a positive effect on both your health and your appearance.

personal assessment: YOUR PERSONAL HEALTH PRACTICES

Read each of the statements below. Record your answer, yes or no, on a separate sheet of paper. For items for which you answered no, explain why you answered as you did. Then read the feedback at the end of the chapter.

1. I am aware of the value of washing my face with soap and water twice a day.
2. I am familiar with the sun's damaging effects on exposed skin.
3. I know when and how often I need to use sunscreen.
4. I know what SPF stands for when describing a sunscreen product.
5. I know what my skin type is and what kind of sunscreen is best for me.
6. I know how to care for my skin in order to prevent and treat acne.
7. I am aware of the health risks of tattooing and body piercing.
8. I know how to care for my teeth and gums to prevent periodontal disease.
9. I am knowledgeable about the proper way to care for my hair.
10. I am aware of things I can do to ensure that I get a good night's sleep.

YOUR SKIN

Skin is your body's protective covering: a sturdy, flexible, mostly waterproof covering that prevents infectious organisms from entering the body. The skin consists of two distinct layers. (See Figure 5-1.) The outer layer, the **epidermis**, is made up of five levels of cells. The outermost layer consists of dead cells that are constantly flaking off. Within the deepest level, there are cells that produce new cells to replace the ones that slough off. In this layer, there are specialized cells that produce a pigment called **melanin**, which is responsible for giving color to the skin. Dark-skinned people have more melanin in their skin than light-skinned people. A suntan is the result of the skin's increasing its production of melanin when it is exposed to the sun.

epidermis

the outermost layer of the human skin

melanin

substance in the skin that contributes to skin color

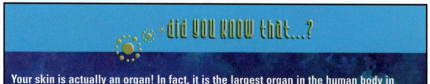

did you know that...?

Your skin is actually an organ! In fact, it is the largest organ in the human body in weight and area. The average person sheds 40 pounds of skin in a lifetime.

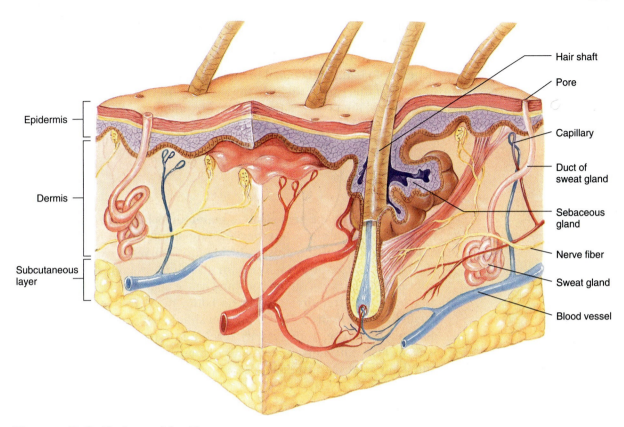

Figure 5-1 The layers of the skin

The inner layer of skin is the **dermis**. The dermis is sometimes referred to as the true skin because it contains the substances that give skin its structure and elasticity. The dermis also contains blood vessels, nerves, sweat glands, and hair follicles.

Caring for Your Skin

In addition to protecting your body, your skin is the part of you that is most exposed to the outer world. Both your general health and your appearance are affected by the condition of your skin. There are a number of things you can include in your wellness plan to help you maintain the health of your skin.

Good Nutrition

Maintaining a healthy diet is important for the skin. Your skin especially likes vitamins A, B, C, and E, which you get from eating fruits and vegetables each day. (You will learn more about good nutrition in Chapter 8.) You don't have to eat special foods to benefit your skin, and it's not necessary to take special vitamin supplements. As long as you

dermis

the inner layer of the human skin

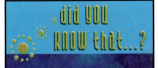

Mosquito repellents don't repel mosquitoes. They hide *you*. The chemicals in the mosquito spray block the mosquitoes' sensors so they don't know you're there.

consume a variety of nutritious foods, your body will send the vitamins and other nutrients where they are needed.

Have you seen ads for skin lotions and creams that describe the benefits of vitamins included in their compounds? There is no clear evidence that these products help the skin any more than a good, balanced diet. In fact, the products themselves are often very expensive and may not be a good value. They may act as a moisturizer, but they cannot provide the skin with vitamins because it can't absorb them when they are applied to its surface.

Bathing

Your skin needs to be kept clean to maintain its health and appearance. Keeping the skin clean is especially important for teens because the changes in the body chemistry during the teen years can contribute to conditions that favor acne. The skin also produces oils and sweat that interact with bacteria on the body and cause body odor. Preventing acne and body odor requires that teens bathe more frequently than they might have as children. How often you should bathe or shower depends on your skin type, your activity level, and environmental conditions such as heat, humidity, and dust. Whether you take a shower or a bath and the type of soap you use are matters of personal preference.

Deodorant

Your body builds up heat when the weather is warm or you are exercising. Overheating can lead to sickness and even death. The purpose of sweat is to help the body cool off. Sweat forms on the skin, and, as it evaporates, the body cools. Body odor does not come from sweat itself, which has no odor, but from the bacteria on the skin and hair that feed on the sweat and produce waste products. Young children sweat, but because of their body chemistry and the lack of the type of bacteria on the skin that cause odor, they don't produce body odor.

Body odor is not considered socially acceptable in our culture. Fortunately, body odor can be reduced by bathing and using a deodorant. A deodorant doesn't actually stop perspiration. It is a scented product that masks the odor associated with perspiration. Antiperspirants, on the other hand, are deodorants that also contain chemicals such as aluminum chlorohydrates that prevent sweating. Whether to use a deodorant or antiperspirant is a personal preference.

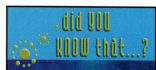

did you know that...?

Your feet have more sweat glands than any other part of the body—nearly 250,000 of them!

Sun Exposure

At the turn of the nineteenth century, it was fashionable to have clear white skin. People with tanned skin were considered laborers without social standing. People of wealth avoided exposure to the sun. By the beginning of the twentieth century, society's attitudes had shifted, and the suntan was a sign that people had leisure time to spend at the beach or other vacation spots.

Young people today continue to seek a tan, and research indicates that a third of teens don't bother to use sunscreen. A tan may give the impression of health, but its effect is actually just the opposite! There is probably nothing more harmful to your skin than sun exposure. People with a lot of sun exposure eventually become significantly more wrinkled than those who have less exposure. Even more serious, it increases their risk of skin cancer. The sun's rays contain harmful ultraviolet (UV) radiation, which would destroy human life if it were not filtered by the earth's **ozone layer**. The ozone layer is located in the stratosphere, about 10 miles above the earth's surface. Ozone is a gas that absorbs some of the UV radiation.

Ultraviolet Radiation. Ultraviolet (UV) radiation arrives at the earth in three forms:

1. UV-A is needed by our bodies to manufacture vitamin D. Too much UV-A, however, can cause toughening of the skin, weakening of the immune system, and, to some degree, cataracts of the eyes and reddening of the skin. UV-A is not absorbed by the ozone layer.

2. UV-B has effects on both plants and animals but is mostly absorbed by the ozone layer. The greatest threats to humans from long-term exposure to the rays that do pass through are reddening of the skin, skin cancer, cataracts, and suppression of the immune system.

3. UV-C is very dangerous to plants and animals, but it is completely absorbed by the ozone layer and does not reach the earth's surface.

Prolonged exposure to UV rays puts one at risk for a number of negative effects on the skin. The strongest UV rays occur between the hours of 10 A.M. and 3 P.M. On a cloudless day during the summer, the rays of the sun can cause second-degree burns on someone with light skin who is not wearing sunscreen or whose skin is not conditioned for the exposure. To protect your skin from sun damage, limit sun exposure during peak hours. In a practical sense, limiting exposure may be difficult to do. At the very least, the best precautions are to use a waterproof sunscreen product with a **sun protection factor** (SPF) rating of 15 or higher and to wear a wide-brimmed hat. Table 5-1 lists skin types and recommended SPF ratings for each. The paler a person's skin, the higher should be the SPF factor in the sunscreen.

Skin Cancer. Sunburn is a harmful short-term consequence of overexposure to the sun. The long-term, very serious consequence is skin cancer. Each year more than 1 million cases of skin cancer are reported, and more than

ozone layer

layer of gas that protects the earth from harmful ultraviolet rays

sun protection factor

ability of a sunscreen to protect the user from ultraviolet radiation; the higher the SPF value, the greater the amount of protection

Sunscreen can help prevent sunburn and skin cancer.

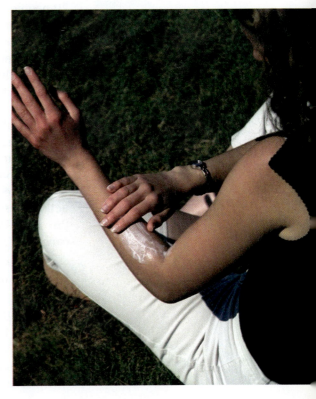

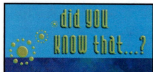

There are 34 substances known to contribute to the depletion of the ozone layer. Some of these substances can last in the atmosphere for many years. Scientists are constantly monitoring the depletion of the ozone layer, and efforts are under way to protect it.

Table 5-1   Skin Type Classifications

Classification	Skin Type	General Physical Characteristics	Skin Care Product
I	Always burns, never tans	Pale white skin, blue eyes, blond hair	SPF 30
II	Always burns easily, tans minimally; may freckle	White skin, blue or green eyes, blond to light brown hair	SPF 20–30
III	Burns moderately, tans uniformly	Light brown to olive skin, green or brown eyes, brown to black hair	SPF 20
IV	Burns minimally, always tans well	Moderately brown skin, brown eyes, brown to black hair	SPF 15
V	Rarely burns, tans profusely	Brown skin, brown eyes, brown to black hair	SPF 10
VI	Never burns	Brown to black skin, brown eyes, black hair	SPF 5–10

actinic keratosis

a precancerous condition in which sores form on the skin as a result of sun exposure

20 people die from skin cancer every day. Several factors increase the risk of skin cancer. The greater the amount of exposure to UV rays, the greater the likelihood of getting skin cancer. A person with skin type I is at greater risk than someone with skin type VI. And the risk is greater for individuals who had at least one sunburn as a child that was serious enough to blister the skin.

Skin cancer can take years of sun exposure to develop in some people, but the medical community is now seeing cases of skin cancer among teens. It is important to understand that, although sunscreens are designed to allow longer exposure time in the sun, they *do not eliminate* the possibility of skin cancer.

A precancerous condition that appears on sun-damaged skin is **actinic keratosis**, in which sores, called actinic keratoses, appear on the skin. These sores can develop into one of the three forms of skin cancer:

1. *Squamous cell carcinoma.* This form of skin cancer occurs in the outer layer of skin cells and is easily treated if detected early.
2. *Basal cell carcinoma.* Basal cell carcinoma forms in the lower levels of the skin. It is the most common form of skin cancer in the United States and, like squamous cell cancer, can be treated if detected early. Because this cancer forms deeper in the skin layers, it not as easily recognized and later detection requires greater levels of treatment.

3. *Malignant melanoma.* This form of skin cancer originates in the lower level of the epidermis (see Figure 5-2). It can spread more rapidly than carcinomas. It is curable, but it can be deadly if not caught early because of its ability to quickly spread to other body parts. Melanoma is related to sun exposure and is becoming increasingly more common. In 1935, risk for melanoma was 1 in 1,500; by 2000, the risk was 1 in 75 and claimed the lives of more than 7,000 people in the United States.

Skin cancer is treated in a number of ways. A physician may use liquid nitrogen to freeze actinic keratosis sores. Patients can also use a prescription cream that destroys the sores over time. Either one of these procedures kills the damaged cells and allows new cell growth to take place. If tests confirm that cancer is present and it has not spread, it may be surgically removed. If the cancer has spread, other treatments may be necessary. (See Chapter 24 for more information about cancer and its treatment.)

Indoor Tanning. Some people use indoor tanning devices to get their tan. The companies that sell the equipment and services for indoor tanning claim that the devices are safe. The bottom line is that indoor tanning is no safer than outdoor tanning. In fact, indoor tanning may be more dangerous because people who use tanning beds *think* they are safe, so they expose themselves too long and don't use sunscreen.

Indoor tanning companies make the claim that indoor tanning is safe because their tanning beds produce "only" UV-A rays. Remember that the production of melanin, which results in a tan, is the body's effort to *protect* itself from harmful radiation. There is no such thing as a safe tan. The best thing to do is to avoid exposing yourself to a harmful situation.

Acne

There is probably no single condition that concerns teens more than acne. Every teen wonders if he or she can grow into adulthood without getting acne. The reality is that very few people go through their teen years without getting acne to some degree. In fact, by the time they reach their midteens, 40% of young people will have acne severe enough to require help from a doctor.

Acne is a skin condition that can occur on the face, neck, shoulders, and back. It is common during adolescence because of the rise of the male hormone **testosterone** in males and females (yes, females produce a little testosterone, too!). This increase in testosterone causes the oil glands in the skin to be more active, and this extra oil creates blockages of the hair follicles. The bacteria present in the follicles produce small infections that then produce pus.

If you care for your skin properly, acne should not create major problems. Here are some recommendations for taking care of your skin:

- Don't squeeze, pinch, or scrape acne sores. Those procedures don't help and may make things worse by increasing the amount of infection and contributing to scarring.

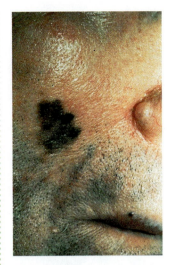

Figure 5-2
Malignant melanoma is a cancerous lesion associated with sun exposure.

testosterone

the primary male hormone

- Wash your face and other affected areas twice a day with soap and warm water. Regular skin soap is fine, but if acne is a problem, your doctor can recommend a cleanser that is best for your skin type. (Cleansing liquids should be used only if recommended by a doctor.)

- Don't scrub hard. Too much friction on the skin can actually worsen the condition.

- Be cautious about using cosmetics. If you feel you must use them, be sure they are oil free.

- See a physician for recommendations if you have problems with excessive amounts of pimpling or infection.

Tattooing

fad

something that is very popular for a short period of time

A current **fad** among some young adults is tattooing. Tattooing involves piercing the skin and inserting a colored ink into the wound. Because piercings are done with needles and create open wounds, the work should be done only by a trained professional under sterile conditions. It is extremely important that tattoos not be done by friends or family members at home because of the high risk of infection.

real teens

Pam and Janna thought it would be fun to get tattoos and decided to talk it over with their parents. Their parents advised them against it, pointing out that the marks would be permanent. They were afraid the girls would be doing something they would later regret.

The two friends waited until they were 19 and off at college. They decided they still wanted to each get a small tattoo, so they investigated the local tattoo shop, which they were told adhered to the "highest standards." Three months after they got their tattoos, they began experiencing stomach pain and feeling tired all the time. They finally went to the doctor, and tests revealed they both had hepatitis C. It turned out they had contracted the hepatitis C virus when they received their tattoos at the commercial tattoo shop with the "highest standards." Pam and Janna were fortunate because the disease was caught early enough to be treated. If hepatitis C is left untreated, liver disease and serious illness can result. But Pam and Janna now warn their friends who are interested in getting tattoos about the risks involved and the need for careful research to determine exactly how well disease-control standards are followed at tattoo shops.

Although the decision to get a tattoo is a personal one, teens under the age of 18 should discuss it with their parents. In fact, most states have laws that prohibit minors from getting tattoos without parental permission, and some states will not allow tattooing if the client is not at least 16 years of age, even with parental permission.

It is important to understand that there are health risks associated with tattooing. These risks increase if the tattoo is applied by an amateur and include the following:

- *Infection.* Tattoos create open wounds that bleed after the procedure. It is extremely important that the wounded area be kept clean and protected from infection.

- *Blood-borne diseases.* Transmission of HIV (human immunodeficiency virus) or **hepatitis C** is possible if the equipment is not properly sterilized.

Anyone considering a tattoo must realize that the coloration of the skin is permanent. Remembering that a tattoo is permanent is especially important when using names of dating or marital partners. The name of someone special tattooed on a visible body part may be romantic at the time, but if the relationship dissolves, the name stays. It is possible to alter or remove a tattoo, but the procedures are painful, time consuming, and expensive.

Laser surgery is the most expensive method of tattoo removal. It can cost much more to get a tattoo removed than it did to get it put on. Laser surgery is popular because it's less likely to have harmful side effects, than are other methods of removing tattoos. The laser pulses simply pass into the outer layers of skin and break the pigment into small pieces that can be absorbed into the body. It usually takes several laser treatments to completely remove a tattoo. The larger and more brightly colored the tattoo, the more treatments it takes to remove.

Surgery works best for small tattoos. The skin around the tattoo is numbed with a local anesthetic, and the tattooed skin is cut away with a scalpel. The edges of skin are then sewn together, leaving a small scar. Larger tattoos may have to be removed in several stages, removing

❃ teen forum ❃

Tattooing

There are young people who wish to get tattoos but are discouraged or prohibited from doing so by adults—parents, legislators, or physicians. Many states have laws that prohibit people under the age of 18 from getting a tattoo without parental permission.

- If you were a parent and your teen came to you and asked about getting a tattoo, what would your reply be?

hepatitis C

a liver disease that is transmitted via the hepatitis C virus when blood products or injection instruments are shared

What's News?

Some studies have shown higher rates of hepatitis C infection among individuals who have received commercial tattoos. A person with a tattoo may have up to a nine times greater chance of getting hepatitis C than a none-tattooed person. The U.S. Centers for Disease Control and Prevention (CDC) is conducting a large-scale study across the United States to learn more about this risk.

small pieces one at a time. Skin grafts may be required, in which skin is taken from another area of the body to replace the skin removed from the tattooed area.

Dermabrasion is a procedure in which the top layers of the skin and the tattoo ink are removed by buffing with a round sanding instrument (or a water-and-salt solution known as Salabrasion). The skin is first numbed with an anesthetic spray and then bandaged because the peeling of skin causes some bleeding. This method can cause skin discoloration, changes in skin texture, or scarring.

Body piercing is another fad some young people have tried. As is tattooing, piercing procedures are risky. The greatest risk associated with piercing is infection. The risk increases if piercing is not performed by a reputable shop. Figure 5-3 offers some cautions for anyone considering tattoos or body piercing.

Perhaps you know someone who has expressed interest in getting a tattoo or a piercing. You may be able to help with the decision if you know some things about the risks involved and how to minimize them.

The Decision
Tattoos should be considered *permanent*. Even with current technology, removal is painful, time consuming, and expensive. Removing a $50 tattoo can cost $1,500 to $2,000. After the procedure, the treated skin will not exactly match the skin around it.

The Facility
Never let friends do the tattooing or piercing. The fact that they are untrained and do not have the proper equipment increases the health risks dramatically.

Tattoo and piercing shops should be investigated. Have your friend go to the shops and talk with the owners about the procedures they use. A good shop will proudly show and tell how they keep their equipment sterile. If they do not want to talk about their procedures, they should be avoided. Watch the artists as they handle materials. They should wear rubber gloves and change the gloves if they are used to handling nonsterile material such as money or telephones.

Leftover ink should be thrown away.

A piercing gun should not be used. There is no way to properly sterilize it. The object that is inserted after the piercing should be made of nontoxic material such as 14-carat gold, surgical steel, or titanium and should be sterile.

Aftercare
The facility that performed the service will tell you what people have to do to care for the tattoo or piercing to prevent infection. Tell your friend to follow the instructions. There are also Web sites where you or your friend can obtain more information related to tattooing and piercing. Use your health literacy skills.

Figure 5-3

Cautions for tattooing and body piercing

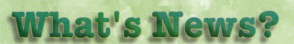

What's News?

Tattoo to monitor diabetes? Scientists in Texas and Pennsylvania are collaborating on the development of a tattoo that contains special compounds that would change chemically to alert patients when their blood sugar level is low. The compounds are known as polyethylene glycol beads that are coated with fluorescent molecules. Low blood sugar causes the tattoo to glow, telling the wearer to care for the condition.

YOUR HAIR

Hair is a characteristic of all mammals. Almost our entire body has hair on it, but not so thick that it would be considered fur. Some hair is very thick, like the hair on your head, and some hair is almost invisible.

Our hair grows from special structures, called hair **follicles**, located in the epidermis. (See Figure 5-4.) It grows in cycles, sometimes growing actively and sometimes resting. The hairs on your head are usually there for three to five years. A hair is shed when a new one is formed in the follicle to replace it. Baldness, which occurs mostly in

follicles

special structures in the skin where hair growth takes place

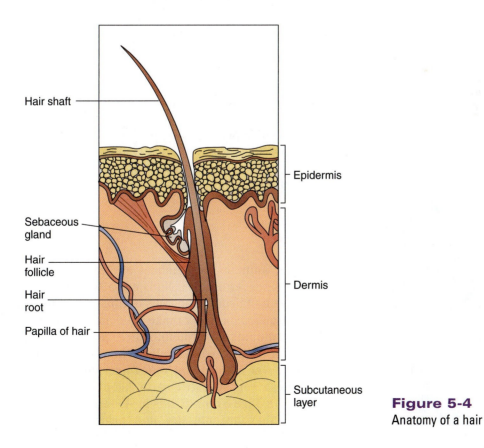

Hair shaft

Sebaceous gland

Hair follicle

Hair root

Papilla of hair

Epidermis

Dermis

Subcutaneous layer

Figure 5-4
Anatomy of a hair

men, is the result of an inherited trait that causes certain parts of the head to stop producing hair.

Genetic factors contribute to hair color and texture, which ranges from straight to tightly curled (kinky). The thickness of hair also varies among individuals, from very thick to very thin. A strand of women's hair is about half the diameter of a strand of men's hair. Hair color is caused by pigments in the hair shaft. The darker the hair, the greater the amount of pigmentation in the hair. Hair without pigmentation is white or gray.

Caring for Your Hair

Proper care is necessary to maintain the health of your hair and scalp. Hair gets dirty when **sebum**, an oily substance produced by the skin's **sebaceous glands**, coats the hair shaft and attracts and holds dirt. The amount of oil produced varies from person to person and from day to day. You should wash your hair when it feels oily, or at least twice a week. If you believe you need to shampoo every day, be sure to use a pH-balanced shampoo; wash your hair only once, and rinse it well. Overcleansing your hair will actually produce more oil. You can get into a cycle of washing too often and creating more oil than if you shampooed less frequently.

To understand why pH balance is important, you need to understand what pH is. Every solution can be classified as either acid or alkaline (base). The pH scale, which ranges from 1 to 14, measures the level of acid or base in a solution. Battery acid has a pH of 1; baking soda (base) has a pH of 12. The chemistry of solutions is interesting. When combined, acids and bases balance each other. If you spilled battery acid, you could use baking soda mixed with water to clean it up. The resulting pH would be about 6. Products that are pH balanced are formulated to have a pH somewhere between 6 and 7, so they work well on the hair and skin, where the pH is slightly acid (between 5 and 6) to protect against infection. Almost all shampoos are pH balanced. If they were not, using them would cause the hair to become very dry and frizzed.

YOUR NAILS

Whereas other animals have hooves and claws, human beings have nails on their fingers and toes. Nails are a type of dead skin cells that grow out of the nail beds at the ends of fingers and toes. Although they are made of protein, you can't make your nails grow or get stronger by eating extra amounts of protein. Some people claim that you can strengthen your nails by eating gelatin, but this claim is not true.

Have you ever noticed that your fingernails grow faster than your toenails? Unless you want them to keep growing, they should be trimmed about a once a month. It is best to trim your nails after bathing because then they are not dry and brittle. Fingernails should be

---

sebum

an oily substance that keeps the skin lubricated

sebaceous glands

glands in the skin by each hair follicle that produce sebum

---

did you know that...?

The record for the longest fingernails belongs to a man from India, who grew the nails on his left hand for more than 50 years. They became twisted and curled as they grew to their final length of more than 20 feet for the combined total of all five fingers.

trimmed so they are rounded at the end. Toenails should be trimmed with the ends more straight across. If you trim them with rounded ends, you increase the likelihood of getting an ingrown toenail, which occurs when the toenail grows into the skin on the side of the toe. You want to avoid ingrown toenails because they are quite uncomfortable and in severe cases require surgical correction.

YOUR TEETH AND GUMS

The teeth are located in special sockets in the upper and lower jaws. The primary function of the teeth is to prepare food for digestion by cutting, tearing, and crushing. In fact, the process of digestion begins when we chew our food and mix it with saliva. Another important function of our teeth is to assist with forming words as we talk. Figure 5-5 illustrates the various parts that make up an individual tooth.

As a teen, you are likely to have between 28 and 32 teeth, depending on whether you have your wisdom teeth (the four molars in the back of the mouth). The wisdom teeth arrive sometime during late adolescence. Many people have their wisdom teeth removed because the teeth are uncomfortable and, in some cases, because the wisdom teeth push the other teeth out of alignment, resulting in biting problems.

Tooth **enamel**, the hardest substance in the body, covers the top part of the tooth. Although enamel is very hard, it can be penetrated by

enamel

the hard outer covering of the tooth

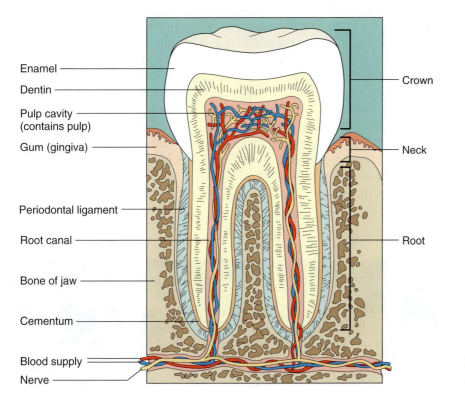

Enamel
Dentin
Pulp cavity (contains pulp)
Gum (gingiva)
Periodontal ligament
Root canal
Bone of jaw
Cementum
Blood supply
Nerve
Crown
Neck
Root

Figure 5-5
Anatomy of a tooth

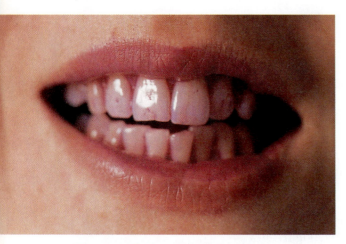

Figure 5-6 Plaque on teeth looks like a soft, white, sticky mass and hardens into tartar if not properly removed.

plaque

a mixture of bacteria and food residue that forms on the teeth

tartar

a hard, scaly substance between the teeth and the gum line caused when plaque is not removed properly

periodontal disease

loss of supporting structures around the tooth caused by bacterial plaque; If left untreated, it leads to tooth loss

the acid produced when bacteria in your mouth react with the sugar and starch in foods you eat. This acid is what causes tooth decay. The foods you eat also combine with bacteria in your mouth to cause **plaque**. (See Figure 5-6.) If plaque is not removed, it will harden into **tartar** within two days. Tartar, once formed, can be removed only by a dental professional. As plaque and tartar accumulate, tooth and gum damage can occur.

Caring for Your Teeth and Gums

Good dental care is largely under your personal control. Taking five minutes twice a day to brush and floss is a very good investment of your time and an important part of your wellness plan. These simple preventive measures can help you avoid discomfort, tooth loss, and costly dental procedures. See Figure 5-7, a guide to the proper way to brush your teeth. In addition to good self-care, it is a good idea to have your teeth examined at least once a year by a dental professional.

Flossing is a good way to remove plaque from between your teeth, in the spaces the toothbrush bristles don't clean well. Flossing is especially important if your teeth are very close together. If your teeth are very close together, it may be a good idea to choose a thin, waxed floss so the floss does not get stuck between the teeth or shred.

Lack of good dental care can lead not only to the development of cavities but also to the development of **periodontal disease**. Periodontal disease is caused by the accumulation of plaque in and around the gum line. If not removed, the plaque will begin to destroy the supporting structures that connect the teeth to the bone, first near the gum line and then deeper into the socket. The pocket eventually gets so deep that the connective structures between the bone and teeth are destroyed and the tooth is no longer supported.

Brushing and flossing twice a day, done properly, should prevent periodontal disease. The following are signs of problems that should be reported to a dental professional:

- Gums that bleed during brushing
- Persistent bad breath
- Red, swollen, or painful gums

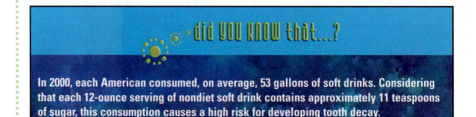

did you know that...?

In 2000, each American consumed, on average, 53 gallons of soft drinks. Considering that each 12-ounce serving of nondiet soft drink contains approximately 11 teaspoons of sugar, this consumption causes a high risk for developing tooth decay.

Equipment and Supplies

Your toothbrush will work best if it has soft bristles. A small brush head is good because it lets you get to hard-to-reach places. Replace your toothbrush every three to six months.

Procedure Steps

1. Grasp the brush and place it so that the bristles are at a 45-degree angle, with the tips of the bristles right at the gum line.
2. Using the tips of the bristles, vibrate the brush back and forth with short light strokes for a count of 10, allowing the tips of the bristles to clean the tooth under the edge of the gum.
3. Lift the brush and continue into the next area or group of teeth until all areas, front and back, inside and outside, have been cleaned.
4. The bristles of the brush can be used to clean the tongue by gently scrubbing it with a vibratory back-and-forth motion.

Brushing your tongue is not necessary. The tongue gets constant motion and is not prone to developing plaque as are the teeth. Brushing the tongue can offer some help with bad breath, but it is not the cure. If you feel comfortable brushing your tongue, there is no harm in doing so.

Figure 5-7
Bass toothbrushing technique

take it on home

Talk with family members about their dental needs. Do the adults in your family have their wisdom teeth? If any do not, find out why the individual doesn't have those teeth. If every adult does have wisdom teeth, it is likely you will be able to keep yours. Does everyone in your household use dental floss as well as their toothbrush twice a day? Do you have all the dental care devices needed to care for your teeth? Prepare a report of your findings, and recommend actions you and your family can take to maintain good dental health. Include your report in your Health Folio.

SLEEP

Sleep is extremely important to our well-being because it is during sleep that we renew our physical and mental energies. Unfortunately, many people don't understand how important it is to get an adequate amount of sleep. Current research shows that Americans are working more and sleeping less.

We don't understand every aspect of the sleep process, but we do know something about our sleep patterns. We know, for example, that our bodies are programmed to sleep twice a day: once at night and again in the early afternoon. This programming is part of the brain complex that regulates the **circadian rhythms** that make up our "biological clock." Have you ever begun to feel a little tired when it starts to get dark? This feeling is caused by a hormone, **melatonin**, that lowers your body temperature and makes you drowsy. Take a look at Table 5-2 for an explanation of the different stages of sleep.

circadian rhythms

daily rhythms, such as sleep, that are created by the body's internal clock

melatonin

a hormone produced in the brain stem that lowers body temperature to produce a sleep state

Table 5-2   Sleep Stages

Stage	Characteristics	Duration	Phase
Waking	Person feels the need to sleep, but muscles are tense and eyes moving erratically when they are closed.	Varies with level of fatigue	Non-REM sleep
Stage 1	Characterized by drowsiness. The eyes may be closed, but the person will be able to hear activity nearby.	May last for 5–10 minutes	
Stage 2	Light sleep. Characterized by alternating periods of muscle tension and relaxation. Heart rate slows, and body temperature drops.	The longest sleep stage for the young adult; approximately 4 hours	
Stage 3	The first of two deep sleep stages. Known as delta sleep. Breathing and heart rates slow.	Approximately 15 minutes	Delta sleep
Stage 4	The deepest stage of delta sleep. Stage during which it is most difficult to rouse the sleeper. Time when sleepwalking could occur. This is when the body produces growth hormone and when the body repairs itself from injuries.	Approximately 1 hour	
REM	REM (rapid eye movement) sleep. Little body movement during sleep, vivid dreaming.	About 2 hours; begins about 2 hours after sleep begins	REM sleep

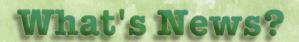

What's News?

Evidence is mounting that sleep — even a nap — enhances information processing and learning. Recent experiments at Harvard University reveal that an afternoon "power nap" of 10–15 minutes reverses daily information overload. The researchers also found that a full night's rest is helpful in consolidating the memories of habits, actions, and skills learned during the day.

Sleep patterns vary throughout our lifetime. Growing children need a lot of sleep, about 10 hours a night. Teens need about 8½ to 9 hours of sleep to be at their best. Ideally, adults should get 7 to 8 hours. Getting too much or too little sleep is not healthy. An important fact about sleep is that you can neither make up for lost sleep nor "bank" sleep to use later. Trying to do so disturbs your circadian rhythms and eventually leads to sleep disturbances.

We have learned from the science of sleep that there are things you can do to develop good sleeping habits. How many of these sleep hygiene practices apply to you?

- Avoid playing video games right before bedtime.
- Leave your bedroom and do a quiet activity such as reading if you can't fall asleep.
- Maintain a regular wakeup time, even on weekends.
- Avoid taking long naps (more than 15 minutes) during the daytime.
- Avoid large meals before bedtime.

BUILDING YOUR Wellness Plan

Your personal grooming habits certainly improve your appearance, but taking good care of your skin, hair, nails, and teeth also contributes to good health. Good habits will also pay dividends during your adult years and will reduce the chances of high medical and dental bills. The following deserve special attention in your wellness plan:

- Practicing good skin care that includes washing your face with mild soap and water every day, especially if you have acne
- Protecting your skin when you go out in the sun, including applying a sunscreen of at least SPF 15 on exposed skin
- Carefully investigating the health and social risks if you are considering a tattoo
- Taking the time to care for your skin, wash your hair, and brush and floss your teeth
- Developing and practicing good sleep habits

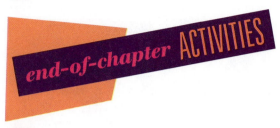

 Weblinks

Flossing

Orbis: **http://www.dentalreference.com** (click on "prevention" then "flossing")

Stuart A. Greene, DDS: **http://www. qualitydentistry.com** (search for "flossing")

Short-Answer Questions

1. Name the substance in the body that helps protect the skin from the sun.
2. Name the vitamins that are best for your skin.
3. Name the vitamin that is helped by UV-A.
4. During what time of the day are UV rays the strongest?
5. State the minimum SPF sunscreen value that someone who sunburns easily should use.
6. Name two disadvantages of tattooing.
7. List three ways that tattoos can be removed.
8. What color is hair that has no pigment?
9. Name two symptoms you might see in your mouth that would make you go to see a dental professional.
10. Explain the risks associated with plaque formation on the teeth.

Discussion Questions

1. List and describe things you can do for the health of your skin.
2. Describe the effect of ultraviolet light on the human skin.
3. Explain how to care for acne.
4. List and discuss the health effects of tattooing.
5. Discuss actions you can take to get a good night's sleep.

Chapter Vocabulary

Using a separate sheet of paper, list and define the following terms:

actinic keratosis	melanin
circadian rhythms	ozone layer
dermis	sebaceous glands
epidermis	sebum
follicles	sun protection factor

Application Activities

Language Arts Connection

Imagine you are a famous newspaper advice columnist who answers questions sent in by people around the country. A father writes asking for your opinion about letting his 17-year-old get a tattoo. Write a response to the father, providing justification for your advice.

Science Connection

1. In this chapter, you learned that ultraviolet rays contribute to skin cancer, that the earth's ozone layer helps filter out ultraviolet rays, and that the ozone layer is thinning. Research some online resources or library references to find out what can be done to reduce shrinkage of the ozone layer. Prepare a report that explains what ozone is and how we can prevent the loss of ozone in the atmosphere.

2. Search on the Web or in your library to obtain information about periodontal disease. Prepare a report on the types of procedures dental professionals use to correct the problem. Include in your report the length of recovery and the expected results with each procedure.

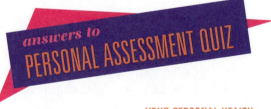

personal assessment: YOUR PERSONAL HEALTH PRACTICES

Hopefully you answered yes to each of the items on the assessment. If you were not able to do so, look at the items to which you answered no, and use the chapter information or other sources like the World Wide Web or the library to get the information that will allow you to make informed decisions about your health knowledge and skills. While not all the items in this assessment present serious health risks, many of them do play a role in your social acceptability.

chapter 6

Safeguarding Your Senses

When Christa was in seventh grade, Paula moved into her neighborhood. It took a while for the girls to become friends because Paula didn't go to Christa's school. Paula has an inherited eye disease that caused her to go blind by the time she was four years old, so she attends a special school for the visually impaired. Christa is happy to have Paula as a friend. As teenagers, they share the same interests in music and reading, although Paula reads books in Braille and listens to books on tape.

Christa has learned so much from her friend. Although she is saddened by Paula's loss of sight, she marvels at how sharp all her other senses are. Paula can hear someone approaching the house long before Christa can, and because Paula uses her fingertips to "see" objects in a room or read a book in Braille, it's almost as if she never needed her eyes. And Paula's companion dog, Taffy, gives her a "view" of the world that is very safe. As a result of her friendship with Paula, Christa has developed a greater appreciation of her own senses and the need to care for them properly.

chapter OBJECTIVES

When you finish this chapter, you should be able to:

- List and describe each of the human senses.
- Describe the structures and functions of the human eye.
- Describe activities that increase the risk for eye damage.
- Describe the structures of the human ear.
- Explain how the hearing mechanism works.
- Explain why the senses of taste and smell work together.
- Discuss the condition of synesthesia.

key TERMS

cones
cornea
iris
malleus, incus, and stapes
olfactory area
power of accommodation
retina
rods
semicircular canals
tympanic membrane

Introduction

You can thread a needle, recognize a friend you see outdoors on a moonlit night, hear the sound of waves hitting the shore, smell the spaghetti sauce in the kitchen, and feel the softness of a rabbit's fur. All of these activities are possible because of the wondrous part of your nervous system known as the senses. The detection of things in your environment—light, color, sound, odors, flavors, and textures—adds pleasure to life and helps keep you safe. Have you ever thought about what it would be like to lose one of your senses? They are so automatic that most of us take them for granted. The truth is, your connection to the world through your senses depends on a complex system of specialized structures, along with nerves and impulses that carry messages to the brain for interpretation into sights, sounds, and smells. This chapter explains how these structures and functions work and how you can best care for your senses to ensure they always function at their best.

personal assessment: WHAT DO YOU KNOW ABOUT YOUR SENSES?

Read each of the following statements. On a separate sheet of paper, write whether it is true or false and explain in a couple of sentences the reason for each of your choices. The answers are located at the end of the chapter.

1. Of all our senses, we depend on vision more than any other.

2. Men are more likely to be color blind than women.

3. Sunlight is harmful to your eyes.

4. You ears are responsible for your sense of balance.

5. The smallest bones in your body are found in your ears.

6. An explosion in outer space cannot be heard.

7. Your middle ear is connected to your throat.

8. Loud music can harm your hearing.

9. Odors help you taste things.

10. Some people can smell sounds.

VISION

Your eyes provide you with a powerful and colorful visual connection to the world. In fact, research indicates that we depend on our sense of sight more than any of our other senses. The eye has the remarkable ability to bring objects, both near and far, into our visual field. Suppose you are sitting outside on a clear summer day reading a magazine. Hearing a roar overhead, you look up from the page and instantly see an airplane that is 25,000 feet–almost 5 miles–up. Then you turn right back and continue reading your magazine, which is only *1* foot away. This process all seems so automatic, you probably take it for granted. But the eye has many functioning parts that allow you to quickly change focus. Just exactly how does it function and enable us to see?

THE STRUCTURE OF THE EYE

The eye is a ball-shaped organ with specialized structures that transmit information to the brain, where the images are interpreted into what we see. (See Figure 6-1.) The **cornea** is the transparent covering of the outer eye. It helps protect the eye and directs entering light rays to the lens. Although the **iris** is the colored part of the eye, the iris is actually a set of muscles that controls the amount of light entering the eye. The iris makes the pupil larger when we enter a darkened area so more light can enter the eye. When the environment is very bright, the iris constricts, causing the pupil to get smaller to reduce the amount of light

cornea

the transparent covering of the outer eye

iris

the colored part of the eye that regulates the amount of light entering the eye

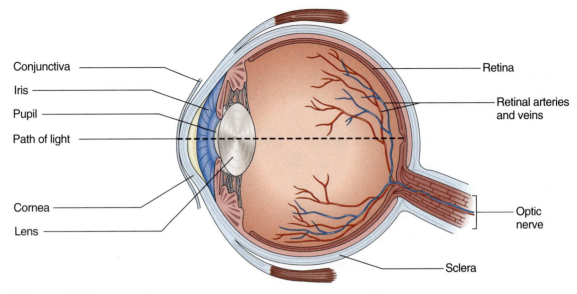

Figure 6-1 Anatomy of the human eye

retina

innermost area of the eye, where the image is received by the rods and cones

rods

specialized cells in the eye that are sensitive to light

cones

specialized cells in the eye that are sensitive to color

power of accommodation

the ability of the eye to focus on objects at various distances because of changes in the shape of the lens

entering the eye. Light passes through the pupil to the lens, where the light rays are redirected as the image that strikes the **retina**. The retina contains two types of specialized cells: the **rods**, which are sensitive to light, and the **cones**, which are sensitive to color. The human adult eye contains 120 million rods and about 6 million cones. Have you ever noticed that you can see objects and shapes outdoors on a moonlit night but that they tend to be colorless? The objects appear colorless because the cones don't function well in dim light. The rods and cones transmit their messages through the optic nerve, which extends from the back of the eye to the brain, where the image is interpreted into something you recognize and see.

POWER OF ACCOMMODATION

Remember the example of sitting outside and looking up at the airplane? The reason you can quickly see objects that are both near and far away is because of your **power of accommodation**, which allows you

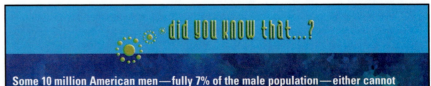

did you know that...?

Some 10 million American men—fully 7% of the male population—either cannot distinguish red from green or see red and green in very different shades than most people! This condition is known as red-green color blindness. You may ask, "How can they recognize traffic signals?" The green signals actually have some blue crystals in them, and the red lights contain some yellow.

to focus on objects both near and far away. Focusing on objects at different distances is done by muscles in the eyes that change the shape of the lenses. The power of accommodation won't work when objects are closer than 6 inches from the eyes. People also find that their power of accommodation diminishes as they age because the lens is no longer elastic enough to change shape. This reduction in the power of accommodation is why some older people need bifocals, or even trifocals, to help them focus on objects that are both close and far away while using the same set of glasses.

Caring for Your Eyes

The eye is surrounded by structures that help protect it from harm. The bony structures around the eye protect the eyeball from being hit. The eyelashes and eyebrows help prevent dust and small objects from directly striking the eye. The eyebrow also shields the eye from direct sunlight. Your wellness plan should include personal behaviors that add further protection, such as:

cataracts

clouding of the lens of the eye, causing blurred vision

1. Avoid prolonged exposure to sunlight without wearing sunglasses. UV-B (ultraviolet-B) rays can contribute to the formation of **cataracts**, regardless of a person's skin type. There are more than 1 million surgeries each year in the United States to correct cataracts of the eye. Although cataracts are often a natural part of aging, they can also occur in younger people as a result of too much sun exposure.

2. Always wear eye protection when working in any situation where there is the possibility of flying debris or splashing of toxic chemicals. Devices such as lawn trimmers and power saws and activities such as cutting wood can throw off fast-traveling particles that can enter and severely damage the eyes. Acids and cleaning fluids can be accidentally splashed and burn the eyes. Purchasing and using a $5 pair of safety goggles can eliminate a lot of expensive agony.

3. If you get something in your eye, do not rub it. A grain of sand, for example, may be irritating, but if you rub your eye, the sand is likely to scratch the cornea. Let tears wash out the particle. If tears don't remove the particle, try lifting the upper eyelid outward and down over the lower lid. If the particle still doesn't wash out, keep the eye closed, lightly bandage it shut, and see a physician.

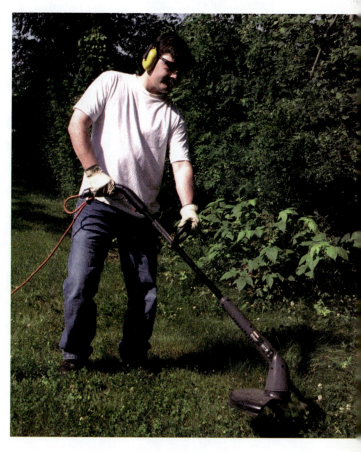

HEARING

Your ears connect you to the sounds of the world. The ear is actually composed of three sections: the outer ear, the middle ear, and the inner ear. (See Figure 6-2.) Each plays an important role in the hearing process.

The Outer Ear

The major structure of the outer ear is the **auricle**, the part of the ears you see. The auricle serves two purposes. The first is to protect the important hearing structures inside your head that make up the middle and inner ear. The second is to act as a funnel to direct sounds through the auditory canal to the **tympanic membrane** (eardrum) inside the ear canal. Have you ever cupped your ear to improve your hearing? Cupping your ear is like having an even larger auricle to better direct the sound into the auditory canal.

The Middle Ear

An important part of the middle ear is the series of three tiny bony structures that are connected to the inner side of the eardrum. These bones are called the **malleus**, **incus**, and **stapes**; they are also known as the hammer, anvil, and stirrup, named after their shapes. When sound waves that enter through the outer ear strike the eardrum, it begins to

auricle

the external part of the ear

tympanic membrane

the membrane that separates the outer from the middle ear; commonly known as the eardrum

malleus, incus, and stapes

three very small bones in the middle ear that transmit sound from the eardrum to the inner ear

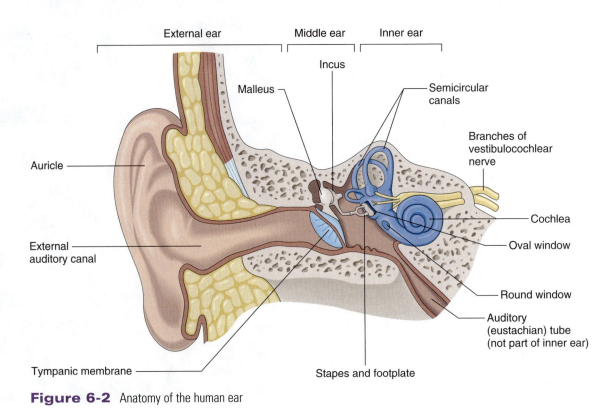

Figure 6-2 Anatomy of the human ear

vibrate. This vibration, in turn, causes the bones on the other side to move and increase the vibrations.

The **eustachian tube** connects the middle ear to the throat. This tube helps equalize air pressure in the middle ear. Have you had the experience of going under water or descending in an airplane and feeling the pressure in your ears? This pressure is relieved by swallowing or gently blowing your nose until the pressure in the middle ear is equalized. Because the eustachian tube connects to the throat, it is sometimes considered part of the respiratory system. Sometimes, infection will develop in the middle ear, known as **otitis media**. The infection gets to the middle ear by way of the eustachian tube and is more common among young children because the eustachian tube of a child lies in a more horizontal direction than it does in an adult.

The Inner Ear

The inner ear contains a series of interconnected tubes. The stapes is connected to the **oval window**, which is a membrane in the wall of the **cochlea**, a snail-shaped structure that helps transmit sound to the brain. The oval window receives vibrations from the stapes and causes the fluid in the cochlea to move. Inside the cochlea, almost 2 million tiny hairlike receptors pick up the vibrations from the fluid and convert the physical energy of the sound waves to electrical impulses that travel to the brain for interpretation.

Other important structures of the inner ear are the **semicircular canals**. These canals contain fluid that moves as the head is turned or tilted. This change in the fluid is picked up by nerves in the canals that send to the brain the message that the body has changed position. These canals are not part of the hearing mechanism but help the body maintain its balance. Have you ever gotten dizzy by spinning around in a circle? The dizziness results from the rapid movement of the fluid in the semicircular canals.

The Nature of Sound

Very simply described, sound is the vibration of some material, such as air, metal, fluid, or wood. Sound travels faster through a solid material such as steel, than it does through a gas, such as air. That's why you can hear a train by putting your ear on the track long before you can hear the sound coming through the open air.

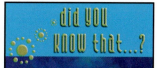

The stapes is the smallest bone in the human body (about the size of a grain of rice).

eustachian tube

passageway connecting the middle ear to the back of the throat

otitis media

infection of the middle ear

oval window

a membrane that connects the middle ear to the inner ear

cochlea

spiral, fluid-filled structure that is the essential organ of hearing

semicircular canals

fluid-filled structures in the inner ear that are responsible for helping to maintain balance

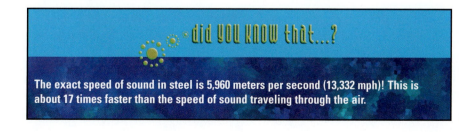

The exact speed of sound in steel is 5,960 meters per second (13,332 mph)! This is about 17 times faster than the speed of sound traveling through the air.

Because sound cannot be produced in a vacuum, an explosion in outer space would not be heard. Sound travels in waves and has two characteristics that are important to the hearing process:

1. *Frequency.* The **frequency** of a sound wave refers to how often the material through which the wave passes vibrates in response to the wave. The frequency of sound is measured in **hertz (Hz)**: 1 Hz is one cycle per second, and 100 Hz is 100 cycles per second. The higher the number, the higher the pitch of the sound. The human ear can hear frequencies between about 10 Hz and 20,000 Hz. Dolphins can hear frequencies up to 120,000 Hz.

2. *Intensity.* Simply put, the intensity of sound is how loud it is. This loudness is measured in units called **decibels (dB)**. The higher the decibel number, the louder the sound. You can learn about the decibel level of common sounds in Table 6-1.

Caring for Your Ears

The sounds we hear can range from very pleasing (soft music) to annoying (loud traffic or road noise) to painful (an explosion). In fact, sound can be so loud that it permanently destroys hearing. Many young people prefer their music loud rather than soft. Rock concerts delivered through huge speakers, personal disk players and home stereo systems are capable of delivering loud music to the listener. The most damaging sounds are probably from loud music delivered through a personal

frequency
how often the material in a medium vibrates when a wave passes through the medium

hertz (Hz)
unit used to measure the frequency of sound

decibel
a measure of the intensity, or loudness, of a sound

Table 6-1 Decibel Levels of Common Sounds

Sound	Decibel Level	Likelihood of Damage
Whispers	40 dB	
Everyday conversation	60 dB	
Restaurant	70 dB	
Heavy city traffic, vacuum cleaner, factory noise	80 dB	
Workshop tools, lawn mower	90 dB	Damage at exposure for 8 hours per day
Jet takeoff	100 dB	Damage at exposure for 2 hours per day
Amplified rock music	110–130 dB	Damage at exposure for 10–30 minutes per day
Shotgun blast, air raid siren, military jet	130 dB	Damage at 5 minutes per day
Pistol shot	140 dB	Danger level

disk player or in a very confined space. As a young person, you may not worry much about loud sounds because your hearing quickly recovers. But you may face problems as you get older. There are two reasons for concern. The first is that habits established during the teen years tend to be carried into adulthood. The second is that every loud assault on the hearing mechanism can leave it slightly damaged. The damage may not be noticeable at first, but an accumulation of assaults over the years is likely to rob older adults of their hearing. Do you ever feel your ears buzzing after listening to loud music? They buzz because your hearing mechanism has been challenged by varied frequencies at high decibels.

Look back at Table 6-1 for examples of damaging sounds. People who work in occupations in which they are exposed to loud noises are required to wear ear protection. Companies must provide ear protection for employees who are exposed to sounds of 90 decibels or higher during an eight-hour period. Many rock stars actually wear earplugs to protect their hearing when they play in concerts.

TOUCH

In Chapter 5, you learned that the skin is the largest organ in the body. In addition to being a covering for the body, skin keeps you in touch with your environment. The feelings associated with the pain of a burn, the softness of fur, or the touch of a friend begin at the skin's surface. Buried within the layers of your skin are many receptors that pick up energy from external sources. The stimulation within these receptors is converted to electrical energy and sent through the nervous system to the brain. There are different types of receptors, each designed to detect specific sensations.

Pressure

Specialized receptors allow you to perceive pressure against the skin's surface. They are sensitive enough to feel the pressure of a soft cotton-ball. Pressure receptors are not distributed evenly throughout the skin. Touch receptors are densest in your fingertips (about 100 per finger) and least dense in your lower back and buttocks. This distribution helps explain why we use our fingertips rather than our elbow to feel a texture.

Vibration

Most of the receptors that detect vibration on the skin are associated with hair follicles. When the wind blows on your skin or a leaf falls in your hair, the hairs on your body begin to vibrate. These vibrations are detected by receptors at the base of the hair shafts. There are also receptors in the deeper layer of the skin (dermis) that detect vibration. Have you ever noticed that you can actually feel the vibration from concert speakers on your skin when the volume is really loud?

✦ teen forum ✦

Whose Noise Is It, Anyway?

Modern sound systems have been engineered to produce an accurate reproduction of sound. But these same systems have also been manufactured to present the sound loudly. These conditions present two problems—one personal and one social. The personal problem is the possible harm to hearing from playing the music too loudly. The social problem is one of playing music so loudly that it can be heard by someone outside the listener's location (house, car, and so on).

- Just how loudly should people be allowed to play music?

- While the listeners have the right to enjoy themselves, others outside the location have the right to listen or *not* to listen. Whose rights should be respected?

- Should there be a limit to how loudly people can play music in their home or car?

- When considering these questions, be sure to place yourself on both sides of the situation.

Temperature

There are separate receptors for detecting hot and cold. Your skin can tell you when you are getting too much sun exposure, and it will also tell you if you are in danger of frostbite. Your skin also works in tandem with the body's internal receptors to sense if your body as a whole is overheating or getting too cold. You normally maintain an internal body temperature of about 99 degrees Fahrenheit but will begin to feel uncomfortable when the temperature outside the body rises above 90 degrees. When warm temperatures are experienced by the skin, sensors cause the pores in the skin to open and produce perspiration to help keep the body cool. Extremely cold temperatures cause the pores in the skin to close to prevent heat from leaving the body.

Pain

The pain receptors in the skin send impulses to the spinal cord, which, in turn, sends them to the brain, where the sensations are interpreted as pain. Pain, which ranges from very slight to unbearable intensity, is experienced by almost everyone at one time or another. There is an entire science dedicated to the study of pain. One thing we have learned is that each individual experiences pain differently. Another is that people handle their pain differently. Some people dwell on it and suffer a great deal; others will it away with their mind. How do you deal with physical pain?

..did you know that...?

The pain receptors in your skin are the same receptors that pick up and transmit pleasurable sensations.

take it on home

Try this experiment on each person at home. While holding two pencils that the subject can see, ask your subject to raise one arm overhead and then cross the middle finger over the top of the index finger. Then, without letting the person see what you are doing, slide only one of the pencils in the V formed by the two crossed fingertips. Now ask how many pencils the person feels touching his or her fingers. The likely answer is two even though you're using only one pencil. Why? Because our receptors are not used to sensing objects in this way. Now have the person look at what you were doing with the pencil. Come back in a day or two, and perform the same experiment. When you ask the person how many pencils he or she feels, the answer will be one. Why not two this time? Write your findings and include them in your Health Folio.

Burns provide an example of pain inflicted directly on the skin. Sunburn can start with the skin feeling hot. Redness and pain, the symptoms of a first-degree burn, can come later. A serious sunburn can result in second-degree burns, in which the skin is blistered and more painful. Third-degree burns, which would not happen with sun exposure, are the most severe. They result in such severe tissue damage that the pain receptors in the skin are destroyed, so the burns themselves are not very painful.

Caring for Your Touch Sensors

The quality of your sense of touch depends on the health of your skin and nervous system. You can't improve your natural sense of touch, but there are things you can do to keep the mechanisms of touch functioning well. One is to eat a balanced diet. If you get the Reference Daily Intake (RDI) of vitamins and minerals, the body will take care of its sensory structures. Protect your skin, which contains the touch sensors, by practicing safety procedures. For example, use good protective equipment when you are skateboarding or rollerblading to prevent bad scrapes and severe skin damage that can affect your touch sensors.

SMELL

The sense of smell is one of our two chemical senses, meaning that the information that stimulates the receptors comes from chemical sources. The odors we receive can be very pleasing—perfume, flowers, and home cooking!—or they can be noxious—rotten food and sewage. For the most part, we learn about smells from our experiences, but it seems we are also born with a sense of which odors are pleasing and which odors are not. Experiments on day-old infants show that babies will make expressions of rejection when presented with unpleasant odors such as the smell of rotten eggs.

Our sense of smell begins in the **olfactory area**, which is located in the upper region of the nasal passage. (See Figure 6-3.) This area contains many sensory structures and specialized cells that detect odors. It is the chemicals in odors that are detected by the receptors. Have you ever found yourself sniffing when you were trying to smell something? Sniffing moves odors up into the nasal passage. The structures in the

olfactory area

region of the nasal passage where odors are detected

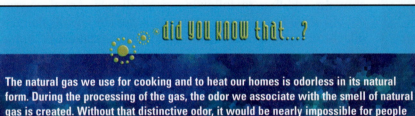

did you know that...?

The natural gas we use for cooking and to heat our homes is odorless in its natural form. During the processing of the gas, the odor we associate with the smell of natural gas is created. Without that distinctive odor, it would be nearly impossible for people to detect gas leaks in their homes.

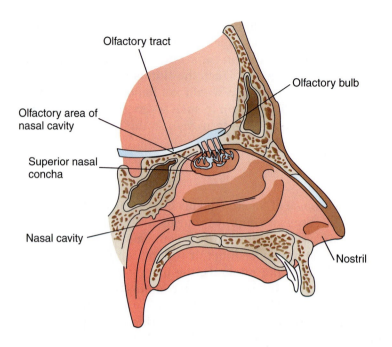

Figure 6-3
The olfactory region

Pleasant fragrances, such as the smell of flowers, can have an effect on our emotions and memories.

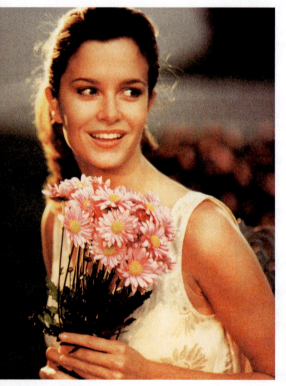

olfactory area then transfer information about the odor to the brain, where it is interpreted. Our sense of smell is closely linked to and supports our sense of taste. Try holding your nose and eating pieces of apple and onion. They will taste the same! Did you ever notice that food does not taste the same when you have a cold?

Our sense of smell serves us in a number of ways. Odors can tell us if our food is safe to eat. You have probably experienced the smell of spoiled food! Pleasant odors, on the other hand, can have a calming effect. The fragrances from flowers or scented candles are relaxing, and some can even contribute to romance and our attraction to others. And odors are strongly associated with our memories. The smell of popcorn, for example, may remind you of a favorite movie experience.

Caring for Your Olfactory Structures

The nerve endings of the olfactory structures lie close to the skin. In addition to following good dietary practices, you should avoid inhaling substances that can chemically damage olfactory structures. For example, the inhalation of fumes from substances such as paint, solvents, and cleaning fluids can assault the nerve endings and disrupt your sense of smell. The inhalation of drugs such as cocaine, heroin, or inhalants can damage the structures. The inhalation of cigarette smoke can also be damaging. If the exposure is over a long period of time, the damage can be permanent.

What's News?

Scientists are keenly aware that fragrances are capable of producing memory recall. The memories are related to the emotions associated with an event rather than the facts of the event itself.

We do not know exactly what causes the memory association to occur. Scientists at the Monell Chemical Senses Center in Philadelphia are searching for the answer.

TASTE

Taste is the second of our chemical senses. The ability to taste comes primarily from the tongue, but the tongue works along with the sense of smell to detect different flavors. When you chew food, it mixes with your **saliva** and breaks down into molecules that are carried over the taste buds on the tongue.

Have you ever wondered why you can taste so many different flavors with only one tongue? Although the approximately 10,000 taste buds on your tongue are similar and react to all sensations of taste, some react more strongly to specific types of flavors, and the taste buds for each type are clustered together in different locations on the tongue. For example, sweetness is tasted most noticeably on the tip of the tongue. If you eat something bitter, you get a stronger sensation when the food gets to the back of the tongue. Until recently, it was believed that there were four taste sensations: sweet, sour, bitter, and salty. Scientists now believe there is a fifth taste, known as **umami**. Umami is a taste that is described as "beefy" and is easily triggered by chemicals such as monosodium glutamate (MSG), which is commonly used in asian cooking.

The sense of taste diminishes as a person enters old age. This diminished sense of taste explains why some elderly people complain that their food has no flavor, and it can have negative effects on health. First, elder adults may oversalt food, and salt may cause an increase in blood pressure, a potential health hazard. Second, if older people's food seems without flavor, they may eat less and suffer the effects of poor nutrition.

Caring for Your Taste Buds

Perhaps the best thing you can do to protect your taste buds is to refrain from smoking. The chemicals in cigarette smoke can damage the taste bud receptors and prevent the smoker from easily distinguishing flavors in food. When people give up cigarette smoking, one of the first things they notice after a period of being tobacco free is the return of their sense of taste.

saliva

digestive fluid that is produced by the salivary glands to aid food digestion

umami

a recently discovered taste sensation described as "beefy"

synesthesia

condition in which stimulation of one sense creates a response in both the stimulated sense and another sense

SYNESTHESIA

Some people (about 1 person out of 25,000) have a hereditary sensory condition known as **synesthesia**. Synesthesia literally means "joined sensation" and has been described as the "sixth sense." It is a rare brain condition in which the people experience a stimulus through multiple senses, something they can't prevent from happening. They may see *and* taste a color or words; they may hear music but also see it as color. One man reported that the word *London* "tasted" like mashed potatoes when he read it. Although scientists can prove that synesthesia exists, they cannot yet explain what causes it. They do know there is a hereditary component, that women in the United States are three times more likely than men to have synesthesia, and that right-handed people are less likely to experience synesthesia than are left-handed or ambidextrous individuals.

real teens

Karen has synesthesia. It wasn't until her sophomore year in high school that she began to enjoy her condition. When she was younger, she quickly found out that she was different from the rest of the kids. In elementary school, when the class was reviewing the alphabet, she would hear a letter and "see" it in color. No matter what she did, the letters always came up in the same colors. Even now, the letter *A* is white; the letter *U* is purple; and *O* is black, but kind of transparent. She recently mapped out the entire alphabet with colored markers. Karen used to think of herself as a freak, but after she had talked to her best friends, Jill and Mira, about her experience, things changed. At first they couldn't believe what she was saying, but as they talked it through and researched on the Internet to learn about synesthesia, Jill and Mira became intrigued by the condition. They wanted to experience it, but as hard as they tried, they couldn't do what Karen does naturally. Now they not only appreciate Karen's view of the world, they are envious of her extra sense. Karen has become so comfortable with her condition that she can smile and feel good as she experiences her special world.

BUILDING YOUR Wellness Plan

This chapter has given you information to help you appreciate your senses and what they can do for you. As remarkable as they are, your sensory structures can diminish in performance if they are continually exposed to certain conditions. With proper care, however, your senses can last a lifetime. There are a number of healthy behaviors you can build into your wellness plan now to safeguard your senses for a lifetime.

- Protect Your Eyes. Flying debris can hit your eye faster than you can blink. An object that punctures the eye can cause permanent damage. Another danger is too much sun exposure. Use the information you learned in this chapter to take care of your eyesight.

- Protect Your Ears. Loud machines, speaker systems, and personal music devices can easily generate enough decibels to harm your hearing mechanism. Your hearing will begin to fail after years of exposure. If the ears' structures are severely damaged, even hearing aids cannot help restore hearing. Limiting your exposure to very loud noise and using protective earplugs when working in loud jobs or playing loud music are two ways you can help prevent hearing loss.

- Protect Your Nose. Avoid exposure to chemical aerosols and, by all means, do not inhale drugs or tobacco or marijuana smoke.

- Protect Your Skin. Be careful that you don't burn your skin: this includes sunburn. Severe burn damage can scar the skin and damage nerves. If you know you are going to be outside, make sure you use a sunscreen to keep your skin from burning.

- Protect Your Taste. Remember, the sense of taste is connected to the sense of smell. Hot liquids and overexposure to heavy spices can have a dulling effect on taste.

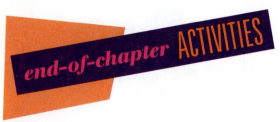

Weblinks

Color Blindness

Color blindness test patterns: **http://webexhibits.org** (search for the article "How Do Doctors Test for Color Vision Deficiency?")

Ear

Nemours Foundation: **http://kidshealth.org** (enter the teen site, then search for "ear")

Eye Injuries

U.S. National Library of Medicine: **http://www.nlm.nih.gov** (click on "Search Our Website," then under Health Information type "eye injuries")

Hearing

Sight and Hearing Association: **http://www.sightandhearing.org** (click on the ear)

Receptors

Society for Neuroscience: **http://www.sfn.org** (search for "nociceptor" then read the article "Nociceptors and Pain." Also search for "brain facts")

Short-Answer Questions

1. Which of our senses do we depend on the most?
2. What is it in the eyes that allows us look up from a book we are reading and clearly see objects outside the house?
3. Name the structures in the eye that help us detect colors and light.
4. Just exactly what is it that produces sound?
5. What is the frequency range of human hearing?
6. Explain the purpose of the three bones in the middle ear.
7. Explain what a decibel is and what it means to your hearing.
8. What are our two chemical senses?
9. Name the recently discovered fifth taste sensation.

10. What happens to people's sense of taste as they enter old age?

Discussion Questions

1. Explain the actions you can take to protect your sight.
2. Describe how sound is transported from the environment to your brain.
3. Describe how noise can cause permanent damage to the hearing mechanism.
4. Explain why we would not be able to hear an explosion in outer space.
5. Explain the interconnectedness between the sense of smell and the sense of taste.

Chapter Vocabulary

Using a separate sheet of paper, list and define the following terms:

cones	power of accommodation
cornea	retina
iris	rods
malleus, incus, and stapes	semicircular canals
olfactory area	tympanic membrane

Application Activities

Mathematics Connection

Animals hear a different range of sounds than humans do. Research the range of hearing for a variety of animals and prepare a graph or chart that lists the names of the animals you investigated and the low and high frequencies those animals can hear.

Science Connection

1. Designate for yourself a "Use the Other Hand Day." Try to go through an entire day using your nondominant hand for everything: opening doors, eating, carrying objects, and so on. (Don't use your opposite hand if you are writing assignments in school unless you have your teacher's permission.) Write a report describing the change and how you handled it. List the various senses you found yourself using to deal with the change.

2. Search the Internet or use the library to find information about visual disorders. Prepare a larger version of the table below and include all the requested information.

Visual Disorder	Symptoms	Causes	Number of People Affected	Treatment
Myopia				
Hyperopia				
Amblyopia				
Astigmatism				
Presbyopia				

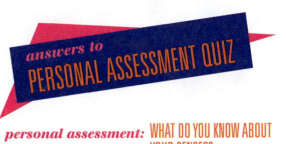

answers to
PERSONAL ASSESSMENT QUIZ

personal assessment: WHAT DO YOU KNOW ABOUT YOUR SENSES?

Each of the statements is true! The correct answers are discussed in the chapter. After completing this chapter, you will be able to explain why each item is true and develop ways of incorporating the information into your wellness plan.

chapter **7**

Understanding Growth and Development

Brenda's younger sister, Michelle, is going through puberty. Michelle has questions about her changing body and the emotional experiences she is having along the way, so she has turned to her older sister, Brenda, to help find answers. Fortunately, Brenda has already experienced these changes that are a natural part of being a teen. Brenda didn't have an older sister to talk things over with. She relied on her mother, the information she learned in health class at school, information from some of her friends, and information from some sites she visited on the Internet. Brenda feels good about having accurate information about reproduction she can share with her sister and use in her own wellness plan to keep herself healthy. She is also looking forward to the possibility of sharing this information with her own children someday.

chapter OBJECTIVES

When you finish this chapter, you should be able to:

- Identify the major endocrine glands and explain the functions of each.
- Describe the endocrine glands that have important roles in human development and reproduction.
- Discuss the onset of secondary sex characteristics of males and females.
- Explain the major changes in the reproductive structures of males and females that are needed for reproduction.
- Explain the relationship between the menstrual cycle and fertilization.
- Discuss the importance of prenatal care during pregnancy.

key TERMS

adrenaline
androgens
endometrium
hypothalamus
meiosis
mitosis
progesterone
semen
testosterone
urethra

Introduction

There is perhaps no other personal health issue as important to you, as a teen, as your physical development into an adult. With this development come the body changes that signify your transition from girl to woman or from boy to man. These changes are also accompanied by emotional changes. Perhaps you remember when you began to experience romantic feelings for someone or felt confused about your role as an adolescent and your interest in being an adult. These changes and feelings are normal for teens to experience. They are part of a series of events that start when you enter puberty, stabilize a few years later, and conclude with your full maturation as an adult. The growth from child to adult involves significant chemical changes that take place inside your body. This chapter will provide information to help take the mystery out of this exciting but perplexing part of the journey to becoming an adult.

personal assessment: WHAT DO YOU KNOW ABOUT REPRODUCTION?

Read each of the statements below and on a separate piece of paper indicate whether you think each statement is true or false. The answers are located at the end of the chapter.

1. There are male and female hormones present in every adult.
2. The pituitary gland controls all other glands in the body.
3. Hormones are very important in the reproductive process.
4. Males develop their secondary sex characteristics earlier than females do.
5. Only one sperm cell will fertilize the ovum.
6. A bone in a man's penis is responsible for his erection.
7. When a woman becomes pregnant, the fetus grows in her uterus.
8. It is possible for a woman to become pregnant without having sexual intercourse.
9. Ovulation generally takes place on the fourteenth day of a woman's menstrual cycle.
10. Both males and females produce estrogen.

PHYSICAL AND CHEMICAL CHANGES OF ADOLESCENCE

From the moment you were born, the growth and development of your body was controlled by the genetic blueprint you received from your parents. As did that of most of your peers, your development followed a standard schedule. The steady controls of childhood are replaced by special changes during adolescence. When young people enter their teen years, they will undergo chemical and physical changes in their bodies that transform them into adults. These changes are all part of a period known as puberty. Puberty is the time when a young person's body is affected by chemical shifts as the teen's genetic code directs the body for reproduction.

There is nothing about puberty that is the same for every teen, except for the fact that everyone goes through puberty. Some teens start changing early in their teen years, some start later; some teens change quickly, some change slowly. When and how an adolescent goes through puberty are largely determined by the genetic conditions established by the teen's parents. These genetic conditions will cause chemical changes among the numerous glands in the body that will in turn effect the physical changes that go with puberty.

The Endocrine System

The chemical changes that play an important part in sexual development are controlled by the endocrine system, a collection of small glands that exert chemical control over many body processes. This control involves a very delicate balance of chemicals through a partnership between the endocrine glands and the nervous system. These interactions are necessary to keep the body in homeostasis, which is the sum of the processes that keep the body's internal environment in balance.

The **hypothalamus**, an area at the very center of the brain, is the information-processing center that coordinates the activities of the endocrine system. The various body organs send information to the hypothalamus through the nervous system and bloodstream. The hypothalamus then processes this information and sends out messages that result in chemical responses by the appropriate endocrine structures to regulate homeostasis.

The Endocrine Glands

The endocrine glands are ductless glands, meaning that the hormones produced by these glands enter directly into the bloodstream. There are eight major endocrine glands in the body. Each gland performs a specific function, but they also work in a coordinated manner to regulate body functions. The major endocrine glands are the pituitary gland; the pineal gland; the thyroid gland; the parathyroid glands; the thymus; the adrenal glands; the pancreas; and the gonads, or reproductive glands, which include the testes and ovaries. (See Figure 7-1.)

The Pituitary Gland. The **pituitary gland** is located in the very depths of the brain. Approximately the size of a pea, the pituitary is known as the "master gland" because hormones from the pituitary exercise control over many other endocrine glands. The front portion of the pituitary produces hormones that, in addition to other functions, regulate growth, the development of male and female reproductive structures during puberty, and the function of the reproductive organs throughout the life span. The back part of the pituitary helps maintain appropriate water balance in the body and produces the hormone that stimulates the birthing process.

The Pineal Gland. The pineal gland is located in the base of the brain. It produces two hormones: **melatonin** and **serotonin**. Melatonin helps regulate sleep cycles, and serotonin assists with the transmission of nerve impulses.

The Thyroid Gland. The **thyroid gland** is located on the windpipe, just below the larynx (voice box). The thyroid produces hormones that regulate the metabolism of carbohydrates, fats, and proteins. You need

hypothalmus

an area in the center of the brain that exerts nervous system control over the pituitary gland and the rest of the endocrine system

pituitary gland

pea-sized gland in the center of the brain that regulates most of the endocrine glands in the body

melatonin

a hormone produced by the pineal gland to help regulate sleep cycles

serotonin

a hormone produced by the pineal gland to help regulate nerve impulses

thyroid gland

gland that produces hormones that influence growth and development by regulating metabolism

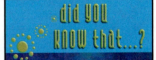

...did you know that...?

A lack of sufficient growth hormone from the pituitary can result in a form of impaired growth called dwarfism. Perhaps the most famous pituitary dwarf was known as Tom Thumb, who worked for the P.T. Barnum Circus. When Tom died in 1888, at the age of 45, he was only about 38 inches tall.

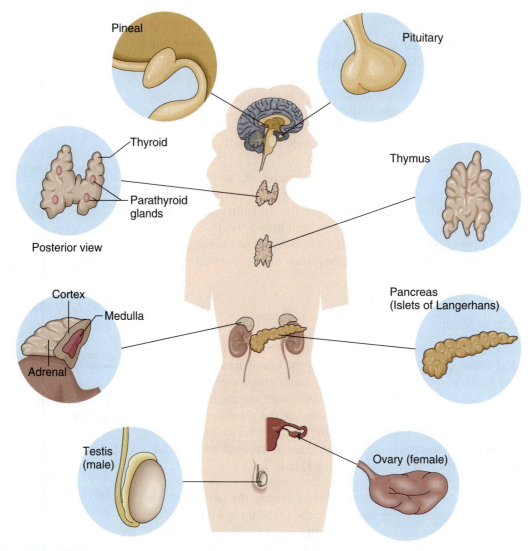

Pineal

Pituitary

Thyroid

Thymus

Parathyroid glands

Posterior view

Cortex

Medulla

Pancreas (Islets of Langerhans)

Adrenal

Testis (male)

Ovary (female)

Figure 7-1 The location of the endocrine glands

to have an adequate amount of iodine in your diet for the thyroid to function properly. The principal source of iodine in the diet is seafood. If you are like most people in the United States, you do not consume a lot of seafood. Have you ever noticed the word *iodized* on salt containers? Iodine is added to common table salt to provide a convenient source of iodine.

parathyroid glands

four very small glands located on the thyroid gland that help regulate calcium

The Parathyroid Glands. The **parathyroid glands** are four pea-sized glands located on the back of the thyroid. The hormone from the parathyroid glands is responsible for regulating the distribution of calcium throughout the body.

The Thymus. The **thymus** is located behind the sternum (breastbone). The purpose of this gland is to assist in the development of a child's immune system. Your thymus will have changed into fatty connective tissue by the time you reach full adulthood.

The Adrenal Glands. The **adrenal glands** are attached to the top of each kidney. Each gland has two parts: the adrenal medulla (inner part) and the adrenal cortex (outermost part). The adrenal medulla produces two hormones: **adrenaline** and **noradrenaline**. These two hormones work together to produce the changes that take place in the body under conditions of stress, such as increased heart rate and blood pressure, the distribution of blood throughout the body, and the production of sugar as a source of energy for the muscles.

The adrenal cortex produces male sex hormones known as **androgens**. Although androgens are male sex hormones, they are produced by both men and women. Androgens are responsible for the development of male sexual characteristics as young males pass through puberty. Lower levels of androgens, which are produced by adult women, are responsible for stimulating sex drive.

The Pancreas (Islets of Langerhans). The islets of Langerhans are scattered throughout the pancreas, an organ found behind the stomach. The islets produce the hormones **insulin** and **glucagon**, which work together to ensure that the level of glucose (sugar) in the blood is in balance.

Testes (Males). The **testes** are a pair of male reproductive structures. These structures do two things: they serve as endocrine glands, and they produce sperm. In their role as endocrine glands, the testes produce **testosterone**, the primary male hormone. Testosterone is produced during puberty and leads to the development of the male's **secondary sex characteristics**. Every young man develops his secondary sex characteristics according to his own inherited biological time line, but, in general, the secondary sex characteristics develop according to the schedule shown in Table 7-1.

Testosterone levels start decreasing after a man reaches age 30. The rate of decline is approximately 10% per decade throughout his lifetime. This decline in testosterone means that muscle strength and sex drive also diminish.

thymus

endocrine gland that helps with the development of a child's immune system

adrenal glands

a set of glands on top of each kidney that produce two types of hormones that regulate the stress response and sexual development

adrenaline and noradrenaline

hormones produced in the adrenal medulla that regulate blood pressure and blood flow under conditions of stress

androgens

male sex hormones produced in the adrenal cortex

insulin and glucagon

two hormones produced in the pancreas that regulate the level of blood sugar

testes

male sex glands that are located in the scrotum and are responsible for male sexual development and sperm production

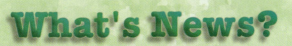

What's News?

Research is beginning to find that lower testosterone levels in older men are related to lower performance on memory tests. Scientists are not encouraging testosterone supplements because of possible health concerns, but research is continuing.

testosterone

the male hormone that is produced in the testes

secondary sex characteristics

changes in the body that occur as someone passes through puberty

Table 7-1 Male Secondary Sex Characteristics

Characteristic	Average Age of Onset
Hormone levels increase	10 years
Penis grows, pubic hair appears	12 years
Sperm are produced	13 years
Weight spurt begins, muscles develop	13 years
Height spurt begins	14 years
Voice lowers	15 years
Facial hair appears	16 years
Full adult height reached	21 years

Ovaries (Females). The reproductive endocrine glands of the female are the ovaries. The primary hormones produced in the ovaries are **estrogen** and **progesterone**. These two hormones are responsible for the development of the secondary sex characteristics listed in Table 7-2. As a young woman passes through puberty, these hormones influence the development of her reproductive structures and the development of her body. These developments include fat deposits on her hips, broadening of the pelvis, and the voice's maintaining its high pitch. Later in this chapter, you will learn how these hormones contribute to pregnancy.

estrogen

the female hormone produced by the ovaries to repair the uterine lining after menstruation and to enhance feminine characteristics

progesterone

the female hormone responsible for developing the uterus during pregnancy

take it on home

You may find it interesting to talk with your parents about their experiences during their sexual development. For some teens and parents, this may not be an easy task, but communication is an important part of being a family. If you have any concern about discussing these issues with your parents, try introducing a related topic such as how to go about dating someone, and eventually introduce issues related to growth and development. You may create your own questions, or you can organize your discussion around such questions as: How old were you when you first noticed you were going through puberty? How long did it take for you to completely develop your secondary sex characteristics? What were some of the feelings you experienced as you went through puberty? Prepare a report for your Health Folio.

Table 7-2 Female Secondary Sex Characteristics

Characteristic	Average Age of Onset
Hormone levels increase	9 years
Internal sex organs enlarge	9 years
Breasts develop	10 years
Pubic hair appears	11 years
Weight spurt begins	11 years
Height spurt begins	12 years
First ovulation, menstruation begins	12 years
Pubic hair and breasts fully grown	16 years
Full adult height reached	18 years

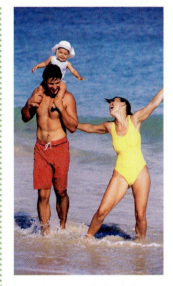

Male hormones during puberty help develop muscles. Female hormones contribute to a feminine form.

MALE REPRODUCTIVE SYSTEM

The male reproductive system consists of both external and internal structures. The external **genitalia** are the penis and the scrotum. The internal structures include the testes, epididymis, vas deferens, seminal vesicles, prostate gland, and bulbourethral gland (Cowper's gland). (See Figure 7-2.)

Penis

There is perhaps no other part of the anatomy that so identifies a man's "maleness" as the penis. When a male child is born, the persons present at the delivery can look at the baby and quickly determine that he is a male. The penis is an external organ that serves two functions. It is a passageway for urine to leave the body, and it is capable of becoming erect and firm in order to perform sexual intercourse and deliver sperm to the uterus in the female.

The penis has two main sections: the shaft and the glans. The **glans** is also referred to as the head of the penis. At birth, the glans is covered with a section of tissue known as the foreskin. The removal of the foreskin is called **circumcision**. In the United States, the decision to have a child circumcised is a personal one. For the past decade, the rate of hospital circumcisions has remained fairly steady, with approximately 60% of male infants being circumcised, according to the National Center for Health Statistics.

The shaft of the penis contains three spongy tissue layers that are rich with blood vessels. Two of these layers are on the top side of the penis. The third is on the underside and has the **urethra** passing through it.

genitalia

the reproductive sex organs

glans

the rounded head of the penis

circumcision

surgical removal of the foreskin

urethra

passageway from the bladder to the outside of the body

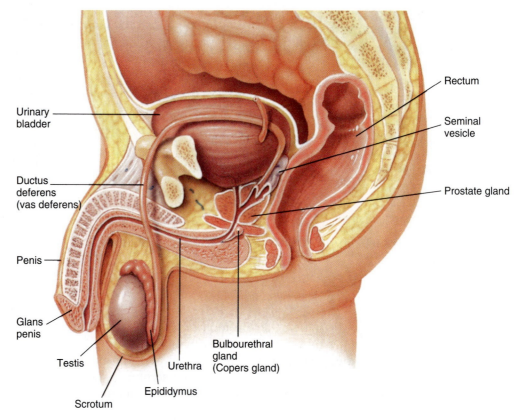

Urinary
bladder

Ductus
deferens
(vas deferens)

Penis

Glans
penis

Testis

Scrotum

Epididymus

Urethra

Bulbourethral
gland
(Copers gland)

Rectum

Seminal
vesicle

Prostate gland

Figure 7-2 The male reproductive system

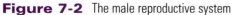

✿ teen forum ✿

Circumcision

The decision to perform circumcision on the penis is not without controversy.
There are a variety of opinions surrounding this procedure. Over the years,
research has disclosed reasons *for* circumcision, only to have later research
report reasons *against* it. The debate continues today.

- Research both the pros and cons of circumcision and prepare to argue
  both sides.

- If you were to have a male child, would you want to have him circumcised?

Scrotum

The scrotum is a pouch that contains the testes, in which sperm cells
are manufactured. Although it may appear to be only a pouch of skin,
the scrotum is much more than that. In fact, it contains layers of tissue
and muscle that enable it to perform a very important function. For the
male to manufacture sperm, the testes must be at a temperature a

did you know that...?

Males are capable of obtaining an erection at any time after they are born. Erection is a physiological process that can occur in infants as well as teens and mature men. In adulthood, males are socialized to have erections only during sexual arousal.

couple of degrees cooler than normal body temperature. The nerves and muscles inside and near the scrotum work together to bring the testes closer to the body under cold conditions or to allow the testes to drop lower from the body when the body is overheated. The scrotum and testes are a very sensitive part of a male's body. To protect these structures from injury, males are advised to wear protective equipment during contact sports and other activities in which a blow to that area might occur.

Internal Sex Structures

The testes serve two important functions. As endocrine glands, they are responsible for producing testosterone and delivering it into the bloodstream. They also serve a reproductive function by manufacturing **sperm** cells. This function begins when a male enters puberty.

The sperm cells are stored in the **epididymis**, just outside the testes, until they are used for reproduction. The **ductus deferens** is the duct system that transports the sperm from the epididymis to the **seminal vesicles** and **prostate gland**. The **bulbourethral gland** sits at the entrance of the urethra. Bulbourethral fluid enters the urethra during conditions of sexual arousal and serves to prepare the urethra for the presence of sperm.

Reproductive Functions

Sometime in his very early teen years, a male enters puberty. Puberty is the time when inherited genetic factors trigger changes in the pituitary gland. The pituitary sends chemical messages by way of various hormones that signal the structures in the reproductive system to mature and become functional for reproduction.

Sperm Production

One of the first changes to take place at puberty is the production of sperm. A male is born with millions of specialized cells (primary sperm cells) in his testes. But not until puberty can the male's body convert these cells into sperm. This conversion is controlled by pituitary hormones that continue this function throughout the life span.

---

sperm
reproductive cells manufactured in the testes

epididymis
structure adjacent to the testes where sperm are stored

ductus deferens
duct that transports sperm from the epididymis to the penis

seminal vesicles
structures that produce a component of semen that nourishes and protects sperm

prostate gland
accessory structure of the male reproductive system that supports movement of sperm

bulbourethral gland
small gland near the base of the urethra that produces a fluid that conditions the urethra for the movement of sperm

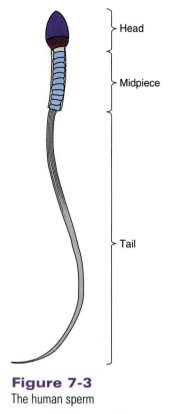

Figure 7-3
The human sperm

Head

Midpiece

Tail

meiosis

the process of reducing chromosome numbers in reproductive cells to one half the original number

mitosis

the process of duplicating living cells

semen

a milky fluid containing sperm and fluids from the seminal vesicles and prostate

ejaculation

the process of ejecting semen from the penis

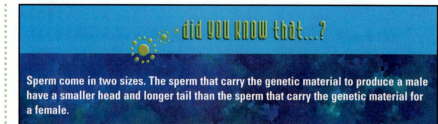

did you know that...?

Sperm come in two sizes. The sperm that carry the genetic material to produce a male have a smaller head and longer tail than the sperm that carry the genetic material for a female.

The primary sperm cells undergo some interesting changes as they become sperm that are capable of playing their role in reproduction. All the cells in the human body contain 46 chromosomes. The male and female each contribute one half, or 23, of the chromosomes necessary for human life. Therefore, the primary sperm cells, which themselves have 46 chromosomes, must reproduce themselves while reducing the chromosome number in each cell to 23. They do this through a process called **meiosis**, or reduction division. (Meiosis should not be confused with **mitosis**, the process by which cells reproduce themselves. Primary sperm cells also go through mitosis in order to maintain their numbers.)

Once the sperm cells have been reduced to 23 chromosomes, they grow tails and are moved to the epididymis, where they are stored as sperm. This entire process continues almost daily throughout the male's lifetime. (See Figure 7-3.)

Sperm play 50% of the role in reproduction. To carry out their function, they must move from the epididymis to the female. During sexual arousal, the sperm are moved from the epididymis through the ductus deferens to the penis. Along the way, fluids from the seminal vesicles and prostate are added to the sperm to produce **semen** (also known as seminal fluid). These fluids help nourish the sperm and ensure they are mobile once they enter the female. The semen then collects at the base of the penis until **ejaculation**.

Erectile Function

A male usually has an erection prior to ejaculation (although it is possible for ejaculation to take place without an erection). The penis becomes rigid when specialized muscles at its base push accumulated

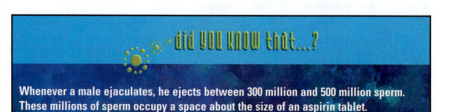

did you know that...?

Whenever a male ejaculates, he ejects between 300 million and 500 million sperm. These millions of sperm occupy a space about the size of an aspirin tablet.

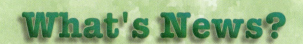

blood into its spongy layers. An erection can result from either sexual arousal or urine retention while sleeping. Either way, the same mechanism causes the penis to become erect.

Care of the Male Reproductive System

Although testicular cancer is not a common form of cancer in general, it is one of the most common cancers among males between ages 18 and 36. If detected early, this cancer is almost 100% curable. Males should know how to do a testicular self-examination so that early detection of testicular cancer is possible. You can learn more about self-examination from the American Cancer Society.

FEMALE REPRODUCTIVE SYSTEM

A woman's reproductive structures serve a number of purposes. Unlike the male's reproductive structures, the female's structures are almost entirely internal. Because everything is on the inside of the body, it can be difficult for a woman to detect any changes or diseases in her reproductive organs. Therefore, it's recommended that women learn as much as possible about their reproductive system so they can properly take care of themselves.

Female Reproductive Structures

The most external parts of the female sex structures are the **labia**. The labia are folds of skin and tissue that appear at the entrance of the **vagina**. The vagina is a muscular, yet flexible, passageway, about 4 inches long, that extends from the labia to the **cervix**. The cervix is the opening between the uterus and the vagina. (See Figures 7-4 and 7-5.)

The **uterus**, or "womb," is a major organ of the female reproductive system. The inner lining of the uterus, the **endometrium**, is where the fertilized **ovum** is implanted to start a pregnancy. This lining develops structures to nourish and grow the fetus. It is in the uterus that the birthing process begins at the conclusion of pregnancy.

labia
folds of skin at the entrance to the vagina

vagina
a muscular, flexible passageway between the labia and the uterus

cervix
opening to the uterus

uterus
a pear-shaped, muscular structure that provides the proper environment where the fertilized ovum develops into a fetus

endometrium
the innermost lining of the uterus, where a fertilized ovum becomes implanted

ovum
the female reproductive cell (the plural is *ova*)

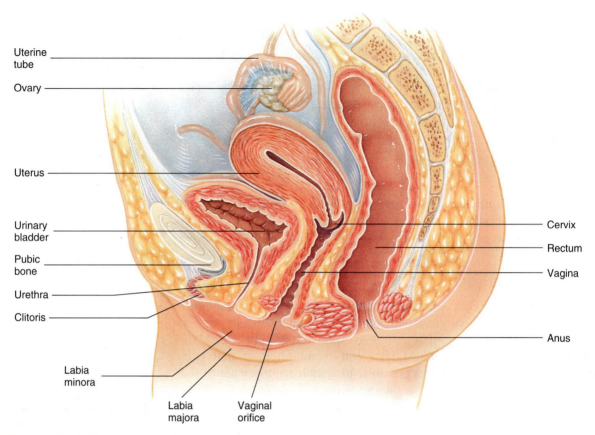

Uterine tube

Ovary

Uterus

Urinary bladder

Pubic bone

Urethra

Clitoris

Labia minora

Labia majora

Vaginal orifice

Cervix

Rectum

Vagina

Anus

Figure 7-4 The female reproductive system, side view

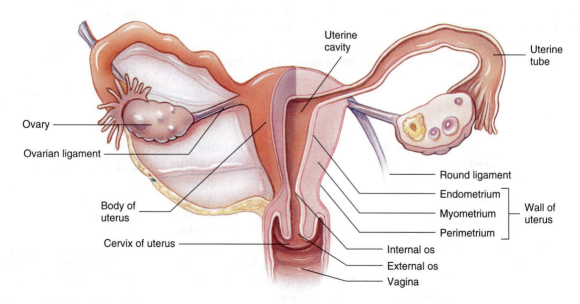

Uterine cavity

Uterine tube

Ovary

Ovarian ligament

Body of uterus

Cervix of uterus

Round ligament

Endometrium

Myometrium

Perimetrium

Wall of uterus

Internal os

External os

Vagina

Figure 7-5 The female reproductive system, front view

An ovum is released, through a process called **ovulation**, from one of the female's two **ovaries** once every month. An illustration of an ovum is presented in Figure 7-6. Keep in mind that the ovum is actually smaller than the period at the end of this sentence. (The sperm cell in the illustration is shown for size comparison to the ovum.) This process begins when a young woman enters puberty and lasts until she reaches middle age, around age 50. By the time a woman reaches age 60, she is likely to have stopped producing ova. The **uterine tubes** (also called fallopian tubes), which extend from each side of the uterus to the ovaries, serve to transport the ovum to the uterus. The journey to the uterus takes about three to five days. Because an ovum is capable of being fertilized by a sperm for about 24 hours, fertilization almost always take place in the uterine tube.

The Menstrual Cycle

A woman's menstrual cycle is a unique and very significant event. (See Figure 7-7.) As a girl approaches puberty, her genetic makeup triggers her pituitary to produce hormones that influence the development of

ovulation

the release of an ovum from one of the ovaries

ovary

structure responsible for producing reproductive cells and female sex hormones

uterine tube

passageway that transports the ovum from the ovary to the uterus

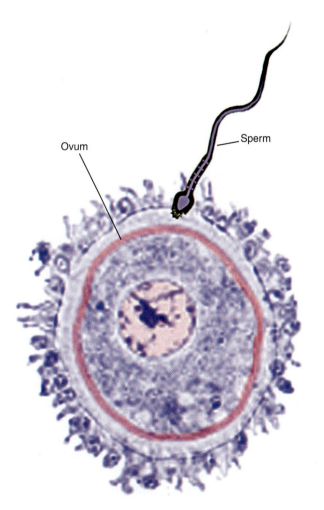
Ovum

Sperm

Figure 7-6
The human ovum and sperm

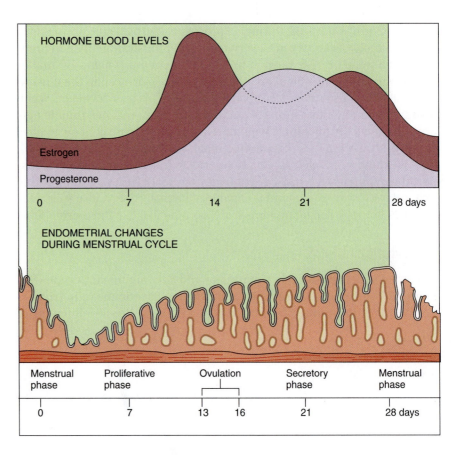

HORMONE BLOOD LEVELS

Estrogen

Progesterone

| 0 | 7 | 14 | 21 | 28 days |

ENDOMETRIAL CHANGES
DURING MENSTRUAL CYCLE

| Menstrual phase | Proliferative phase | Ovulation | Secretory phase | Menstrual phase |

| 0 | 7 | 13 | 16 | 21 | 28 days |

Figure 7-7
The menstrual cycle

her secondary sex characteristics. One of the most significant changes is her ability to produce reproductive cells, or ova.

The ova are produced in the ovaries at the rate of about one each month. When a female is born, each of her ovaries contains almost 200,000 immature ovum cells. On entering puberty, the young woman's pituitary gland begins producing FSH (follicle-stimulating hormone), which directs her ovaries to cause an ovum to mature. At the same time, her pituitary will produce LH (luteinizing hormone), which stimulates the endometrium of the uterus to prepare to receive a fertilized ovum.

Once an ovum is mature, it is released from the ovary and enters the uterine tube to begin its journey to the uterus. At the same time, at the location where the ovum left the ovary, another important hormone called progesterone is produced. Progesterone is responsible for developing the endometrium to receive a fertilized ovum. Once it implants in the endometrium, the fertilized ovum will need blood and nutrients so it can grow.

If an ovum is not fertilized by a sperm cell on its way down the uterine tube, it will not implant properly on the endometrium. The failure to implant causes a hormone message to be sent to the ovary to halt the production of progesterone. Without progesterone, the lining of the endometrium sloughs off during a 3- to 5-day period of bleeding. This bleeding period is known as **menstruation**. Doctors have labeled the first day of blood loss as Day 1 of the menstrual cycle as a convenient way to describe it.

Many textbooks and materials about reproduction portray the menstrual cycle as being 28 days long. This is done as a matter of convenience. But the following facts provide a more complete picture of the relationship between ovulation and reproduction:

1. Not all women have menstrual cycles that are 28 days long. It is important to recognize that 28 days represents an *average* number among all women. Not everyone is average.

2. Menstrual cycles, especially for teens and young women, are not regular. It is not uncommon for a teenager's cycles to vary from 3 to 5 days from cycle to cycle.

3. Ovulation generally takes place about 14 days *before* the next menstrual cycle begins. We have no way of accurately predicting when the next cycle will begin, so we can't predict ovulation either.

FERTILIZATION

An ovum is released from the ovary once every month or so. If sperm are present in the uterine tube when the live ovum arrives, they will gather around the ovum and attempt to enter it. Each sperm cell is equipped with an enzyme that enables it to weaken the wall of the ovum to make it easier to enter. As soon as one sperm enters the ovum, another type of enzyme is released from the ovum that stops the remaining sperm cells from trying to enter.

Once the sperm is inside the ovum, the head breaks down and the 23 chromosomes from the sperm blend with the 23 chromosomes from the ovum to form a nucleus containing 46 chromosomes. The cells in this mass then begin to reproduce as the fertilized ovum tumbles down the uterine tube to the uterus. Figure 7-8 illustrates ovulation, fertilization, and implantation. In the early stages of pregnancy, the cells reproduce approximately every 20 minutes. When the mass of cells arrives in the uterus, the mass (now known as a **blastocyst**) implants itself on the endometrium, generally in the upper third of the uterus. Once implantation occurs, the messenger hormone (human chorionic gonadotropin, or HCG) is released into the bloodstream for transport to the ovary, which is then signaled to continue producing progesterone. This feedback loop of HCG and progesterone continues until the pregnancy is well established, and then the placenta takes over the maintenance of the pregnancy.

The site where the blastocyst has implanted eventually develops into the **placenta**, which serves as the point of exchange of oxygen and nutrients with carbon dioxide and waste materials between the mother and the fetus.

menstruation

a cyclical shedding of the uterine lining in response to changes in hormone levels

blastocyst

a mass of cells that implants in the uterus after fertilization of the ovum

placenta

an organ that forms in the uterus to control the movement and exchange of nutrients and wastes between the fetus and the mother

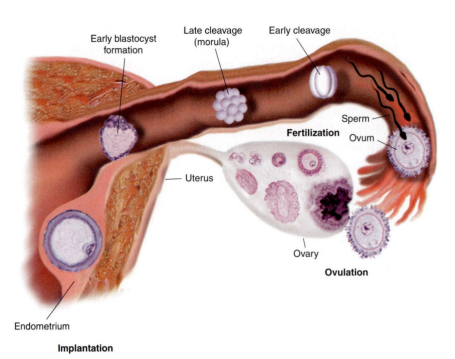

Figure 7-8 Ovulation, fertilization, implantation

Prenatal Care

Prenatal care (*prenatal* means "before birth") refers to all the medical attention a woman receives and personal actions she takes to protect the health of her unborn child during the course of her pregnancy. Prenatal care during the first three months of pregnancy is especially important because this is the time when many organs and structures are formed in the fetus.

Good prenatal care includes having regular medical checkups, getting physical exercise, and eating well. It is also important for the mother to remember that anything she consumes that can make its way into her bloodstream will also enter the fetus. That's why she should avoid tobacco, drugs, and alcohol, all of which can negatively affect the development of the fetus.

A pregnant woman's exposure to environmental hazards such as environmental tobacco smoke, certain metals (such as lead, mercury, cadmium, and arsenic), pesticides, and organic solvents can also cause problems for the developing fetus. For example, if a fetus is exposed to lead through the mother, it may slow mental and physical development depending on the level of exposure. During pregnancy, a woman should be very careful to avoid environmental hazards that can affect the fetus.

prenatal care

all the things done to safeguard the health of the mother and fetus throughout pregnancy

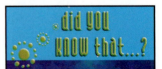

When a man and woman conceive a child, each partner contributes 23 chromosomes to the child. But each chromosome contains many genes. Given the numbers of chromosomes and genes, scientists have calculated that there are over 69,949,000,000,000 different combinations of chromosomes that can result from fertilization!

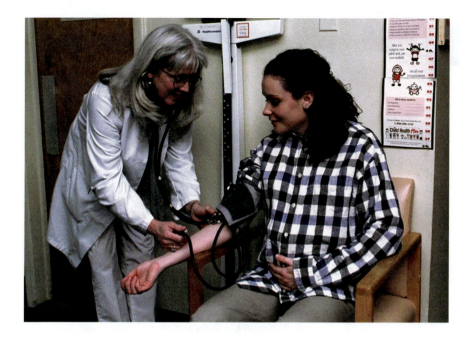

Regular visits with a health care provider throughout pregnancy are important for ensuring a healthy pregnancy.

BUILDING YOUR Wellness Plan

This chapter discussed the special aspects of human development and reproduction. It is important to learn about the reproductive systems of both genders, not just your own. If you have knowledge about the opposite sex, you will better understand their health conditions, needs, and interests. And if you have children someday, this information will help you understand their physical and emotional needs as they mature, regardless of their gender. To ensure good reproductive health in your own wellness plan, you can:

- Follow good nutritional practices to ensure the healthy development of your endocrine system.

- Avoid the use of tobacco, alcohol, and other drugs. These products can impair performance of the endocrine system, and they can interfere with healthy development of any future offspring.

- Understand that environmental hazards, such as lead and noise, have a harmful effect on fetus development, so you and your spouse can provide a safe environment if you decide to have children someday.

- Practice using your health literacy skills to seek out scientific and medical knowledge to help you make educated decisions about your reproductive health.

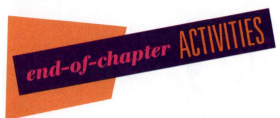

end-of-chapter ACTIVITIES

Weblinks

Pregnancy and Childbirth

Childbirth.org: **http://www.childbirth.org**
iVillage: **http://www.parentsplace.com**

Testicular Self-Examination

American Cancer Society: **http://www.cancer.org**
   (search for "testicular self-examination")

Short-Answer Questions

1. Name the structure in the endocrine system that is known as the "master gland."
2. What substance is needed in order for the thyroid gland to function properly?
3. State the two functions of the testes.
4. What is the process whereby reproductive cells are formed so they contain 23 chromosomes?
5. Name the structure where the fetus develops during pregnancy.

Discussion Questions

1. Describe the changes that occur in males and females during puberty.
2. List and describe the major structures of the male and female reproductive systems.
3. Discuss the conditions that need to be in place before an ovum can be fertilized.
4. Explain why prenatal care is important for the mother and the fetus.
5. Describe the relationship between the menstrual cycle and fertilization.

Chapter Vocabulary

Using a separate sheet of paper, list and define the following terms:

adrenaline	mitosis
androgens	progesterone
endometrium	semen
hypothalamus	testosterone
meiosis	urethra

Application Activities

Language Arts Connection

Use the Internet or research in the library to gather information about prenatal care. Using this information, create a brochure that could be used to educate pregnant women about the importance of prenatal care.

Science Connection

Use the Internet or research in the library to learn more about fertilization and pregnancy. Put the mind mapping technique you learned in Chapter 3 to work and create a mind map of the facts and processes that are related to fertilization and pregnancy.

Mathematics Connection

All human beings start out as a single cell. This cell divides into two cells, and these two cells divide into four cells. Use your math skills to calculate how many cells there would be if the fertilized ovum and its subsequent cells divided 30 times. This exercise will give you a sense of how one cell develops into a human being that is composed of trillions of cells.

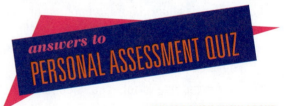

answers to
PERSONAL ASSESSMENT QUIZ

personal assessment: WHAT DO YOU KNOW ABOUT REPRODUCTION?

1. True	6. False
2. True	7. True
3. True	8. True
4. False	9. False
5. True	10. True

unit 3 | Physical Health

Introduction

When you think about being healthy, you are likely to think first about your physical health. Although your physical health is only one aspect of your health, it is a very important one. The decisions you make during your teen years will affect your health both now and throughout your future. The material in this unit will help you understand how to care for your physical health now and increase the likelihood that you will have good physical health throughout your life.

When you are young, it's easy to take your health for granted. Yet if you think about the adults you know, you will recognize that many of them are not as healthy as you are now. If you learn and practice good physical health habits as a teen, you will not only be a healthier teen, you are more likely to continue these healthy habits as an adult. In this unit, you will learn how eating well and managing your weight in a healthy way can protect your health. You will learn about the importance of staying physically active both as a teen and as an adult and how to prevent injury so that you can enjoy a long and healthy life.

chapter 8

Eating for Wellness

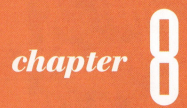

Jerry really likes Thanksgiving at his grandparents' house. Many of his relatives travel a long distance to attend. He gets the opportunity to catch up with the whole family. Everyone always has a great time, and there is always a lot of good food. Sometimes they eat seconds or even thirds of their favorites, but Jerry sometimes wonders if he's eating the right kinds of foods.

Last year, his grandfather had heart surgery to clear blocked arteries. Jerry learned in his health class that heart disease can run in families, and diets high in fats can be harmful.

As Jerry looks over the foods on the Thanksgiving table and tries to decide what to eat, he thinks about the fat content of the foods. He wants to make smart choices and, at the same time, enjoy a good meal.

chapter OBJECTIVES

When you finish this chapter, you should be able to:

☀ List and discuss the major classifications of nutrients.

☀ Explain the relationship between foods and metabolism.

☀ Describe the significance of the essential amino acids.

☀ Discuss the significance of fats in the diet.

☀ Describe the difference between water-soluble and fat-soluble vitamins.

☀ Explain the rationale for the food pyramid.

☀ Demonstrate how to read a food label.

☀ Explain how to handle food safely to prevent diseases.

key TERMS

amino acids
antioxidant
basal metabolism
essential amino acids
essential fatty acids
hydrogenation
polyunsaturated fats
saturated fats
trans fats
unsaturated fats

Introduction

Food is an important part of human existence. People need food to live. But food is more than a necessity; it also plays a very important social function. Food is often used to help celebrate special occasions. In fact, virtually every culture has special dishes to mark holidays and other important occasions.

In the United States, most people don't have to worry about starvation. In fact, in the United States, our most serious nutrition problems are caused by too much, rather than too little, food. Most of us get plenty to eat. The key is to eat what is best for our health.

As a young adult, you are in a position to make many of your own food choices. With these choices comes the responsibility to make good ones. And the evidence indicates that teens, in general, are not well nourished. Why do you think this is true? Maybe it's because many young people tend to choose popular, high-fat fast foods and high-sugar snack foods instead of healthier foods.

In the years to come, you will be making many more independent choices about food and other factors that affect your health. If you have children, you will be responsible for making food choices for them until they are old enough to make their own. Now is the time to develop your nutrition wellness skills and start practicing eating habits that will result in a lifetime of good, healthy eating.

personal assessment: YOUR EATING HABITS

Think about the foods you might eat on an average day. Then on a separate piece of paper, answer the questions below as accurately as you can. Feedback is located at the end of the chapter.

1. How often do you eat breakfast?
   a. I don't eat breakfast.
   b. I eat breakfast some days.
   c. I eat breakfast most days.
   d. I eat breakfast every day.

2. On an average day, how many portions of fruit and vegetables do you eat?
   a. I don't eat fruit or vegetables.
   b. 1 or 2 portions
   c. 3 or 4 portions
   d. More than 4 portions

3. On an average day, how many portions of meat do you eat?
   a. More than 5 portions
   b. 4 or 5 portions
   c. 2 or 3 portions
   d. 1 portion

4. How many portions of dairy products (milk, cheese, yogurt, ice cream) do you eat?
   a. More than 7
   b. 6 or 7 portions
   c. 4 or 5 portions
   d. 2 or 3 portions

5. How many portions of pasta, bread, or grain products do you eat?
   a. Fewer than 2 portions
   b. 2 or 3 portions
   c. 5 or 6 portions
   d. 6 to 10 portions

6. With respect to your eating habits, what would you say about your weight?
   a. I am way underweight.
   b. I am way overweight.

    c. I am gaining weight.

    d. My weight is about right.

7. If you had to choose one of the following snack foods to eat, which would you choose?

    a. Cheese puffs

    b. Artificially flavored apple pie

    c. Salted nuts

    d. Canned fruit

NOURISHMENT

Active, growing teens are often hungry. In this country, teens are fortunate because they usually have food available at home or enough money to buy food when they're on the go. Americans take having sufficient food for granted, and we often satisfy our hunger with what we *like* to eat instead of what is *best* to meet our nutritional needs. Eating what we like may be satisfying at the time, but poor eating habits can eventually result in negative consequences later on. The eating patterns you establish now will persist later in life, so you might want to be sure they fit into a wellness lifestyle.

Being well nourished is not the same as being well fed. A person whose diet largely consists of fast food and high-calorie snacks probably consumes enough food (too much, in fact!) but is not well nourished. Good nutrition is important so the body can function at its best. Research indicates that teens are not all that well nourished. In fact, of all age groups in the United States, teens are the most poorly nourished. And, among teens, females are the least well nourished. Poor eating habits put young people at risk for a number of health problems, including obesity, delayed sexual maturation, and failure to reach their potential height. The continuation of poor eating habits into adulthood increases the risk for thin and brittle bones (osteoporosis) and high levels of blood fat that can lead to heart disease.

NUTRIENTS

Nutrients are the substances in food that the body must have to function properly. There are six basic nutrients the body must have: carbohydrates, protein, fats, vitamins, minerals, and water. Along with satisfying hunger, providing nutrients is the real purpose of food. Nutrients are extracted from foods during the digestive process, which takes place in the stomach and small intestine as the food passes through the **alimentary canal** (also known as the gastrointestinal tract). See Figure 8-1 for an illustration of the digestive system.

Acids, enzymes, and other secretions in the alimentary canal break the food down into molecules that can be absorbed into the

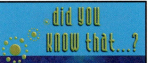

did you KNOW that…?

Osteoporosis is a condition that affects older women. Current research indicates that one out of every two females exhibits some form of osteoporosis and that prevention actually needs to start in the teen and young adult years. It is important for young women to consume sufficient calcium and to participate in weight-bearing exercises such as aerobics, walking, and jogging. The risk for osteoporosis is increased if there is a family history of osteoporosis. In these cases, preventive habits are especially important.

nutrients

various substances that are needed for the body to function

alimentary canal

the tubular passage from mouth to rectum that functions in digestion, the absorption of food and water, and the elimination of waste

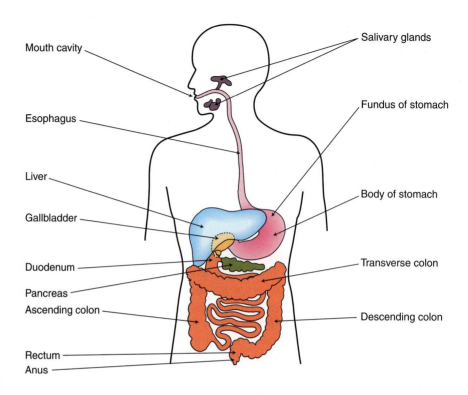

Figure 8-1
The digestive system

Labels: Mouth cavity, Esophagus, Liver, Gallbladder, Duodenum, Pancreas, Ascending colon, Rectum, Anus, Salivary glands, Fundus of stomach, Body of stomach, Transverse colon, Descending colon

bloodstream. The blood then carries the molecules to the body's cells, where they are used to provide energy and maintain various bodily functions. Nutrients come in many forms, and each serves a specific purpose in the body.

Carbohydrates

Carbohydrates are perhaps the single most important nutrient because carbohydrates provide energy for the body. Energy is needed for all body functions, even sleeping. Energy is used to support many functions such as maintaining your heartbeat, processing your food through digestion, and growing new cells. Energy is even necessary for thinking. An active person needs more energy than someone who is inactive. Can you imagine why?

The amount of energy needed to carry out the basic body functions when you are at rest is known as **basal metabolism**. When you exercise, your heart beats faster than normal, you breathe harder, and your muscles work harder. All of these processes require extra energy and, therefore, use more calories. That's why someone who is active needs more energy sources than someone who is not active. As a teen, your energy requirements are just about at your lifetime high. The amount of energy needed to maintain basal metabolism gradually decreases with age, starting at about age 20. At the same time, many people begin decreasing their level of physical activity. This is one

take it on home

Our food choices and preferences are often related to the family in which we are raised, and our family's preferences are based on the preferences of the family in which they were raised. These preferences are part of our family histories. Talk with your family and find out what food preferences have been handed down from generation to generation. See if you can find out what food preferences originated with the racial or cultural background of your family. Write a report of your findings and keep it in your Health Folio.

carbohydrates

food substances that provide energy for the body

basal metabolism

the amount of energy needed to maintain body functions at rest

reason why people tend to gain weight as they get older if they maintain the same eating habits they had when they were younger.

Energy is measured in calories. A **calorie** is a scientific measure of the amount of energy needed to raise the temperature of 1 kilogram (a little more than 1 quart) of water 1 degree centigrade (about 1.8 degrees Fahrenheit). The number of calories a person should consume each day depends on how much energy is needed to live. This amount is determined by body weight, lean muscle mass, activity level, and age.

Carbohydrates come in two forms: simple carbohydrates and complex carbohydrates. Simple carbohydrates are sugars. Examples of simple carbohydrates are table sugar, known as sucrose, and fruit sugar, called fructose. Simple carbohydrates are first converted into glucose during digestion. Glucose is the simplest form of sugar–the form that is actually used by the body cells for energy.

Simple carbohydrates provide a quick source of energy because they are rapidly processed by the body and absorbed into the bloodstream. Foods composed of simple carbohydrates are what you need if you are participating in an athletic event, such as gymnastics or track and field events, that are of short duration and require short, powerful bursts of energy.

Complex carbohydrates are known as starches. They have larger molecules and take longer to be digested than simple carbohydrates, and they release their energy over longer periods of time. The large molecules must be broken down into simple carbohydrates before their energy becomes available. Beans, wheat bread, oatmeal, and tortillas are examples of complex carbohydrates. An athlete who is

calorie

a measure of the amount of energy needed to raise the temperature of 1 kilogram of water 1 degree centigrade; scientists burn foods to measure the number of calories they contain

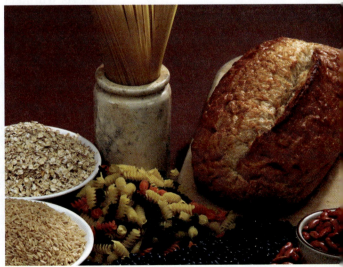

playing in a soccer match or running a marathon should eat a lot of complex carbohydrates before the competition. Because complex carbohydrates take longer to release energy, the athlete will have a constant supply of energy during the event.

Protein

Protein is the nutrient needed to build and repair tissue in the body, to help regulate some body functions by helping to build hormones and enzymes, and to provide energy for the body in times of starvation. There is some protein in almost all the foods you eat, but animal products are especially high in complete protein. As food is digested, the protein compounds are broken down into **amino acids**, the building blocks of protein. The amino acids are then combined in the body to form the kinds of proteins the body can use.

The human body needs approximately 20 amino acids. Many of these can be manufactured from foods eaten. There are 9 amino acids, however, that the body cannot manufacture. These are known as **essential amino acids** because they must be present in the foods we eat. Foods that contain all nine of these amino acids are known as **complete protein** sources. Complete protein sources come from animal tissue such as that found in eggs, meats, cheese, milk, and fish. If you eat foods that contain **incomplete proteins**, you can still get all the essential amino acids if the protein sources are complementary. This means that they combine to become complete. Here are some examples of complementary protein combinations:

- Peanut butter and bread
- Soybeans and rice
- Beans and tortillas
- Tofu and rice

Young adults who are quite physically active or who participate in sports will need more protein than those who are less active. Because most Americans consume more protein than they normally need, there

protein

nutrient used by the body to build and repair tissue and to manufacture enzymes

amino acids

organic compounds that are the building blocks of protein

essential amino acids

the amino acids that humans must get in their diet and that cannot be manufactured by the body

complete protein

protein source that contains all nine essential amino acids

incomplete protein

a protein source that does not contain all nine of the essential amino acids

did you know that...?

People in many countries have been consuming complementary proteins for centuries. In some areas, the use of complementary proteins is due to the scarcity of meat products, but in some countries it may be for religious reasons. Here are some common complementary dishes in other cultures:

- Lentils and wheat is a common dish in India.
- Peas and wheat are common combinations in the Middle East.
- Beans and corn are favorite complements in Mexico and Central and South America.

is no real reason for teens to consume large amounts of protein or to take protein supplements. Some young people who are involved in weight lifting mistakenly believe that if they eat more protein or take supplements, they can build more muscle tissue. The truth is that eating extra protein cannot cause muscle to grow. Muscle growth and strength come from training and an adequate diet. The athlete who consumes very large amounts of protein runs the risk of **ketosis**. Ketosis is an accumulation of acids in the bloodstream produced during metabolism of the fat in the protein source.

Fats

Fats, also known as **lipids**, are greasy food materials that are concentrated sources of energy. A tablespoon of butter contains 100 calories, whereas a tablespoon of sugar has only 45 calories. Fats are usually the part of the meal that makes us feel full.

Some fats are necessary for good nutrition. In addition to giving you energy, fats carry certain vitamins through the body and help develop certain hormones. When stored in the body, fat helps cushion and support the organs. It is only when you eat too many fats that they are unhealthy. The best recommendation is that you should receive *no more than 30%* of your total daily calories from fat sources.

There are three major types of fat in our diet: **saturated fats**, **monounsaturated fats**, and **polyunsaturated fats**. Saturated fats are found in animal fat sources. Butter, cream, cheese, fat on meat, palm oil, and lard are examples of saturated fats. These fats are firm at room temperature. Saturated fats tend to raise the **cholesterol** level in the blood. The body needs some cholesterol to build cells and produce certain hormones, but too much cholesterol can be harmful. You may have heard the expressions "bad cholesterol" and "good cholesterol." Bad cholesterol is low-density lipoprotein (LDL). High levels of LDL can accumulate in the arteries and lead to heart disease and other health problems. Good cholesterol is high-density lipoproteins (HDL) and act as cholesterol sponges that help keep cholesterol from clinging to the walls of the arteries. It is desirable to have low levels of LDLs and high levels of HDLs. In addition to eating habits, the following wellness practices affect cholesterol levels:

- Exercise tends to increase the level of HDL and lower the level of LDL.
- Smoking tends to lower the level of HDL.
- Too much sugar in the diet tends to lower the level of HDL.

The American Heart Association recommends that you consume no more than 300 milligrams of cholesterol each day. One egg contains approximately 215 milligrams.

Unsaturated fats are found in plant oils. Some oils, such as corn oil and safflower oil, are polyunsaturated. They are better for you than saturated fats because they do not significantly raise cholesterol levels.

ketosis

buildup of ketone bodies, potentially poisonous by-products of protein metabolism

lipids

fatty compounds in foods that provide energy and transport certain vitamins

saturated fats

fats from animal sources that are firm at room temperature

monounsaturated fat

types of oils containing fats that contribute very little to the development of heart disease

polyunsaturated fats

fats that come from plant sources that are better for heart health than saturated fats

cholesterol

a waxy, fatlike substance in the body an excess of which may contribute to heart disease

unsaturated fats

fats that come from vegetable oil sources

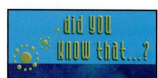

hydrogenation

the addition of hydrogen molecules to liquid fats to make them firm at room temperature

trans fats

liquid fats that have been intentionally enhanced with hydrogen to make them firm at room temperature or more suitable for frying

essential fatty acids

fats needed by the body that must be consumed in the diet because the human body cannot manufacture them

Even better are the monounsaturated fats, such as peanut oil, olive oil, and canola oil. These oils are actually called "heart healthy" fats because they have a favorable effect on cholesterol levels. These fats are liquid at room temperature, unless they have had hydrogen added during processing to make them more solid. This process, known as **hydrogenation**, converts the unsaturated oils into **trans fat**. Food products that contain trans fats are margarine, commercially prepared pie crusts, baked goods, fried foods, and to a lesser degree, butter. Research has shown that a number of health problems are associated with the consumption of trans fat. Trans fat can increase LDL levels and decrease HDL levels. Trans fat consumption by mothers has also been linked to low-birthweight infants. Low birthweight is a leading risk factor for infant deaths during the first year of life.

Americans do not knowingly consume large amounts of trans fat, but trans fat is unknowingly consumed because it is in many processed foods such as cookies, pie crust, processed cheese, peanut butter (unless it is naturally prepared, in which case the oil separates from the peanuts). It would be almost impossible to eliminate all trans fat from your diet. The best advice is to avoid eating large quantities of foods that contain hydrogenated or partially hydrogenated oils. Read your food labels and look for oils that are "hydrogenated" or "partially hydrogenated" oils.

Among the fats we need from our diet, **essential fatty acids** are probably the most important and most overlooked. Essential fatty acids (EFAs) are important because they are present in every cell of the body and are critical for normal growth and development.

Deficiencies in EFAs contribute to a number of health problems, including reduced growth rates, decreased immune function, and skin changes that include dryness and scaliness. Basically, there are two forms of EFA: omega-3 fatty acids and omega-6 fatty acids. Omega-3 fatty acids are found in cold-water fish such as salmon, tuna, mackerel, and flounder, but they are also present in nuts, vegetables, beans, and fruit. Omega-3 fatty acids are very good for the heart. Omega-6 fatty acids are found in safflower, sunflower, and corn oils. Studies indicate that Americans eat 30 times more omega-6 fatty acids than omega-3

What's News?

The National Academy of Science (NAS) in the U.S. Institute of Medicine has confirmed the need to moderate the consumption of trans fatty acids in the diet. The NAS report in 2002 validated previous reports implying that trans fatty acids were a culprit in the formation of heart disease. Check the labels on your favorite snack products. Do they contain hydrogenated oils? If they do, you may want to cut back on how many of them you eat.

did you know that...?

It is estimated that 68% of American deaths are related to excessive fat consumption and poor diet, including heart disease (44% of deaths), cancer (22%), and diabetes (2%).

fatty acids. The reason is that we consume more foods fried in oils that contain omega-6 fatty acids (french fries and potato chips) or made with omega-6 oils (cookies, pies, and packaged snack foods) than foods that contain omega-3 fatty acids such as fish, nuts and vegetables.

Vitamins

Vitamins are compounds that are necessary in small amounts for a number of body processes. Contrary to popular belief, vitamins themselves do not give you energy. Rather, they enable the body to produce energy from the foods you eat. Select dietary vitamin requirements are expressed as **Reference Daily Intakes** (RDIs). The RDIs for various nutrients have been set according to research on humans and animals. There are no RDIs for fat, sodium, cholesterol, or carbohydrates. The recommendations for these and certain other foods are expressed as **Daily Reference Values** (DRVs). The DRV for protein is determined by both age and gender. Keep in mind that RDIs have a cushion built in to help ensure that sufficient amounts are consumed. For example, if you get 70% of the RDIs, you are likely to prevent deficiency symptoms. See Table 8-1 for a listing of nutrients and their corresponding RDIs and DRVs.

Although vitamins are important, they should not be overused. In fact, **megadoses** can be toxic (poisonous) if taken for long periods of time. For example, taking megadoses of vitamin A can lead to bone pain, decreased appetite, and hair loss. Excessive doses of vitamin C can lead to the development of kidney stones. Keep in mind that "if a little is good, a little is good enough." There is no need to take higher doses than the minimums recommended.

There are two classifications of vitamins, water soluble and fat soluble. Water-soluble vitamins are easily destroyed by air, light, and cooking, so it is important to properly store and prepare the vegetables that contain them. For example, one spear of raw broccoli contains 141 **milligrams** of vitamin C, but a cooked spear contains only about 110 milligrams. If it is overcooked, the spear will contain even fewer. One way to recover lost vitamins is to make soup from the cooking liquid.

Reference Daily Intake (RDI)
the level of a vitamin or mineral recommended to be included in the diet each day

Daily Reference Values (DRVs)
reference values of eight selected nutrients for a 2,000-calorie diet; the basis of nutrition labels

megadose
dosage that is much larger than what is recommended, approximately 5—10 times the RDI

milligram
a unit of metric weight that is 1/1,000 of a gram; 100 milligrams is equal to 0.0035 of an ounce — about the same weight as a pinch of salt

Table 8-1 Reference Daily Intakes and Daily Reference Values for a 2,000-Calorie Diet

Nutrient	Reference Daily Intake (RDI)	Nutrient	Reference Daily Intake (RDI)
Vitamin A	5,000 international units (900 micrograms for men; 700 micrograms for women)	Vitamin E	22 international units
Vitamin B$_6$	2.0 milligrams		
Vitamin B$_{12}$	6 micrograms	Calcium	1.0 gram
Vitamin C	75 milligrams	Copper	900 micrograms
Thiamin	1.5 milligrams	Folic acid	0.4 milligram
Pantothenic acid	10 milligrams	Iodine	150 micrograms
Riboflavin	1.7 milligrams	Iron	18 milligrams
Biotin	0.3 milligrams	Magnesium	400 milligrams
Niacin	20 milligrams	Phosphorus	1.0 gram
Vitamin D	400 international units	Zinc	11 milligrams

Nutrient	Daily Reference Values (DRVs)	Nutrient	Daily Reference Values (DRVs)
Total carbohydrate	300 grams	Cholesterol	300 milligrams
Protein	50 grams	Fiber	25 grams
Fat	65 grams	Sodium	2,400 milligrams
Saturated fatty acids	20 grams	Potassium	3,500 milligrams

antioxidant

compound that interferes with the damaging effects of certain compounds in the body; may help lower LDL in the blood and prevent certain cancers

Fat-soluble vitamins are not lost in cooking. When eaten, they are transported through the body by lipids in the bloodstream. Unlike water-soluble vitamins, which do not remain in the body, excess amounts of fat-soluble vitamins are stored in the liver and can be used later. This is why fat-soluble vitamin deficiencies are slower to appear than are water-soluble vitamin deficiencies. See Table 8-2 for a list of fat-soluble and water-soluble vitamins and their sources, functions, and deficiency problems.

We used to believe that if people ate a balanced diet, they didn't need a vitamin supplement. But recent evidence indicates this is not necessarily true. Taking a vitamin supplement has been shown to add health benefits, especially if you add to it an extra **antioxidant** such as vitamins A, C, or E. A well-balanced diet for a teen will usually provide the vitamins needed each day, but supplementation is okay as long as it is not overdone.

Table 8-2   Fat-Soluble Vitamins and Water-Soluble Vitamins

Name	Food Sources	Functions	Deficiency Problems
Fat-soluble vitamins			
Vitamin A	Liver, whole milk, butter, cream, cod liver oil, dark green leafy vegetables, deep yellow or orange fruit, fortified margarine	Maintenance of vision in dim light Maintenance of healthy skin Growth and development of bones Reproduction Healthy immune system	Respiratory infections Cessation of bone growth
Vitamin D	Eggs, fortified milk, oily fish, sunlight	Regulation of calcium and phosphorus absorption Building and maintenance of normal bones and teeth Prevention of tetany	Osteoporosis Poorly developed teeth and bones Muscle spasms
Vitamin E	Green and leafy vegetables, salad dressing, wheat germ and wheat germ oils, vegetable oils, nuts	Antioxidant (prevents diseases) Considered essential for protection of cell structure, especially of red blood cells	Destruction of red blood cells
Vitamin K	Liver, milk, green leafy vegetables, cabbage, broccoli	Blood clotting	Prolonged blood clotting/ hemorrhaging
Water-soluble vitamins			
Thiamin (vitamin B_1)	Lean pork, beef, eggs, fish, whole and enriched grains	Metabolism of carbohydrates and some amino acids Maintenance of normal appetite and functioning of nervous system	Gastrointestinal tract, nervous system, and cardiovascular system problems Beriberi
Riboflavin (vitamin B_2)	Liver, kidney, heart, milk, cheese, green leafy vegetables, cereals, enriched bread	Aids release of energy from food Health of the mouth tissue Healthy eyes	Eye sensitivity Skin irritation Sensitivity to light
Niacin	Milk, eggs, fish, poultry, enriched breads and cereals	Energy metabolism Healthy skin and nervous and digestive systems	Pellagra—dermatitis, dementia, diarrhea
Pyridoxine (vitamin B_6)	Pork, fish, poultry, milk, eggs, whole-grain cereals, legumes	Conversion of amino acid to niacin Release of glucose from glycogen Protein metabolism and building of nonessential amino acids	Skin irritation Confusion Depression Irritability
Vitamin B_{12}	Seafood, poultry, red meat, eggs, milk, cheese	Making red blood cells Treatment of anemia Using folic acid	Anemia Sore mouth and tongue Anorexia Nerve disorders
Folate (folic acid)	Red meat, green leafy vegetables, spinach, seeds, broccoli, cereal fortified with folate, fruit	Making red blood cells Developing DNA	Anemia Birth defects

continues

Table 8-2 *continued*

Name	Food Sources	Functions	Deficiency Problems
Biotin	Milk, egg yolks, soy flour, cereals, fruit	Aids in carbohydrate and amino acid metabolism Converting amino acid to niacin	Skin irritation Nausea Anorexia Depression Hair loss
Pantothenic acid	Eggs, salmon, poultry, mushrooms, cauliflower, peanuts	Metabolism of carbohydrates, lipids, and proteins Making fatty acids, cholesterol, steroid hormones	Rare: burning feet syndrome, vomiting, fatigue
Vitamin C (ascorbic acid)	All citrus fruits, broccoli, melons, strawberries, tomatoes, potatoes, green peppers	Prevention of scurvy Formation of tissue Healing of wounds Release of stress hormones Absorption of iron Antioxidant Resistance to infection	Scurvy Muscle cramps Ulcerated gums Tendency to bruise easily

There are number of misconceptions that surround vitamin use. Perhaps you have heard some of these:

- ***"Vitamins in food are better than vitamins from food supplements."***
  Not true. The body recognizes vitamins for what they are able to do, not for where they come from. The chemical composition of vitamins in foods and in pill form is the same.

- ***"Organically grown foods contain superior vitamins."***
  Not true. It doesn't matter how the plants are grown. In fact, even if the plant is grown under very poor conditions, and the fruits and vegetables are sparse or small, they will still contain vitamins and minerals.

- ***"Some vitamin supplements are better than others—you get what you pay for."***
  Not true. Read the labels. If the product advertises a certain percentage of the Reference Daily Intake, you can rely on the nutrients being available. According to the U.S. Food and Drug Administration policy, the label must accurately reflect the product being sold.

Myths about vitamin use

Minerals

Minerals are elements that are found in the earth. Our bodies need them in small amounts, but we cannot manufacture them. They must come from our food. Most of the minerals in your diet come from plant sources. Foods from animal sources indirectly supply small amounts of minerals. As do those for vitamins, the RDIs for minerals vary according to age and gender.

There are two classifications of minerals. Major minerals are those needed in amounts greater than 100 milligrams per day. Minor minerals are those needed in amounts less than 100 milligrams per day. See Tables 8-3 and 8-4 for a list of the minerals we need.

Table 8-3 Major Minerals

Name	Food Sources	Functions	Deficiency Problems
Calcium	Milk, cheese, salmon, some dark green leafy vegetables	Development of bones and teeth Transmission of nerve impulses Blood clotting Normal heart action Normal muscle activity	Osteoporosis Rickets Poor tooth and bone formation
Phosphorus	Milk, cheese, lean meat, poultry, fish, whole grain cereals, nuts	Development of bones and teeth Maintenance of normal blood Component of all body cells Necessary for effectiveness of some vitamins Metabolism of carbohydrates, fats, and proteins	Poor tooth and bone formation Weakness Anorexia General weakness
Potassium	Oranges, bananas, dried fruits, vegetables, milk, cereals, meat	Contraction of muscles Maintenance of fluid balance Transmission of nerve impulses Regular heart rhythm Cell metabolism	Muscle weakness Confusion Abnormal heartbeat
Sodium	Table salt, beef, eggs, poultry, milk, cheese	Maintenance of fluid balance Transmission of nerve impulses	Nausea Exhaustion Muscle cramps
Chloride	Table salt, eggs, seafood, milk	Gastric acidity Fluid balance Acid-base balance Formation of hydrochloric acid	Imbalance in gastric acidity Nausea Exhaustion
Magnesium	Green leafy vegetables, whole grains, avocados, nuts, milk, legumes, bananas	Transmission of nerve impulses Activation of metabolic enzymes Component of bones, muscles, and red blood cells Necessary for healthy muscles and nerves	Possible mental, emotional, and muscle disorders
Sulfur	Eggs, poultry, fish	Maintenance of protein structure Building hair, nails, and all body tissues Component of all body cells	Unknown

Table 8-4 Trace Minerals

Name	Food Sources	Functions	Deficiency Problems
Iron	Red meat, poultry, shellfish, liver, dried fruits, whole grain or enriched breads and cereals, dark green and leafy vegetables	Transports oxygen and carbon dioxide Component of red blood cells Component of cellular enzymes essential for energy production	Iron deficiency anemia characterized by weakness, dizziness, loss of weight, and pallor
Iodine	Iodized salt, seafood	Regulation of basal metabolic rate	Thyroid problems
Zinc	Seafood, especially oysters, liver, eggs, milk, wheat bran	Formation of tissue Wound healing Taste acuity Essential for growth Immune reactions	Loss of appetite Skin changes Impaired wound healing Decreased taste acuity
Selenium	Seafood, red meat, grains	Component of most body tissue Needed for fat metabolism Antioxidant functions	Unclear, but related to Keshan disease (weak heart muscle) Muscle weakness
Copper	Liver, shellfish, oysters, nuts, whole grains	Essential for formation of red blood cells Component of enzymes Wound healing Needed metabolically for the release of energy	Anemia Bone disease Disturbed growth and metabolism
Manganese	Whole grains, nuts, fruits, tea	Component of enzymes Bone formation Metabolic processes	Unknown
Fluoride	Fluoridated water, seafood	Increases resistance to tooth decay Component of bones and teeth	Tooth decay Possibly osteoporosis

fiber

the indigestible material in food

DIETARY FIBER

Fiber is the indigestible plant material in food. It cannot be digested because it is composed of materials that cannot be absorbed into the bloodstream. Complex carbohydrates are high in fiber content. Although fiber is not a nutrient, it is an important component of your diet and has many health benefits. In addition to helping move waste materials through the digestive tract, it gives a feeling of fullness without adding calories. This benefit can assist in weight management and reduce the chance of obesity. A high-fiber diet can help prevent weight gain and promote weight loss. It also is believed to slow fat absorption. As a result of these benefits, research indicates that fiber may be helpful in preventing diabetes, cancer, and heart disease.

The average American consumes about half the recommended amount of fiber each day. If you don't eat much wheat bread or consume several servings of fruits and vegetables each day, you are probably not getting enough fiber. If you want to increase your fiber intake, it is best to do it gradually and drink lots of water with meals. Consuming too much fiber in a short period of time can cause intestinal discomfort.

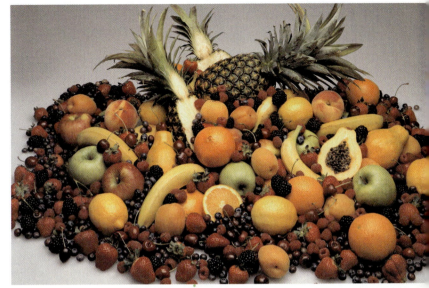

WATER

Water has no direct nutritional value but is essential to our survival. Depending on conditions, a person can live about one week without water. Approximately 60% of your body weight is water, although the exact percentage varies from person to person. Water contains no calories. In fact, your body will burn 100 calories as it processes 16 ounces of water.

real teens

Corina likes water and knows that it's good for her. She carries a water bottle with her all day long. She used to bring bottled water from home or buy it from the snack machine at school. Corina believed that drinking bottled water was healthier than drinking directly from the tap.

A few weeks ago she heard something on the news that caught her attention. The reporter said that bottled water may not be as healthy as we've been led to believe. It seems that bottled water goes through a series of filtrations or it comes from springs where the water has no fluoride in it. In junior high, Corina had learned that fluoride is good for your teeth. After hearing the news report, she decided that she needed more information. She began some research of her own. Doing this research worked out well because she had to do a report for science class anyway and now she had a good topic.

Corina used the Internet to find out what kinds of chemicals and other components are in bottled water. She also contacted her local water plant and requested a report on the city water. To her surprise, Corina learned that not all bottled water is the same and that there is actually more fluoride in the city water than in any brand of bottled water. As a result of her research, Corina decided not to continue buying bottled water. Now she fills her water bottle at the school fountain. Not only does she get her fluoride, she doesn't have to pay for the water.

Water serves several functions in the body:

- It is a component of all body tissues.
- It helps regulate body temperature.
- It helps lubricate the joints.
- It transports nutrients and cellular waste.

It is recommended that you consume eight glasses of fluid a day to maintain good health. Some of this can come from liquids other than water, such as juice, milk, sports drinks, and soup, but half of your fluid needs should come from water alone. Exercise increases your need for fluids. And the hotter and more humid the environment, the more water you need.

PLANNING TO EAT WELL

Knowing about nutrients is a proper first step in developing good eating habits, but the information must be applied to contribute to wellness. Applying the information means making healthy choices about what you eat. We have so many foods available to us that the greatest challenge may be combining eating for wellness with eating for enjoyment. If you look around, you will see many people in this country who are "overfed." In fact, overweight and obesity are becoming major health problems because they contribute to a variety of serious diseases and conditions, such as heart disease and diabetes.

The Food Guide Pyramid

The Food Guide Pyramid was developed in 1984 to make it easier to select the right types and amounts of foods to stay healthy. The pyramid categorizes food into five major groups and shows the number of daily recommended servings from each group. The latest version was created in 1996 to reflect new discoveries about how food contributes to wellness. Look at the guide in Figure 8-2 and you'll see the emphasis on breads and cereals at the base of the pyramid. The group with the fewest recommended servings is at the top and includes fats and sweets.

The specific nutritional needs of teens are listed in Table 8-5. You can see that the recommended servings per day are different for teen males and females. And the number of servings corresponds to activity level. If you follow the guidelines in the food pyramid, you can be assured that your nutritional needs will be met. Even if you don't follow the guide every day, you can make good wellness decisions by keeping the basic principles in mind. For example, if you are in doubt about what to eat when you're hungry, choose vegetables, fruits, or grains.

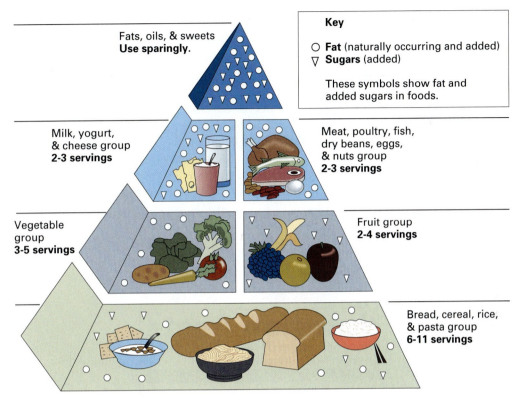

Key

○ **Fat** (naturally occurring and added)
▽ **Sugars** (added)

These symbols show fat and added sugars in foods.

Fats, oils, & sweets
Use sparingly.

Milk, yogurt,
& cheese group
2-3 servings

Meat, poultry, fish,
dry beans, eggs,
& nuts group
2-3 servings

Vegetable
group
3-5 servings

Fruit group
2-4 servings

Bread, cereal, rice,
& pasta group
6-11 servings

Figure 8-2   The Food Guide Pyramid

Table 8-5   Daily Nutritional Needs of Teens

Food Group	Examples	Older Children, Teen Girls, Most Women (2,200 Calories)	Active Teens, Men (2,800 Calories)
Grains group (one serving: ½ cup rice or 1 slice bread or 1 roll)	Bread, pasta, tortillas, rice	9 servings per day	11 servings per day
Vegetable group (one serving: 1 cup raw vegetables or ½ cup cooked vegetables)	Carrots, broccoli, squash, green beans	4 servings per day	5 servings per day
Fruit group (one serving: 1 piece fruit or ½ cup juice)	Apples, pears, oranges, pineapple, melon	3 servings per day	4 servings per day
Milk group	Milk, cheese, yogurt	2 or 3 servings per day	2 or 3 servings per day
Meat and beans	Chicken, fish, beef, pork, beans (pinto, kidney, etc.)	2 servings per day	3 servings per day

Reading Food Labels

The U.S. Department of Agriculture and the Food and Drug Administration require that most foods (meat and poultry are excluded) be clearly labeled with nutritional information for the consumer. The nutrient information required by law includes what makes up a serving size, the number of servings per container, and the number of calories per serving. Look at the typical food label shown in Figure 8-3. Note that all the values listed on the label are *per serving*. This fact is important; a person who didn't know this might eat a whole package of food thinking the total calories are for the entire package! In addition, the label must contain the amounts per serving of the following nutrients:

- Fats: total calories and the amounts of saturated fats and cholesterol
- Sodium
- Total carbohydrates
- Dietary fiber

Nutrition Facts

Serving Size 1/2 cup (114g)
Serving Per Container 4

Amount Per Serving

Calories 90   Calories from Fat 30

	% Daily Value
Total Fat 3g	5%
Saturated Fat 0g	0%
Cholesterol 0mg	0%
Sodium 300mg	13%
Total Carbohydrate 13g	4%
Dietary Fiber 3g	12%
Sugars 3g	
Protein 3g	

Vitamin A	80%	•	Vitamin C	60%
Calcium	4%	•	Iron	4%

• Percent Daily Values are based on a 2,000 calorie diet. Your daily values may be higher or lower depending on your calorie needs:

	Calories	2,000	2,500
Total Fat	Less than	65g	80g
Sat Fat	Less than	20g	25g
Cholesterol	Less than	300mg	300mg
Sodium	Less than	2,400mg	2,400mg
Total Carbohydrate		300g	375g
Fiber		25g	30g

Calories per gram:
Fat 9   •   Carbohydrate 4   •   Protein 4

Figure 8-3
A typical food label

take it on home

Look at some of the foods in your cupboards at home. Try to find products that are very similar, such as different cereals or canned vegetables. Read the labels and compare food values. Use the information you have about food labels to draw conclusions regarding the nutritional value of the various foods. You may want to take the activity a step further and find out how much the products cost. Paying more for each serving of a product does not necessarily mean it's more nutritious. Keep track of your findings and place them in your Health Folio.

- Sugars
- Protein
- Vitamin A
- Vitamin C
- Calcium
- Iron

When you shop for packaged foods, it is a good idea to compare nutrients among products and brands to ensure that you are getting the nutrients you want and need.

Vegetarianism

People who choose to eat foods only from plant sources are known as **vegetarians**. These individuals follow a vegetarian diet for a variety of reasons. Some people object to killing animals; some are concerned about all the land needed to raise meat sources compared with the amount of land needed for vegetarian sources. Some people eat plants and vegetables to avoid the fat in meat. There are many personal reasons that may influence one's choice to be vegetarian.

If planned correctly, a vegetarian diet can be very nutritious, reduce obesity, and prevent heart disease and some cancers. Although most vegetarians avoid eating all types of meat, there are actually three forms of vegetarianism.

1. *Lacto-ovo vegetarians* eat plants and dairy products (cheese, milk, yogurt, and so on) and eggs but consume no meat, poultry, or fish.
2. *Lacto-vegetarians* use dairy products with their plant foods, but eat no meat, poultry, fish, or eggs.
3. *Vegans* avoid all animal products. Vegans eat plant foods only.

vegetarianism

the practice of consuming foods only from plant sources, except eggs or dairy products in some instances

If you have any interest in vegetarian eating, be sure to research the topic well before you begin. Vegetarian diets are not perfect. For example, a strict vegan diet tends to be very low in calcium and iron. As a growing teen, it is important that you plan your menus correctly to ensure that you get all the nutrients you need for proper growth and wellness. It will take some planning on your part.

EATING SAFELY

We sometimes take the safety of our food for granted. Although we have many laws and procedures in place to protect our foods, we still need to be careful to handle them correctly and safely. Even with inspections, packaging, and refrigeration, improper handling of food can cause serious illnesses and even death. There are two ways in which food can do damage:

1. Organisms invade food products and alter them by releasing toxic (poisonous) chemicals. These organisms can grow inside improperly prepared or damaged cans. See Chapter 23 for more information about organisms that contribute to food poisoning.

2. Organisms that cause illness enter the body, using foods as a means of transport.

Organisms that cause illnesses can be present in the air, on preparation surfaces, or on the hands of the food preparer. There are some important basic rules you should follow to prevent food-borne illnesses:

- When you shop, try to purchase frozen and refrigerated items last. If you buy them first, they have more time to be exposed to warm temperatures that could encourage the growth of disease-causing organisms.

- Read labels. Don't buy foods that have passed their expiration date. Expired foods are likely to spoil.

- *Never* buy or attempt to eat vegetables in a can that has a bulging top. The cans bulge from the poisonous gas that comes from organisms that were not destroyed during canning.

- Always wash your hands before and after handling food. Your hands contact germs on surfaces all day long. If you get sick from your food, it is most likely because of the germs on your hands.

- Be careful of cutting boards, especially wooden boards. Germs can get caught in the cut marks and become transferred to your food. Occasionally sanitize the board with 1 teaspoon of bleach in 1 quart of water, and thoroughly wash it with soap and hot water after each use.

- Do not thaw meats at room temperature. The outside of the meat will thaw first and become a place for germs to multiply. Defrost food in the refrigerator overnight.

- Cook meats thoroughly. Doing so will ensure that the germs are destroyed all the way through the food.

BUILDING YOUR Wellness Plan

Eating well is one of the best and easiest things you can do for yourself. You eat several times a day, and, almost every time, you get to make decisions about what you eat and how much food you consume. As you develop your wellness plan for nutrition, there are a few essential things to keep in mind:

- Develop a basic working knowledge of the food nutrients. Understand what specific nutrients do for you and what quantities are necessary for good health. This knowledge will enable you to understand food labels and to make healthy decisions when you select what foods you will eat.

- Identify nutrients, such as trans fat, cholesterol, and sugar, that in excess may be harmful to your health. Learn what foods contain large amounts of these nutrients and plan ways to avoid consuming large quantities of them.

- Make an effort to develop good eating patterns at each meal. This does not mean planning every meal on paper. It does mean remembering to follow the food pyramid when making food choices and not eating in excess.

- Use the safe food-handling practices discussed in this chapter whenever you are preparing food.

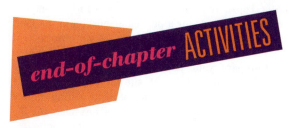

end-of-chapter ACTIVITIES

Weblinks

Food Guide Pyramids

U.S. Department of Agriculture:
  http://www.nal.usda.gov:8001/py/pmap.htm

U.S. Department of Agriculture:
  http://www.nal.usda.gov/fnic/etext/000023.html

Food Labels

U.S. Food and Drug Administration:
  http://www.cfsan.fda.gov/~dms/foodlab.html

Safe Food Handling

U.S. Department of Agriculture:
  http://www.fsis.usda.gov/OA/pubs/facts_basics.htm

Vegetarianism

Beyond Vegetarianism: **http://www.beyondveg.com**

U.S. National Institutes of Health:
  **http://www.nlm.nih.gov/medlineplus/
  vegetarianism.html**

Short-Answer Questions

1. What is a simple carbohydrate? What is a complex carbohydrate?

2. Name two complementary sources of protein that you could eat in combination to provide complete protein.

3. List three things water does for the body.

4. Name the food group in the food pyramid from which you should get the most daily servings.

5. Name a major nutrient category that is not required on a food label.

☀ Discussion Questions

1. Explain how our bodies use the two types of carbohydrates.
2. Discuss the problems associated with eating too much protein.
3. Explain the benefits and problems associated with fats in the diet.
4. Discuss the misconceptions associated with vitamin use.
5. Explain how to safely handle food in the home.

☀ Chapter Vocabulary

Using a separate sheet of paper, list and define the following terms:

amino acids	hydrogenation
antioxidant	polyunsaturated fats
basal metabolism	saturated fats
essential amino acids	trans fats
essential fatty acids	unsaturated fats

☀ Application Activities

Math Connection

How many calories do you need each day? Do the math and find out. Prepare a worksheet that includes the following and fill in the missing information.

How much do you weigh?	_____
1. Calculate your basal metabolism. Each day, you need about 10 calories per pound. How many calories is that for you?	_____
2. Calculate the number of calories you need for normal activities. That would be 3 calories per pound.	_____
3. Calculate the number of calories you need for each hour of exercise. If you don't have access to tables that give you the exact calories needed per pound per exercise, you can use averages. Light exercise = 200 calories per hour Moderate exercise = 300 calories per hour Strenuous exercise = 400 calories per hour	_____
4. Total the first three solutions.	_____

After you have completed the Science Connection exercise, compare the energy values (calories) you totaled there with your total from this exercise. How do they compare?

Social Studies Connection

Several U.S. agencies oversee foods, food testing, and food packaging. These agencies create laws and regulations that ensure food safety. For example, there are laws that protect the consumer by regulating how food products are labeled. Using your health literacy skills, research and write a report about the laws pertaining to these regulations and explain why these laws are needed.

Science Connection

Keep track of all the things you eat and drink for a day. Do the best you can to estimate the portion sizes. Develop a worksheet containing a table on which you list all the foods and their serving sizes along the left side column. Across the top row, list the following nutrients to head columns that create a table:

Energy Protein Fat Fiber Vitamins Minerals

Now, go to the Web site for the U.S. Department of Agriculture (USDA), specifically **http://www.nal.usda.gov/fnic/cgi-bin/nut_search.pl.** There you will find a box where you can enter the name of a food or beverage. You will not be able to enter a brand name. Instead, just name the product. For example, "cola" instead of Coca Cola or Pepsi. You can search the site to uncover the amount of nutrients for a particular portion of the food you entered. Complete the sections of your worksheet using the information you get from the site.

Compare your table with the Reference Daily Intakes from the USDA Web site for your gender and age group. Write a summary of your eating habits and whether you would recommend any changes for yourself. Place your summary in your wellness folio.

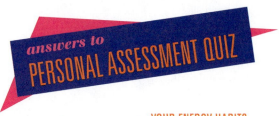

answers to
PERSONAL ASSESSMENT QUIZ

personal assessment: YOUR ENERGY HABITS

Scoring: For each of the items, d = 4 points; c = 3 points; b = 2 points; a = 1 point.

The more points you score, the better your dietary habits are. You can consider yourself eating well if you have more than 24 points!

chapter 9

A Healthy Approach to Weight Management

Keisha has never really paid much attention to how much she weighs, but lately every time she and her girlfriends get together, it seems all they talk about is what they eat and whether they're getting too fat. Every time they eat, there is a discussion of what everyone is eating, how much they're eating, and whether it is fattening. Keisha is beginning to feel guilty about eating and enjoying it. When she talked with her best friend, Tiffany, about how she felt, Tiffany replied, "Well, Keisha, some people *care* about how they look." Keisha cares about how she looks, but she doesn't think about it all the time. She thought she looked okay, but after Tiffany's remark, she's no longer sure. When she asks her older brother if he thinks she's too heavy, he tells her, "I don't get it. Girls always think they're too fat when they're not. Guys always think of themselves as 'too wimpy.' Why can't people just be who they are and be okay with that?" Keisha is more confused than ever.

How can she determine whether she weighs too little or too much or if her weight is just about right?

chapter OBJECTIVES

When you finish this chapter, you should be able to:

- ☀ Discuss historical and social perceptions regarding weight.
- ☀ Identify the factors that affect body image.
- ☀ Describe the relationship of overweight and obesity to health.
- ☀ Identify the four main factors that affect weight management.
- ☀ Describe healthy techniques and strategies to manage weight.
- ☀ Describe three types of eating disorders and identify the factors that contribute to them.
- ☀ Develop a personal plan for healthy weight management.

key TERMS

anorexia nervosa
binge-eating disorder
body composition
body image
bulimia nervosa
dieting
eating disorders
ideal body weight
obese
overweight

Introduction

Today's society places a great deal of emphasis on how people look. For females, "thin is in," whereas for males, the focus is on being muscular and "built." Teens want to fit in and be the "right" size and weight. They often compare their size and weight with the size and weight of friends or the teenagers they see on television and in the movies. But how can you know what is healthy for *you*?

Americans seem to be obsessed with diet, exercise, nutrition, and weight loss. Yet the majority of Americans weigh more than is considered healthy. Medical professionals are encouraging Americans to eat better, exercise more, and lose weight. At the same time, unhealthy eating patterns are on the rise. How can you make sense of all this confusing information and create a healthy weight management plan that works for you? In this chapter, you will have the opportunity to learn some of the information and skills you need to make healthy choices about managing your weight.

personal assessment: WEIGHT MANAGEMENT QUIZ

Before reading this chapter, see how much you already know about weight management. Read the questions below and, on a separate sheet of paper, answer True or False. The answers are located at the end of the chapter.

1. About 25% of all Americans weigh more than is considered healthy.

2. The American cultural "ideal" size for women is much thinner than it was 100 years ago.

3. Eliminating 500 calories a day from your diet will lead to a weight loss of 2 pounds per week.

4. Fat deposited around the abdomen ("apple" shape) is more dangerous to your health than fat deposited in the hips and thighs ("pear" shape).

5. Obesity can increase the risk of diabetes and coronary heart disease.

6. People who are the same height should weigh the same amount.

7. There are almost three times as many overweight adolescents today as there were in 1970.

8. For safe and healthy weight loss, most experts recommend losing no more than 2 pounds per week.

9. About 50% of all people who diet are successful in losing weight and maintaining their new weight.

10. Images of extreme thinness in women promoted by the advertising and entertainment industries may be a factor in the rise in eating disorders.

AMERICAN VIEWS ABOUT WEIGHT

For much of American history, it was desirable to be overweight. Attractive women were "round and plump." Extra weight on men was an indication that they were successful and wealthy. It was not until the 1890s that these cultural ideals began to change. For the first time, weight became a matter of public concern and discussion. As the culturally ideal figure became thinner, disgust for those who had excess body weight began to appear. Restricting food intake for the specific purpose of losing weight became popular. The word *diet*, which had previously referred simply to the food that a person consumed, now began to be associated with weight loss.

A curious thing has happened over the past 100 years. While the focus on weight control has increased, Americans have gotten fatter. We now weigh more on average than at any other time in our history. The result is that what we want to weigh and what we actually weigh are moving in opposite directions.

✿ teen forum ✿

Real versus Ideal

Today the average woman in the United States wears a dress size of 12–14. Yet the typical store mannequin is a size 6, and many models and actresses claim to wear a size 4 or smaller.

- How do you feel about this difference between reality and the ideal?
- How does it affect you?
- How does it affect the way people in our society look at the female body?
- If you are a male, how does it affect your feelings about the females you know?
- What are your feelings about the differences between the real and ideal male body?
- Are men made to feel the same way about their size as women are?

INFLUENCES ON IDEAS ABOUT WEIGHT

> **media**
>
> methods of mass communication such as radio, television, movies, magazines, and newspapers

The **media** are a powerful influence on our ideas about weight. We are constantly bombarded by advertisements, magazine articles, television programs, and movies that suggest that if we are a certain size, weigh a certain amount, or look a certain way, we will be popular and happy. The message is that what you look like determines how successful you will be and how well people will like you. In reality this is not true. Although your appearance may contribute to your success in school, business, or interpersonal relationships, it is not the most important factor in determining your value and quality of life.

The media have created ideal images of men and women as part of a sales strategy. The masculine ideal is portrayed as strong, powerful, and muscular. The feminine ideal is tall, very thin, and strikingly beautiful. In real life, our appearances are much more diverse. If we all fit these ideal images and looked the same, life would be pretty boring.

Advertisements try to appeal to our emotions and to create needs. For example, if we don't look like the people in the ads, we may feel the need to buy the products and services offered in order to look like the ideal. What the ads don't tell us is that the ideal does not really exist. They show people made to look their best with the help of makeup

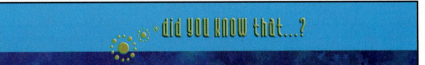

did you know that...?

Although the focus on thinness involves both men and women, women are affected the most. In a 1997 survey conducted by the magazine *Psychology Today*, 24% of women and 17% of men said they would give up more than three years of their lives just to be thin! Many women believe they must be thin in order to be happy.

artists, hairstylists, clothing consultants, lighting experts, and physical trainers. The images may even be computer generated, electronically edited, or airbrushed to achieve a certain effect. But to us, they look like "the real thing." Most of us don't have the time, money, or even the desire to spend that much to create a temporary image, but we may feel pressured to look like the ideal anyway.

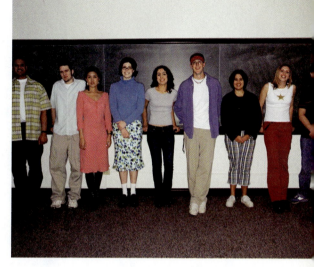

You can become a more critical viewer of the many media messages you are exposed to each day. The next time you see an advertisement, remind yourself that the "perfect" person you see has been created in order to persuade you to buy something. Ask yourself, "What are they trying to sell me?" Being aware of the motives of advertising can help you make conscious decisions about whether to accept what is being promoted. This awareness can help you develop a more realistic and healthy view of yourself.

EXPLORING BODY IMAGE

Body image is the way you see yourself when you look in the mirror or when you picture yourself in your mind. Body image is influenced by your beliefs about your appearance, such as how you feel about your height, shape, and weight. Some people have an image of themselves that is very close to reality. But many people, especially girls and women, have a distorted body image and do not see themselves as they really are.

In one study, 50% of young women who were actually underweight classified themselves in the overweight category. In other words, they saw themselves very differently from the way they actually looked. People who have a negative body image often feel ashamed, self-conscious, and uncomfortable about the way their body looks or moves. These feelings can affect the way they feel about themselves and the way they relate to other people.

Many factors contribute to your body image: past experiences, family, friends, and the influence of the media. You may have been teased about your weight or the shape of your body in the past. Or you may compare yourself with others or with unrealistic media images. A poor body image can lead to an obsession with weight and body shape. Most of us know someone who is constantly counting calories and fat grams. Constant worry and obsession about weight wastes valuable time and energy that can be devoted to achieving more important goals.

The first steps toward achieving a positive body image are recognizing and respecting the natural shape of your body and appreciating the many ways your body works for you. People who have a positive body image feel comfortable and confident in their bodies and refuse to spend an unreasonable amount of time worrying about their appearance. Figure 9-1 contains a list of helpful ideas to help you create a positive body image.

body image

the way you see yourself when you look in the mirror or when you picture yourself in your mind

1. Begin treating your body—the way it is—with respect and kindness.

2. List all the things your body is able to do.

3. When you wake up in the morning, thank your body for resting and preparing you to enjoy the day.

4. Put a sign on each of your mirrors that reminds you, "I'm beautiful, inside and out."

5. Don't let your weight or shape keep you from doing activities you enjoy.

6. Wear comfortable clothes that you like and that feel good to you.

7. Find a physical activity that you enjoy and can do regularly.

8. Surround yourself with people and things that make you feel good about yourself and your abilities.

9. Keep a list of at least 10 things that you like about yourself that aren't related to your appearance.

10. When you go to bed at night, thank your body for all that it helped you accomplish that day.

Figure 9-1
Ten steps toward a positive body image

HOW MUCH SHOULD I WEIGH?

You will hear many recommendations about how much you should weigh. Some of the oldest methods for estimating "ideal weight" are based on the relationship of weight to height. Others are based on the increased likelihood for specific health problems if you weigh more than a certain amount. The simplest way to define your **ideal body weight** is the weight at which you feel strong and energetic and are able to lead a healthy, normal life. Although formulas, charts, and expert recommendations can help guide you in determining how much you should weigh, your ideal body weight is the weight at which *you* are healthy and feel good.

It is important to remember that "healthy weight" doesn't mean the current societal ideals about thinness. It is natural to have a great deal of diversity among people. Every *body* is different. Discovering your own healthy weight is part of developing your individuality as a human being.

Defining Overweight and Obesity

Guidelines to describe different levels of excess weight have been developed to help people determine if they are at increased risk for health problems. **Overweight** is a term to describe body weight that is too high

ideal body weight

the weight at which you feel strong and energetic and are able to lead a healthy life

overweight

a term to describe body weight that is too high in relation to height

in relation to height. **Obese** is a term to describe an excessively high amount of body fat in relation to height.

The United States leads the world in the percentage of its population that is overweight or obese. In 1999, the Centers for Disease Control and Prevention (CDC) estimated that 61% of all adults in the United States were overweight. About 21% of all adult men were obese. Among women, obesity rates among minority women were higher than the national average. Whereas 26% of all adult women were obese, 39% of African American women and 36% of Hispanic women were obese. Of growing concern is the rising number of overweight and obese children and teenagers. Older children and teenagers who are overweight are at increased risk for becoming an overweight or obese adult. Results from the National Health and Nutrition Examination Survey (NHANES) in 1999 showed that about 13%–14% percent of children and adolescents were overweight. The percentage of overweight adolescents (12–19 years of age) had increased from 5% in 1970 to 14% in 1999.

obese

a term used to describe an excessively high amount of body fat in relation to height

Body Composition

Body composition is one method of determining whether you are at a healthy weight. **Body composition** is the relationship between fat-free mass (muscle, bone, and water) and fat tissue in the body. The body needs a certain amount of fat tissue. This is known as **essential body fat**. It is the minimum amount of body fat needed by the body to provide insulation, cushion body organs, and maintain normal bodily functions. Essential body fat requirements are estimated to be about 3%–7% in males and about 13%–15% in females. Females need a higher percentage to support pregnancy if it occurs.

Additional body fat is known as **storage fat**, which results when excess calories are stored by the body. Because of the differences in the amount of essential body fat, ideal body composition varies between

body composition

the relationship between fat-free mass (muscle, bone, and water) and fat tissue in the body

essential body fat

the amount of fat necessary for use by the body to provide insulation, cushion body organs, and maintain normal bodily functions

storage fat

body fat that is a result of excess calories stored by the body

teen forum

"Weight Alert" Letters: Too Heavy?

Recently, as the problem of overweight and obesity in children and teenagers has increased, some schools have started sending "weight alert" letters to parents when a health examination reveals that their child or teenager is overweight or obese. Some parents have been offended by these letters. They believe that weight is a personal issue and not something that schools should be concerned about. Schools respond that if a school health examination reveals vision or hearing problems, the parents are contacted. They question why a weight problem should be any different. They suggest that overweight and obesity are major health concerns and parents should be warned of the potential dangers.

- What do you think? Record your reasons for your opinion in your Health Folio.

males and females. For males, the approximate percentage of total body fat should be 12%–15%. For females, the approximate percentage of total body fat should be 18%–21%.

Weight gain usually occurs when a person consistently consumes more calories than the body uses. The way this extra weight is distributed differs between males and females. Most males store extra body fat in what is called an "apple" pattern. This means it is concentrated around the middle of the body in the abdominal area. In contrast, most females store extra body fat in the hips and thighs in what is called a "pear" pattern. Although females are quick to complain about the tendency to acquire this pear shape, it is actually not as dangerous to health as storing extra body fat in an apple pattern. The extra fat concentrated in the abdominal area has been linked to an increased risk of heart disease. Figure 9-2 shows how extra body weight is stored on men and women.

Assessing Body Composition

There are many ways to determine how much body weight is lean mass and how much is fat tissue. Traditional height-weight charts have been

Figure 9-2
Males tend to store extra body weight in an apple shape, whereas females tend to store it in a pear shape.

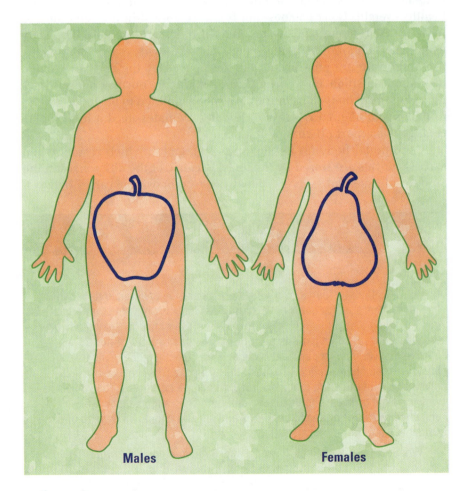

Males   **Females**

used for many years to suggest ideal weights. But they cannot accurately estimate body composition. A better indicator is the **body mass index** (BMI), which measures the relationship (or ratio) of weight to height using a mathematical formula. BMI is more closely correlated to percentage of body fat than is any other height-weight indicator. It has become the most common standard for assessing overweight and obesity because it is reasonably accurate and easy to use. See Figure 9-3 for instructions on how to calculate your own BMI.

According to health experts, a BMI of 18.5–25.0 represents a weight at which a person is unlikely to experience health problems due to excessive weight. If BMI falls below 18.5, there is a risk that weight is too low to be healthy. If BMI is above 25.0, there is an increased risk for health problems related to excess weight. According to government guidelines, people who have a BMI of 25–29.9 are classified as being overweight. People who have a BMI of 30 or above are classified as obese. Notice the range of acceptable BMIs. This provides evidence that there is not one single ideal weight for an individual.

Another mathematical formula used to predict health risks calculates the waist-to-hip ratio. A ratio of 1.0 or higher indicates a higher level of risk for health problems for both men and women. Ideal ratios are 0.9 or lower for men and 0.8 or lower for women. See Figure 9-4 for instructions on calculating the waist-to-hip ratio.

A third method for determining body fat is the skinfold caliper pinch test. A skinfold caliper is used to measure skinfolds at designated points on the body. To ensure accuracy, the person doing the test should be well trained and experienced. The results are then correlated with standardized body fat measures to estimate the actual percentage of body fat.

body mass index

a commonly used measure of the relationship (or ratio) of weight to height expressed in a mathematical formula

---

Calculate your body mass index (BMI):

1. **Multiply your weight in pounds by 703.**

2. **Divide the result by your height in inches.**

3. **Divide that result by your height in inches again.**

Figure 9-3
Method for calculating body mass index

Calculate your waist-to-hip ratio:

1. **Measure waist circumference in inches.**

2. **Measure hip circumference in inches.**

3. **Divide waist circumference by hip circumference.**

Figure 9-4
Method for calculating waist-to-hip ratio

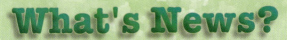

According to a study conducted by Steven Blair, director of research at the Cooper Institute for Aerobics Research in Dallas, Texas, previous studies linking obesity and death from heart disease and other major killers may have missed the important influence of exercise. Blair's study followed more than 30,000 men and women for 10 years. The results show that populations of obese people who exercise enough to be fit have *half* the death rate of populations of people who are slender but not fit. Blair says people who are both thin and active are more accepted by society. But in terms of lowering health risk for heart disease and diabetes, his study shows that it is a low fitness level, rather than excess weight, that is the most important risk factor.

Weight and Health

Although obsession with weight is not healthy, it is also true that excess weight can contribute to serious health problems. The Centers for Disease Control and Prevention (CDC) estimates that excess weight and physical inactivity combine to account for more than 300,000 premature deaths each year in the United States, second only to deaths related to smoking. The risks for heart disease, stroke, diabetes, and certain types of cancer are all higher in adults who weigh too much. The more overweight a person is, the greater his or her chances are for having weight-related health problems.

FACTORS THAT AFFECT WEIGHT MANAGEMENT

It is not fully understood why some people struggle so much to maintain a healthy weight and others maintain a healthy weight without even thinking about it. What is known suggests that there are four main factors that influence whether a person will become overweight or obese: genetics or heredity, food intake, physical activity, and psychological factors. A complex interaction of these factors accounts for individual differences in body weight. Let's look at how these four factors affect body weight.

Genetics/Heredity

Have you ever noticed how family members often have similar body types and shapes? One reason may be that family members have similar eating and exercise patterns. But experts in weight management have consistently documented that genetics influences body shape, size, and weight. For example, your genetic heritage can affect your metabolic rate, the speed at which your body burns energy. Some people burn energy (calories) at a higher rate than others. Suppose that two people start at the same weight. Even if they eat exactly the same foods and exercise the same amount, it is unlikely that they will have the same weight at the end of a year.

Not everyone can achieve the same weight goals regardless of their efforts. This does not mean that if you have a genetic predisposition for gaining weight or being too thin you cannot do anything about it. It simply means you will have to put forth more effort to achieve and maintain a healthy weight.

take it on home

Which of the shapes in Figure 9-5 most resembles your body shape? Do the members of your family have a similar shape, or is it different from yours? Ask the adult members of your family if their body shape is the same now as it was when they were your age. What conclusions, if any, can you reach on the basis of this information? Give reasons for the conclusions you reach and record them in your Health Folio.

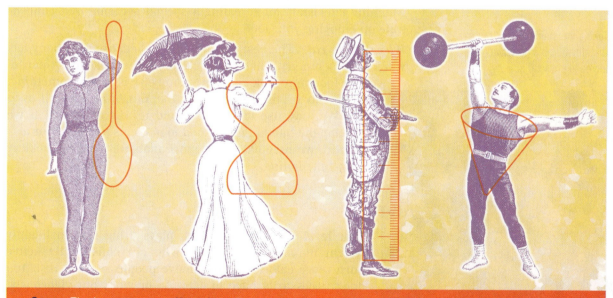

Spoon: The bottom part of your body is heavier than the top part of your body.

Hourglass: The top part of your body is about the same size as the bottom part of your body, but your waist is narrower.

Ruler: Your body is fairly straight up and down.

Cone: The upper part of your body is heavier than the bottom part of your body.

Figure 9-5 Four typical body shapes

Food Intake

There's no way of denying it: what you put in your mouth plays a big role in your body size and weight. The fact is that about 3,500 calories equals 1 pound of body fat. A general guideline is that we gain weight when we take in more calories than we burn up. Here are some of the things to consider about your food intake:

- *What kinds of food do you eat?* Do you eat mostly fruits and vegetables or mostly hamburgers, fries, and pizza? There's nothing wrong with eating hamburgers, fries, and pizza, but a steady diet of these items can add too many calories and too much fat to your diet, especially if you aren't burning the extra calories with physical activity. This type of diet makes it hard for you to manage your weight and get enough of the nutrients your body needs to function well.

- *When do you eat?* Do you eat most of your calories early or later in the day? Several studies indicate that eating the majority of your calories early in the day, while your body is most active, helps to avoid weight gain. Consuming a high number of calories in the evening may make it easier for your body to store the excess calories as fat.

- *Where do you eat?* It's easy to consume a lot of calories very quickly if you're not paying attention to what you are eating. Avoid eating while you are doing something else such as driving or watching television. Make eating a special occasion and concentrate on enjoying your food.

- *Why do you eat?* The best reason to eat is because your body lets you know it's hungry. But often, we eat for other reasons. A particular food may look good, everyone else is eating something, or we rely on the clock rather than our hunger to tell us to eat. We may use food to respond to our emotions. If we develop the habit of using food to make us feel better or as a reward, we may eat much more than we need for healthy body functioning.

Physical Activity

Your level of physical activity plays a big role in healthy weight management. People who are consistently active burn more calories than inactive people, even at rest. You don't necessarily have to exercise or work out vigorously; even moderate activity burns calories. Whenever you have a choice, *choose to move*. For example, take the stairs instead of the elevator. Walk instead of driving in the car or riding on the bus. Physical activity alone won't keep your weight at a healthy level, but it is certainly a key part of an effective weight management plan. You'll also feel better and have more energy if you're physically active.

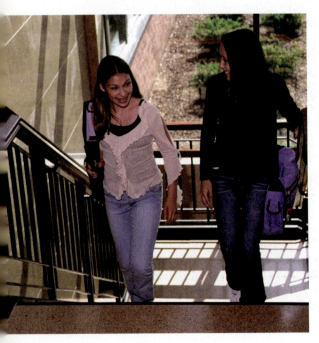

Taking the stairs instead of the elevator is a good way to increase physical activity.

Psychological Factors

Do you use food to cope with stressful and emotionally upsetting situations? Many people do. Think back to when you were a small child. It's likely there were times when you were offered special foods when you were upset about something. Foods become associated with comfort. Can you remember what those foods were? When you feel a certain way now, do you use food to make yourself feel better? Eating because you are bored, lonely, sad, nervous, or frustrated, instead of because you are truly hungry, can add calories quickly. And eating is usually not an effective way to solve the problem that's upsetting you in the first place. When you are stressed or emotionally upset, think of ways that you can make yourself feel better without using food, such as going for a walk or talking to a friend.

DIETING

How often do you hear someone say, "I can't eat that. I'm dieting"? **Dieting** has become a national obsession in the United States. It is estimated that at any given time, about one-half of all American women are trying to lose weight. For adolescent and young adult females, the percentage is even higher. Although American males are not as obsessed with dieting as American females, a substantial number of males eat an unbalanced diet in order to achieve a certain body size or shape. The dietary restrictions are often so severe that people do not regularly get enough of the nutrients their bodies need. Without proper nutrition, physical and mental performance can suffer.

The biggest problem with dieting for weight loss is that *it usually does not work*–at least not over the long term. Several studies have shown about 95% of people who lose weight by dieting regain all the pounds they lost (and sometimes more) within a year. Some experts believe that this weight loss and gain ("yo-yo effect") can lead to changes in the body's metabolism that make it even more difficult to manage weight effectively.

Despite the thousands of weight-loss books and products sold, the long-term success rate for dieting is quite low. That is one reason there is always some new **fad diet** on the market. People who have failed with one diet continue their search for the magic pill, potion, or formula to solve their weight problems. Most fad diets overemphasize one particular food or type of food and contradict the guidelines of good nutrition. At best, they are ineffective; at worst, they can be downright dangerous.

When we go on a diet, the assumption is that we will also eventually go off a diet. Attaining and maintaining a healthy weight takes time. There are no quick and easy ways to lose weight. Healthfully managing weight requires the formation of new habits. You can make eating healthy a new way of life. It may take longer to achieve the results you want, but you are much more likely to keep the weight off permanently.

dieting

temporary patterns of eating that restrict calories for the purpose of losing weight

fad diets

eating regimens that overemphasize one particular food or type of food and contradict the guidelines of good nutrition

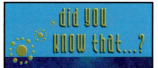

did you know that...?

Americans spend more than $40 billion a year on dieting and diet-related products. That's about the same amount the U.S. federal government spends on education each year. Do you think this money is being spent wisely? Think about all the other things Americans could choose to do with $40 billion a year.

HEALTHY TECHNIQUES AND STRATEGIES TO MANAGE WEIGHT

If dieting doesn't work, then what *can* you do to manage your weight? First, weight management must be approached as a long-term commitment. You must also be willing to change some lifestyle and eating habits. Figure 9-6 shows some suggestions to increase your chances for success. Read on for more information on these techniques.

Keep Your Weight in Perspective

Managing your weight is an important goal that can help keep you healthier throughout your lifetime. But it's not the only thing that's important in your life. Focus on your overall health and well-being, not just on your weight.

Listen to Your Body

A good technique for healthy weight management is learning to listen to your body. This means eating when you are truly hungry and stopping when you are full. Every day you are bombarded by cues to eat: what kind of foods to eat, how often to eat, and how much to eat. Food is readily available in vending machines, fast-food restaurants, and convenience stores. Sometimes people eat because they are bored, stressed, lonely, or restless. It takes some effort to recognize true hunger signals from your body. The same is true for learning to stop eating when you are full.

Eat Breakfast

Although it is tempting to skip breakfast, studies indicate that people who are successful at losing weight and maintaining that weight loss regularly eat breakfast. Eating a nutritious breakfast gives your body

Figure 9-6
Checklist of healthy techniques and strategies to manage your weight

✔ **Keep your weight in perspective**

✔ **Listen to your body**

✔ **Eat breakfast**

✔ **Eat a wide variety of foods**

✔ **Pay attention to portion sizes**

✔ **Practice mindful eating**

what it needs to start the day. It also prevents excessive hunger and overeating later in the day.

Eat a Wide Variety of Foods

Eating a wide variety of foods helps ensure that your body has the fuel it needs to perform at its best. You should try to get most of your calories from foods that are healthy for you, but don't fall into the trap of labeling foods as good or bad. A well-balanced weight management plan can include all types of food in moderation.

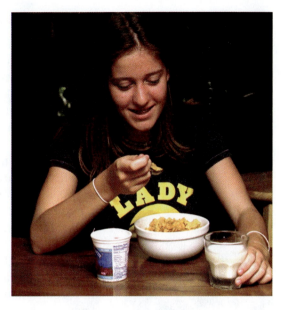

Pay Attention to Portion Sizes

American portions are much larger than portions in other countries. We have biggie-size fries and drinks and two-for-one "value" meals. Foods that are high in calories or fat, such as potato chips, are often packaged with several servings in a single container. Check food labels to make sure you are eating a single serving. You don't have to finish food left in the bag or on your plate if you are no longer hungry.

Practice Mindful Eating

Mindful eating means paying attention to the food you are eating and enjoying its tastes, smells, and textures. Mindful eating can help you learn to recognize your body's cues for when to start and stop eating. Too often, we eat while we are doing something else and don't pay attention to the amount we are consuming. For example, people who watch television while they eat often consume much more than they intended. It's easy to go through most of a bag of potato chips or cookies without being aware of how much you have eaten.

mindful eating

paying attention to the food you are eating and enjoying its tastes, smells, and textures

UNDERSTANDING EATING DISORDERS

Eating disorders are problems related to food, weight, and body image that are harmful to physical or psychological health. There are several types of eating disorders, but they all cause significant health problems. Eating disorders are much more common in females than in males. About 90% of eating disorders occur in females, with only about 10% of eating disorders occurring in males.

Identifying eating disorders early and getting proper treatment are the keys to preventing serious health problems and death. Without treatment, up to 20% of people who have serious eating disorders die. Of those who receive treatment, only about 2%–3% die. Let's take a look at the major eating disorders in the United States today.

eating disorders

problems related to food, weight, and body image that are harmful to physical or psychological health

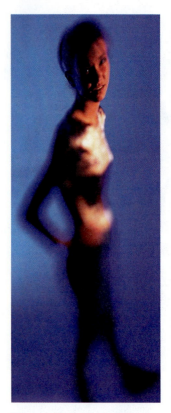

People suffering from eating disorders such as anorexia nervosa have a distorted body image.

Anorexia Nervosa

Anorexia nervosa is considered the most serious of all the eating disorders because of the high rate of death associated with it. People who have **anorexia nervosa** do not eat enough to maintain body function at a healthy level. Weight may fall to 85% or less of what is expected for their age and height. Despite dramatic weight loss and extreme thinness, anorexics view themselves as fat and continue to deny themselves enough food.

Anorexia nervosa is most common in adolescent and young adult females. Research suggests that about 1% of female adolescents have anorexia. As many as half of all cases of anorexia seem to have a genetic component. Without treatment, persons with anorexia gradually starve themselves to death. Of all the psychiatric disorders, anorexia has the highest rate of mortality (death).

Successful treatment focuses on restoring the lost weight; providing psychotherapy to treat the distortion of body image, low self-esteem, and relationship difficulties; and sustaining long-term recovery. Anorexia requires treatment from medical personnel for both physical and psychological issues. Early treatment for anorexia focuses on restoring body weight so that the person does not die. Resolving underlying psychological issues is also a part of the treatment plan. It is not unusual for full recovery from anorexia nervosa to take at least five years.

Bulimia Nervosa

Bulimia nervosa is an eating disorder in which a person eats a great deal of food and then vomits or uses other methods, such as laxatives or overexercising, to avoid gaining weight. This effort to rid the body of food that has been consumed is called **purging**. It is estimated that about 4% of adolescent and young adult females in the United States are bulimic. In contrast to those with anorexia, most people with bulimia have normal or nearly normal body weight, so other people may not realize they have an eating disorder. Because the condition is not obvious, treatment may be delayed or may not occur at all.

Bulimics describe themselves as feeling out of control while eating and unable to stop themselves. Because they believe their self-worth depends on their being thin, they become caught in the cycle of overeating and then purging to get rid of the food they consumed to avoid gaining weight. Psychologically, bulimics often report feeling depressed, lonely, ashamed, and unworthy, although these conditions may not be obvious to other people. It appears that psychological distress contributes to the development of bulimia in the first place, rather than being a result of the disorder.

About half of all cases of bulimia nervosa appear to have a genetic component. With proper treatment, most bulimics are able to recover and return to a more normal pattern of eating. Successful treatment often includes the use of antidepressant drugs and psychotherapy. In contrast to anorexia nervosa, the primary focus of treatment is directed toward resolving psychological issues.

Binge-Eating Disorder

Binge-eating disorder is a condition in which a person eats large amounts of food frequently and repeatedly. Persons with this disorder describe themselves as feeling out of control and unable to stop eating during binges. Because they feel guilty and ashamed of these binges, they often eat in secret so that no one can see how much food they are consuming. In contrast to persons with bulimia, binge eaters do not regularly vomit, overexercise, or abuse laxatives. They usually have a long history of unsuccessful dieting and tend to be obese. It is estimated that about 1% of females in the United States have a binge-eating disorder. About 30% of women who seek treatment to lose weight admit to being binge eaters. Our society tends to consider binge eating more abnormal and inappropriate for women than for men. Men also seem to experience less guilt related to their binge-eating behavior.

Disordered Eating Patterns

Disordered eating patterns occur when concerns about dieting, food restriction, fear of becoming overweight, and dissatisfaction with body image interfere with normal daily life. Disordered eating patterns may lead to the development of an eating disorder, although this does not occur in all cases. More commonly, the person becomes so focused on dieting, food, weight, and body image that all other goals and activities are cast aside. If you find yourself giving dieting, food, weight, and body image a great deal of your attention, you may want to think about ways to find a better balance in your life. If you are unable to stop focusing on food on your own, you should consider seeking professional assistance. There is so much more to life than eating!

CREATING A HEALTHY WEIGHT MANAGEMENT PLAN

You may decide to apply what you have learned in Chapters 8 and 9 to create a personal weight management program. The first step is to determine realistic goals. What do you want to accomplish? Do you want to gain weight, lose weight, or maintain your current weight by eating a healthier diet?

The next step is to identify ways to help you make slow, steady progress toward your goals. Each person will have a different plan. When losing weight, some people prefer to increase their physical activity to burn up extra calories. Others would rather eat less to decrease the number of calories they consume. Still others may need to learn to recognize their body's hunger signals and how to limit eating

purging
removing undesirable substances; in the case of bulimia nervosa, it refers to vomiting or using laxatives or exercise to remove excessive amounts of food consumed

binge-eating disorder
a condition in which a person eats large amounts of food frequently and repeatedly

disordered eating patterns
conditions in which dieting, food restriction, fear of becoming overweight, and body image dissatisfaction interfere with normal daily life

to only those times when they are truly hungry. A combination of these actions may result in a plan that is just right for you. It helps to be patient with yourself as you try to adopt new habits. Remember, truly successful weight management requires a plan that you can stick to over an extended time.

Actions That Increase Your Chances of Success

It's important to develop a weight management plan that you can maintain for the rest of your life. The following actions will increase your chances of success in managing your weight.

Have Realistic Expectations

Many people start with unrealistic expectations about losing weight. They think that if they just eat less, they will be able to lose weight at a rapid pace, such as 5 pounds a week or more. Losing 5 pounds in a week, without increasing activity level, would require consuming 17,500 fewer calories than your body needs! That's a reduction of about 2,500 calories a day—more than many people normally eat in a day. Cutting too many calories leaves too few to carry on normal bodily functions. Your body metabolism slows down because it thinks food is scarce, and it responds by trying to protect its fat stores. Rapid weight loss is unhealthy and makes it difficult to maintain the weight loss. Weight management experts believe that a loss of approximately 1 or 2 pounds per week is the most that should be attempted. So if you're thinking about trying a fad diet to lose 10 pounds for some big event next weekend, think again. There is no healthy way to do that. Instead, focus on progressing slowly over a longer period of time.

Be Committed and Consistent

Once you have created a healthy weight management plan, the best way to ensure success is to be committed to the plan and consistent in following through with your intentions. Small changes, carried out consistently, can make a big difference. For example, if you have decided to reduce the amount of sweets you eat, simply eliminating 250 calories a day (about the number of calories in a chocolate bar) will result in lowering your caloric intake by about 1,750 calories a week. This is the same as half a pound. Maintained consistently, this one behavior adds up to a loss of more than 25 pounds in a year!

Find a Support Buddy

A positive way to help you stay committed to your weight management plan is to find someone who is willing to support you in your efforts. This might be someone who is trying to lose weight as well, or it might be someone who cares about you and is willing to help motivate you to stay on track. Do you have a family member or close friend who could be your support buddy? You may want to ask more than one person. Different people may be able to offer different kinds of support. For example, a family member might be willing to cook meals that are healthier and less fattening. Your best friend might encourage you by reminding you of your goals and doing little things to let you know how important you are. Maybe there's a classmate who exercises regularly who will work out with you. Having several support buddies to keep you focused on your goals can help you avoid the temptation to quit before you see the results.

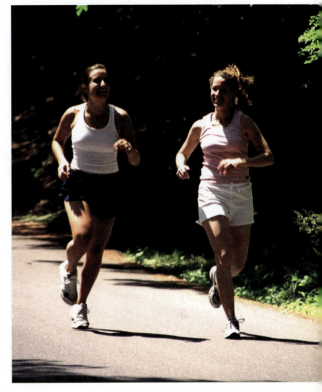

Record Your Progress Regularly

Keeping track of your progress in a weight management journal can help keep you motivated and focused on attaining your goals. Recording the times you eat, the foods you eat, and how you are feeling at the time you eat can help you identify your eating patterns and understand what is working and what is not in your weight management plan. It can also help you stay committed to your goals. Reviewing your journal can also help you see if your plan is helping you achieve your goals. You may discover that something is not working for you and that you need to try something new. It may take some time, but eventually you will discover a plan that works well for you.

take it on home

Are there members of your family who would be willing to support you in your weight management efforts? Talk to them about your plans and tell them what you want to accomplish. What kinds of actions would make you feel supported? Make a list of these actions and then ask members of your family if they would be willing to do some of those things. Be sure they understand that helping you doesn't mean nagging, trying to make you feel guilty about eating, or making fun of you to make you stick to your plan. You might discover that other members of your family are interested in joining your efforts and you can achieve success together! You can use your Health Folio to keep track of your progress.

BUILDING YOUR Wellness Plan

Maintaining a healthy weight is one of the most important things you can do to achieve maximum wellness. It is also something over which you have personal control. This chapter provided information you can apply to develop a successful, lifelong weight management plan. For your personal wellness plan:

- Determine a healthy weight and appropriate body image for *you*.

- Explore the different factors that affect your weight. Learn which ones might be problems for you and steps you can take to control them.

- Stay informed about why maintaining a healthy weight is important for achieving a high level of wellness. Use your health literacy skills to learn about the diseases and conditions that can be prevented by avoiding excess weight.

- Learn to recognize the signs of eating disorders. Be prepared to help both yourself and others who may suffer from these conditions.

- Create a personal weight management plan you can live with permanently.

end-of-chapter ACTIVITIES

Weblinks

Overweight and Obesity

U.S. Office of the Surgeon General: **http://www.surgeongeneral.gov** (search for "overweight and obesity")

U.S. National Heart, Lung, and Blood Institute: **http://rover.nhlbi.nih.gov** (search for "Obesity Education Initiative Website")

Managing Your Weight

First Gov for Consumers: **http://www.consumer.gov** (click on "Partnership for Healthy Weight Management")

U.S. National Institute of Diabetes and Digestive and Kidney Diseases, National Institutes of Health: **http://www.niddk.nih.gov** (click on "Weight Loss and Weight Control" under "Health Information," then click on "Take Charge of Your Health")

Eating Disorders

Anorexia Nervosa and Related Eating Disorders, Inc.: **http://www.anred.com**

National Eating Disorders Association: **http://www.nationaleatingdisorders.org**

Short-Answer Questions

1. Name three diseases that are related to overweight and obesity.

2. List several factors that influence body image.

3. Identify four factors that can cause overweight and obesity.

4. Briefly describe at least three ways of assessing body composition.

5. List several reasons why weight loss is difficult to maintain.

☀ Discussion Questions

1. Describe the current state of overweight and obesity in the United States.

2. Discuss the influence of the media on body image.

3. Describe the differences between anorexia nervosa, bulimia nervosa, binge-eating disorder, and disordered eating patterns.

4. Describe the components of a healthy personal weight management plan.

5. List and explain four actions you can take to help your personal weight management plan succeed.

☀ Chapter Vocabulary

Using a separate sheet of paper, list and define the following terms:

anorexia nervosa	dieting
binge-eating disorder	eating disorders
body composition	ideal body weight
body image	obesity
bulimia nervosa	overweight

☀ Application Activities

Language Arts Connection

1. On the basis of information you have learned about weight management, construct a personal weight management plan.

2. Write a letter to your body expressing your feelings about it. Then pretend that your body is writing a letter back to you. What would your body say to you?

3. Write a personal essay expressing how you feel about your body image.

Math Connection

1. Using the formula given in your text in Figure 9-3, calculate the BMI for the following people:

   Casey is 5 feet 4 inches tall and weighs 100 pounds. Kevin is 5 feet 8 inches tall and weighs 200 pounds.

   Carey is 6 feet tall and weighs 180 pounds. Michelle is 5 feet 6 inches tall and weighs 120 pounds.

   Which of these four individuals is most likely to experience health problems associated with his or her weight?

2. Using the formula given in your text in Figure 9-4, calculate the waist-to-hip ratio for the following people:

   Tom has a waist of 40 inches and hips of 37 inches. Carissa has a waist of 24 inches and hips of 32 inches.

   Micah has a waist of 44 inches and hips of 40 inches. Tonya has a waist of 35 inches and hips of 45 inches.

   Which of these four individuals has a waist-to-hip ratio that indicates an elevated risk for health problems?

3. Calculate your own BMI and waist-to-hip ratio. How do you feel about your results? Include this information in your Health Folio.

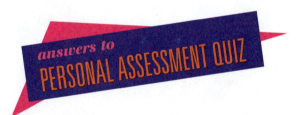

answers to PERSONAL ASSESSMENT QUIZ

personal assessment: WEIGHT MANAGEMENT QUIZ

1. False	6. False
2. True	7. True
3. False	8. True
4. True	9. False
5. True	10. True

Enjoying a Physically Active Lifestyle

Wendy's boyfriend, Jason, rides his bicycle practically everywhere he goes. He rides it to and from school and work. He rides it to hang out with Wendy at her house. He also likes riding his bicycle just for fun. At first Wendy couldn't believe he liked going for long bike rides on the weekends, but now she has seen how much he enjoys it. Jason has tried to convince Wendy that she should start riding her bicycle too. He pointed out that if she would start riding her bicycle, they could ride together to a park about 10 miles away and take a picnic lunch. Wendy likes Jason's idea, and she knows she needs to be more physically active. She decides that it would be a good idea to get her bicycle out of the storage shed, and she is looking forward to all the places she and Jason can go.

chapter OBJECTIVES

When you finish this chapter, you should be able to:

- ☀ Explain the benefits of being physically active.
- ☀ List and describe the diseases associated with physical inactivity.
- ☀ Identify the various components of health-related physical activity.
- ☀ List and describe the major types of injury caused by physical activity.
- ☀ Develop a personal fitness plan.

Introduction

Our bodies are created to move and participate in physical activity. Just like machines with moving parts, bodies function best when they are used regularly. Joints that go too long without moving can get "rusty" and be easily injured. The fact is, the more we demand of our bodies, the stronger and fitter they become.

In the past, daily living required the performance of physically demanding tasks. There were no cars for transportation, and most labor had to be done by a person rather than by a machine. Most people got a lot of physical activity just in accomplishing their daily tasks. Today, however, we often have to make a special effort to get enough physical activity to stay healthy and perform well. This chapter looks at what it means to be physically active, why it is important, and what you need to know to make smart decisions about physical activity.

key TERMS

body composition
cardiorespiratory fitness
FITT formula
flexibility
health-related fitness
muscular endurance
muscular strength
physical activity
skill-related fitness
target heart rate range

personal assessment: PHYSICAL ACTIVITY QUIZ

Before reading this chapter, test how much you already know about physical activity. Read each statement and, on a separate sheet of paper, answer True or False. The answers are located at the end of the chapter.

1. American teenagers are more physically active now than they were 25 years ago.

2. The most important type of health-related fitness is cardiorespiratory fitness.

3. The only way to be physically fit is to play some type of competitive sport.

4. In general, people who are physically active live longer than those who are inactive.

5. Teenagers exercise more often than adults who are over the age of 55.

6. You can die of a heat-related illness such as heatstroke.

7. Research shows that being physically active may help you learn better.

8. You can develop and maintain good flexibility by stretching once or twice a week.

9. If you do strength training, you should exercise the same muscle group every day.

10. Research shows that regular physical activity may be just as effective as drugs or therapy for treating depression.

THE BENEFITS OF BEING PHYSICALLY ACTIVE

There are so many benefits of being physically active that, as physician and author Robert N. Butler said, "If exercise could be packed in a pill, it would be the single most widely prescribed and beneficial medicine in the nation." Physical activity not only helps prevent chronic diseases such as heart disease and diabetes but also increases your level of energy. When you take part in physical activities you enjoy, you're a triple winner. First, when you're doing the activity you're having fun. Second, you gain extra energy to participate more fully in the other aspects of your life. Finally, you build habits that prevent chronic diseases. Being physically active on a regular basis makes you a big winner!

Physiological Benefits

Research has shown that people who engage in regular physical activity are much healthier physically than are those who are not regularly active. The 1996 Surgeon General's report *Physical Activity and Health* noted that people who are usually inactive can improve their health by participating in even moderate levels of activity on a regular basis. The activity does not have to be strenuous in order to achieve health benefits, although the higher the level of activity, the greater the benefits.

The International Consensus Conference on Physical Activity Guidelines for Adolescents recommends that all adolescents should be physically active daily, or nearly every day. This physical activity does not have to be "exercise"; it can be a part of play, games, sports, work, transportation, recreation, or physical education classes. The guidelines further recommend that adolescents have at least three sessions per week of activities that last 20 minutes or more and require moderate to vigorous levels of exertion.

Let's look at some of the specific physical benefits of exercise:

- ***Improved function of the heart, lungs, and circulatory system.*** During exercise, these organs and systems are forced to work harder to meet the body's oxygen demands. The heart muscle gets stronger and begins to pump more blood with each beat. As a result, it doesn't have to work as hard at rest or during lower levels of activity.

- ***Increased resting metabolic rate (the rate at which the body burns calories while at rest).*** An individual who exercises regularly burns more calories when at rest than one who doesn't exercise, so you benefit from exercise even when you're reading, watching television, or sleeping.

- ***Increased muscle mass from strength training.*** Increasing muscle mass also increases the resting metabolic rate because it takes more calories to maintain muscle mass than fat. Strength training also improves body composition. Low levels of body fat help prevent diseases such as **type 2 diabetes**.

- ***Increased levels of HDLs (high-density lipoproteins), the "good" cholesterol, and decreased levels of both LDLs (low-density lipoproteins), the "bad" cholesterol, and triglycerides.*** High levels of LDLs and triglycerides are one of the six major risk factors for heart disease. (See Chapter 8.)

- ***Reduced chance of hypertension.*** Hypertension is abnormally high blood pressure, which is another risk factor for heart disease and stroke.

- ***Decreased risk of colon cancer and possibly lower risks for breast and prostate cancer.*** Colon cancer is the second leading cause of cancer death for men and women combined. Prostate and breast cancers are the second leading cause of cancer deaths for men and women individually.

- ***Reduced risk of osteoporosis, a thinning of the bones.*** Weight-bearing activities, such as running or walking, are necessary to reduce this risk.

type 2 diabetes

a condition in which the body cannot transport enough glucose (sugar) to the cells to be converted into energy

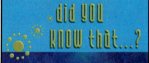

did you know that...?

Weight-bearing exercise during the teenage years may be one of the best ways for women to help prevent osteoporosis later in life. Results from the ongoing Penn State Young Women's Health Study show an association between adult hip bone density (important for preventing hip fractures in older women) and sports-exercise patterns from ages 12–18. The activity you engage in now can help ensure that you are able to be active later!

• *Improved immune function.* People who participate in regular, moderate physical activity have fewer colds and upper-respiratory infections than do inactive people.

Psychological Benefits

In addition to the many physiological benefits, there are great mental and emotional benefits to be gained from physical activity. Doing something active that you enjoy is a great way to relieve stress. Even something as simple as going for a walk can be helpful in getting rid of anger and frustration.

Longer sessions of activities, between about 45 and 60 minutes, trigger physiological changes in the body that help improve mood. Although researchers have not yet determined exactly how exercise affects our mood, studies show that people who are physically active feel less stressed, experience less anxiety, and are less likely to be depressed than are inactive people. There are several theories about how physical activity affects moods. One is that the rhythmic motion of the body during exercise stimulates an area of the brain associated with mood. Another theory is that certain neurotransmitters (chemicals in the brain) that influence mood are affected by activity.

Another advantage of participating in physical activities is that they provide opportunities to meet new people and do fun things with friends. Participation may also increase creativity, and there is new evidence from brain-based research that physical activity helps us learn better!

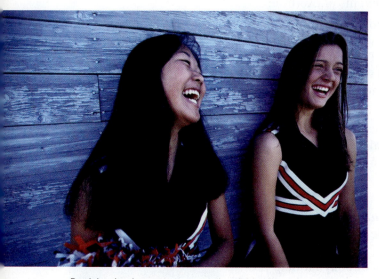

Participating in group sports and activities is a great way to make friends.

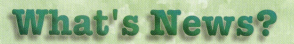

New findings in brain-based research have shown that daily physical activity gives students an advantage for learning. Subjects who engaged in vigorous activities improved their short-term memory, creativity, and reaction times. In other studies, students performed activities that required movements that crossed an imaginary line down the center of the body. This activity seemed to help increase blood flow in all parts of the brain, making the brain more alert and ready to learn. Does this mean that a quick game of catch with your buddy before your math exam might help improve your test score? Well, more research still needs to be done before we can say for sure, but if you can use a bit of extra help on that next math exam, try a game of catch before the exam and judge the results for yourself!

did you know that...?

Some studies show that regular physical activity can be just as effective as therapy or drug treatment in treating depression. If a person doesn't have any health insurance, talking to a therapist or taking a prescription drug may not be an option. In addition, medications to treat depression can have negative side effects. But any side effects from physical activity are likely to be positive, not only physically but mentally and emotionally as well.

PHYSICAL FITNESS

What does it mean to be physically fit? There are actually two major types of physical fitness: skill-related fitness and health-related fitness. **Skill-related fitness** includes power, **agility**, coordination, speed, and balance. This type of fitness enables you to be successful in many kinds of sports. Learning new skills and participating in competitive sports can be both enjoyable and rewarding, adding to your sense of well-being.

The second type of fitness is even more important. This is **health-related fitness**, which is the type of fitness necessary to gain health benefits and prevent certain diseases. Even mild physical activities help develop health-related fitness. Health-related fitness has five major components:

1. Cardiorespiratory endurance
2. Muscular strength
3. Muscular endurance
4. Flexibility
5. Body composition

skill-related fitness

the type of fitness required for participating in sports or other skill-related activities; includes such components as power, agility, coordination, speed, and balance

agility

the ability to move easily, quickly, and lightly

health-related fitness

the level of fitness necessary to gain health benefits

☆ teen forum ☆

Physical Activity in Schools

Even though we have a lot of evidence that regular physical activity has important physiological and psychological benefits, many schools have found it difficult to include time for physical activity during the school day. It seems that students are spending less time than they used to in physical education classes.

- What's happening in your school? Do you think there is sufficient time devoted to physical activity?
- Are you involved in physical activities outside of school?
- In your opinion, is school the best place for teens to get physical activity? Or should they be responsible for arranging physical activities on their own time?

Cardiorespiratory Fitness

cardiorespiratory fitness

the ability of the respiratory and circulatory systems to provide enough oxygen to sustain moderate levels of activity for long periods of time

aerobic activities

activities that require a continual supply of oxygen during the activity

anaerobic activities

activities that require short bursts of energy that cannot be sustained for long periods of time because the body cannot supply enough oxygen quickly enough to keep up with the demand

aerobic capacity

the maximum amount of oxygen that can be delivered to and used by the cells of the body during vigorous workouts

target heart rate range

the percentage of the predicted maximum heart rate that must be reached to obtain improvements in aerobic capacity

Cardiorespiratory fitness is the ability of the circulatory and respiratory systems to provide enough oxygen to sustain moderate levels of physical activity for long periods of time. It is often considered to be the most important component of health-related physical fitness. A strong heart, lungs, and circulatory system help you perform physical activities. When you have good cardiorespiratory fitness, your heart and lungs function efficiently and don't have to work too hard during times of rest.

The best way to increase cardiorespiratory fitness is to participate in activities that increase your heart rate above your normal resting rate for a sustained period of time. Activities that use the large muscle groups of the body in continuous motion for an extended period of time increase cardiorespiratory fitness. Walking, running, cycling, and swimming are examples of these activities. Activities such as these that require a continual supply of oxygen are called **aerobic**. Activities that require short bursts of energy and cannot be sustained for long periods of time are called **anaerobic**. Examples include sprinting, racquetball, and weight lifting. Anaerobic activities are not very effective for increasing cardiorespiratory fitness because they do not require sustained periods of exercise.

Aerobic Capacity

Aerobic capacity is the maximum amount of oxygen that can be delivered to and used by the cells of the body during vigorous workouts. If aerobic capacity is high, the heart, lungs, and circulatory system are able to deliver more oxygen to the body with fewer heartbeats per minute. Aerobic capacity can be measured by a treadmill test, in which you walk or run on a treadmill while heart rate and respiratory function measurements are taken. Aerobic capacity can also be estimated by field tests, such as a 12-minute walk/run test.

Aerobic capacity can be improved by participating in regular aerobic activities. The heart rate must reach a certain level, known as the **target heart rate range**, to obtain improvements in aerobic capacity. The target heart rate range is a percentage of a person's predicted maximum heart rate.

Components of a Cardiorespiratory Fitness Program

Developing cardiorespiratory fitness is important for everyone, not just athletes. Designing a program to increase your cardiorespiratory fitness is not difficult, once you understand the four components of the program. You can remember these by using the FITT acronym:

F = frequency

I = intensity

T = time

T = type of activity

Your fitness goals will determine how much emphasis to give to each component. Do you want to develop just enough cardiorespiratory fitness to receive health-related benefits? Or do you want to attain a high level of fitness so you can participate in a competitive sport?

Frequency. **Frequency** is the number of times each week that you engage in a physical activity. You can engage in mild or moderate levels of activity every day. For more strenuous activities, you may want to rest for a day or two during the week. At a minimum, you should engage in some type of aerobic activity three to five times a week.

If your goal is to achieve health-related fitness, you can choose low to moderate levels of activity such as walking or cycling and do them daily. To achieve a high level of fitness, you will need to work out at least five times a week at a higher level of **intensity**. As intensity and time increase, frequency may be decreased.

Intensity. Intensity is how much effort you expend, or how hard you work, during a typical workout. It is calculated using a formula based on your predicted maximum heart rate, which is 220 minus your age. For example, if you are 15 years old, your predicted maximum heart rate is 205. Taking a percentage of this predicted maximum heart rate gives an estimate of your target heart rate range, which is the level of physical activity necessary to increase your cardiorespiratory fitness. The Karvonen Formula provides a more accurate way of calculating your target heart rate range. See Figure 10-1 for instructions on calculating your target heart rate range according to this formula.

frequency
the number of times each week that you engage in an activity

intensity
in reference to exercise, how much effort you expend, or how hard you work, during a typical workout

The Karvonen Formula for Calculating Target Heart Rate Range

Predicted maximum heart rate is calculated by subtracting your age from 220. Resting heart rate is calculated by taking your pulse before getting out of bed in the morning. Exercise intensity is a percentage of 100%. In the following example, the target heart rate range is calculated for a 15-year-old with a resting heart rate of 70, and exercise intensity is calculated at 60% and 80%.

minus age	220 15 205	predicted maximum heart rate
minus resting heart rate	70 135	135
times percentage of exercise intensity	.60 81	.80 108
plus resting heart rate	+ 70 151	+ 70 178 heartbeats per minute (target heart rate range)

Figure 10-1
The Karvonen Formula can be used to calculate target heart rate range.

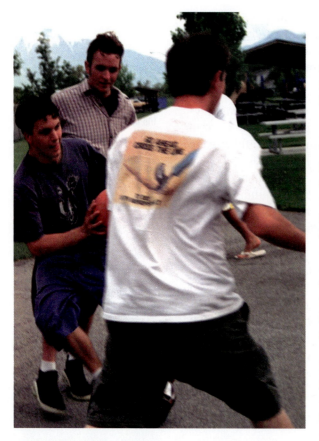

If you are just beginning to participate in aerobic activity, starting at an intensity of 50%–60% of your predicted maximum heart rate is usually about right. If you cannot carry on a normal conversation while working out at this level, you should decrease the intensity.

As your fitness increases, you should be able to work out at an intensity level of between 70% and 85%. Working out at intensity levels higher than 85% is not necessary unless you are training for a competitive activity or want to achieve a very high level of cardiorespiratory fitness. Working out at intensity levels that are too high can make it difficult to participate in the activity long enough to achieve benefits. It can also discourage you from regular participation in the activity because it will feel like too much work. Keep in mind that you can achieve the health-related benefits of physical activity at a moderate level of intensity.

duration

the number of minutes you engage in an activity at one time

Time. Time (sometimes called **duration**) is the number of minutes you engage in an activity at one time. You should spend 20–60 minutes at a moderate level of intensity almost every day to gain health-related benefits. In most cases, as intensity increases, the length of time you need to spend performing the activity decreases. And the 20–60 minutes can be divided into several sessions throughout the day, as long as each session is at least 10 minutes long and allows you to reach your target heart rate range.

Type. Selecting an activity you enjoy is key to the success of your cardiorespiratory fitness program. If you don't like what you are doing,

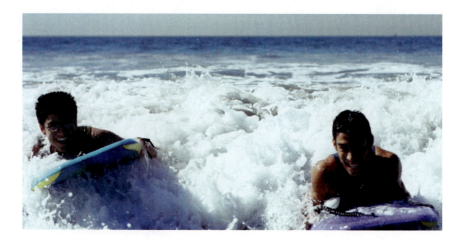

Having several types of physical activities you like to do can keep you interested and motivated.

chances are you won't stick with it. Some people enjoy team activities such as volleyball and basketball. Others enjoy activities they can do alone, such as running or bicycling. Even if you prefer team activities, you should find some activities you can do alone so that you can get exercise even when no one is available to join you.

Warm-up and Cool-down

Although not components of the FITT formula, properly warming up and cooling down are important actions that give the body time to adjust to and recover from the demands of physical activity. The ideal warm-up is a low-intensity activity. You can follow this with some gentle stretching to loosen up. When you have completed your workout, take some time to cool down. During workouts, much of the blood supply of the body is directed to the muscles. The cooling-down period allows the body to redirect the blood back to the rest of the body. A good time to do more substantial stretching is after this cooling-down period.

real teens

On December 6, 1998, a 17-year-old Australian named Jesse Martin began a 27,000–nautical–mile, solo, nonstop, unassisted sail around the globe. Jesse planned to use only solar and wind generators on board and the yacht's sail to take him around the world. He wanted his voyage to highlight our overreliance on and overuse of fossil fuels (coal, oil, and natural gas). To finance his trip, Jesse put together a budget proposal and went looking for sponsors. He was able to convince his major sponsor to commit $200,000 to the trip, and his mother remortgaged the family home to get the additional funds he needed. On October 31, 1999, Jesse became the youngest person ever to sail around the world, single-handed, unassisted, and nonstop. Jesse faced incredible physical and mental demands during his voyage. Have you ever wanted to do something that would really challenge you? If you have, what was it?

Muscular Strength

Muscular strength is the amount of force a muscle is capable of exerting against a resistance with a single maximum effort. You need muscular strength to perform many everyday tasks, such as lifting a heavy box off the floor.

The most common way to measure the strength of a muscle is to determine the maximum amount of weight it can move at one time. This is known as the one repetition maximum. Muscular strength is increased by resistance training (also called strength training). Resistance can be provided by the weight of the body, elastic bands, or weights. In resistance training, the amount of weight is similar to intensity in cardiorespiratory fitness. If your primary goal is to achieve maximum muscular strength, your strength-training program should include heavy weights lifted a few times.

Working a muscle group against an object that doesn't move is known as isometric exercise. Pushing against a wall is an example of an isometric exercise. Isometrics, however, do not provide strength through a range of motion and so are not widely used. Isotonic exercises are those in which the muscle group works against a movable

muscular strength

the amount of force a muscle is capable of exerting against a resistance with a single maximum effort

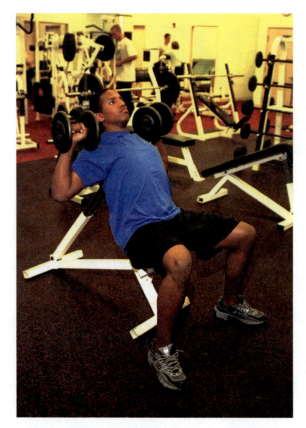

object. Push-ups, pull-ups, and lifting weights are examples of isotonic exercises.

The body is composed of many muscle groups. Each group must be exercised to develop strength throughout the body. But it is important not to overuse the muscles. The same muscle group should not be worked two days in a row because muscle tissue should be given at least 48 hours between workouts to repair itself. The American College of Sports Medicine recommends that weight training for a particular muscle group should be done two to three times a week.

Muscular Endurance

Muscular endurance is the ability of a muscle to contract over and over again without becoming fatigued. We need muscular endurance for all types of daily activities such as walking, climbing stairs, and participating in recreational sports.

Muscular endurance is measured by the number of times you can move a weight using a particular muscle. These movements are known as repetitions. If your goal is to increase muscular endurance, you will want to choose lighter weights and do more repetitions than when you are training to develop muscular strength. To increase muscular endurance, you have to continue the activity for a longer period of time.

Flexibility

Flexibility is the ability to move the joints of the body through a full range of motion, meaning the various directions that a joint can move. The joints throughout the body have different types and ranges of motion. Developing flexibility involves stretching the muscles and **tendons** that surround each of the joints.

Flexibility is probably the most frequently overlooked component of health-related fitness. We are naturally flexible as infants and children, but flexibility begins to decline as we grow older, especially for people who don't regularly engage in activities that require stretching. Many back and joint problems are caused by lack of flexibility. Maintaining good flexibility can help you avoid injuries during work, play, and competitive sports.

To be most effective, stretching exercises to maintain flexibility should be performed daily. The best time to stretch a muscle group is when it has been warmed up by exercise. Although it is good to stretch lightly before an activity, most stretching should be done at the end of a workout.

muscular endurance

the ability of a muscle to contract repeatedly without becoming fatigued

flexibility

the ability to move the joints of the body through a full range of motion

tendon

dense connective tissue that attaches muscle to bone

Chapter 10 Enjoying a Physically Active Lifestyle

There are two main types of stretching exercises: static and ballistic. Static stretching is slow and controlled. The muscle is stretched for 10–30 seconds to a point of mild discomfort and then returned to its original position. This process allows the muscle to relax and then stretch to a greater length than normal. This is the type of stretching currently recommended to increase flexibility.

The second type is ballistic stretching. This is a jerky, bouncing stretch that fitness experts no longer recommend because of the risk of injury to the muscles and tendons.

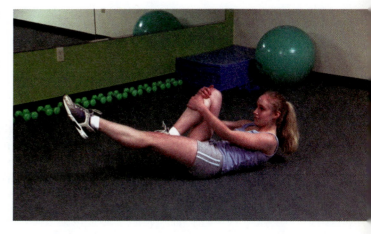

Body Composition

Body composition is the relationship between fat-free mass (muscle, bone, and water) and fat tissue within the body. It was discussed in Chapter 9. Recall that, for males, the approximate amount of body fat should be 12%–15%; for females, 18%–21%. Research shows that as body fat increases above these recommended levels, health risks also increase. Therefore, increasing muscle, or decreasing body fat, or both are important aspects of being fit.

AVOIDING INJURY

Many people who begin fitness programs injure themselves and cannot continue. There is always some risk when participating in physical activities, and some activities have more risk than others. You can lower your risk of injury in several ways:

- Properly prepare your body for the activity.
- Learn how to perform the activity correctly.
- Practice proper safety precautions.
- Know your own limitations.

There are two main types of injury related to physical activity: overuse injuries and traumatic injuries.

Overuse Injuries

Overuse injuries involve the muscles and joints. They occur when you try to do too much too fast. Shin splints are an example of a common overuse injury. Perhaps you have experienced the ache and pain during walking that can occur when you do a vigorous activity you're not used to, such as running or playing basketball. Overuse injuries are not usually serious, but they can take a long time to heal, especially if you continue exercising.

When you start a physical fitness program, it's easy to be overly enthusiastic and set your goals too high. As you push to accomplish

> **body composition**
> the relationship between fat-free mass (muscle, bone, and water) and fat tissue within the body

these goals, your body doesn't have enough time to adapt, and you could suffer an overuse injury. The best way to prevent this type of injury is to start your workout program slowly and then gradually increase your activity level. Be sure that any increases in frequency, intensity, or time are added slowly. Good footwear, with good arch support, appropriate to the particular activity, is also critical for preventing overuse injuries.

If you feel pain in a joint or muscle when you exercise and believe it may be an overuse injury, rest the painful area and avoid any activities that cause pain. Rest usually allows the body's tissues to repair themselves and prevents the need for further treatment. Once the pain is gone, you can resume activity. But begin slowly and cut back again if the pain returns. If the pain continues, you may need to see a physician.

Traumatic Injuries

The second main category of injury is traumatic injuries. These are usually sudden and accidental. Examples of traumatic injuries include a sprained ankle, strained knee, broken arm, and head injury. Traumatic injuries can be serious, even life threatening. It is best to try to prevent them rather than have to treat them once they occur. Effective prevention techniques include:

- Learning the proper skills needed to safely perform an activity
- Using caution while engaging in the activity
- Using appropriate safety equipment

Safe cycling, for example, involves knowing how to properly ride a bicycle, following the rules of the road, watching out for cars or pedestrians that may not be paying attention to you, and wearing a helmet at all times. Wearing a helmet and safety pads also helps to prevent serious injury while skateboarding or riding a scooter. Racquetball players should always wear protective eyewear. Eye injuries from a speeding ball can result in permanent loss of vision. Working out alone at night is a risk you don't need to take. Find a buddy to go with you, and always be aware of your surroundings. Be sure to wear reflective clothing so you can be easily seen.

The treatment for a traumatic injury will depend on the nature of the injury. If you have a serious traumatic injury, such as a broken bone, you need to seek medical assistance immediately. For less serious injuries, you may be able to do some initial treatment yourself. If you have a traumatic injury to soft tissue, such as a strain or sprain, using the RICE formula may help reduce swelling. RICE stands for the four components of the treatment:

R = rest

I = ice

C = compression

E = elevation

Apply ice in 10- to 20-minute intervals immediately after the injury. Place a towel or other cloth between the ice and the skin surface to avoid damage from the cold. Applying a compression wrap that is not too tight and elevating the injured area can also help keep the swelling down.

Traumatic injuries can be serious, so it is best to consult medical personnel for proper treatment. Proper treatment may prevent further damage to the injured part.

Safety Considerations

In addition to avoiding injury, there are other considerations to ensure your safety when you are participating in physical activities. For example, you should always wear reflective clothing if you exercise at night. Never exercise outdoors when lightning is present or in stormy weather. Be aware of hazardous conditions and use common sense to keep your fitness program healthy and enjoyable.

Hot Weather

You must take extra care when exercising in hot weather because your body may not be able to get rid of the extra heat it is generating. A combination of high humidity (the amount of moisture in the air) and high temperature presents an even more dangerous situation. Overheating and failing to take in enough fluids can result in heat exhaustion and heatstroke.

Heat exhaustion occurs when the body begins to overheat because of loss of fluids. Heatstroke is even more serious. It occurs when the body is generating heat so rapidly that its cooling mechanism can't keep up with the demands on it. Heatstroke is a life-threatening emergency and can result in death very quickly. A person with suspected heatstroke needs immediate medical attention.

To prevent heat-related illnesses, avoid vigorous activity during the hottest part of the day or at times when both heat and humidity levels are high. Always get enough fluids to replace what you are losing. Drink at regular intervals; don't wait until you feel thirsty.

Cold Weather

Prolonged exposure to freezing or near-freezing temperatures can result in frostbite or hypothermia. Frostbite is an external freezing of the skin from prolonged exposure to cold temperatures. It can occur more rapidly if it is windy or if you get wet or damp. Fingers, toes, ears, and the facial area are particularly susceptible to frostbite. Keep these areas dry and protected from cold and wind. Frostbite should not be taken lightly. This condition can be serious and can result in the death of the injured tissues.

Hypothermia is a potentially fatal condition in which the body is losing heat faster than it can produce it. This imbalance results in an

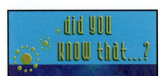

abnormally low core body temperature. If you are participating in a physical activity in cold and windy or wet conditions, wearing proper clothing is important. Choose layers and fabrics that will help "wick" the moisture away from your body. A great deal of heat escapes from the head, so always wear a hat. Pay particular attention to protecting the face, fingers, and toes. In extreme conditions, taking the day off from an outdoor activity may be a good idea.

Illness

Participating in physical activity during a mild illness, such as a cold, is usually okay if you feel like doing it. If you don't, it's a good idea to wait until you're feeling better. It is especially important to minimize physical activity if you have a fever; are being treated with prescription drugs; or feel weak, dizzy, or faint. If you do participate, you may want to decrease the intensity of the activity and not push yourself too hard.

Fluid Replacement

You can avoid many problems by drinking enough fluids to replace those that you are losing because of physical activity. The rule of thumb is to "drink before you're thirsty." By the time you feel thirsty, your body is already experiencing the effects of not having enough fluids.

A general guide is to drink at least 8 ounces of water for every 30 minutes of activity and more if the weather is hot or humid. If your workout is less than 60–90 minutes long, water alone is sufficient to replace the fluids your body has lost. For intense exercise over 60–90 minutes, a commercial energy replacement drink may help replace some of the electrolytes the body is losing and supply simple carbohydrates for energy. Inadequate fluid intake can cause your performance in an activity to suffer. It can also contribute to serious problems such as heat exhaustion and heatstroke.

Nutritional Supplements

The use of nutritional supplements to enhance performance is a controversial subject. There is no quick, easy way to become stronger and fitter. Physical conditioning requires consistent, steady effort over a period of time. Many of the well-advertised supplements have little proof to support their claims. There have also been few studies conducted to determine how safe these supplements are. Remember, if it sounds too good to be true, it probably isn't true!

DEVELOPING A PERSONAL FITNESS PLAN

There are two steps in developing a personal fitness plan: (1) determining your goals and (2) designing a plan to achieve them. To get started, ask yourself these questions:

- What do I want to accomplish?

- What activities do I want to engage in?
- What facilities and equipment will I need?
- Is there anything I'll need to buy?
- How much time do I have to devote to physical activities?
- What will help me stay motivated?

Designing Your Plan

When designing your plan, keep in mind that there are various levels of **physical activity**. Some physical activities don't require much expenditure of energy, such as washing the car, raking leaves, and playing Frisbee. Other physical activities may use a little more energy, although the energy required may not be constant. Activities that fall into this category include walking to school with friends, riding your bike to work, and playing softball. Then there are activities that consistently require a high expenditure of energy. Examples include hiking, biking, running, playing basketball, and swimming. These activities use the large muscle groups.

Even mild to moderate physical activities help develop health-related fitness. Participating in fast-moving, vigorous sports is not necessary. And some people have limitations that must be considered. For example, you may have a medical condition such as asthma or diabetes, or you may have a unique characteristic or physical challenge that makes it difficult to find an appropriate activity. Many activities can be adapted so that people of all abilities can participate and enjoy themselves. Wheelchair basketball and tennis are examples of adapted activities. Regardless of individual limitations, almost everyone can benefit from some type of physical activity. You can prepare a personal activity plan using a format like the one shown in Figure 10-2.

Increasing Your Chances of Success

Many people who start a personal fitness program don't stay with it very long. Starting any new routine can be difficult. It can be tempting to quit if you don't see immediate results. The results will come over time. The first month is the most difficult. After that, you have developed a habit of physical activity, and it will become easier to maintain it. Starting now, as a teen, to be physically active will give you benefits for years to come. The habits you develop now are likely to determine how physically active you will be as an adult. Many people who have been physically active all their lives remain active in their seventies, eighties, and beyond. You are laying the foundation for your future.

There are several things you can do to increase your chances of sticking with your fitness program and being successful. Following these suggestions can help you continue your fitness program and accomplish your goals without getting injured.

physical activity

any activity performed by the skeletal muscles (muscles concerned with body movement) that requires the body to use more energy than it does when it is at rest

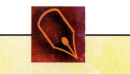

take it on home
Ask other members of your family if they were physically active as children and teenagers. If they were, find out what activities they did during those times and how their activities in their younger years affected the physical activities they engage in today. If other members of your family are not physically active, find out what keeps them from being physically active. What family tradition do you want to begin or continue regarding physical activity? What will you do to start that tradition now? Write your findings in your Health Folio.

PERSONAL ACTIVITY PLAN				
My Overall Goal:				
My Plan to Achieve My Goal:				
	Frequency	**Intensity (if applicable)**	**Time**	**Type**
Cardiorespiratory fitness	(Example: Four times per week)	(Example: 65%)	(Example: 30 minutes)	(Example: Walking)
Muscular strength				
Muscular endurance				
Flexibility				
Body composition: Current body fat percentage: Body fat percentage goal:				
People who will support me in my efforts:				
How I'll reward myself for my progress:				

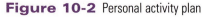

Figure 10-2 Personal activity plan

Start Out Slowly

Remember that your body needs time to adjust to new activity levels. Starting slowly also prevents overuse injuries. Depending on the type of activity, it will take your body about three to six weeks to adjust to your new activity level. Being patient and starting slowly increase your chances of avoiding injury and being able to continue your planned workout schedule.

Have Reasonable Expectations

It is also important to have reasonable expectations. It is *not* reasonable, for example, to think that you can run three miles seven days a week if you have not been exercising. The current condition of your body has developed over years. It will take time and consistent effort to make the changes you want.

Be Committed and Consistent

Success requires being committed to your program and not giving up easily. On some days, you will be excited and eager to work out. On other days, you may not feel very enthusiastic. When you don't feel like doing your planned activity, sometimes the only thing you can do is to follow the Nike slogan and "Just Do It." Sometimes, just getting started is the hardest part! The important thing is to do something active every day, even if only for a short period of time. Regular, consistent activity over time is the best way to achieve all the health-related benefits of physical activity.

Find an Activity Buddy

Finding someone who has goals similar to yours and who wants to work out with you can make the difference in whether you continue with your fitness program or drop out. Knowing that someone is counting on you to show up makes it more likely that you will too. It's also more fun to work out with a buddy. You should, however, have a plan for individual activities in case your buddy can't join you. An alternative is important, too, if you participate in group activities. Have a backup plan in case the group is not available. Don't become dependent on others to make sure you follow your plan.

Regularly Record Your Progress

Keeping track of the physical activities you engage in can help keep you motivated. Recording the time, distance, and number of days a week can help you determine if you are achieving your goals. Some people prefer simple systems, such as "gold stars," if they work out. Others are willing to devote extra time to keep more complicated records that give them a clear picture of their improvement. Just getting into the habit of writing down your activities every day can help you maintain your commitment to your goals. Review your activity journal periodically to see if you should make changes in your fitness plan.

Consider Cross-Training

In recent years, cross-training has become very popular. **Cross-training** involves participating in two or more different activities to achieve cardiorespiratory fitness. It helps prevent the boredom of doing the same activity over and over. Cross-training can also help avoid overuse injuries by

take it on home

Is there someone in your family who would be a good activity buddy? You might not know unless you give it a try! Look for something that you and another family member might enjoy doing together. Walking, for example, is a great activity that the whole family can be involved in.

cross-training

participating in two or more different physical activities to achieve cardiorespiratory fitness giving the various muscle groups time to rest. One of the more popular types of cross-training is triathlon-style training, which includes running, swimming, and bicycling. Even if you don't plan to compete in a triathlon, the combination of these activities can produce high levels of cardiorespiratory fitness and minimize the chances of boredom or injury.

BUILDING YOUR Wellness Plan

In this chapter, you learned about the benefits of physical activity and the ways to plan a program to increase your physical fitness. Exercise is one of the single most important things you can do to prevent disease and live a long, high-quality life. The following actions will help you take advantage of the many benefits of physical activity:

- Assess your own fitness needs.
- Set personal fitness goals.
- Investigate various physical activities and choose some you think you might enjoy.
- Learn the proper skills for the activities you have chosen.
- Learn and apply the safety guidelines appropriate for your activities and local conditions.
- Consider finding a fitness buddy you can enjoy some of these activities with.
- Create a plan for using your chosen activities to achieve your goals.

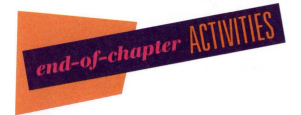

end-of-chapter ACTIVITIES

Weblinks

FITT Formula (Cardiorespiratory Fitness)

TeenHealth:
   http://www.healthnet.com/adap/getfitnow

Jesse Martin

Jesse Martin: **http://www.jessemartin.net**

Organizations for Athletes with Disabilities

Paralympics: **http://www.usparalympics.org**
Special Olympics: **http://www.specialolympics.org**

Personal Fitness Goals

American Heart Association:
   http://www.justmove.org

⚛ Short-Answer Questions

1. Name three diseases that are related to physical inactivity.
2. List the major physiological benefits of physical activity.
3. List the major psychological benefits of physical activity.
4. Briefly describe the five components of health-related physical fitness.
5. Describe the two major types of injury related to physical activity.

⚛ Discussion Questions

1. Describe the current level of physical activity practiced by Americans in various age groups.
2. Explain several reasons why a teenager should be physically active.
3. Construct a personal fitness plan that includes the five components of health-related fitness.
4. List and explain five actions you can take to help your personal fitness plan succeed.
5. Explain the actions you should take to avoid injury during physical activity.

⚛ Chapter Vocabulary

Using a separate sheet of paper, list and define the following terms:

body composition	muscular endurance
cardiorespiratory fitness	muscular strength
FITT formula	physical activity
flexibility	skill-related fitness
health-related fitness	target heart rate range

⚛ Application Activities

Language Arts Connection

Collect information about the Special Olympics or the Paralympics. Write a paper describing some of the ways these organizations encourage people of different abilities to become and stay physically active.

Math Connection

Refer to the instructions given for the Karvonen Formula in Figure 10-1. Use the Karvonen Formula to calculate the target heart rate range for each of the following individuals:

Name	Age	Resting Heart Rate	Intensity Level
Jack	14 years old	70	60%–80%
Alicia	17 years old	60	70%–90%
Kim	20 years old	80	45%–65%
Jose	30 years old	50	75%–85%
Micah	50 years old	75	40%–60%

What conclusions can you draw about the influence of resting heart rate on target heart rate range? How does intensity level affect heart rate range?

Social Studies Connection

Select four or five countries. Research in your library or on the Internet and describe the types and levels of activities the people in those countries typically engage in. Compare and contrast your findings. How are they different from or similar to the habits of Americans? Are people of these countries more or less active than Americans?

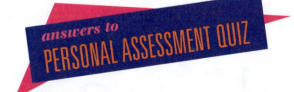

answers to PERSONAL ASSESSMENT QUIZ

personal assessment: PHYSICAL ACTIVITY QUIZ

1. False
2. True
3. False
4. True
5. False
6. True
7. True
8. False
9. False
10. True

chapter 11

Preventing Injury

Three weeks ago, Shelley asked her parents for permission to go to a concert with her boyfriend, Kirk, who is a year older than Shelley, and another couple. Kirk has had his driver's license for about a year. The concert was in a large city about 30 minutes from the small town in which Shelley lives. Shelley's parents knew her boyfriend well and believed that he was a good driver but that he lacked experience driving in the city. After gathering some information about the concert and asking Kirk's parents about his driving record, they reluctantly agreed to let Shelley go to the concert. On the day of the concert, it began to snow, lightly at first and then a little harder. When Shelley's parents got home from work, they discussed it and decided that Shelley could not go to the concert because the snow and bad weather had made the roads too hazardous. Shelley was furious because they had already promised her she could go.

Do you think Shelley is able to accurately assess the risk in this situation? Why or why not?

chapter OBJECTIVES

When you finish this chapter, you should be able to:

- Explain the difference between unintentional and intentional injuries.
- List the four major categories of unintentional injuries.
- Explain the major causes of motor vehicle injuries.
- Identify the top three causes of death for young people ages 15–24.
- Describe the relationship of age and gender to unintentional and intentional injuries.
- Develop a personal and family safety plan.

key TERMS

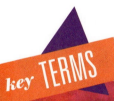

date rape
Heimlich maneuver
homicide
intentional injuries
sexual assault
statutory rape
unintentional injuries
violence
violent victimization statistics
years of potential life lost

Introduction

Living an interesting and active life includes learning to handle the risks you may encounter. Although it is impossible to avoid all types of risks, you can make choices that decrease your risk for injury. Injuries range from mild bumps and bruises to injuries severe enough to cause death.

Many injuries, including those that are most serious, can be prevented if you learn about their causes and follow techniques to prevent them. This chapter presents information to help you develop strategies for safe living. You will also be challenged to determine what level of risk for injury you are willing to accept for the kind of lifestyle you want.

personal assessment: PREVENTING INJURY QUIZ

Before reading this chapter, test how much you already know about keeping yourself and others safe from injuries. Read each statement and, on a separate sheet of paper, answer True or False. Then see the answers found at the end of the chapter.

1. Motor vehicle crashes are the leading cause of death in the United States for all age groups.

2. It is estimated that 75% of all motor vehicle crashes occur on interstate highways.

3. The fatality rate for 16-year-old drivers is much higher than for drivers who are 20–24 years old.

4. The number of teenagers involved in fatal crashes that are alcohol related has decreased in recent years.

5. Most home injuries and deaths are caused by unintentional discharge of firearms.

6. Most deaths related to fires are due to smoke inhalation rather than to burn injuries.

7. The number of violent acts in the United States is at the lowest rate in almost 30 years.

8. Rates of violence are higher among persons over the age of 25 than among those younger than 25.

9. Murder deaths are the leading cause of work-related deaths for employees under the age of 18.

10. Most cases of sexual assault involve an attack by a stranger.

CHOICES AND CONSEQUENCES

As a teen, you may feel that you don't get to make as many of your own decisions as you would like. It may seem as if your parents or other adults make most of the important choices in your life. As you continue progressing on the path to adulthood, however, you will have more and more opportunities to make your own choices. But each of these choices has consequences. As you are allowed to make your own choices, you will also be expected to understand and be responsible for their consequences.

Deciding how much risk you are willing to accept is part of this process. Think about how much risk you are willing to accept in exchange for the way you want to live. For example, if you really enjoy driving a car at high speeds, are you willing to risk getting a traffic ticket and having your car insurance rates increase? Are you willing to accept the risk that you might be killed or severely disabled? Or that you might kill or disable someone else?

Your safety is important to the adults who care about you. They may believe that you aren't yet able to recognize the consequences involved with potentially risky behaviors. Some teens seem to believe they are immortal and invincible. They have an attitude that "It can't happen to me." Many teens, however, can calculate the risks and make healthy choices. They know how to gather information and are willing to get input from trusted adults so that they can make informed decisions.

UNINTENTIONAL INJURIES

Unintentional injuries are injuries that happen when no harm was intended to occur. They are sometimes called accidents, but the word *accident* suggests that nothing can be done to prevent harm or injury. In fact, most unintentional injuries can be prevented.

The four major categories of unintentional injuries are:

1. Motor vehicle crashes
2. Injuries that occur in the home
3. Recreational or leisure-time injuries
4. On-the-job injuries

Unintentional injuries are the leading cause of death and disability among children, teens, and young adults. They are also the reason for more **years of potential life lost** than any other cause of death. Young people have their whole lives ahead of them, up to 70 or 80 years. Preventing death from unintentional injury helps ensure that young people will live out their expected life span, rather than having it cut short before they even reach adulthood.

Motor Vehicle Injuries

According to the National Safety Council, motor vehicle crashes are the leading cause of death for people ages 1–33. Motor vehicle crashes are also the leading cause of severe brain injury in the United States as well as the cause of most cases of paralysis due to spinal injuries. Many of these deaths and injuries occur when the person is a passenger in a vehicle. It makes good sense to be concerned about the safety of teenagers any time they are in an automobile, whether they are drivers or passengers.

It is estimated that 75% of motor vehicle crashes occur within 25 miles of home at speeds less than 40 miles per hour. This is exactly the type of driving that teens do most often. Although young drivers represent only about 7% of the nation's licensed drivers, they are involved in 15% of all fatal crashes. Driver inexperience behind the wheel plays a big part in these crashes. Think about the first time you tried to ride a

> **unintentional injuries**
> injuries that happen when no harm was intended to occur; formerly called accidents

> **years of potential life lost**
> the difference in years between an individual's life expectancy and that individual's age at the time of death

bicycle. Chances are you were wobbly and probably even "crashed" several times. Learning to drive is no different. As with any skill, it takes time and practice to learn to drive well. Driving is a complex skill that requires attention to many factors at once. Teen drivers often make errors in judgment. In fact, it is estimated that most motor vehicle crashes are a result of human error. Five of the most common reasons for motor vehicle crashes are (1) excessive speed, (2) aggressive driving habits, (3) driver distraction, (4) alcohol and other drugs, and (5) improper use and nonuse of safety equipment.

Driving at the posted speed limit based on road conditions, being courteous to others who share the road, and paying attention at all times can help minimize the likelihood that you will be involved in a motor vehicle accident.

Excessive Speed

Excessive speed is cited as a cause of approximately two-thirds of all crashes. The faster you are driving, the less time you have to react to an unexpected situation, and the longer it takes to bring the vehicle to a stop. Think for a moment about speed limits in neighborhoods. Assume that the posted speed limit is 25 miles per hour. Your friend insists on obeying the speed limit and going only 25 miles per hour. You, on the other hand, always push it to at least 35 miles per hour. You may think that 25 miles per hour is "crawling" and that the police never monitor this street anyway. If a child suddenly runs into the roadway, who will be most likely to be able to stop before hitting the child—you or your friend? Is this a risk that you are willing to take in order to drive faster?

Aggressive Driving Habits

Reports of aggressive driving incidents have increased approximately 7% per year since 1990. Even so, most aggressive driving incidents still go unreported. As roadways become more crowded, drivers are more likely to find themselves in situations that are annoying or irritating. People also seem to be in more of a hurry these days. Some drivers deal with their frustrations by weaving in and out of traffic and making numerous lane changes in order to save a few seconds. Others try to make it through a yellow light that is sure to turn red

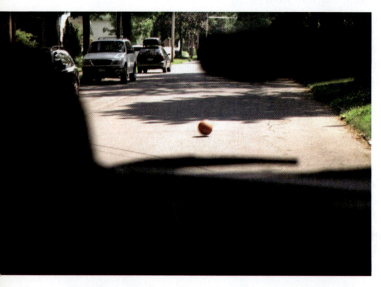

If a child runs in front of your car while you are speeding, will you be able to stop in time?

before they completely cross the intersection. These are examples of aggressive driving behaviors that are, in fact, *habits*. The good thing about habits is that they can be changed. Becoming aware of your driving habits can be a good first step to changing them.

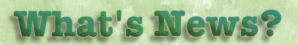

What's News?

Road rage is an exaggerated form of aggressive driving that has received increased attention in the past few years. People who drive too aggressively may violate traffic laws, but those who exhibit road rage behaviors are guilty of criminal behavior. Road rage is demonstrated by uncontrolled anger that results in violence or threatened violence on the road. Road rage is often provoked by something trivial, such as someone driving too slowly or music that is too loud. Although road rage has many possible causes, it is commonly linked to personal attitudes about other drivers and a high stress level that the person lacks the skills to handle appropriately. Both males and females can exhibit road rage, but it is most common among male drivers ages 18–26.

Driver Distraction

Driver distraction can be caused by fatigue and sleepiness, as well as by the use of cellular phones, passengers in the vehicle, and performing other tasks at the same time as driving. Fatigue is a major contributor to motor vehicle crashes. Fatigued drivers are not as alert to situations occurring on the roadway and have slower reaction times than well-rested, alert drivers. Some drivers even fall asleep while driving!

Traffic safety experts are becoming more and more concerned about the dangers of the increased use of cellular phones while driving. Talking on the phone is just one of the many possible distractions that drivers encounter each day. It seems, however, to be among the most potentially dangerous. The National Highway Traffic Safety Administration suggests that the distraction of using a cell phone can be blamed for 20%–30% of all traffic collisions. A study published by the National Safety Council found no significant difference in response time between users of handheld and hands-free phones. It is important to know the laws in your state regarding the use of cellular phones. In some states, a driver can be ticketed for using a handheld phone while driving.

In crucial driving situations, response time is a critical factor for avoiding a collision. Driving safely is a skill that requires continual complex reactions. Any type of distraction can increase the likelihood of a crash. Unrestrained pets, changing the radio station, inserting a CD, or reaching for food or a drink are some of the many distractions that have led to motor vehicle crashes. For teenagers, one of the biggest distractions is having other teenagers in the vehicle. Talking to or trying to impress a group of friends can take your attention from the roadway and increase your risk for a crash.

Alcohol and Other Drugs

According to the National Safety Council, alcohol-related fatalities in 1989 represented about 50% of all traffic deaths. Ten years later, in

1999, that percentage had dropped to 38%. Among teenagers, the number of young drivers involved in fatal crashes that were alcohol related decreased 61% from 1982 to 1998. Raising the minimum legal drinking age to 21 and passing zero-tolerance-for-alcohol traffic laws are thought to have been partially responsible for this decrease.

Although we have seen a substantial drop in alcohol-related traffic deaths, there is still a lot of room for improvement. Even when the amount of alcohol in the bloodstream is below the legal limit, which varies by state, driving ability can be impaired. Reason, judgment, and response time are all affected by even small amounts of alcohol. Combining alcohol with driving is taking a big risk that has life or death consequences—don't chance it!

Improper Use and Nonuse of Safety Equipment

Over the past few decades, the safety equipment installed in motor vehicles has become more advanced. In addition to lap safety belts, new vehicles now have lap and shoulder belts, front airbags, and sometimes even side airbags. Many motorists, however, don't take advantage of these devices. It is estimated that about one-third of all occupants of a motor vehicle either do not use a safety belt or use it incorrectly. Studies show that you are twice as likely to be injured in a motor vehicle crash if you are not wearing a safety belt. In fatal crashes, an estimated 60%–70% of those killed could have survived if they had been wearing a safety belt.

Airbags are a recent innovation in safety equipment. It seems likely that airbags reduce the chance of injury and death. As airbags inflate, however, they can injure or even kill a child or small adult in the passenger seat. Children 12 years of age and under are always safest

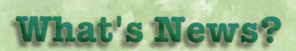

What's News?

Recognizing that teenagers' youth and inexperience are major contributors to motor vehicle crashes, many states have adopted a process known as graduated driver licensing (GDL). This process phases in teenage driving privileges over two or more years. Thirty-one states and the District of Columbia have already passed full-scale graduated licensing laws. Under an ideal GDL program, the minimum age for a learner's permit is 16. The first stage lasts for at least six months, during which parents must verify that they have provided 30–50 hours of supervised driving. The second stage lasts until at least age 18. Depending on the state, this stage may include two major provisions: (1) a nighttime driving restriction, in which a licensed adult must be in the vehicle beginning at 9 or 10 P.M. and (2) a teenage passenger restriction, in which no additional teenagers, except family members, are allowed in the car without the presence of a licensed driver, 21 years of age or older. Full, unrestricted driving privileges then become effective at age 18.

in the backseat. Infants and young children are required to be restrained in a safety seat. Following specific instructions for installation of an infant or child safety seat is critically important. Many inspections of safety seat installation have shown that the seats are installed incorrectly and are not providing proper protection. It is the driver's responsibility to make sure that all children and passengers in the vehicle are safely and properly restrained.

Motorcycles

One in 10 traffic fatalities among those who are 15–34 years old involve a motorcycle. Motorcycles share the road with cars, trucks, recreational vehicles, and 18-wheelers that are much larger and heavier. A motorcyclist involved in a collision with one of these larger vehicles is almost always the loser. After an accident, a frequent comment from the driver of one of these larger vehicles is, "But I never even saw it." If you decide to operate a motorcycle, it is critically important that you make sure you are easily visible to other drivers. Loss of control is another factor in many motorcycle accidents. This is often associated with excessive speed or skidding from improper braking. Riding a motorcycle is a risky behavior. It is up to the motorcyclist to take all necessary precautions.

Participating in a motorcycle safety training program can alert you to important safety precautions, yet fewer than 1 in 10 motorcyclists have received formal training. Another way to increase your chance of survival in case of an accident is the consistent use of an approved motorcycle helmet at all times.

Bicycles

Bicycles are usually included in statistics regarding motor vehicles because they are considered to be moving vehicles with all the rights and responsibilities of an automobile. Most injuries to bicyclists occur as a result of a collision with a motor vehicle. One of the major safety concerns for bicyclists is related to confusion regarding the place of a bicyclist when sharing the road with other vehicles. Many motorists believe that bicyclists should get out of the way or stay on the sidewalk. On the other hand, many bicyclists act as if they have a privileged status that allows them to cut through stopped traffic, run through stop signs and red lights, and switch from road to sidewalk depending on their mood. These attitudes and behaviors create dangerous situations in which neither motorists nor bicyclists know what to expect of each other.

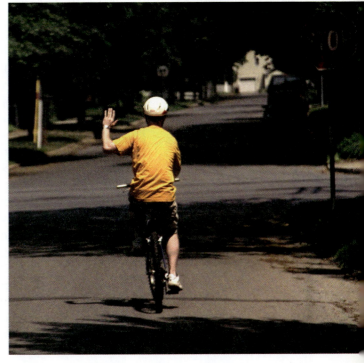

Safety campaigns to help both bicyclists and motorists understand the rules of the road can make automobile-bicycle collisions less likely. As are motorcyclists, bicyclists are difficult to see. Wearing brightly colored, reflective clothing and riding defensively can reduce the risk of a collision.

The single most important factor in reducing deaths among bicyclists is wearing an approved safety helmet at all times. About two-thirds of all deaths of bicyclists are a result of head injuries, and it is estimated that helmet use reduces the risk of death by 85%. Yet less than half of bicyclists consistently wear a helmet. Even just a short ride around the block can turn into tragedy if there is a fall or collision. Wearing a helmet *every single time you ride* might save your life. Are you willing to risk dying just to let your hair fly free in the breeze?

Injuries in the Home

According to the National Safety Council, there is a fatal injury every 18 minutes and a disabling injury every 4 seconds in homes across America. The four leading causes of fatalities in the home are falls, fires and burns, poisonings, and suffocation by an ingested object. Most of us feel safer at home than anywhere else. We don't often think about the dangers that exist there. Many injuries in the home can be prevented, however, by becoming aware of potential dangers and then taking simple safety precautions.

Falls

Although we usually think of a fall as something that occurs from a height, many falls occur as a result of tripping or slipping at ground level. Tripping over a toy or other object left on the floor and slipping on icy or snowy sidewalks are common examples of falls that result in injuries and sometimes even death. It may be hard to imagine that a simple fall can cause death, but in the year 2000, falls caused or led to 15,400 deaths. About half of those falls occurred in the home. Even slipping in the shower can lead to death if you strike your head against a hard or sharp object.

When we talk about assessing risk and determining consequences, most of us could agree that even though there is a risk of death from falling in the shower, we would still choose to take regular showers. This is an example of a situation in which we assess the risk and the likelihood of consequences and decide that the benefits outweigh the risks. At the same time, we can take actions to lower our risk of danger, such as using nonskid mats. Other actions that can lower the risk of falling in the home include making sure that stairs and living areas are well lighted, installing handrails in stairways and bathrooms, and keeping the floor and walkways clean and clear of clutter.

take it on home

What can you do to make your home safer? Does your family have a plan to prevent and deal with the major causes of injuries and deaths in the home? If not (or if your family safety plan needs additions or revisions), request a family meeting to create one. Having a plan for what to do, before an emergency occurs, can mean the difference between life and death. Some of the items in a family safety plan might include a first aid kit, a fire exit plan, and a list of emergency phone numbers. What other items should be included?

Fires

It is estimated that residential fires claim a life every two hours. Most of these deaths are a result of smoke inhalation rather than burns. Maintaining working smoke detectors in key areas of the home is the best way to prevent smoke inhalation deaths. Fire deaths are twice as high in homes without working smoke detectors. Too often, smoke detectors have been installed but do not function correctly. Batteries in smoke detectors should be tested at least once a month to make sure they are still able to sound an alarm in the event of a fire.

Another key aspect of home fire safety is having an established escape plan for every member of the family from every room in the house. Your local fire department can provide guidelines for establishing an escape plan. It is important to practice the plan, preferably at night, which is the time when most fires occur. Designate a pre-arranged meeting place for all members of the family once they have exited the house so you will know that everyone is safe.

Poisonings

Poisoning from both solids and liquids is another major cause of death in the home. Young children are particularly vulnerable to death by poisoning because of their curiosity and lack of knowledge about the harmfulness of common products. Even common, over-the-counter drugs such as aspirin can cause death if too much is consumed. Cleaning agents, houseplants, and prescription and over-the-counter drugs should all be kept out of the reach of children.

In the event of a poisoning, the best action is to call the Poison Control Center. Keep your local Poison Control Center number next to the phone. Treatment varies, depending on the type of poisoning, so it is important to call for advice. Inducing vomiting, for example, is recommended for some types of poisoning. For others, vomiting can make the problem worse.

Suffocation and Choking

Half of all suffocation deaths involve children. Many of these deaths occur when children are too young to recognize the dangers involved and adequate action has not been taken to protect them. Infants can suffocate if they become tangled up in bedding that obstructs their breathing. Other potential dangers for young children are plastic bags, which, when placed over the face, can block the mouth and nostrils, and window blind cords, which can strangle a child.

Young children are also particularly susceptible to suffocation and choking deaths by airway obstruction. The airway can become obstructed when a child inhales food particles, pieces of a balloon, coins, or small

take it on home

Perform a home safety check to see if smoke detectors and fire extinguishers are present in key areas of your home, such as the kitchen and hallways. Work with your family to set up a schedule for regularly testing your smoke detectors (such as on the first day of each month) to make sure they are operating correctly. Keep some extra batteries on hand in case they need to be replaced. Make sure all the members of your family know where the fire extinguishers are located. You may want to map out an emergency plan that includes escape routes, important numbers to call in emergencies, and a place for all family members to meet in the case of a fire, such as the lawn of a neighbor's house. Write out your emergency plan and keep a copy of it in your Health Folio.

Heimlich maneuver

the use of abdominal thrusts to dislodge items that are causing choking; it is named after the physician who invented the technique, Henry Heimlich

toy pieces. Many teenagers like to talk and eat at the same time, but doing so can put you at risk for food particles or candy pieces getting sucked into the windpipe.

Many lives have been saved by prompt use of the **Heimlich maneuver**, a relatively simple action that uses abdominal thrusts to dislodge items that are obstructing breathing. For information on how to use the Heimlich maneuver, see Figure 11-1.

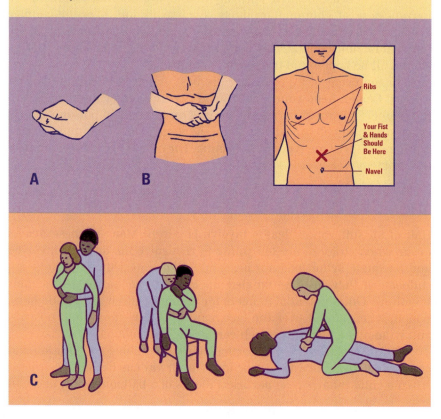

1. **Ask the person if he or she is choking.**
2. **If the person starts to cough, wait.**
3. **If the person cannot speak, cough, or breathe, but is conscious:**
   a. **Stand behind the victim and wrap your arms around the victim's waist.**
   b. **Make a fist, keeping thumb straight (see A).**
   c. **Place the thumb side of your fist against the victim's upper abdomen, below the rib cage and above the navel (see B).**
   d. **Grasp your clenched fist with the other hand and press into the victim's upper abdomen with a quick upward thrust. Do not squeeze the rib cage or "hug" the victim (see C).**
   e. **Repeat the upward thrusting of your hands until the object is expelled.**

Ribs

Your Fist & Hands Should Be Here

Navel

A

B

C

Figure 11-1
The Heimlich maneuver

Unintentional Discharge of Firearms

Although unintentional discharge of firearms is not one of the top four causes of death in the home, it is the cause of many preventable deaths every year. This often occurs when young children find and play with guns without the knowledge of an adult. Some adults believe the firearms they keep in the home are not loaded. More often, however, adults know the firearm is loaded but believe they have put it where the children can't find or reach it.

Even teens are sometimes tempted to play foolish games if they find a firearm. The careless use of a firearm, whether it is believed to be loaded or not, can result in tragedy. Never point a gun at someone or something you don't intend to shoot.

You can also protect yourself and teach others to do the same by understanding the dangerous and unpredictable nature of guns. A firearm in the hands of someone who has no sense of how guns operate or knowledge of what a discharged bullet can do is very dangerous. The best advice for anyone is to leave the area as soon as a gun appears. Do not stand around and watch while someone else is handling a gun. Your life is too important.

Many states require people to attend gun safety classes before they can purchase a handgun. These classes teach people to respect the power of weapons and to use guns safely. This information helps reduce accidental shootings. Non-gun users can do some things to protect themselves:

- Never attempt to handle guns without proper training.
- Avoid situations where untrained people are handling guns.
- Never challenge or threaten someone who has a gun.
- Avoid situations where you know there will be unsupervised teens with guns.

Can you think of any other strategies for protecting yourself against guns and weapons?

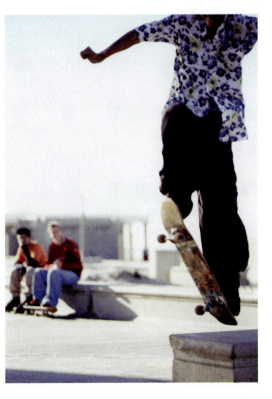

Skateboarding and in-line skating without proper safety equipment can lead to head, knee, arm, and wrist injuries.

Recreational Injuries

Numerous safety hazards are associated with recreational or leisure-time activities. Americans are spending more time engaging in recreational activities, so it is important to be aware of the potential risks. With all recreational activities, the keys to preventing unintentional injuries are to:

- Use safety and protective gear properly.

- Avoid the use of alcohol and drugs.

- Be aware of your actions and the actions of others.

Water sports are potentially hazardous. Carelessness in swimming and boating can result in drowning deaths. These are often caused by a combination of carelessness and alcohol use. Household pools should always be fenced and locked to keep unattended young children from wandering into the pool. Skateboards, in-line skating, and scooters are frequent causes of injuries to the head, wrist, arm, and hand. Proper and consistent use of safety equipment, including a helmet, can help prevent many of these injuries.

Work-Related Injuries

Time spent at work is actually safer than time spent driving, at home, or engaging in recreational activities. Work-related injuries and deaths have declined as job safety procedures have become stricter. Employers want to protect their workers, and they also recognize that job-related injuries can cost the employer a lot of money.

Employees sometimes feel as if safety precautions are a waste of time. These attitudes must be changed so that employees and employers can work together to create a safe workplace. Some employees lack the knowledge or skills to perform their jobs safely. Training in proper techniques can prevent many injuries. Back injuries, for example, are responsible for about 20% of all work-related injuries. Teaching individuals the best way to lift heavy objects and requiring the use of back supports have led to a decrease in back injuries.

Stress and fatigue can contribute to carelessness and result in injuries. Environmental conditions in the workplace can also be a source of injuries or illness. Work-related deaths and injuries are particularly high for laborers and agricultural workers. Although laborers make up less than half of the overall workforce, they represent 75% of all work-related injuries and illnesses. Some keys to preventing work-related injuries and deaths are to:

- Be sure you have received proper workplace safety training.
- Always follow safety guidelines for your workplace.
- Exercise caution when engaging in any potentially risky activities.

INTENTIONAL INJURIES AND VIOLENCE

Intentional injury is any harm, injury, or death that is caused deliberately. **Violence** is the use of physical force with the intent to inflict harm, injury, or death. A variety of violent crime statistics are compiled by different organizations in the United States. The FBI Uniform Crime Reporting Program keeps statistics for all murders in the United States. The U.S. Department of Justice, through its National Crime Victimization Survey (NCVS), collects statistics on all nonfatal violent crimes against persons 12 years of age and older. **Violent victimization statistics** include rape, sexual assault, robbery, aggravated assault (assault with a weapon), and simple assault. Although the statistics gathered are not exact, they give a good estimation of violent crimes other than murder. According to the NCVS, violent victimization fell 15% from 1999 to 2000,

intentional injury

any harm, injury, or death that is caused deliberately

violence

the use of physical force with the intent to inflict harm, injury, or death

violent victimization statistics

statistics for rape, sexual assault, robbery, aggravated assault (assault with a weapon), and simple assault; statistics do not include murder the greatest annual percentage decline since data began to be collected for this survey in 1973. The overall violent victimization rate in 2000 was the lowest in almost three decades. This is good progress, but many forms of violence still exist and much work needs to be done to further reduce violence.

Homicide

Homicide is the second leading cause of death among young people aged 15–24, second only to motor vehicle crashes. Males, teenagers, young adults, and persons of color are most likely to be victims of homicide.

In most homicides, the **perpetrator** is male. Females do kill, but they do not initiate violence as often as males and they kill for different reasons, often in self-defense. Homicides are frequently the result of an argument that gets more and more intense and leads to angry and aggressive behavior. If a person decides to use force and a firearm is available, all too often the argument ends in a homicide.

In 2000, about two-thirds of all homicides involved the use of a firearm. Contrary to popular opinion, you are unlikely to be killed by a stranger. Only 15% of homicide victims were murdered by strangers. Pay attention to potentially violent behavior in people with whom you associate. For example, it might not be safe to be closely involved with a person who gets angry easily and threatens or seems capable of violence.

Gang-Related Violence

Gang-related violence was once thought to be a problem only in urban, inner-city neighborhoods. Today, however, gangs exist not only in urban areas but also in suburban and rural areas. Gangs tend to develop when teens and young adults perceive the need to "stick together" to protect themselves or establish dominance over another group. All humans need companionship, support, security, and a way to gain self-esteem. Gangs provide a way of belonging to a specific group. Conflicts over territory, the need to establish dominance, and the need to experience excitement and victory are some of the most common reasons for rival gangs to fight. Gang violence tends to spread beyond the gang itself, sometimes resulting in family members or innocent bystanders being injured or killed.

Hate Crimes

Hate crimes are acts of violence committed against an individual because of his or her race, ethnicity, national origin, religion, or sexual orientation. Hate crimes occur when people are unable to accept the differences that exist between individuals and groups in our society.

homicide

the deliberate killing of one human being by another

perpetrator

a person who commits an act of violence

Sometimes persons who lack the knowledge and skills to deal effectively with those differences feel as if violence is the only way to express their dissatisfaction or frustration with people who are different.

Hate crimes can be directed at either individuals or groups. They can also be focused on the disfigurement or destruction of property, such as painting graffiti or burning a church or place of worship. In 1999, the motivation for just over half of the hate crimes was racial or ethnic bias. Disagreement about religion and sexual orientation were the next two most frequently cited reasons for hate crimes.

School Violence

School violence has received a lot of attention in the past few years because of several school mass shootings that resulted in the deaths of teachers and students. Statistics show, however, that teenagers are actually safer at school than they are at home, in the workplace, or on the road. In 1999, among 12- to 18-year-olds, serious violent crime was almost three times more likely to occur away from school than during time spent at school.

Despite these figures, the threat of violence in schools today is common. In a survey of students in grades 9–12, about 8% reported they had been threatened or injured with a weapon, such as a gun, knife, or club, in the past 12 months while on school property. About 7% surveyed reported that they had carried a weapon to school in the past 30 days. These statistics are evidence that weapons are often present on school campuses. Many schools have now adopted school safety plans to deal with both unintentional injuries and intentional violence. Do you know if your school has any kind of safety plan to help students deal with injuries and violence?

Workplace Violence

Although relatively few deaths occur in the workplace, approximately 40% of those that do are homicides. Homicide is the second leading cause of death on the job, second only to motor vehicle crashes that occur on the job. It is the number one cause of death on the job for women. Even so, men are three times more likely to become workplace homicide victims than are women.

Approximately three-fourths of all work-related homicides in 2000 were related to a robbery. About three-fourths of all workplace homicides were committed using a firearm. In contrast to homicides in other situations, the majority of workplace homicides involve perpetrators and victims who don't know each other. Although the media give a lot of attention to violent acts by someone employed in the workplace, only 9% of all work-related homicides involved a coworker or former coworker.

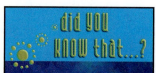

did you know that...?

Homicide is the leading cause of work-related death for employees under the age of 18. Interacting with the public, exchanging money, delivering services or goods, working late night or early morning shifts, and working alone are all factors that increase the risk of work-related homicide. If you have a job, consider the potential risks associated with the job responsibilities and take precautions to protect yourself to the greatest extent possible.

Family and Intimate Violence

Women are most frequently the victims of violent acts committed by family or **intimate partners**, accounting for approximately 90%–95% of cases of violence by intimate partners. Nearly one in three adult women report at least one physical assault by an intimate partner during adulthood. In fact, about 28% of *all* violence against women is committed by an intimate partner.

The majority of perpetrators of family violence have two characteristics in common: (1) they are male, and (2) they witnessed family violence while they were growing up. Abusive partners have a need to control their partner and are unable to communicate, negotiate, and compromise to get their needs and desires met. Figure 11-2 presents the four-phase cycle of violence that most acts of family violence follow.

In one survey, two-thirds of victims who suffered violence by an intimate partner reported that alcohol was a factor; three-fourths of spousal victims said alcohol was involved. Many women stay with abusive partners because they lack the financial resources to leave or have low self-esteem and don't believe they can make it on their own.

When children are involved, the situation is even more difficult. Children, as well as women, are at risk when family violence occurs. According to one study, in homes where there is partner abuse, children are 1,500 times more likely to be abused than in families where partner violence is not present.

Violence against Children

Violence against children can take many forms: physical, emotional, sexual, or simply neglect. A violent act committed by a parent is one of the five leading causes of death among children ages 1–18. Parenting is a difficult and demanding task, even under the best of circumstances. Parents who lack the knowledge and skills to cope effectively with the demands of parenthood may become angry and frustrated with their

intimate partners
current or former spouses and boyfriends or girlfriends

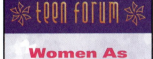

Women As Victims

Women aged 16–24 are more likely to experience violence from an intimate partner than any other age group.

- Why do you think this is true?

- If you are a female, what actions can you take to keep from becoming a victim of intimate partner violence both now and in the future?

- If you are a male, what actions can you take to reduce the chances that you will be involved in a relationship with an intimate partner that turns violent?

2. The tension explodes into some form of violent behavior.

1. Tension builds between the partners, often over a relatively minor problem.

3. The abuser begs for forgiveness and promises that the violence will never happen again.

4. If the victim forgives the abuser, a "honeymoon" period of calm follows, but chances are high that the cycle will soon be repeated.

Figure 11-2
The cycle of violence

children. If they cannot express this anger and frustration appropriately, they may take it out on the children.

Sometimes one child is singled out as the target for the parent's frustration. Trying to work, take care of children, and manage all the details of a household can put a big strain on all parents, but the strain can be especially severe for single parents. Single parents who don't have adequate support from others are at risk for acting violently toward their children.

If you are involved in a violent situation at home or are a witness to violence, confide in a trusted adult who can assist you in finding the help you need. Getting help early before the situation gets out of hand can prevent more serious problems later.

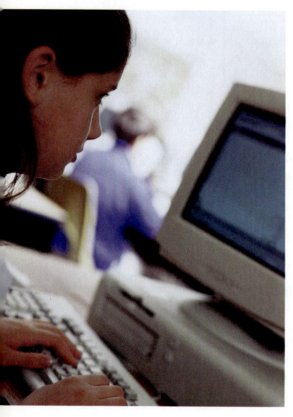

Cyberviolence

With the rapid growth in the use of the Internet, new concerns have surfaced over "virtual" violent acts that are the result of Internet interactions. Concern has been raised about the violent content of some Web sites and electronic messages. There is more concern, however, about the possibility of a "real-life" violent act committed against someone after an Internet relationship has been established through e-mail or chat rooms.

The anonymity of the Internet allows people to pretend to be someone they are not. For example, a man might convincingly pretend to be a 13-year-old girl and establish an online friendship with a young girl. He might then make arrangements to meet the young girl in an attempt to harm her. Because it is almost impossible to be absolutely sure about the identity of people you "meet" on the Internet, you should never reveal anything about yourself that could allow the other person to identify and locate you. Don't ever give out your last name, home address, school, or workplace. It may seem harmless to talk to people on the Internet, but the risk for danger should always be considered.

Sexual Assault

Sexual assault is a violent crime involving the use of force or threat of force to have sexual relations with someone without that person's voluntary consent. Acts of sexual violence can be directed toward both males and females, although it is more common for them to be directed toward females. Although many females fear sexual assault by a stranger, women are most at risk of being assaulted by men they know.

In the vast majority of cases of sexual assault, a weapon is not used. In 2000, only 6% of sexual assaults involved a weapon, such as a gun or knife. The lack of a weapon, however, does not mean that it is not sexual assault. Verbal threats and physical intimidation can be used to force the victim into submitting to a sexual act.

Experts have different opinions about whether a victim should fight back when being sexually assaulted. If the perpetrator is a stranger rather than someone the victim knows, there is a greater likelihood that the person will be physically injured or killed, especially if the victim tries to fight back. Victims of sexual assaults should never be criticized for their decision about how much to resist or the type of resistance they used. They are not at fault for being assaulted.

Acquaintance and Date Rape

About 60% of all sexual assault victims report that a current or former spouse, boyfriend, or date was the perpetrator. This crime is known as **date rape** or **acquaintance rape**. Many of these incidents are never reported to legal authorities. The woman often feels that the incident may have been her fault because she was attracted to the man. There may have been no weapons, direct verbal threats, or strong use of force. Nevertheless, if a woman is coerced into having sexual relations without her consent, she was the victim of sexual assault.

Date rapes are frequently alcohol related. Alcohol can affect the judgment and reasoning ability of both the perpetrator and the victim. The effects of alcohol may make it impossible to determine if there was consent. Sometimes drugs are used to produce temporary amnesia so that the victim will not remember the incident clearly. Use of these so-called date rape drugs is a criminal act, whether or not sexual assault actually occurs.

Engaging in any type of sexual behavior without establishing clear and direct verbal consent is a risky behavior for both males and females. Males can later be accused of rape, even if they thought the sexual activity was agreeable at the time it occurred. Sexual boundaries should be communicated clearly and directly early in the situation. Once boundaries have been established, follow through by enforcing those boundaries.

Sexual Harassment

Sexual harassment is a milder form of sexual violence than sexual assault, but it can still have many negative consequences for the parties involved. Unwelcome sexual advances, requests for sexual favors, or any other conduct that is sexual in nature and creates an intimidating atmosphere can be considered sexual harassment.

Sexual harassment often occurs in situations in which there is an imbalance of power, such as between a teacher and student or an employer and an employee. Sometimes, sexual favors are demanded in exchange for a passing grade or maintaining employment. If you find yourself in a situation in which you feel that sexual harassment is occurring, tell the person clearly and directly that you find the sexual

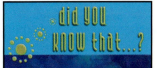

did you know that...?

If the victim is younger than the state's legally defined age of consent, a sexual relationship is considered statutory rape regardless of whether there was mutual consent. For this reason, an older teen who engages in a sexual relationship with a younger teen can be charged with statutory rape, even if the sexual relationship was agreeable to both parties.

statutory rape

any sexual relations with an individual who is under the legal age of consent

date rape or acquaintance rape

any forced sexual activity in which the victim is acquainted with or is dating the rapist

sexual harassment

any unwelcome sexual advances, requests for sexual favors, or other conduct that is sexual in nature and creates an intimidating atmosphere in an academic or work environment comment or action inappropriate. Tell him or her to stop the objectionable behavior immediately. If the individual continues the behavior, file a formal complaint with the person's supervisor, employer, or the school administration.

Factors That Contribute to Violence

Recent rates of violence and intentional injury in the United States have declined. However, they are still higher in the United States than in other similar countries, particularly for murder. Many factors contribute to this situation. Understanding those factors can help you avoid being a victim of violence.

Population Characteristics

Rates of violence are not consistently distributed across the United States. The geographic area of the country that you live in, your gender, your age, and your socioeconomic status all affect the amount of violence to which you are likely to be exposed. For example, rates of murder (especially those involving guns) are higher in western and southern states than in northern and eastern states.

Most perpetrators of violent acts are male. Although females do commit violent acts, including murder, they do not do so nearly as often as males. In fact, males are nine times more likely to commit murder than are females. Males are also more likely to be victims of violent acts. Three-fourths of all murder victims are males.

Rates of violence are higher among young people than among older adults. One-half of all persons arrested for violent crimes are under the age of 25. Teenagers and young adults are also victims, as well as perpetrators, of violence. Those 12–24 years of age have historically had the highest levels of violent victimization of any age group. An estimated one in eight people murdered is less than 18 years of age.

Violence occurs in all racial and ethnic groups, as well as all socioeconomic levels, but it is highest among minority groups with low socioeconomic status. Living in an area in which the majority of residents lack status, power, and economic resources puts you at risk for experiencing some type of violence.

Interpersonal Relationships

Although you may hear warnings about being careful around strangers, the fact is that most victims of violence know their attacker. Victims and perpetrators are usually similar to each other in gender, ethnicity, educational level, and socioeconomic status. Women, especially, are often the victims of attack by someone who is known to them. In cases of murder, 60% of the women knew their attacker. The rates for sexual assault are even higher: 80% of the women knew their attacker. Men are less likely to know their attacker; about 50% of male victims of violence identified a stranger as the perpetrator of the violence.

Use of Alcohol and Other Drugs

Use of alcohol and other drugs is closely related to violent behavior. Many individuals behave much more aggressively when they are under the influence of alcohol or other drugs than they normally would. Judgment and reason are among the first things affected. A simple argument, fueled by alcohol, can turn into an angry confrontation that leaves someone injured or dead. More than one-third of convicted offenders had been drinking at the time of the offense.

Violence in the Mass Media

Graphic images of violent acts appear frequently in the mass media. Dozens of television programs and movies focus on various aspects of crime. News reports also contain detailed reports of crime and violence.

In most cases, violent incidents are shown in great detail. Receiving a constant dose of violent images through the media can make real-life violence seem more common and acceptable. What are often left out are the consequences of violent acts: the suffering of victims and the punishment faced by perpetrators. This unbalanced presentation may give the false impression that there are no real consequences of violence.

Availability of Firearms

In the United States, many different types of firearms are easily available. It is easier to obtain handguns in the United States than in any other industrialized country. Many people believe that the easy accessibility of handguns is one of the reasons that the rate of homicide is as much as 10 times higher in the United States than in other industrialized

---

Tips for Avoiding Weapons

With images of violence and weapons appearing frequently in the mass media, what can you do to avoid dangerous situations?

- Never carry a gun, knife, or other weapon. If you feel threatened, find a trusted adult and talk with them about the situation. Or contact the police and report your concerns. If you feel reporting the problem to authorities will make things worse, consider an anonymous tip. Confronting a situation with a weapon of any kind greatly increases the chance of serious injury.
- Stay away from individuals who carry weapons, and avoid dangerous areas.
- Travel with a group of friends to avoid being alone in the wrong place at the wrong time.
- Learn conflict resolution skills to help keep conflicts from becoming violent. Start a conflict resolution program in your school or community to help others learn to avoid violent conflict.
- Get involved in a crime-watch program to help keep your school or community free from weapons, violence, and crime.
- Use the Internet to find more strategies for avoiding weapons, violence, and crime.

❖ teen forum ❖

Violence in the Mass Media

There is a great deal of debate about whether seeing frequent graphic images of violent acts in television programs, cartoons, video games, and movies makes people more likely to act violently themselves.

- What do you think?
- Would your opinion change depending on how old the person viewing the violent act is?
- Does it matter what kind of violent act is shown?
- Is the violence in "fantasy," such as in a cartoon, different from "reality," such as in a news program or dramatic movie?
- Do you think the media should show people how to react safely when a gun is present?

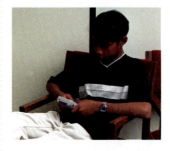

Video games often show violent acts without any consequences.

suicide

the deliberate killing of oneself

countries. The rate of homicides that occur as a result of firearms is eight times higher in the United States than in other industrialized countries.

Perhaps the main reason that firearms increase the homicide rate is because firearms are so effective in causing death. Other weapons may cause serious injury, but the injuries are less likely to result in death. In the United States in 2000, about two-thirds of all homicides were committed using a firearm.

Easy availability of firearms is also a major contributor to **suicide** in the United States. Suicide is the third leading cause of death in persons age 15–24. Over half of all suicides are carried out with a firearm. If there is a gun available in a household, the risk of a person's committing suicide is five times higher than in households where no gun is present. Suicide will be discussed more completely in Chapter 15.

BUILDING YOUR Wellness Plan

Although it is impossible to guarantee that you can always stay safe, certain actions can help you increase the likelihood. After reading this chapter, you should understand the importance of the following concepts and be able to incorporate them into your personal wellness plan.

- Become a skilled driver and take all possible precautions in driving situations.
- Always wear a seat belt and never drink and drive.
- Create an emergency plan for your home and make sure the smoke detectors are working and your family has a first aid kit.
- Learn the facts about the causes of unintentional and intentional injury so you can make decisions about the level of risk you are willing to accept.
- If you participate in high-risk activities, make sure you have—and use—the proper safety equipment every time.
- Understand what cyberviolence is and be careful when communicating with strangers on the Internet.
- Identify actions you can take to decrease the likelihood of being the victim of an unintentional or intentional injury.
- Describe actions you can take to avoid injury from handguns and other weapons.

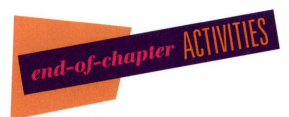

Weblinks

Aggressive Driving

AAA Foundation for Traffic Safety:
http://www.aaafoundation.org (search for
"aggressive driving quiz")

Graduated Driver Licensing

National Highway Traffic Safety Administration:
http://www.nhtsa.dot.gov (search for "saving
teenage lives")

Short-Answer Questions

1. List the four major categories of unintentional
   injuries and give an example of each.
2. Identify three actions bicyclists and motorcyclists
   can take to reduce their chances of injury.
3. List four population characteristics factors that affect
   rates of violence.
4. Identify two types of violence in which males are the
   most likely victims.
5. Identify two types of violence in which females are
   the most likely victims.

Discussion Questions

1. Explain several ways that you can protect yourself
   from motor vehicle crashes.
2. Explain the benefits and drawbacks of graduated
   driver licensing.
3. Discuss the ways age and gender are related to violence and intentional injury.
4. Describe the ways in which firearms contribute to
   violence.
5. Discuss your personal attitude regarding risk and
   how you make decisions about what risks to take.

Chapter Vocabulary

Using a separate sheet of paper, list and define the following terms:

date rape	statutory rape
Heimlich maneuver	unintentional injuries
homicide	violence
intentional injuries	violent victimization statistics
sexual assault	years of potential life lost

Application Activities

Language Arts Connection

Write a poem or essay from the viewpoint of the victim
of a violent crime.

Math Connection

Research homicide rates in the United States and in
three other industrialized countries. Construct a bar
graph to illustrate your findings. Do the same for suicide
rates. What differences did you discover? What do you
think the reasons are for any differences you find?

Social Studies Connection

Research and discuss how social environment affects
attitudes toward violent behavior. For example, if it is
socially acceptable for television programs and video
games to have graphic acts of violence, how does that
affect attitudes toward real-life violence? Consider how
income level might affect a person's attitudes toward
violence. What other sociological factors might influence attitudes toward violence?

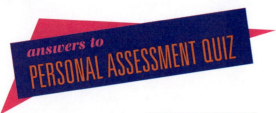

personal assessment: PREVENTING INJURY QUIZ

1. False
2. False
3. True
4. True
5. False

6. True
7. True
8. False
9. True
10. False

unit 4

Mental Health

Introduction

In earlier units, we focused a great deal of attention on ways that you can take care of your physical body. But you can't be truly healthy without being mentally healthy as well. Just as there are actions that help you stay physically healthy, there are things that you can do to keep yourself mentally healthy as well. As a teenager, you face many challenges on your way to becoming an adult. Dealing effectively with these challenges is a lot easier if you have a good wellness plan in place.

One thing is certain about being a teenager: you will encounter lots of changes during the next few years of your life. Often these changes can be very stressful. Learning how to cope with these changes in a healthy way can make your life (and the lives of those around you) much more satisfying. In this unit, you will find out how you can manage stress and develop good mental and emotional health. You will also find information that will help you find resources to help with your mental health needs and the needs of friends and family members who may need support to improve or maintain mental wellness.

chapter 12

Managing Stress

Kim has always considered herself very lucky. Even though she just moved to a new town and started school at East Central last fall, she found it easy to make friends and get involved in school activities. Her family is very supportive, and she usually does well in her classes. Lately though, Kim has been feeling really stressed out, and life just isn't as much fun as it used to be. Her algebra class this semester is really hard, and she's not doing very well. Besides that, most of her friends have a different lunch schedule than she does this semester, and she hasn't really made friends with anyone she feels comfortable eating lunch with. When she was selected as a "special news" reporter for the high school paper at the end of last semester, she was thrilled. But now, between trying to stay on top of all the work for her classes and writing her stories for the paper, she feels as if she has no free time at all. One of her friends just got a job at the local video store, and she wants Kim to apply for a job there, too. Kim talked to her family, and they said the decision was up to her. Kim thinks it would be fun to work at the video store, and she'd like to have the extra spending money. But she's barely getting everything done as it is. She really doesn't know how she could take on anything else.

chapter OBJECTIVES

When you finish this chapter, you should be able to:

- Explain the terms *stress*, *stressors*, *eustress*, *distress*, and *stress response*.
- Describe how stress affects your body and your immune system.
- Explain the health risks associated with continuous stress.
- List and describe the most common categories of stressors for teens.
- List and describe healthy techniques and strategies to manage stress.
- Create a personal plan for successfully managing stress.

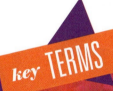

key TERMS

distress
eustress
fight-or-flight response
general adaptation syndrome (GAS)
hardiness
social support
stress
stressors
stress response

Introduction

Being a teenager can be hard. When you try to tell adults how you feel, it often seems as if they don't really understand. "What do you mean being a teenager is hard?" they ask. "This is the best time of your life! You'll never have this much free time and so little responsibility again. Enjoy it!" Some days you probably agree with what they say. Other days, you certainly don't feel very free. In fact, you may feel just the opposite. You feel pressure to perform well at school. Your feelings about your relationships with your family and friends are often like a roller-coaster ride. They can be up one day and down the next.

Many teens' lives are packed with activities. You might be in the band, on a sports team, and involved in other extracurricular activities at school. Perhaps you have a job after school or on the weekend. You might even have responsibilities most of your teachers and friends aren't aware of, such as helping a parent who's sick, or taking care of younger brothers and sisters.

You may wonder at times if there's something wrong with you because you feel so stressed out all the time. Your friends seem to handle life's challenges without getting upset. But you're having a hard time. Although learning to manage the challenges of life is a normal part of adolescence and even adulthood, at times it can be very confusing and frustrating. In this chapter, you'll learn what contributes to stress, how stress affects your body and your health, and what you can do to manage your stress so you can enjoy your life.

personal assessment: STRESS MANAGEMENT QUIZ

Before reading this chapter, see how much you already know about stress and managing stress. Read the questions below and, on a separate sheet of paper, answer True or False. The answers are located at the end of the chapter.

1. We would be healthier if we could avoid all types of stress.

2. Even something positive, such as being selected for an award, can be stressful.

3. The amount of stress you feel depends on how you perceive (view and interpret) a situation, not on the situation itself.

4. Your body responds differently to an imagined stressful situation than it does to an actual stressful situation.

5. The endocrine system controls breathing, heart rate, and blood pressure.

6. Stress hormones that circulate in your bloodstream can damage the body over a period of time.

7. At least two-thirds of all visits to health care providers may be for stress-related illnesses.

8. Feeling depressed, anxious, or upset causes immune system function to become stronger.

9. High levels of stress hormones in the body can increase learning and memory.

10. Getting plenty of sleep, eating a healthy diet, and exercising regularly can help you manage stress.

WHAT IS STRESS?

We hear about stress all the time. Chances are, you can't go through a day without hearing someone complain about stress. "I am so stressed!" or "I'm just so stressed out." You may even find yourself saying or thinking these words.

What do we really mean when we say we're "stressed"? Are we worried? Fearful? Nervous? Actually, **stress** refers to the physical and emotional states that we experience as a result of changes and challenges in our lives. These changes and challenges, which trigger a response in us, are called **stressors**. Stress can affect us physically, mentally, and

stress

the physical and emotional states experienced as a result of changes and challenges in our lives

stressors

situations that trigger physical and emotional reactions in our bodies emotionally. It can cause physical symptoms such as headaches, stomachaches, and difficulty sleeping. It can also disrupt mental functions, making it more likely that you will forget things or have difficulty concentrating. Stress can also affect your emotions. When you're feeling stressed, you may become more moody or be upset more easily than usual.

We usually think of stress as occurring only in response to a negative situation, such as getting a low grade or having a fight with a friend. But the same physical response can happen to us when something good happens. This type of stress is called **eustress**. For teens, eustress can occur when learning to drive, receiving an award, going to a big concert with friends, or going on a date. You can probably think of some times when you felt excited and had "butterflies" in your stomach. This is an example of experiencing eustress.

The negative form of stress also has a special name: **distress**. Distress can be caused by something that's not very important, such as losing your sunglasses when you're in a hurry. Or it can be a result of something major, such as the death of a grandparent or being arrested. An interesting and important fact is that the body responds physically in the same way to both eustress and distress.

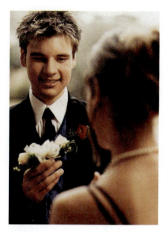

Dating can be a source of eustress for teens.

eustress

a form of stress that occurs in reaction to something we perceive as good

distress

a negative form of stress that occurs in reaction to something we perceive as bad

STRESSORS

What makes something a stressor? It is our *perception*—our attitude and the picture we create in our mind about a situation—that determines whether something is a stressor. Perceptions vary from one individual to another. The same event can be considered eustress by one person and distress by another. Let's look at an example. Terry is the pitcher for his high school baseball team. The bases are loaded and there are two outs. Terry must strike out the next batter, Jason, to win the game. Both Terry and Jason are likely to be experiencing some stress. Each may see the situation as either positive or negative—as an opportunity to win the game or to lose it. Depending on the outcome of the next pitch, one of them is likely to experience eustress while the other will probably experience distress.

Teens face many situations that can cause a variety of emotional responses. Suppose there is a final exam in math. Each student in the class will have a different view of this situation. Some students will feel completely prepared and experience little stress about the exam. Others will feel unprepared and very anxious. A few students will think they know the material well but will be afraid they'll forget everything when the test starts. A small number of students will be completely unprepared but will know they can't do anything about it now. They might decide to relax and not worry about the exam. The situation is exactly the same for all students; there is an important exam in math. But each student reacts according to his or her own individual perception of the circumstances.

Other factors also influence how we experience a possible stressor. These include our past experiences with similar situations, how we are feeling physically and emotionally, and even the timing of the situation. For example, a red light is not usually a major stressor for most people. But if you are late for work, the red light that delays you becomes a stressor.

Other important factors that influence your level of stress are your self-confidence and how prepared you are to handle life's events. Stress is greatly reduced when you have the necessary resources to prevent stressors from developing. Suppose you've agreed with your parents to pay your own car insurance. If you have enough money to pay the bill when it's due, you can take care of it without a second thought. If you don't have the money, however, the bill will become a stressor.

Major Categories of Stressors

Many life events can be stressors. There are three main categories of stressors: (1) personal, (2) interpersonal, and (3) environmental and societal.

Personal Stressors

There are many personal circumstances that teens might consider to be stressful. Being aware of potentially stressful circumstances can help you be prepared to respond to them. Figure 12-1 shows some of the personal stressors teens may experience.

Physical and Emotional Changes during Adolescence. Adolescence is a time of many rapid changes, both physical and emotional. Sometimes these changes occur so rapidly, you feel as if you're a stranger in your own body. Growing 4 inches in a few months or feeling happy one minute or sad the next can leave you feeling confused and stressed.

Academic Pressures and Demands. Many teens feel a great deal of pressure to perform well academically. This is true whether you're a student at the top of your class trying to do your best every time, a student near the bottom of the class just struggling to pass, or somewhere in between. It may feel as if you're always faced with homework and tests. The pressure to perform academically can create lots of stress. You may also be experiencing the stress of knowing that what you do now can affect your future college and career choices.

Competitive Pressure in Sports, Organizations, or Jobs. In almost every area of a typical teenager's life, there is some kind of competitive pressure. You may be a member of a sports team that competes each week. Or you may enter a project in a science fair to compete for a prize or submit a poem to the school paper. But competition may also be less

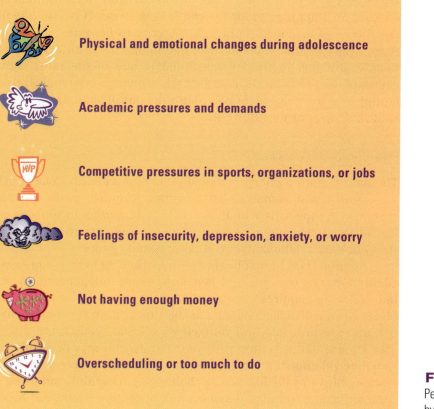

Figure 12-1
Personal stressors experienced by teens

obvious, such as competing for grades at school or attention at home. Competition can cause a great deal of stress, both when you win and when you lose.

Feelings of Insecurity, Depression, Anxiety, or Worry. Adolescence is a time when your emotions can be very unpredictable. One moment you're on top of the world and the next you're down in the dumps. You may feel insecure about the way your body looks, your physical coordination, or your academic performance. You may feel depressed or anxious about your social relationships. You may be worried you will disappoint important adults in your life. All these feelings are normal, but they can be quite stressful and can take the fun out of life.

Not Having Enough Money. How much money is enough for you? Many teens feel confused about money. Your parents may think you have too much money or that you don't spend it wisely. You, on the other hand, may think you don't have enough money to do and buy the things you want. This is an example of the importance of perception. In the case of money, your stress level is determined by your perception of your financial situation, not by how much money you actually have.

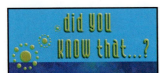

Overscheduling or Too Much to Do. Effective time management is one of the most important skills for controlling stress. It is also one of the most difficult to put into practice. It's easy to become involved in so many activities that you run from one to another with barely enough time to breathe. Being overscheduled is one of the most common causes of long-term stress. Learning when enough is enough and maintaining a balanced lifestyle will help you control your stress levels and contribute to your overall wellness.

Interpersonal Stressors

The most common interpersonal stressors for teens are related to family, friends, and romantic relationships. Conflicts with the people around you, especially with those who are important to you, can create lots of stress. During adolescence, many teens experience increased stress in their relationships with parents and siblings.

An important part of being a teen is learning to take more responsibility for your own life and becoming more independent. Increased independence requires changes in your relationships with your family. Moving toward independence can be threatening for both teens and parents. You probably find yourself wanting to spend more time with your friends and less time with your family. You may be involved in a romantic relationship for the first time. Balancing new and changing relationships in your life can be challenging. Learning and using good communication techniques and conflict resolution strategies (discussed in Unit 5) can help decrease the stress associated with relationships.

Another source of interpersonal stress is feeling lonely and isolated from other people. Sometimes it may seem as if you don't really fit anywhere. Humans are social beings. Feeling connected to the people around us is important for our emotional well-being. Developing the necessary emotional and social skills to make good connections with others is important for teens. Sometimes you may feel as if your friends are pressuring you to make choices that you know are not good for you, such as smoking, drinking alcohol, or taking drugs. Learning to take a stand for what you want, while still getting along with others, is an important task of adolescence.

Environmental and Societal Stressors

Some of the stressors we encounter are not directly related to us as individuals. These stressors affect everyone. Examples of environmental stressors include heat, cold, air pollution, overcrowded spaces, and noise. These factors exist in the background of our lives. We may not even notice them most of the time, but they can develop into major stressors. Think about what happens when the weather gets hot and humid. People tend to become more irritable, and tempers flare up more easily. Have you ever noticed how people act when there is overcrowding, such as in a bus or subway at rush hour? Or maybe you've been in a very noisy restaurant and don't notice how stressful it is until you walk out onto a quiet street. Think about the kinds of environmental stressors that you personally experience.

Living among other people means we're also exposed to societal stressors. One major societal stressor is discrimination. Being a target of discrimination can be very stressful because it affects many aspects of an individual's life. Discrimination can be based on race, religion, or even the way someone looks or dresses. Often, people make judgments about other people on the basis of what they see or think about them without ever getting to know them. People who are discriminated against in this manner may feel sad, depressed, or hopeless. They may also feel irritated and angry that they are being unfairly judged.

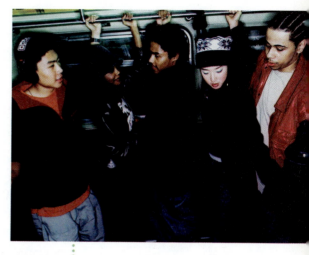

Violence is another major societal stressor. Teens may experience violence at school or in their community. Even if you have not personally been the victim of violence, you constantly receive news reports about national and world problems on TV and the radio and in magazines and newspapers. Sometimes it seems as if the news is nothing but a steady stream of wars, murders, kidnappings, floods, fires, and children who have been neglected or abused. Even when you don't know the people who experience these events, you may be affected by the news reports. It's natural to begin to wonder if the same terrible things might happen to you or the people you care about. Threats of terrorist attacks or war add to our stress levels, even if they never occur to us. Limiting your exposure to reports about distressing events that you can't do anything about is a healthy way to decrease stress. It's important to be informed about current events, but it's also important to take care of yourself and minimize your stress level.

Personally experiencing a traumatic event can result in **post-traumatic stress disorder**, or **PTSD**. When this occurs, memories of the original event are played over and over in the mind. It is as if the person relives the event again each time it is remembered. The traumatic event may have happened to the person directly or been witnessed by the person. The event can even be a natural disaster that happens to an entire community, such as a tornado, or a violent act, such as a shooting.

post-traumatic stress disorder (PTSD)

a mental disturbance that results from experiencing or witnessing a traumatic event, which is replayed over and over in the mind after the event is over

---

✤ teen forum ✤

Societal Stressors

How do you think societal stressors like discrimination and threats of violence affect teenagers? If discrimination or threats of violence occur in a school setting, how do you think teachers and administration should handle them? Is there anything teenagers themselves can do to reduce or eliminate these stressors? If so, what could they do? Do you think teenagers in most schools in the United States have experiences similar to yours about discrimination and violence? Can you support your opinion with any facts?

real teens

Kevin had a summer job as a lifeguard at the local public swimming pool. He was on the lifeguard stand in the shallow end of the pool when suddenly there was a lot of commotion at the other end of the pool. He saw two other lifeguards pulling a young girl out of the water at the deep end. He immediately blew his whistle and got everyone out of the pool. As he was trying to control the crowd of curious swimmers, he could see the lifeguards performing CPR on the girl. The emergency medical services team finally arrived to take over the rescue efforts. Unfortunately, the girl could not be revived. Kevin was not on duty at the deep end of the pool, nor did he actively participate in the CPR efforts. But three months later, he still has nightmares about the drowning. He wakes up in a cold sweat wondering if there was something he could have done to prevent the girl's death.

---

homeostasis

the state of the body during relaxation when the body is functioning normally in a stable, balanced state

stress response

the physiological reactions that occur in the body when a stressor is experienced

general adaptation syndrome (GAS)

the body's physiological response to continuous stress; it includes three phases: alarm, resistance, and exhaustion

HOW STRESS AFFECTS YOUR BODY

When your body is at rest and there are no special challenges, difficulties, or exciting events to deal with, it is in **homeostasis**. During homeostasis, the body has plenty of resources to maintain normal body functions and responses. But when you experience a stressor, a chain of reactions begins to take place in your body. This is known as the **stress response**.

One of the early stress researchers, Hans Selye, suggested that the body's response to a stressor occurs in three phases. He called this response sequence the **general adaptation syndrome (GAS)**, shown in Figure 12-2.

1. *Alarm.* The brain alerts the body that extra resources are needed to deal with a challenge to homeostasis. Various body systems respond quickly to provide the needed resources. If the stressful situation doesn't last long, the body returns to homeostasis.

2. *Resistance.* If the stressful situation continues, the body doesn't return to homeostasis. Physiological changes take place to allow it to continue to respond to the stressor. The body is remarkable in its ability to cope with extended stress, but it can't continue to produce enough resources to meet extra demands indefinitely.

3. *Exhaustion.* The body gradually becomes exhausted from trying to keep up with the increased demands and it eventually breaks down. How long it takes for this breakdown to occur and what specific form it takes vary from individual to individual. All individuals, however, experience a decline of immune system function. This is serious because an individual with an impaired immune system is less able to resist disease.

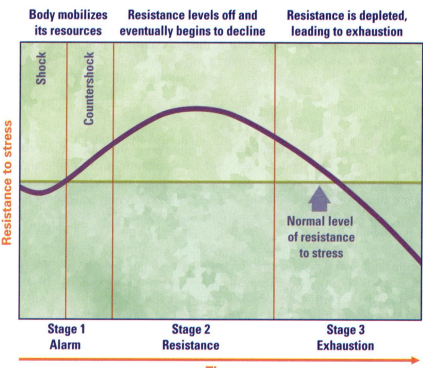

Figure 12-2
General adaptation syndrome

During the alarm reaction phase of GAS, the body prepares for a **fight-or-flight response**. This response was the kind needed by our ancient ancestors. Their stressors, such as wild animals, required them to either fight for their lives or run from the scene. We may no longer face wild animals, but our bodies respond to stressors in the same way they have for centuries.

Two major systems influence the physiological reactions of the body under stress: the nervous system and the endocrine system.

fight-or-flight response

the response of the nervous and endocrine systems to supply the body with energy to fight back or escape from a stressor

take it on home

Interview members of your family about what they consider to be their most common stressors. Into what categories do the stressors fall? Is there a difference between the type of stressors experienced by the adults in your family and those experienced by the teenagers and children? Are there actions you and your family can take to help reduce the stressors?

Together, they prepare you for whatever action is needed to face a stressor. An important fact is that stressors cause the same physiological response in the body whether they are real or imagined. This is why constant worry and negative thoughts can be just as unhealthy as real events.

The Nervous System

Your brain acts as the signal-caller for the rest of the body. It interprets every situation you encounter and decides how your body should respond. If an emergency response is needed, the brain immediately alerts the rest of the body that special action is required. The nervous system relays these messages from the brain to the various parts of the body.

The **autonomic nervous system** plays an important role in stress responses. This part of the nervous system controls basic functions such as breathing, heartbeat, blood pressure, and digestion. These are involuntary actions, actions that happen automatically without our thinking about them.

The autonomic nervous system has two main branches, the **sympathetic nervous system** and the **parasympathetic nervous system**. The role of the sympathetic nervous system is to "rev up" the systems of the body and prepare them to respond to the challenges of stressors. When the sympathetic nervous system is activated, all the energy resources of the body are put on alert and made ready to respond.

The role of the other branch, the parasympathetic nervous system, is to "cool down" the body after the challenge has passed. This system is in control when our bodies are in a relaxed state of normal functioning.

The Endocrine System

The **endocrine system** consists of glands, tissues, and cells that produce hormones. **Hormones** are chemical messengers that help regulate bodily processes. When the sympathetic nervous system responds to a stress alert, it triggers actions in the endocrine system. Certain hormones are associated with the stress response. These hormones target specific cells in the body and provide them with "instructions" for the necessary response. The pituitary, thyroid, and adrenal glands, with the assistance of other parts of the endocrine system, produce most of the so-called stress hormones. When we are confronted with a stressor, these hormones cause a number of changes in the body:

- Faster heartbeat
- Faster breathing
- Narrower blood vessels
- Slower digestion
- Tensed muscles

autonomic nervous system

the division of the nervous system that controls basic body processes that are largely involuntary, such as breathing, heartbeat, blood pressure, and digestion

sympathetic nervous system

the branch of the autonomic nervous system that responds to a stressor by accelerating body processes

parasympathetic nervous system

the branch of the autonomic nervous system that slows down body processes and returns the body to homeostasis after a stressful situation has passed

endocrine system

a system of glands, tissues, and cells that produce hormones to help regulate bodily processes

hormones

chemical messengers produced by the endocrine system to help regulate bodily processes

These physical changes are preparing the body to fight or run. Figure 12-3 illustrates how the body responds in a fight-or-flight situation. You may have heard of adrenaline. This is one of the stress hormones that enables people to do some amazing things in an emergency, such as lift a heavy object off a loved one or run a long distance for help.

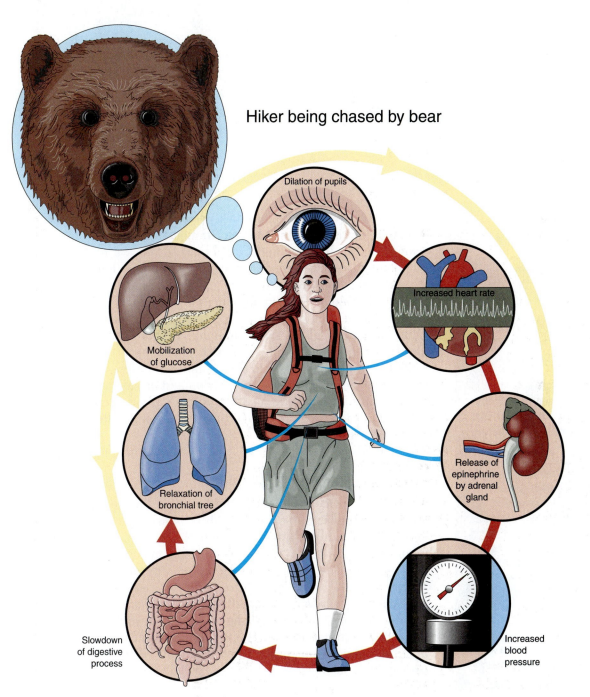

Hiker being chased by bear

Dilation of pupils

Increased heart rate

Mobilization of glucose

Release of epinephrine by adrenal gland

Relaxation of bronchial tree

Increased blood pressure

Slowdown of digestive process

Figure 12-3 Fight-or-flight response: how the body reacts to stressful situations

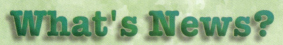

What's News?

Studies have shown that high levels of stress hormones can kill brain cells in the hippocampus (a portion of the brain) that are critical to learning and memory. In one animal study, rats exposed to continuous stress for six months lost as much as 50% of all brain cells. This was twice as many lost cells as occurred in rats that were not exposed to stress. Other studies report that high levels of stress hormones seem to interfere with memory. Normal memory function returns when the levels of stress hormones return to normal. This may be one explanation for test anxiety. The rise in stress hormones causes students to temporarily forget information they actually know. Relaxing and staying calm might be good ways to "study" for a test!

HOW STRESS AFFECTS YOUR HEALTH

The stressors our ancestors faced may have threatened their survival, but they were resolved rather quickly. Today our stressors are different. Although they may not threaten our immediate survival, many are continuous. In fact, continuous stressors are so much a part of our daily lives that we barely even notice them. And it is these long-term, continuous stressors that are most likely to affect our health.

The hormones the body produces in the presence of a stressor are designed to help us respond quickly to short-term stressors. But these same hormones can do serious damage to the organs and systems if they stay in the body too long. One of the systems most affected by stress is the immune system. The stress hormones interfere with its function, making us more susceptible to infection and disease. A weak immune system can make existing health problems worse, increase the likelihood of catching the common cold, and even increase the risk of a heart attack and cancer.

Stress As a Medical Problem

Stress has become a major medical problem in the United States. It is a leading contributor, either directly or indirectly, to the major causes of death and to many illnesses and diseases. Effective stress management could play a big role in decreasing medical costs, increasing work productivity, and improving the quality of life for millions of Americans.

Research shows that not only major stressors—such as the death of someone close to you, personal illness, or severe financial difficulties—cause health problems. The small hassles of daily living also result in stress-related problems. A series of small stressors can add up until something quite insignificant makes the load seem more than a person can handle.

...did you know that...?

It is estimated that between two-thirds and three-quarters of all visits to primary care physicians in the United States are due to an illness related to stress. Some medical experts say the actual number might be closer to 90%! It is estimated that the medical costs of treating stress-related illnesses in the United States are more than $1 billion per year. This estimate doesn't even include job-related costs such as high absenteeism, stress-related work injuries, and reduced productivity on the job. It also doesn't include the personal and emotional costs to the people who experience the problems and to those close to them.

What's News?

An exciting new field called **psychoneuro-immunology**, or **PNI** for short, studies the inter-relationships among the emotions, the brain and nervous system, and the immune system. PNI is still in its infancy, but through research in this area, we are learning about the direct connections between the brain, the emotions, and the immune system. According to Candace Pert, one of the leading researchers, chemical messengers called peptides communicate with cells throughout the body as a result of feeling an emotion. Your body systems actually talk among themselves in response to emotions. Early indications are that stress associated with negative emotions interferes with proper immune system function. The good news is that experiencing positive emotions may improve immune system function.

PROTECTING YOURSELF FROM THE EFFECTS OF STRESS

It is impossible to avoid stress completely. In fact, we wouldn't want to, even if we could. A certain amount of stress keeps life interesting, challenging, and fulfilling. If we never experienced stressful situations, we would almost certainly be bored and would miss opportunities to learn and grow.

The optimal amount of stress varies from person to person. The question is, How much stress is best? We know that too much stress over a long period of time can seriously damage our bodies. It can also result in our feeling annoyed, frustrated, irritable, and unhappy with our lives. Finding the optimal amount of stress means balancing life's challenges with the resources you have to meet those challenges.

There are certain factors that can protect you from experiencing more stress than you can handle. They don't help you avoid stressors, but they can help you cope with them when stress does occur. Three of the most important protection factors are social support, specific personality traits, and a set of characteristics called hardiness.

Social Support

Social support is one of the best protections against feeling overwhelmed by stressful circumstances. Having good social support means having a network of family, friends, and acquaintances who care about you and will provide assistance if you need it. You don't have to face stressful events alone. And, through other people, you have access to more resources. Good social support appears to reduce the likelihood that reactions to stressful events will result in illness. People who have good social support seem to have better health and well-being, whether or not they experience much stress, than do people without much social support.

psychoneuroimmunology (PNI)
the study of the interrelationships among the emotions, brain, nervous system, and immune system

social support
aid or assistance provided by people who care about you

✧ teen forum ✧

Getting Connected

Sociologists and health experts are concerned about the state of social connectedness in the United States. Compared with previous generations, Americans today are more likely to live alone and less likely to have close family ties, be married, or belong to a social organization. People in countries that have close family ties and strong social connections, such as Greece, Spain, and Italy, have higher life expectancies than people in the United States. This difference in life expectancies is despite the fact that in the United States we spend far more money per person on health care than any other country.

- Do you think it's possible that having good social support and feeling a sense of connection and belonging is the best health insurance we can have?
- Do you believe there is a lack of social connectedness in the United States?
- Do you think connectedness affects physical health? If you do, what could you do to help build stronger connections with your family, friends, and community?

Personality Traits

Certain personality traits are believed to put people at increased risk for stress-related problems. Other traits seem to offer protection against stress-related problems. Falling into the first group are people with what are called Type A personality traits. These include being results oriented, a perfectionist, and strongly motivated by the need to succeed. People with Type A personalities are often in a hurry and can be controlling. They are usually very competitive and may exhibit impatience, anger, and hostility, especially if they don't get their way or are hampered in their efforts to achieve.

In contrast, people with Type B personality traits have a more relaxed attitude about life. They usually work and play at their own pace and don't feel the need to compete with others. They tend to take life as it comes and "go with the flow." It isn't surprising that, given the same situation, a Type A may find it a major stressor while a Type B hardly notices it.

Some studies show that the Type A personality traits of anger, cynicism, and hostility are linked to an increased risk of heart disease. Personality traits are at least partly a result of experiences and learned behaviors. Consequently, individuals can learn to reduce their Type A personality traits and become better at handling stress. Even if they can't change their basic personality type, they can make an effort to adopt behaviors to decrease stress in their daily lives.

Hardiness

Psychologist Suzanne Kobasa identified certain attitudes and beliefs that protect us from the negative consequences of stressful situations.

She used the term **hardiness** to describe the resilience or "bounce-back" quality some people display in the face of stressors. Kobasa identified three key characteristics of these individuals, which can be remembered as the 3 Cs:

1. *Challenge.* Hardy individuals don't feel overwhelmed by potentially stressful situations. Instead, they view them as challenges they can handle.

2. *Control.* Hardy individuals believe they have some control over situations. They don't feel helpless in the face of a challenge. They accept responsibility for their own behavior and believe they can make a difference with their own actions.

3. *Commitment.* Hardy individuals are committed to something outside of themselves. This might be a person, religion, community group, or cause that's important to them. They believe their lives have meaning and purpose.

MANAGING STRESS

When you encounter a situation that routinely causes stress for you, there are several ways you can respond. Start by asking yourself these questions:

- Is it possible to reduce or eliminate my exposure to the stressor?
- What do I have control over?
- What do I have to accept?
- Is there anything I can do to change the situation?
- Can I change my perception of the situation?
- What coping mechanisms and resources do I have available to deal with the situation?
- With my available coping mechanisms and resources, what action can I take?

You can prepare yourself to handle unavoidable stress by having a variety of coping strategies available. Coping strategies are habits and behaviors that help you manage stress and make the best of any situation. You might want to think of these strategies as tools you store in a stress-reduction toolbox. When faced with a stressor, you select the best tool to deal with the situation. All the strategies discussed in the next sections are simple and inexpensive. They would be good additions for your stress-reduction toolbox.

Practice Good Self-Care

Practicing good self-care reduces the chance you will perceive situations as stressors. It also helps your immune system function at its best when faced with stressors. Three important self-care activities are getting enough sleep, eating nutritiously, and participating in regular physical activity.

hardiness
resilience when confronted with stressors identified by the characteristics of challenge, control, and commitment

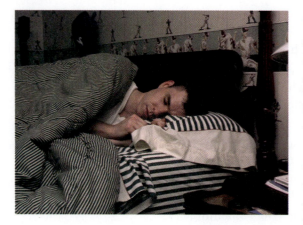

Sleep

Studies have revealed that many Americans are sleep deprived. It is especially important for teens to get adequate sleep in order for their bodies to function well. It's amazing how much better you'll feel, both emotionally and physically, when you get enough sleep. Try it!

Healthy Eating Habits

When you're busy and feeling stressed, you may eat too much without thinking, or you may even forget to eat. It's easy to grab whatever food is available and not pay much attention to what you're putting in your body. But food provides the fuel our bodies need to function effectively. By eating healthy foods, you give your body high-performance fuel to get you through your daily activities. Watch your caffeine intake too; a little caffeine won't hurt you, but too much can add to your feelings of stress.

Physical Activity

Putting your body in motion is a good way to release stress. Physical activity gives you time to unwind and relax. Try taking a 10–20 minute walk when you're feeling stressed. In addition to releasing stress, exercise gives you a "time-out" so you can reframe a stressful situation in a more positive light and develop an effective response.

Learn to Relax

There are a number of strategies you can use to help yourself relax. Some methods require physical actions; others have you focus on your mental and emotional state.

Deep Breathing

One of the simplest stress management tools is to pay attention to your breathing. Taking slow, deep breaths and concentrating on inhaling and exhaling can produce a calming effect on your entire body. Many of us are in the habit of breathing shallowly and have to retrain ourselves to breathe deeply. You can tell if you are taking a deep breath by placing your hand on your abdomen. Does it rise and fall with each breath? If it doesn't, your breathing is too shallow. Taking 10 to 20 deep breaths can increase your ability to cope with a stressful situation.

Progressive Relaxation

Progressive relaxation requires a bit of practice, but it is quite simple to learn. It involves tightening and then relaxing the various muscle groups. Begin with your head, face, and neck. Tighten the muscles, hold for a count of five, and then relax. Do the same thing with your shoulders, arms, and fingers. Gradually work your way down through the remaining muscle groups to your toes, tightening and then relaxing them one by one.

Visualization and Guided Imagery

Visualization is the creation of a mental picture to calm and focus yourself. Picture yourself in a pleasant environment or succeeding at something important to you. Visualization is something that you control yourself. In guided imagery, you visualize a mental picture as it is described aloud or "guided" by someone else. Athletes often use visualization and guided imagery to improve their performance. Suppose you are a tennis player who gets really stressed during a match. You could use visualization to see yourself moving through the match successfully and easily. Or your coach could lead you through a guided imagery to help you focus and concentrate on maintaining good form during each stroke.

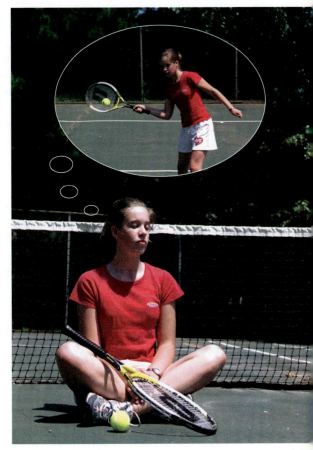

Meditation

The goal of meditation is to produce a state of relaxation, inner peace, and harmony. It usually involves sitting quietly and focusing on a word or image of your own choosing, while taking slow, deep breaths. Other meditative practices involve concentrating on relaxed breathing combined with a physical action repeated in a specific way, such as the practice of yoga or tai chi.

Enjoy Life

There is a bumper sticker with the slogan "Enjoy life. This is not a dress rehearsal." We often rush through life as if simply getting to the end of the day is our only goal. Someone once commented that 99% of people go through life like rats in a maze. The other 1% go through life amazed. We can enjoy our lives much more fully, and reduce our stress levels at the same time, if we choose to be among the 1% who go through life amazed. Try the following techniques to help you enjoy life more.

Mindful Awareness

Have you ever noticed how you can go through a good part of the day without ever really noticing your surroundings? Mindful awareness is really paying attention to each thing you experience and being aware of the present moment. For example, when you're eating, give your full attention to the food. When you're talking to a friend, pay careful attention to what your friend is saying. When you are outside, notice the sights, smells, and sounds around you. Practicing mindful awareness helps you experience life more fully.

Time Management

Good time management is a key factor in avoiding stress. Start by identifying your priorities. What is most important to you? Arrange your schedule so you spend time on the things most important to you, and allow yourself some free time, as shown in Figure 12-4. You may discover that you prefer spending more time with family and friends and less time watching television and playing video games. When the way you spend your time is in balance with your priorities, you will feel less stressed.

Time-outs

Sometimes we just need a time-out. This is when you should take a break. Spend some time with a friend. Do an activity you enjoy just for the pleasure of it. Even breaks as short as five minutes can make a

Friday		Saturday	
8 am	School	8 am	
9 am		9 am	Ballet class
10 am	Biology test	10 am	
11 am		11 am	Mow the lawn
12 pm		12 pm	
1 pm	Meet w/ guidance counselor	1 pm	Library with Rob to work on English report
2 pm		2 pm	
3 pm	Workout with Sarah	3 pm	
4 pm		4 pm	
5 pm	Dinner with Mom	5 pm	RELAX!
6 pm	Babysit for the Smiths	6 pm	
7 pm		7 pm	
8 pm		8 pm	
9 pm		9 pm	

Figure 12-4 Managing your time effectively and giving yourself time to relax may take a little work but can help reduce stress.

major difference in your attitude and increase your enjoyment of life. They give you a chance to relax and return refreshed and ready to face new challenges.

Humor and Laughter

Many studies have shown that laughter increases the efficiency of the immune system and lowers the levels of stress hormones. Laughter is even good exercise for your heart, lungs, and muscles. Try this activity: Pair up with a friend and just start laughing. It doesn't matter what you're laughing about, just concentrate on each other's faces and laugh for at least one full minute. Then notice how you feel when you finish.

BUILDING YOUR Wellness Plan

From the information you learned in this chapter, you can see that stress has a major effect on your health. Learning to manage stress effectively is one of the most beneficial things you can do to improve your health both now and in the future. When stress is reduced, life is more fun. Use the information in this chapter to develop a personal stress management plan:

- Identify your own stressors.
- Think about how you perceive life's problems and challenges. How can you approach them more positively?
- Learn some new behaviors to protect yourself from the negative effects of stress.
- Select coping strategies for your stress reduction toolbox.

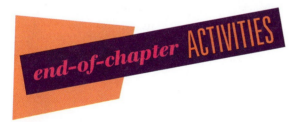

end-of-chapter ACTIVITIES

🖱 Weblinks

Humor and Laughter

The Humor Project: **http://www.humorproject.com**

Personality Traits

Discovery Health:
   http://discoveryhealth.queendom.com (click on
   Type A Personality Test)

Stress

American Psychological Association:
   http://www.apa.org (search for "stress")

Teen Health Interactive Network:
   http://library.thinkquest.org (search for "stress")

☀ Short-Answer Questions

1. Define the terms *stress*, *stressors*, *eustress*, *distress*, and *stress response* and give examples of each.
2. List the major physiological effects of stress on the body.
3. Describe the three phases of the general adaptation syndrome.
4. Identify the major categories of stressors and give an example of each.
5. List several ways to reduce stress or manage it more effectively.

☀ Discussion Questions

1. Discuss the effects of stress on Americans in today's society.
2. Explain several reasons why continuous stress can be harmful to your health.
3. Discuss the most common personal stressors for teenagers in America today.
4. Explain how environmental and societal stressors might affect adolescents.
5. Construct a personal plan for managing stress successfully.

☀ Chapter Vocabulary

Using a separate sheet of paper, list and define the following terms:

distress	hardiness
eustress	social support
fight-or-flight response	stress
general adaptation syndrome (GAS)	stressors
	stress response

☀ Application Activities

Language Arts Connection

1. Imagine you have been selected to write an article in a teen magazine about psychoneuroimmunology. Research and write an article about this subject that includes the most important information readers should know. Write in a style that will both interest and inform a teen audience.
2. Select a situation you currently find stressful. Write an essay about the situation, including the actions you could take to help resolve the situation or make it less stressful.

Social Studies Connection

Research the societal stressors a particular group of teenagers is likely to experience. Possible groups to consider are physically challenged teens, mentally challenged teens, minority teens, overweight teens, economically disadvantaged teens. Suggest ways of reducing the impact of the societal stressors on these individuals.

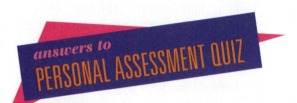

answers to PERSONAL ASSESSMENT QUIZ

personal assessment: STRESS MANAGEMENT QUIZ

1. False	6. True
2. True	7. True
3. True	8. False
4. False	9. False
5. False	10. True

13

Mental and Emotional Health

Deanna has been moody and withdrawn for the past few days. Her parents have asked her what's wrong and have tried to get her to talk about what's bothering her. But she just says, "It's nothing," and goes to her room and closes the door. The truth is she's faced with a big problem, and she doesn't know what to do. She's been close friends with three other girls since elementary school. They've always gotten along well and enjoyed doing the same things. But lately her friends don't seem to be the same. This coming weekend they want Deanna to sneak out of the house after her parents go to sleep and meet them at the apartment of some guys they met at the mall. Her friends don't really know these guys, and besides, Deanna's town has a teen curfew. The whole situation makes Deanna really uneasy. She knows her parents would be disappointed and furious if they found out. For the most part, Deanna gets along with her parents, and she doesn't want to get into trouble. But her friends are saying she's just "chicken" and say, "You never want to do anything fun with us anymore."

What should Deanna do?
How would a mentally and emotionally healthy teenager respond?

chapter *OBJECTIVES*

When you finish this chapter, you should be able to:

- Define mental and emotional health.
- Explain how mental and emotional health are related.
- Identify several factors that affect mental and emotional health.
- Describe Maslow's hierarchy of needs.
- Describe several characteristics of mentally and emotionally healthy individuals.
- Describe several commonly used defense mechanisms.
- Create a list of ways you can improve your mental and emotional health.

key TERMS

defense mechanisms
emotionally healthy
identity
Maslow's hierarchy of needs
mentally healthy
resiliency
self-actualization

Introduction

If you ask a group of teenagers what they want most in life, a common answer is "I just want to be happy." If you ask a group of parents what they want most for their children, they are likely to answer, "I just want them to be happy." But what is happiness? And how can you take actions in your life that will lead to happiness?

Happiness has a different meaning for each of us. We often discover it when we are least focused on finding it. We might say happiness comes from living life in ways that are meaningful and satisfying. We know that our mental and emotional health have a lot to do with how much pleasure and enjoyment we get from our daily lives. Everything is just much more fun when we're mentally active and alert, when we feel good about ourselves, and when our relationships with other people are going smoothly. And good mental and emotional health can have a major effect on our physical health as well.

So just what does it mean to be mentally and emotionally healthy? It's much easier to determine when people are *not* mentally or emotionally healthy than it is to determine when they *are* healthy. This chapter explores questions such as, What are the characteristics of a mentally and emotionally healthy individual? and What actions can you take to become more mentally and emotionally healthy?

personal assessment: MENTAL AND EMOTIONAL HEALTH QUIZ

Before reading this chapter, use a separate sheet of paper to respond to the statements below according to the following scale: Strongly Agree, Agree, Disagree, Strongly Disagree. See the interpretation of results at the end of the chapter.

1. I am realistic about a situation and whether it can be changed.

2. I make decisions about people on their own merits, instead of by their race, religion, or style of dress.

3. I spend a lot of my time worrying about what other people think about me.

4. I make my own decisions and do not rely on my friends to decide things for me.

5. I feel lonely when I am by myself.

6. For the most part, I like myself.

7. When I do poorly at one thing, I feel as if I am a failure at everything.

8. Some people are creative and some are not—I'm not.

9. I like to be involved in things that make me feel as if I have a purpose.

10. My basic needs of food, water, shelter, safety, and security are met.

DEFINING MENTAL AND EMOTIONAL HEALTH

What is the difference between the terms *mental health* and *emotional health*? A person who is **mentally healthy** perceives reality in terms of facts and can respond appropriately to the challenges that life presents. Being mentally healthy means being able to evaluate a situation and interpret its meaning. Mentally healthy people can solve most of the problems of everyday life. People who are **emotionally healthy** are in touch with their entire range of feelings. They can express those feelings appropriately even when they are upset. Their feelings don't interfere with their ability to think clearly. Although mental and emotional health are not exactly the same, the terms are often used interchangeably, and they are used interchangeably in this chapter.

Being mentally and emotionally healthy does *not* mean that you never feel angry, sad, depressed, lonely, or frustrated. And it doesn't mean that you never need help and support from other people. We all have times when we feel overwhelmed by the demands of life. We may be faced with a difficult situation we've never encountered before. Sometimes our emotions are unpredictable. This is especially true for teens. Experiencing a wide range of feelings, including negative ones, is normal for everyone. It doesn't mean that a person is not emotionally

mentally healthy

refers to a person who has the ability to perceive reality in terms of facts and can respond appropriately to the challenges that life presents

emotionally healthy

refers to a person who is in touch with his or her entire range of feelings and can express those feelings in an appropriate way healthy. What counts is being able to manage your feelings so they don't interfere with problem solving, decision making, and your ability to enjoy life most of the time.

Both internal and external factors contributed to creating the person you are today. Internal factors include genetics, personality, and physical health. External factors are the experiences that you've had as you've progressed on your life journey. Some factors are within your control; others are not. You may live in a situation in which you are safe and well cared for by the adults in your life. Unfortunately, not all teens experience this ideal environment.

Regardless of your past experiences or current situation, you can still become mentally and emotionally healthy because many of the characteristics of mentally and emotionally healthy people can be learned. Researchers have been studying a characteristic they call resiliency. **Resiliency** is the ability to bounce back after experiencing distressing or traumatic events. Resilient individuals are able to trust and form caring relationships, have good problem-solving skills, are independent and persistent, and believe their lives have meaning and purpose. Experts believe that each of us has a natural capacity for resiliency that can be strengthened with training.

MASLOW'S HIERARCHY OF NEEDS

Human beings have various needs that must be met in order for them to enjoy physical and mental well-being. Psychologist Abraham Maslow researched these needs and ranked them in order of importance for our survival. These are organized in the shape of a pyramid called **Maslow's hierarchy of needs**, as shown in Figure 13-1. Maslow believed that people must satisfy their most basic needs before they can fully satisfy higher-level needs. Basic physical needs—such as food, water, and shelter—form the base of the pyramid. Once those needs are satisfied, an individual can focus on developing a sense of safety and security, a sense of love and belonging, and good self-esteem. At the top of the pyramid is a quality Maslow called **self-actualization**. He defined this as functioning at or near one's optimal level of mental and emotional health.

Have you ever thought about what it would be like to be homeless? You would probably spend lots of time trying to meet your basic needs for food, water, and shelter. Where would you get your next meal? Would there be a place to stay out of the weather? Where could you use the bathroom? Is there someplace you could take a shower? Most of us take our basic needs for granted. But in many places around the world and even in this country, there are people who face these problems daily. Struggling to meet basic needs doesn't leave much time for addressing the needs on the higher levels of the pyramid.

As you move toward adulthood, you will have increasing responsibilities for meeting the needs Maslow described. Eventually you will

resiliency

the ability to bounce back after experiencing distressing or traumatic events

Maslow's hierarchy of needs

a well-known representation of human needs progressing from most to least urgent; these needs include physical needs, safety and security, love and belonging, self-esteem, and self-actualization

self-actualization

the highest level in Maslow's hierarchy of needs, representing an optimal level of mental and emotional function

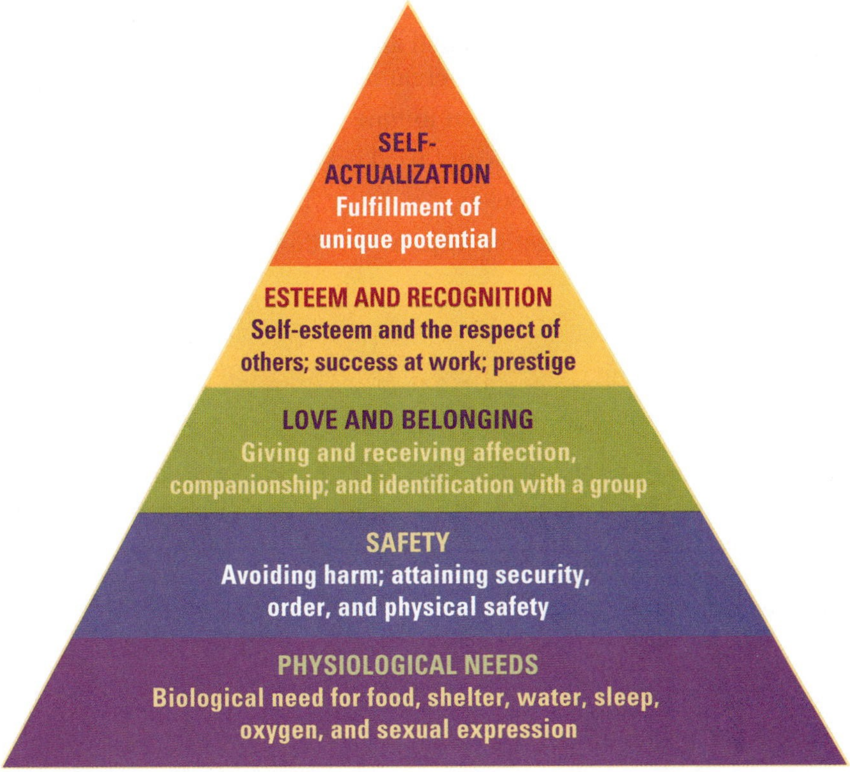

SELF-ACTUALIZATION
Fulfillment of unique potential

ESTEEM AND RECOGNITION
Self-esteem and the respect of others; success at work; prestige

LOVE AND BELONGING
Giving and receiving affection, companionship; and identification with a group

SAFETY
Avoiding harm; attaining security, order, and physical safety

PHYSIOLOGICAL NEEDS
Biological need for food, shelter, water, sleep, oxygen, and sexual expression

Figure 13-1
Maslow's hierarchy of needs. Maslow argued that if basic needs are not met, individuals are unlikely to be able to meet higher-order needs.

have to provide your own food, water, and shelter. You will have to find ways to ensure your safety and security. You will be on your own to establish relationships to meet your needs for love and belonging. Your self-esteem will be related to your success in taking care of your own needs as well as to what you accomplish and contribute to others. As you move closer to an optimal level of mental and emotional health, you will be well on your way to achieving self-actualization.

DEVELOPING YOUR IDENTITY

Identity refers to all the characteristics that make you who you are. Your early identity was influenced by family members and other people who played significant roles in your life. These people served as models for your thoughts, attitudes, and behaviors. As a result, your identity as a child was probably largely a reflection of how other people related and responded to you. It was also shaped by your personal experiences and the physical and social environment in which you lived.

As a teen, you have more control over the continuing development of your identity. You are now shaping your own attitudes, beliefs, and values and are determining your purpose for living. And your identity will continue to develop as you enter adulthood. It will reflect the

identity

the recognition and expression of your uniqueness as a person, including your attitudes, beliefs, and behaviors experiences you have and the choices you make. A strong, healthy identity plays an important role in mental and emotional health. Some of the most important tasks involved in creating your identity include:

- Recognizing what makes you unique
- Identifying your strengths and weaknesses
- Defining your role in society
- Learning to form relationships with others without losing your sense of self

CHARACTERISTICS OF THE MENTALLY AND EMOTIONALLY HEALTHY PERSON

Maslow and other researchers have identified characteristics of people who are mentally and emotionally healthy. Think of people you know who appear to be mentally and emotionally healthy. As you read through the next sections, think about whether those people possess the qualities listed in Figure 13-2.

Realistic

People who are realistic see the world in terms of facts. They understand what they can change and what they must accept. Suppose you were badly injured in a car accident. You were fortunate to survive, but now you walk with a limp. This fact cannot be changed. It's something

✔	Realistic
✔	Accepting
✔	Autonomous
✔	Authentic
✔	Capable of intimacy
✔	Creative
✔	Good self-esteem
✔	Have value and purpose for living
✔	Optimistic
✔	Comfortable being alone

Figure 13-2
Characteristics of mentally and emotionally healthy people

you must accept. People sometimes stare at you, but you have learned to remind yourself about how fortunate you are to be able to walk. You have decided not to let the actions of others spoil your day.

Accepting

Being accepting means having positive but realistic feelings about yourself and others. People who are accepting don't demand perfection in themselves or in others. They understand that not everything in life will be to their liking. They can handle it when things don't go their way. Suppose a group of your friends wants to spend time at the music store, but you really want to go see a baseball game. You can accept the fact that not everyone wants to do the same thing at the same time. You feel free to choose between going with your friends to the music store or going to the baseball game by yourself. Either way, you aren't upset about the situation. People who are accepting also respect differences and value diversity among people. Their opinions about people are based on individual characteristics, not on group stereotypes.

Autonomous

Autonomous means being inner directed and not controlled by the desires or wishes of other people. It is making choices on the basis of your own values and beliefs rather than following the crowd or trying to please other people. In a few years, you'll be making choices about your future. You might decide to attend college. Or you might choose to go right to work. You might even decide to move to another state or country to pursue a dream that's important to you. You can take advice from others, but the choice will be yours. Suppose you have an uncle who really wants you to stay in your hometown and work for him in his furniture store. The money would be good, but you really want to move to the West Coast, work at a restaurant to support yourself, and try to develop a career as a musician. Making good decisions for yourself in such situations will depend on your ability to develop a strong inner compass that you trust.

Authentic

Authentic people are not afraid to be themselves. They are genuine and able to express their thoughts and feelings honestly. We might describe them by the phrase "What you see is what you get." Being authentic means being "real" and not pretending to be someone you aren't just to gain approval from others. Although it is normal for teens to be somewhat self-conscious, people who are authentic don't spend much time worrying about what other people think of them. A wise person once said, "We would spend less time worrying about what other people think about us if we knew how seldom they think about us!" Although it may seem as if everyone is focused on you, they probably aren't.

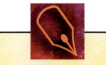

take it on home

Is there someone in your family who seems to be very happy and satisfied with life? Spend some time talking with this person. Ask for permission to conduct an informal interview and find out what qualities he or she believes are most important for happiness and mental and emotional health. Write a summary of what you learn from this experience and include it in your Health Folio.

Capable of Intimacy

People who are comfortable with themselves are capable of establishing appropriate physical and emotional intimacy (closeness) with other people. They have something to offer a relationship. They are able to express their feelings and are willing to take the risks necessary to create a relationship. They respect both themselves and others. Because establishing emotional intimacy can be quite threatening and challenging, teens are sometimes more comfortable with physical intimacy than with emotional intimacy. But physical intimacy without emotional intimacy can lead to shallow relationships that are not respectful of the individuals involved.

For many people, intimacy is defined only as sexual contact. Actually, intimacy is developed while communicating and sharing feelings. Abstinence from sexual activity provides time for a couple to develop their level of intimacy. A sexual encounter that results in a pregnancy or transmission of a sexually transmitted infection can actually have a harmful effect on intimacy, not to mention a person's emotional health. For teens, it is important to abstain from sexual activity to allow for healthy emotional development and maturation.

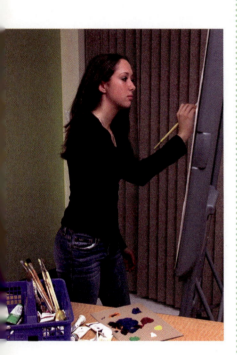

Creative

You may not think that you're the creative type, but all of us are the artists of our own lives. Being creative means being open to new experiences. Instead of staying safe and secure in what they already know, creative people are curious and adventurous. Even if they don't demonstrate great talent in a particular area, they may participate in it just for the enjoyment. Think about how you would feel if you were given a box containing the following items, all brand-new: fingerpaints, Play-Doh, a box of 64 colorful crayons, 24 markers, assorted colors of pipe cleaners, scissors, assorted colors of construction paper, and a tablet full of blank white paper. Would you want to play?

Good Self-Esteem

Self-esteem is your own opinion of your value and worth as a human being. If you have good self-esteem, you generally like yourself despite what others might say and do. Self-esteem continues to develop throughout life and is based on both our own experiences and feedback from others. Sometimes our self-esteem is threatened. Suppose you've always taken pride in your athletic ability. So far, you've mastered every sport you've attempted. Other people always comment on what a great athlete you are. Your confidence in your athletic ability contributes to your self-esteem and how you see yourself. Last week a friend invited you to go snowboarding for the first time. You were confident you wouldn't have any trouble learning. But after a whole day on the beginner slope, you still spent more time picking yourself up out of the snow than actually snowboarding. It was a real blow to your ego. People

❃ teen forum ❃

Finding Your Purpose

Many young people don't believe they have anything important to accomplish while they are teenagers. They believe significant accomplishments come later, when they're in college or have a career. We sometimes hear adults describe teenagers as lazy, self-centered, and unmotivated. Yet time and time again, individual teenagers or groups of teenagers make important contributions to their families and communities. It is well-documented that in cases of natural disaster, such as fires, floods, tornadoes, and hurricanes, teenagers work long and hard without any tangible reward to assist those whose lives have been affected. What's interesting is that they seem to enjoy helping and describe it as a fulfilling, satisfying experience.

- Search for examples of teenagers who have made a difference for others and read their stories.
- Do you think teenagers are capable of finding a purpose?
- Give examples of how these experiences made a difference to the people involved, including the teenagers themselves.

with good self-esteem are able to accept that they won't automatically succeed at everything they try.

Have Value and Purpose for Living

People who are mentally and emotionally healthy value life and have discovered a purpose for living. In other words, they know why they are here on this earth. Sometimes it takes many years to develop a clear sense of your purpose in life. A good first step to finding your purpose is to consider all the things you have to be thankful for in your life. Take some time to consider how your actions affect others and how you can contribute to the good of others and to society as a whole. We all have opportunities to make a difference in the world.

Optimistic

Optimism is a way of looking at life. You have probably heard the question "Is the glass half empty or half full?" For people who are optimistic, most often the glass is half full. They see the possibilities and opportunities in life as opposed to the barriers and pitfalls. If something bad happens, they assume it's temporary and won't last forever. They also believe that one unfortunate event is simply one event, and they don't complain that "everything is always going wrong." According to Martin Seligman and other researchers, there may be a genetic predisposition toward optimism or pessimism. But we can all learn to approach life in a more optimistic way.

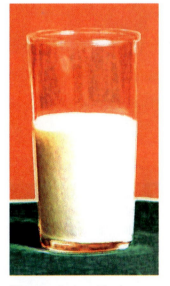

When you look at this glass of milk, is it half full or half empty? What does your answer tell you about your level of optimism?

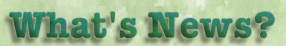

What's News?

Several years ago, Daniel Goleman, a psychologist and science writer, wrote a book titled **Emotional Intelligence**. In this book, he reports on new discoveries in brain research that show emotional intelligence to be more important than standard measures of intelligence, such as IQ tests, in determining an individual's success in life. It seems that when an event occurs, emotional memories are stored for future use. If the memories are mostly positive, such as self-awareness, self-restraint, hope, optimism, and empathy, we develop an "emotional intelligence" that serves us well in meeting future challenges.

If the memories are mostly negative, such as fear, anxiety, frustration, anger, and depression, we may find ourselves reacting to future situations with similar negative responses. Goleman believes that emotional intelligence can be taught, both at home and in schools, to help children learn to identify and manage their emotions in positive ways. For more information on emotional intelligence, check out the 6 Seconds Emotional Intelligence Network Web site at http://www.6seconds.org. It includes an explanation of emotional intelligence, as well as related stories, articles, and cartoons.

Comfortable Being Alone

People with good mental and emotional health are comfortable spending time alone as well as with others. They don't feel helpless. They can satisfy many of their own needs without depending on others. For example, imagine you've had a hectic week and have been looking forward to spending Friday night relaxing on your own listening to music and reading or drawing. You want to relax quietly. Then your friend calls on Friday afternoon and wants you to go to a party. You feel comfortable saying that you really just want to hang out on your own tonight. On the other hand, you may decide to accept the invitation because you really want to go, but not because you're worried about being alone.

DEFENSE MECHANISMS

defense mechanisms

mental strategies and behaviors used to protect ourselves from situations that cause conflict or anxiety

Defense mechanisms are mental strategies and behaviors used to avoid painful feelings caused by difficult situations. They provide a distraction or escape from having to directly confront and deal with events or circumstances we find upsetting. They also serve as protection when we are faced with unpleasant thoughts, emotions, or situations that threaten our self-esteem or contradict our perception of reality. The occasional use of defense mechanisms is common. But using them as a regular means of dealing with life is unhealthy. They may help us escape temporarily from our bad feelings, but they also prevent us from doing something about solving the problems that caused those feelings.

Some of the most common defense mechanisms are repression, denial, rationalization, daydreaming and fantasy, humor, projection, and displacement. People usually have favorite defense mechanisms that they use when they feel threatened. Reflect on whether there are any of these that you use often to try to protect yourself.

Repression

Repression involves pushing upsetting thoughts, feelings, or circumstances from conscious memory. When an individual represses an event, he or she may not even remember it happened. This is particularly true if the situation was extremely traumatic.

Denial

Denial is a favorite defense mechanism for many people. It means consciously rejecting an obvious truth or reality. For example, if someone close to you is seriously injured in a car accident and is not expected to live, you may refuse to believe the seriousness of the situation in order to protect yourself from feeling upset.

Rationalization

Rationalization involves creating a possible, but false, reason to explain a situation. For example, if you want to buy a new pair of shoes you know you don't really need, you might rationalize your purchase by telling yourself, or someone else, that your current shoes are too small and no longer fit.

Daydreaming and Fantasy

Daydreaming and fantasizing are ways to escape from your real life into an imaginary, more pleasant world. It is another of the most commonly used defense mechanisms. All of us engage in daydreaming and fantasizing from time to time. This can be a healthy and creative way to add pleasure to our lives. But daydreaming can be destructive if it gets out of hand and becomes a habitual way of responding to any situation we find disturbing.

Humor

Using humor and laughing are two of the best things we can do for ourselves. But they can also be misused. Sometimes we poke fun at others in a way that is hurtful. Then if they get upset, we protest, "But I was only joking!" Humor that takes advantage of another person in order to get a laugh is unkind. Sometimes we use humor to make fun of ourselves. This can be a coverup for our true feelings when we're upset about something. For example, a student who failed an important exam might make fun of another student who did well by saying, "Well, it's a good thing you're smart and don't have to depend on your looks." Or they might make fun of themselves by saying, "I guess I must have been at the back of the line when brains were handed out."

Projection

Projection is attributing your own thoughts and feelings to someone else. For instance, suppose you really want to see a particular movie, but you don't want to take responsibility for expressing your feelings directly. Instead, you might say, "Let's go see that new movie that started this week. It's supposed to have great special effects. Luis really wants to see it and I know he'll be mad if we don't see it this weekend."

Displacement

Displacement occurs when you transfer an emotion from what caused it to something or someone else. If you've had a bad day at school, you may come home and argue with your parents or your brother or sister. They are not the cause of your frustration, but you use them as the target for your frustration.

Using Defense Mechanisms

Everyone uses defense mechanisms at one time or another. However, regularly relying on defense mechanisms to avoid dealing with what's bothering you is not healthy, nor does it resolve the original problem. Table 13-1 offers some examples of common defense mechanisms and how they may be used by teens.

How have you used defense mechanisms in the past? In some ways, using them may have been useful to you. In some ways, using them may have caused problems for you. When you are faced with a difficult situation, try to identify a healthier way to resolve daily problems than using your favorite defense mechanisms.

DEVELOPING COMMUNICATION SKILLS

Identifying and clearly expressing your thoughts, feelings, and emotions are important skills for maintaining good mental and emotional health. Developing and using good communication skills will be discussed more thoroughly in Unit 5. In this section, we will look at some aspects of communication that support good mental and emotional health.

Table 13-1 Major Defense Mechanisms

Defense Mechanism	Definition	Example
Daydreaming and fantasy	Escape from boring or unpleasant circumstances by imagining more pleasant situations	A student in a difficult math class daydreams about getting a high-paying job as a computer whiz.
Denial	Refusal to admit to a painful reality, which is treated as if it does not exist	The boy whose girlfriend breaks up with him denies that their relationship is over and continues to call her or to give her gifts as if she still were his girlfriend.
Displacement	Redirection of negative urges or feelings from an original object to a safer or neutral substitute	The girl who has an argument with her best friend at school comes home and treats her younger siblings rudely.
Humor	Use of humor to make fun of, demean, or belittle oneself or another person	A boy who feels uncomfortable about his height teases his friends who are shorter.
Projection	Attributing one's own feelings or thoughts to someone else	The girl who doesn't get the part in the school play tells others that the rest of the cast thinks she should have been chosen
Rationalization	An effort to replace or justify acceptable reasons for feelings, beliefs, thoughts, or behaviors for real ones	A boy who wants to skip band practice tells himself that he will use the extra time to study for a test.
Repression	Unconscious or purposeful forgetting of painful or dangerous thoughts (the most basic defense mechanism)	A girl whose father died in a car accident says she doesn't feel sad about it one year later.

Honesty

Emotionally healthy people are honest with themselves and with others. Sometimes it's easy to communicate honestly; sometimes it's difficult. It's often difficult to be honest when we don't want to hurt someone's feelings or we aren't sure how to deliver bad news. For instance, suppose you've been dating someone exclusively for several months, but now you find yourself attracted to someone new. You want to break off the relationship, but you don't know how to do it. Being honest and straightforward means talking to the other person and explaining as kindly as possible that you no longer want to be involved in an exclusive relationship. It may seem easier just to ignore this person or to act badly and hope that he or she will end the

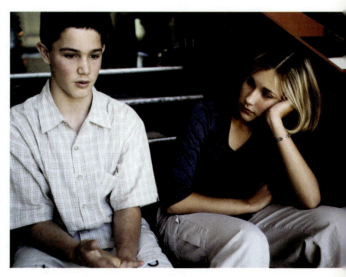

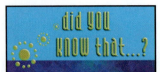

...did you know that...?

We usually think about communication as something that takes place between two or more people. But have you ever thought about the way you communicate with yourself? It's called self-talk, and many of us say things to ourselves we would never say to someone we care about. When we're talking to ourselves (and this "talk" can be out loud or just our internal thoughts), we tend to be harsh and critical, focusing on our flaws and failures. You can learn to change your self-talk to be more encouraging and positive toward yourself. You'll be surprised at what a big difference it makes in the way you feel about yourself.

relationship. But that's not an honest way of handling the situation. It is fairer to others to tell the truth, as painful as it might be for both of you.

Self-Reflection

Sometimes it's difficult to even identify exactly what you're feeling, let alone express the feeling to someone else. Self-reflection means looking into yourself to discover your true feelings. This is a necessary first step before meaningful communication can take place. Let's say you just lost your campaign for election to office in a school organization. It might take some time and self-reflection to determine what you're really feeling. Are you disappointed? Embarrassed? Angry? When you can identify your innermost feelings, you have a better chance of communicating them clearly to someone else. You may have to tell friends, "You know, right now I think I'm just really disappointed and I don't feel like talking about it. Could we just talk about something else? I'll let you know later when I feel more like talking about it."

Assertiveness

Assertiveness means respecting yourself and letting others know what you need. It also means respecting the rights of others, even when you disagree. When you communicate assertively, you try to find the balance between giving up your own rights (being too passive) and forcing your beliefs or desires on others (being too aggressive). Suppose you're in a restaurant with friends and they start making fun of someone at the next table who is very overweight. You believe this behavior is cruel. Being assertive means letting your friends know you think they are being unkind, but doing so without insulting them or putting them down.

MANAGING YOUR FEELINGS

It's normal and healthy to have a wide range of feelings. Managing our positive feelings is usually not a problem for us or for others. People rarely complain because we are happy or excited, even if we're overdoing it a bit. But managing our negative feelings can be more difficult. Even though feeling sad, anxious, depressed, or angry is completely normal, most people aren't as comfortable with these feelings as they are with more positive feelings. Our negative feelings can also be upsetting to the people around us.

Many studies show it's best to acknowledge your feelings rather than hide them or pretend they don't exist. An important wellness skill is learning to express your feelings without overreacting and behaving inappropriately. Although it's not possible to handle your feelings well all the time, you can work toward recognizing and managing them well most of the time.

Anger

Anger is one of the most difficult feelings to manage because it often catches us off guard. We may find ourselves angry before we're even aware of what's happening. In the heat of the moment, it's hard to step back and think clearly about the best way to respond to a situation.

Anger usually occurs when we face an actual or imaginary situation that may cause us to experience harm, loss, or blame. Catching yourself before your anger gets out of control is a skill you can learn. Strategies for managing anger and handling conflict are discussed more fully in Chapter 18.

Depression

Depression is another feeling that can be difficult to manage. Sometimes we can identify the factors that contribute to depression, but it's common for teens to feel blue without any specific reason. Part of depression is feeling unable to cope with the problems of daily life. Another symptom is feeling paralyzed and unable to take any action to resolve life's problems. Depression is one of the most common mood disorders in the United States. It is discussed more fully in Chapter 14.

Anxiety and Fear

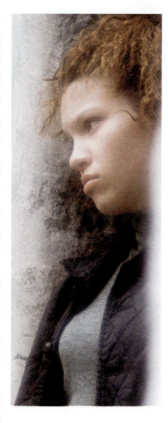

Anxiety and fear are useful when they help us avoid potentially dangerous or harmful situations. But sometimes we spend a lot of time worrying about things that aren't actually harmful or that never happen. Fear of an unpleasant outcome can keep us from taking a risk that might turn out well. Suppose you want to try out for a part in the school play, but you are afraid of failing or, worse yet, of making a fool of yourself. Just thinking about the tryouts causes you anxiety. When faced with this kind of situation in which there is something to gain, it might be helpful to ask yourself these questions:

- What's the worst thing that can happen?
- How will I respond if that happens?
- How will I feel if it turns out well?
- Am I willing to take the risk?

Effectively managing anxiety and fear means learning when to pay attention to what your feelings tell you and when to take action despite them.

Loneliness

Everyone feels lonely at one time or another. No matter how close we are to our family or how many friends we have, part of the human experience is to occasionally feel all alone in the world. Loneliness can be an indicator that we need to spend more time developing a good relationship with ourselves. It can also be an indicator that we need to spend more time developing our social connections with other people.

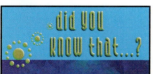

did you know that...?

A large number of research studies show that regular exercise can lower depression and anxiety. Researchers believe that exercise increases the levels of serotonin, a brain neurotransmitter. Serotonin is one of the brain chemicals responsible for positive mood. In some of the studies, exercise was just as effective as psychotherapy and antidepressant drugs in relieving depression.

Although loneliness is not always negative, it can be quite painful. When you experience loneliness, ask yourself what would make you feel more connected to yourself or to others. For example, if you find yourself eating lunch alone and you feel lonely, develop a plan to make some new friends at school with whom you can share the lunch hour. You could start by inviting a couple of classmates from the class that meets right before lunch to join you.

BUILDING YOUR Wellness Plan

Many factors influence mental and emotional health. Some factors are genetic; others are the result of life experiences. Some teens have developed a sound foundation for creating and maintaining good mental and emotional health. Other teens have already experienced some roadblocks or bumps in the road. The good news is that regardless of your past experiences, you can begin now to create a plan that contributes to mental and emotional wellness. The information in this chapter can help you to:

- Understand the characteristics of good mental and emotional health.
- Identify the characteristics you'd like to develop more fully.
- Explore ways you can make these improvements.
- Review Maslow's hierarchy of needs to see if you are meeting these needs for yourself.
- Evaluate your communication skills and see if they include the characteristics described in the chapter.

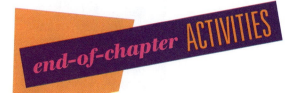

end-of-chapter ACTIVITIES

Weblinks

Resiliency

Resiliency in Action: **http://www.resiliency.com**

Self-Talk

Meaningful Living: **http://www.meaningfulliving.com** (click on "Living/Wellness" then click on "Creating Emotional Wellness")

Short-Answer Questions

1. Explain the concept of resiliency and give an example.
2. Name the five levels of Maslow's hierarchy of needs.
3. List at least five characteristics of people who are mentally and emotionally healthy.
4. List and briefly describe three defense mechanisms.
5. Define the concept of self-talk and give an example.

Discussion Questions

1. Explain the factors that contribute to the development of identity.
2. Create a scenario to describe one of the characteristics of good mental and emotional health.
3. Create a scenario to demonstrate the use of one of the defense mechanisms.
4. Discuss your opinion of the term *emotional intelligence* as used in your text.
5. Describe three actions you could take to improve your mental and emotional health.

Chapter Vocabulary

Using a separate sheet of paper, list and define the following terms:

defense mechanisms	mentally healthy
emotionally healthy	resiliency
identity	self-actualization
Maslow's hierarchy of needs	

Application Activities

Language Arts Connection

1. Write an essay about a time you felt angry, depressed, or lonely and how you managed your feelings. If you would handle the situation differently now, include an explanation.
2. Choose one of the following options and write a short story:
   a. A nonfictional story about a person who exhibits good mental and emotional health
   b. A fictional story about a person who is trying to improve his or her mental and emotional health
   c. A nonfictional story about someone who demonstrates resiliency

Social Studies Connection

Go to your library or go online and research the influence of nature (genetics) versus nurture (environment) on the development of mental and emotional health. On the basis of your findings, how much control do you believe you have over your mental and emotional health? In a written report, provide evidence to support your opinion.

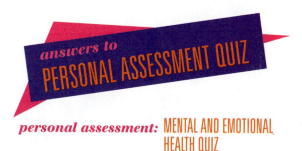

answers to **PERSONAL ASSESSMENT QUIZ**

personal assessment: **MENTAL AND EMOTIONAL HEALTH QUIZ**

- Answering Strongly Agree or Agree to questions 1, 2, 4, 6, 9, and 10 indicates positive mental and emotional health. Answering Strongly Disagree or Disagree to these questions indicates potential roadblocks to mental and emotional health.
- Answering Strongly Agree or Agree to questions 3, 5, 7, and 8 indicates potential roadblocks to mental and emotional health. Answering Strongly Disagree or Disagree to these questions indicates positive mental and emotional health.

chapter 14

Understanding Mental Illness

Starting in junior high school, Rob noticed he was feeling more and more anxious about things in his life. At first he thought he was just worried about the increased responsibilities that came with being a teen. For the past couple of years, though, he seemed to worry about everything. Then Rob began to notice some physical symptoms. He had difficulty sleeping; he was restless much of the day; he couldn't concentrate; and his school grades began to go down. After a meeting with his school counselor and his parents, Rob learned he may be experiencing mental health problems and would benefit from seeing a mental health counselor. Rob has been meeting with a counselor for three weeks now, and he's noticing some improvement in how he feels.

chapter OBJECTIVES

When you finish this chapter, you should be able to:

- Describe in general terms how the nervous system works.
- Understand mental disorders as a form of illness.
- Identify various forms of mental illness that can affect teens.
- List and describe the various forms of anxiety disorders.
- Explain what phobias are.
- Explain how eating disorders are problems for teens.
- Discuss ways you can help people you care about who have mental health disorders.

Introduction

Our health status is related to the quality of our mental and emotional health. Unfortunately, mental health problems are quite common. In fact, at least one person in 20% of all American families will be affected by a mental health problem. It's important to understand that mental disorders can be treated. Teens should be able to recognize common disorders and be prepared to seek help, if necessary, for themselves or for people they care about. Mental disorders should not be suffered in silence, nor should they prevent teens from enjoying their lives now and when they are adults. This chapter will give you information about common mental disorders and their treatment.

key TERMS

compulsion
neuron
neurotransmitter
obsession
phobia
psychiatrist
psychotherapist
psychotic

personal assessment: YOUR KNOWLEDGE OF MENTAL ILLNESS

Read each of the statements below and answer True or False on a separate sheet of paper.

1. Only crazy people have mental illness.

2. Mental illness is something that happens only to adults.

3. Everyone with a mental illness must be treated in a mental hospital.

4. People with mental illness are not in touch with reality.

5. You can treat mental illness yourself if you just work through the problem.

6. People with mental health problems are usually violent.

7. You can prevent someone from committing suicide by telling the person you don't care if they do it.

THE HUMAN BRAIN

The brain is the most complex organ in the body. It contains more than 100 billion nerve cells, or **neurons**. Whereas the other organs are composed of a few different cell types, the brain contains *thousands* of different types of cells. These cells are organized in different parts of the brain to control the functions needed to carry on daily life. These functions include thought, memory, speech, vision, hearing, and muscle movement. Adding to the complexity, each neuron has thousands of connections with other neurons, which enable the cells to communicate with each other. This communication takes place because of chemicals called **neurotransmitters**, which provide complex electrical pathways for impulses to move within and among neurons. These connections allow communication to take place so rapidly, we aren't even aware of the process. Figure 14-1 is a photo of a magnified neuron.

Let's look at an example. Suppose you enter a room and discover a fire. In an instant, you *see* and *smell* smoke coming from a trash can. You *remember* where the fire extinguisher is in the kitchen, so you turn to the hallway, and *yell* to your sister in the kitchen to bring the extinguisher to you quickly! The neurons in your brain work together to take in and process information, take advantage of what's stored in memory, and suggest the appropriate action. And your brain can do all this in less time than it's taking you to read about it!

Mental illness is related to brain function. The complexity of the brain that allows us to do amazing things can also be the cause of problems when these complex

neuron

specialized body cell that is the basic unit of nerve tissue

neurotransmitter

chemical substance that enables transmission of information among neurons

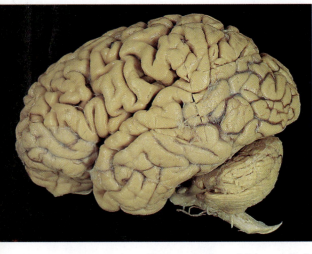

Photograph of an adult human brain

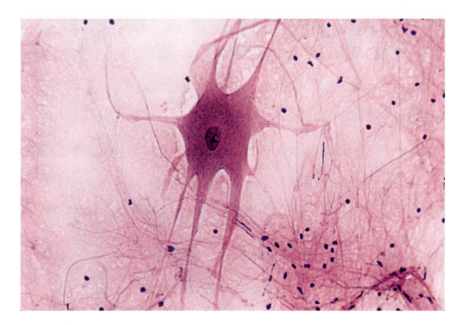

Figure 14-1
The brain contains more than 100 billion nerve cells like this, called neurons.

functions are disrupted. Many of us take the brain for granted and believe we can control both our thoughts and other brain functions. The truth is, our brain function depends on a complicated arrangement of structures, **receptors**, and chemicals that are constantly performing billions of functions. Malfunctions in this complicated system can result in mental illness.

RECOGNIZING MENTAL ILLNESS

Mental illness has always been part of human existence. In the past, mental illness was viewed as less acceptable than physical illness. In fact, as late as the 1700s it was believed to be caused by devil worship and immoral practices. The mentally ill were confined to institutions called asylums. Their confinement was designed not to cure them but to separate them from those who were not mentally ill. The conditions in asylums were very poor, with some "patients" being chained to the walls. Others lived in cells in which three or four people shared a bed.

During the 1800s, interest developed in providing more humane treatment for the mentally ill. Following World War I, mental illness began to be considered a health problem with medical causes. We now have a better picture of what mental illness is, although we still don't have a clear understanding of what causes it. Since 1950, mental health experts have been trying to define mental illness and describe the characteristics of specific mental health conditions.

In 1952, the American Psychiatric Association began publishing the *Diagnostic and Statistical Manual of Mental Disorders* (DSM). The DSM is now in its fourth edition (DSM-IV) and contains classifications of many varieties of mental illness. The purpose of the DSM-IV is to

receptor

nerve ending that receives stimuli, as from the sense organs

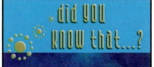

did you know that...?

A recent study disclosed that approximately 29% of the people in the United States have a serious mental illness. The surprising feature of this study was that more than 3 out of every 10 of these people with mental illness were not getting treated for their illness.

❊ teen forum ❊

Factors Affecting Mental Health

Mental health problems can range from almost unnoticeable to severe. Some of these problems are related to chemical changes in the body; some may be influenced by things you experience in your environment. In the same regard, there may be circumstances that encourage good mental health.

- Make a list of environmental factors that you think affect your mental health in both good and bad ways.
- Do you think your classmates would have the same items on their list if they created one?
- Talk to the other students in your class about the items they would list.
- Create a summary of your reactions and findings to include in your Health Folio.

stigma

something not considered normal; a mark of disgrace

out-patient

refers to treatment given to a patient during periodic visits to a health care facility or physician's office

in-patient

refers to treatment given to a patient who has been admitted to a health care facility

help professionals diagnose mental conditions. It does not include suggestions for treatments.

In addition to suffering from mental illness, a problem for patients is the **stigma** many people attach to it. Even today, there are people who regard persons with mental illness as abnormal. This attitude sometimes makes it difficult for people who believe they may have a mental disorder to seek treatment. People with mental health problems may avoid seeking treatment because they think treatment is difficult or hard to find. They may also believe the mental health problems they are experiencing will go away on their own. It is important to understand that mental disorders are *illnesses* and not conditions that are "bad" and carry a stigma. We have concern for someone who has the flu and needs to stay in bed. We have compassion for the person with cancer who undergoes chemotherapy. The same level of concern and compassion should be given to the person with mental illness.

People must know that as are other forms of illness, mental illness is treatable with counseling or medication or both. Some mental health problems can be treated very well on an **out-patient** basis with periodic visits to the health care provider. More serious mental illness may require **in-patient** treatments.

CAUSES OF MENTAL ILLNESS

It is believed mental illness is somehow related to poor functioning among the brain's neurotransmitters. Other factors may also contribute to mental illness.

- *Heredity.* Mental illness is not inherited, but a person may inherit the predisposition for mental illness. The role of genetic factors in mental illness is very complex. Characteristics such as gender, age, and race can play a part in genetic influence. Current research suggests it is the interaction among many genes that contributes to the development of mental health problems.

- *Physical health problems.* Some physical conditions have been associated with mental illness. For example, many children who had a certain bacterial infection of the throat in the 1980s later developed a mental illness known as obsessive-compulsive disorder. There are other disease conditions, such as HIV infection, syphilis, and measles, that may leave a person vulnerable to mental illness.

- *Injury.* Head injuries resulting from accidents and violence can damage the brain and create conditions for impaired mental functioning.

- *Environmental conditions.* Exposure to toxic materials can lead to mental impairment. House paint, for example, used to contain lead. Small children sometimes chew on painted surfaces and swallow the flakes. In older houses that contain leaded paint, this behavior can result in brain damage from lead.

- *Stress.* A vulnerable person, under stress, may develop some form of mental illness. Stress, however, is not itself the primary cause.

- *Drugs.* Use of illegal drugs can contribute to the onset of mental health problems. A cycle of drugs such as speed and depressants that stimulate and then depress the nervous system is especially dangerous.

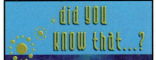

A recent study published in the *British Medical Journal* reports that infants with a low birth weight (smaller than normal) are more likely to suffer stress as adults than are infants with a normal birth weight.

FORMS OF MENTAL DISORDERS

People suffering from mental disorders often overlook the symptoms because they are not as obvious as the symptoms associated with physical health. It's easier to know you are suffering from a throat infection than to recognize you have clinical depression. The DSM-IV lists diagnostic information for more than 450 mental conditions. Some of the conditions, such as "major depression" and "mental retardation," are well known. But there are also lesser known disorders, such as "identity problem" and "pathological gambling." The following sections discuss conditions most likely to affect adolescents.

Anxiety Disorders

There is nothing wrong with feeling anxious. It happens to everyone from time to time. It's natural to experience the "butterfly feeling" in your stomach when you'll be meeting someone new, getting ready for a big test, or starting a new job. Mental health problems arise when feelings of anxiety become more frequent or even permanent. It is also considered a problem when the feelings are not associated with stressful events, or when the feelings are so intense they interfere with daily activities.

Anxiety disorders are real medical illnesses that affect approximately 19 million adults in the United States. Anxiety disorders represent the most common mental health problems among adolescents. One study of 9- to 17-year-olds found that 13% of the subjects in the study had experienced an anxiety disorder in a given one-year period.

There is no clear, single cause of anxiety disorder. In fact, there appear to be both biological and psychological causes. Anxiety disorders tend to run in families, and it appears that excessive stress can trigger anxiety disorder. The conditions come in a variety of forms.

Phobias

phobia

overwhelming, illogical fear of an event or object

Phobias are overwhelming fears related to specific events or things. Phobias are currently the most common psychiatric disorder in the United States. They are also the most common psychological disorder among females of all ages. In young males, they are the second most common psychological disorder.

People with phobias experience both physical and emotional reactions to an object or situation. These reactions may include feelings of panic, dread, or horror; a rapid heartbeat; and an intense desire to flee the situation or avoid the object. People with phobias realize their feelings go beyond what might normally be expected.

Phobias come in many forms. The DSM-IV describes three main types of phobias:

1. *Agoraphobia.* The intense fear of being in open or public places. It is characterized by the specific fear of being in a place where escape would be difficult and help would not be readily available. The condition is worsened by the fear of behaving publicly in an embarrassing manner, such as fainting or displaying excessive fear. People can become so affected by this phobia they won't leave their homes.

2. *Social phobias.* Intense, excessive fears of being observed in one or more social situations, such as performing, speaking in public, or going to a party alone. People with social phobias are afraid they will perform the particular activity in a way that will cause them embarrassment or humiliation.

3. *Specific phobias.* The extreme fear of a specific object, such as a snake, or of a situation, such as being in an enclosed space. Medical and psychiatric journals contain descriptions of many phobias. Some you might find very familiar; others might be unknown to you. Here a are few examples:

    Acrophobia: fear of heights

    Arachnophobia: fear of spiders

    Ergophobia: fear of work

    Hydrophobia: fear of water

Pedophobia: fear of children

Scriptophobia: fear of writing in public

Are you surprised by the kinds of things people find frightening?

Phobias are usually treated in one of two ways: behavioral therapy or medication. A mental health professional recommends the most appropriate method of treatment after examining the patient. In behavior therapy, the patient meets with a trained therapist and learns to control the physical reactions caused by the fear. The patient gradually confronts the phobia in a carefully structured way; each confrontation with the phobia trigger is followed by relaxation techniques. The patient first imagines the feared object or situation. The next step is to look at pictures of the object or situation. Finally, the patient actually comes into contact with the feared object or experiences the situation. By facing rather than fleeing the source of fear, the patient eventually becomes free of the anxiety and dread associated with it.

Medication may be prescribed to control the extreme anxiety or panic experienced during a phobic encounter by reducing the anxiety associated with just thinking about dealing with the object or situation. For patients suffering from agoraphobia or social phobia, medication tends to be the first choice. With treatment, the vast majority of phobia patients can be relieved of their fears and live a symptom-free life.

Post-Traumatic Stress Disorder

Post-traumatic stress disorder (PTSD) can happen after a person is involved in or witnesses an extremely frightening event such as a car accident or sexual abuse. The experience leaves a deep impression that results in mental reactions taking place weeks, months, or years after the event took place.

The person does not have to be physically injured in the event to suffer PTSD. Even people who are not directly involved, but witness a traumatic event, can be affected. As you can imagine, many people of all ages have experienced post-traumatic stress as a result of the terrorist attacks that occurred on September 11, 2001.

Post-traumatic stress disorder is a serious condition that can interfere with a young person's ability to do everyday activities at home and at school. Signs that a teen may be experiencing post-traumatic stress disorder include:

- Nightmares and sleep disorders
- Frightening memories of the event
- Difficulty concentrating
- Not wanting to be with friends
- Discomfort with situations related to the traumatic event

The effects of PTSD can last for years. For example, a person who was abused as a child may be fearful of engaging in a normal intimate relationship as an adult and may need counseling to overcome his or her fear.

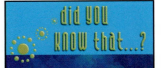

did you know that...?

There is even a phobia describing the fear of going to school! It is called didaskaleinophobia.

The serious symptoms of PTSD can be reduced by using the following coping strategies, but keep in mind that treatment for PTSD must include professional counseling:

- Spend time with other people.
- Talk with others about how you feel, and listen to what others are saying.
- Take time to grieve, and don't be afraid to cry if you need to.
- Get involved in everyday routines.
- Set small goals to tackle big problems.
- Eat healthy foods and get some exercise.

Generalized Anxiety Disorder

Generalized anxiety disorder is characterized by excessive worry about a variety of things over a period of at least six months. This mental health condition develops during childhood or the teen years. Young people with generalized anxiety disorder may also suffer physical symptoms such as headaches, tiredness, and muscle tension. They may complain of having difficulty sleeping or feeling a lump in their throat. Generalized anxiety disorder usually runs in families and can become worse when a young person is stressed. The condition can be treated with medication or counseling. In any case, the symptoms tend to go away as the person gets older.

Panic Disorder

Panic disorder is characterized by unexpected and repeated feelings of fear. The attacks become full-blown in about 15 minutes and can include physical symptoms such as rapid heartbeat, sweating, and dizziness. Panic disorder is relatively rare in children. It is most likely to develop during adolescence or young adulthood. Research indicates that both heredity and stressful experiences may play a role in causing panic disorder. Knowing an attack can happen at any time adds to the fear and stress and may actually contribute to future episodes.

Panic disorders can be treated in a couple of ways. Depending on the level of intensity experienced by the patient, the mental health professional can treat the disorder with counseling, drug therapy, or both.

Separation Anxiety

Separation anxiety is a disorder that involves feelings of distress, worry, and physical symptoms when a young person is separated from someone to whom he or she is attached. The anxiety is more likely to develop when the teen is someplace where he or she cannot easily leave and return home. The worry and anxiety most often are caused by fears that some harm will come to the person from whom the teen is separated. This condition affects about 4% of adolescents.

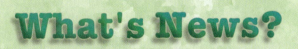

What's News?

Evidence is mounting that sleep — even a nap — improves information processing and learning. Recent experiments at Harvard University reveal that an afternoon "power nap" reverses daily information overload. The researchers also found that a full night's rest helps consolidate the memories of habits, actions, and skills learned during the day. At the same time, research on American teens has discovered that high school students are not getting enough sleep and that teens who get the least amount of sleep are the most likely to suffer from depression and anxiety disorders. Their schoolwork suffers as well. The problems seem most likely to appear if the teen is getting six or fewer hours of sleep each night.

Obsessive-Compulsive Disorder

Obsessive-compulsive disorder (often called OCD) is characterized by repeated disturbing, seemingly senseless thoughts (**obsessions**) or ritual behaviors (**compulsions**) that cannot be easily controlled or stopped. For example, someone who has an uncommon fear of germs (obsession) may constantly wash his hands (compulsion). Another example is someone who repeatedly checks the lock on the door (compulsion) from a fear that someone will try to enter the room or home (obsession).

obsession

an unwanted and distressing thought or impulse that occurs repeatedly

compulsion

a repetitive behavior that is performed in response to obsessive thoughts

Mood Disorders

Mood refers to emotions over a period of time. Our mood influences our attitudes and how we view the world. Mood disorders are characterized by a disturbance of normal mood, which results in symptoms such as depression and hyperactivity.

Mood disorders are the source of much human suffering. They are the cause of lost productivity and many suicides. They rank among the top 10 causes of disability *worldwide*. When mood disorders are not recognized and treated, they can cause physical symptoms. The physical symptoms caused by untreated mood disorders result in unnecessary health care expense and, worse, may prevent the patient from being treated for the real cause of the symptoms.

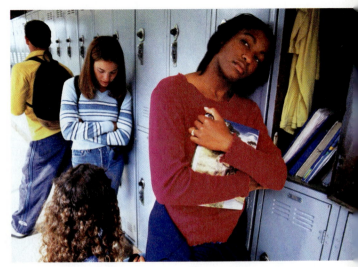

Depression

One thing is very natural about the mental states of human beings; they are not consistent. We are capable of experiencing a wide variety of emotions.

Sometimes we are happy, sometimes angry, and sometimes sad. These emotional states are usually temporary, and it's normal to feel sad or depressed from time to time. What is not normal is depression that is extreme and lasts for a long period of time.

A number of large research studies reveal that up to 8% of adolescents in the United States suffer from depression. In fact, severe depression tends to begin in the teen years, with females twice as likely to be depressed as males. The studies also suggest that the number of cases of depression has risen sharply among children and teens. There is evidence that many young people who suffer from depression continue to suffer from depression as adults.

Depression can interfere with normal development, school performance, and social activities. Identifying and treating depression as early as possible is important so the teen can live a full life now and in the years to come.

Depression is a treatable disorder. It is important for teens to seek help from a mental health professional as soon as they suspect they may be suffering from depression. If you or anyone you know has some of the following symptoms for more than a couple of weeks, it's a good idea to visit with a health care professional who has expertise in mental disorders.

- Withdrawal from friends, family, and normal activities
- Violent actions, rebellious behavior, or running away
- Feelings of hopelessness
- Drug and alcohol use
- Persistent boredom
- Difficulty concentrating
- A decline in the quality of schoolwork
- Frequent complaints about physical symptoms, often related to emotions, such as stomachaches, headaches, and fatigue
- Loss of interest in what were previously pleasurable activities
- Not dealing well with praise or rewards

What's News?

For the 1.5% of the U.S. population who suffer major depression, there may be help on the horizon. About a third of all patients diagnosed with severe depression do not respond to medication. A device already approved by the U.S. Food and Drug Administration (FDA) to help control seizures is now being tested to see if it is effective in treating severe depression. The device is implanted under the skin much as a heart pacemaker and gives off electrical signals every 30 seconds. The impulses stimulate the brain and improve mood.

We don't have a clear picture of what causes depression. It appears that biological and social factors interact to play a role. Because the exact causes are unknown, there is not one specific treatment. Teens who suffer from major depression are usually treated with counseling or medication, or both. In some cases, counseling interventions are combined with medications that address the biological causes. The medications now used to treat adolescent depression are different from those prescribed for adults.

Bipolar Disorder

Bipolar disorder is a serious mental illness that includes extreme shifts in mood ranging from depression to **manic** highs (excited, mostly happy episodes) and mixed conditions. For this reason, the condition has been commonly referred to as manic depression. Everybody has ups and downs in their lives. It is when these episodes become constant and interfere with everyday functions that bipolar disorder can be suspected. The condition represents a special problem among adolescents because bipolar disorder affects teens differently than it does adults. It appears that bipolar disorder increases the risk of suicide. Moreover, the risk of suicide is higher among adolescents than among adults. The higher risk among adolescents is partly explained by involvement in drug abuse.

Suicide

The suicide rate for adolescents has risen dramatically in recent years and is now the third leading cause of death among teens. All suicidal individuals have some form of mental illness underlying their desire to end their lives. It is not surprising that the most significant mental disorder associated with suicide is depression. Because suicide is a serious problem that affects many teens, it is the subject of Chapter 15, where it is discussed in more detail.

Helping Prevent Suicide. If you have a close friend or family member who appears to be suffering from deep depression, you can help. Your role is not to take responsibility for curing the depression. You can help by being caring and supportive until the person gets to speak to a professional. The most important thing is to let the person know you care and are there for him or her. See Figure 14-2 to get more information about the things you should or should not do to help someone who may be suicidal.

manic
referring to mania, excessive mental and physical energy often associated with mood disorders

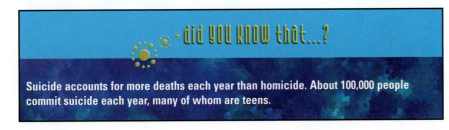

did you know that...?

Suicide accounts for more deaths each year than homicide. About 100,000 people commit suicide each year, many of whom are teens.

- **Prepare to help** by learning about suicide and gathering information about suicide prevention resources in your community.

- **Use your communication skills** and talk with the person. Listen actively and let the person know you and other people care about what happens to him or her.

- **Help** him or her understand that even deep depression is temporary and can be treated.

- **Let the person know** you want to help connect him or her with a medical professional.

- *Do not* issue a challenge. Daring people to follow through on suicide will *not* cause them to think twice about doing it.

- *Do not* tell the person you don't care if he or she commits suicide.

- *Do not* leave the person alone if you think he or she is about to attempt suicide.

Figure 14-2
How to help a suicidal person

schizophrenia

a brain disease that is perhaps the most severe of the mental illnesses

psychotic

referring to a mental disorder in which the patient loses touch with reality by way of hallucinations, paranoid behavior, and fantasy thoughts

Schizophrenia

Schizophrenia is a persistent, serious, and disabling **psychotic** brain disorder. It affects about 1% of the population. Schizophrenia usually appears in adolescence or young adulthood. Symptoms of the disorder are many and varied. In fact, many psychological experts believe schizophrenia is not one condition, but many.

Some of the symptoms can be terrifying, such as hearing internal voices not heard by others. Schizophrenic patients may believe that people are reading their minds, controlling their thoughts, or plotting to harm them. The condition can cause patients' speech and behaviors to become so disorganized that they are incomprehensible and frightening to others. Many patients also experience hallucinations, disturbances of sensory perception in which they believe they see things that don't really exist, and delusions, which are false beliefs held despite obvious evidence they aren't true.

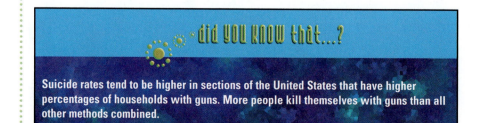

did YOU KNOW that...?

Suicide rates tend to be higher in sections of the United States that have higher percentages of households with guns. More people kill themselves with guns than all other methods combined.

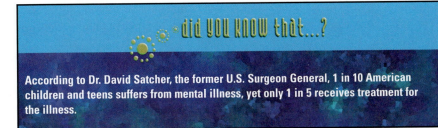
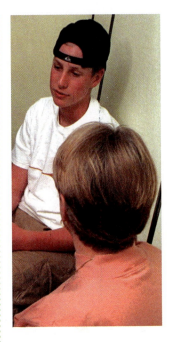

We don't fully understand what causes schizophrenia. It appears there is a genetic link because a teen from a family with a history of schizophrenia is 10 times more likely to exhibit the symptoms of schizophrenia than is someone from a family that has no such history. There is no single treatment for schizophrenia because the disorder may include more than one condition. It is often necessary to prescribe antipsychotic drugs, so schizophrenia is best treated by a psychiatrist.

Eating Disorders

The relation of eating disorders to weight management is discussed in Chapter 9. Although less than 1% of teens may have an eating disorder, it is important to understand that eating

real teens

When she was a sophomore in high school, Anne weighed 135 pounds. That year, many people began to tease her or make comments about her weight. She was even told that no one asked her to the school dance because she was too fat. Even though these kids were just teasing, Anne took the comments seriously and started counting calories. In the beginning, she stopped eating lunch. Her friends commented on her weight loss and told her she was looking better. When swimsuits appeared in the stores in April, she felt she needed to lose more weight. She started skipping breakfast, too. She became obsessed with counting calories and exercising. By summer, she was consuming only 300 calories a day (the equivalent of three slices of Swiss cheese or a ham and cheese sandwich with mayonnaise) and had lost a lot of weight. Then, when she got to 93 pounds, her family and friends began to worry and told her she was nothing but skin and bones. But Anne was horrified by the ripples of fat she imagined on her legs and stomach.

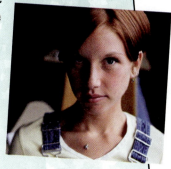

Almost everyone tried to encourage her to seek medical help, but she refused to see a doctor. One day, she fainted while getting on the bus and hit her head on the pavement. The emergency room physician recognized that Anne had anorexia nervosa, a serious eating disorder, and immediately admitted her to the hospital. After a lengthy stay in the hospital and 14 months of therapy, she still struggles with her eating disorder. With the help of her family and friends, however, she is on the road to recovery.

disorders are symptoms of an underlying psychological condition. The person develops an unrealistic obsession to be thin. The obsession for thinness for females may be driven by the unrealistic images of females portrayed by the media. Not all women should have the perfect figure pictured in magazines and portrayed in movies. Males may develop their eating disorder because they diet to restrict their weight because they are wrestlers or jockeys. Because of the underlying psychological aspects of eating disorders, the most effective and long-lasting treatment is some form of psychological counseling, combined with careful attention to the medical and nutritional needs of the patient. People with eating disorders who enter treatment in the early stages can be treated on an out-patient basis. If the disorder has progressed to the point at which physical health is at risk, treatment will be done on an in-patient basis.

TREATMENT PROFESSIONALS

Just as there are many types of mental health disorders, there are many types of treatment. Getting effective treatment for a mental disorder starts with realizing that help is needed. Recognizing that help is needed may sound very simple, but it is not. All too often, the signs of mental illness are not recognized, or the person with the disorder refuses to admit there is a problem. It is common for people to believe their symptoms will take care of themselves and go away. Some people are reluctant to seek treatment because of the stigma associated with mental illness. Still others are afraid of the discomfort they might experience as they go through the changes necessary to correct the disorder.

There are two main types of mental health treatment experts. **Psychotherapists** are trained to diagnose and treat mental disorders using special counseling techniques. **Psychiatrists** are medical doctors with special training to treat mental disorders. They use counseling techniques and are also able to prescribe medications because they have a medical degree. Both psychotherapists and psychiatrists must be licensed by the state in which they practice.

psychotherapist

a mental health professional who is trained to treat mental disorders using psychological counseling techniques

psychiatrist

a medical doctor who specializes in treating mental illnesses

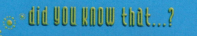

did you know that...?

Treating mental health problems is costly in both human and financial terms. Statistics show mental illness to be the second most burdensome health condition after heart disease. This burden is measured in years of life lost to premature death as well as years of living with a disabling condition. The financial costs of treating mental illness are high. In the United States, we spend about $70 billion annually to treat mental illness; and this figure does not include the costs of drug abuse treatment.

BUILDING YOUR Wellness Plan

Unlike other aspects of health and wellness, mental wellness depends more on your genetic makeup and the biochemical condition of your body than on what you can do for yourself. However, there are some things you can do to increase the likelihood that you and the people around you will enjoy good mental health.

- Practice behaviors that maintain your general wellness level, such as eating well, exercising, and getting enough sleep.
- Monitor your feelings and reactions to stressful conditions. Develop a plan to seek assistance from a trusted adult when needed.
- Learn the signs and symptoms of mental disorders.
- Demonstrate compassion for people who have mental problems.
- Know where mental health caregivers can be found and how to contact them.

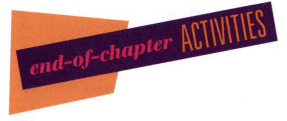

end-of-chapter ACTIVITIES

Weblinks

Phobias

Phobia List: **http://phobialist.com**

Separation Anxiety

Keep Kids Healthy: **http://www.keepkidshealthy.com**
  (search for "infant separation anxiety")

Short-Answer Questions

1. What is the DSM-IV used for?
2. List four types of anxiety disorders.
3. What is ergophobia?
4. Give two examples of social phobias.

5. What do we call a special health professional who treats mental disorders with special counseling techniques?

Discussion Questions

1. List and discuss at least five factors related to the development of mental disorders.
2. Explain how phobias are treated.
3. Describe what steps you would take if you strongly suspected a friend was considering suicide.
4. Describe at least five symptoms of depression.
5. Explain the difference between a psychotherapist and a psychiatrist, and name a mental health disorder best treated by each type of professional.

☀ Chapter Vocabulary

Using a separate sheet of paper, list and define the following terms:

compulsion	phobia
neuron	psychiatrist
neurotransmitter	psychotherapist
obsession	psychotic

☀ Application Activities

Language Arts Connection

Imagine you have a good friend or family member you suspect has an eating disorder. Compose a letter to the person explaining how much you care about him or her, and present some reasons why you would recommend getting a medical evaluation to determine if there is a problem. Research in the library or visit Web sites on eating disorders to gather information to use in your letter.

Social Studies Connection

Use a city resource guide or your local phone directory to locate organizations that help with mental disorders. Choose two of the mental disorders discussed in this chapter and collect information from one of the facilities about how an individual gets into treatment for these disorders.

Science Connection

In this chapter, the concept of neurotransmitters was introduced. Search the Web to find out how neurons work and the role chemicals in your body play for sending "messages" through the nervous system. Prepare a report about what you learn, and draw a diagram of a neuron and neurotransmitter.

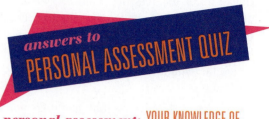

answers to
PERSONAL ASSESSMENT QUIZ

personal assessment: YOUR KNOWLEDGE OF MENTAL ILLNESS

1. False. Mental illness, like many other forms of illness, can range from mild to severe, and the term *crazy* has no place in reference to mental illness.

2. False. Mental illness, like most other illnesses, can occur at any age.

3. False. The vast majority of psychological disorders are treated without the person's ever being admitted to the hospital.

4. False. People with mental illness are in touch with reality unless they are troubled with severe mental illness.

5. False. Psychological problems almost always require the help of a health care professional.

6. False. People with mental problems may exhibit the characteristics of their particular illness, but in general their behaviors are not violent.

7. False. Never challenge a person to commit suicide, nor should you tell the person you do not care. Only by listening and offering support can you help the person with his or her problem.

chapter 15

Understanding and Preventing Suicide

Jake finally has a plan to deal with all the stress, frustration, and pain he's felt for so long. It's not as if anyone would miss him anyway. He's been feeling very depressed for the past few months. Just getting up and getting through the day takes all the energy he can manage. He never hangs out with his guy friends anymore because it's just too hard to pretend everything's okay. His girlfriend, Sandy, was really the only person he wanted to be around. But two weeks ago, she told him she didn't want to be with him anymore. She said he always seemed to be in a bad mood, and he wasn't fun anymore. Sandy told him he needed to get a life, and the new life wasn't going to include her. He pretended he didn't care. But the truth is, Sandy was the only person he could talk to about his feelings. His parents have noticed he just stays in his room listening to music, and they keep asking him what's wrong. But Jake doesn't think they'll understand. Now he's thinking Saturday might be the day to finally do it. His parents are going out, so he'll be alone. And last week he found his dad's gun. Now he just has to do it, and all the pain will be gone. Just like that—wiped out forever. Maybe he'll get drunk and call Sandy just to say goodbye before he really does it.

When you finish this chapter, you should be able to:

- Give current statistics on suicide in the United States.
- List and describe the factors that contribute to suicide.
- Describe the relationship between guns and completed suicides.
- Explain how mental disorders and substance abuse are associated with suicide.
- List and describe the warning signs for suicide.
- Describe what individuals, families, schools, and communities can do to prevent suicide.
- Develop a suicide prevention plan.

Introduction

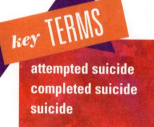

key TERMS

attempted suicide
completed suicide
suicide

Sometimes people come to feel that life is no longer worth living. People might reach this conclusion for a variety of reasons. They may feel so depressed they don't believe they'll ever be happy again. Perhaps they've suffered a great loss and don't think they can live through it. Or maybe they've been so bitterly disappointed they don't feel they'll be able to bounce back. Fortunately, even in the most desperate situations, there is always a way out if we only give ourselves the time to find it. Preventing suicide is possible if we learn the skills to face hopelessness and despair, identify resources to get help, and then give ourselves enough time to figure out solutions to our problems.

Teenagers have one of the highest rates of suicide of any age group in the United States. You may have heard the saying, "Suicide is a permanent solution to a temporary problem." A person who is facing a serious problem may not believe it is temporary, but it really is. Developing the ability to cope with serious problems and understanding that they *are* temporary can mean the difference between life and death, not only for you but also for people who are important to you. In this chapter, we will explore the reasons people consider taking their own lives and what can be done to prevent this tragic loss of life.

personal assessment: SUICIDE AND SUICIDE PREVENTION QUIZ

Before reading this chapter, test how much you already know about suicide and suicide prevention. Read each statement below and, on a separate sheet of paper, answer True or False. Answers are located at the end of the chapter.

1. If someone tries to talk to you about suicide, you should change the subject. Talking about suicide makes it more likely the person will attempt suicide.

2. Depression is one of the major factors that contributes to suicide.

3. Everyone who attempts suicide is mentally ill.

4. The same percentage of males and females actually die from their suicide attempts.

5. The use of alcohol or other drugs increases the risk for attempting suicide.

6. Suicide is the third leading cause of death among young adults aged 15–24.

7. Easy availability of a method of suicide, such as a gun or pills, does not increase the risk of suicide.

8. Low levels of serotonin may increase the risk for attempting suicide.

9. If someone really wants to commit suicide, there is no way to keep that person from doing it.

10. An overwhelming majority of people who eventually commit suicide give some warning of their intentions.

UNDERSTANDING SUICIDE

Suicide is a deliberate, intentional, self-inflicted act that results in one's own death. It is probably not possible to fully understand why a person decides to end his or her own life. There are usually many factors that contribute to this decision. The underlying reason most people decide to commit suicide is that they don't believe they can continue living with the emotional pain they're feeling. It doesn't seem as if the pain will ever pass, and they don't believe they'll ever feel any better. Although this is the way the person feels at the time, there are really many ways to resolve emotional pain without ending one's life. Understanding this pain and identifying options for hope for the future are keys to preventing suicide.

Although suicide affects all age groups, it is a major cause of death for teens. According to the Centers for Disease Control and Prevention

suicide

a deliberate, intentional, self-inflicted act that results in one's own death

attempted suicide

a deliberate, intentional, self-inflicted act that is intended to cause death but does not

completed suicide

a term used to describe a suicide attempt that results in death

(CDC), in the year 2000, suicide was the third leading cause of death for young people aged 15–24 and the fifth leading cause of death for young people 5–14 years old. It is estimated that a far greater number of teens seriously consider suicide or make a suicide attempt. An **attempted suicide** is a deliberate, intentional, self-inflicted act that is intended to cause death but does not. **Completed suicide** is a term used to describe a suicide attempt that results in death.

According to data from the CDC Youth Risk Behavior Surveillance System for 2001, about 19% of teens reported they "seriously considered attempting suicide during the past 12 months." Almost 15% of teens indicated they had "made a plan about how they would attempt suicide during the past 12 months." Data from the National Household Survey on Drug Abuse in 2000 indicated that more than a third of teens aged 12–17 who said they had thought about suicide in the past 12 months actually attempted suicide. These statistics show that thoughts of suicide are not uncommon among teens, and the high number of completed suicides tells us that these thoughts should be taken seriously. They also prove that, although a teenager thinking about suicide may feel very alone, there are many other teens out there who are struggling with the same thoughts and feelings.

It's not possible to know for certain whether someone who attempts suicide really wants to die. We *can* be certain that *all* attempted suicides are cries for help. The person is in such intense emotional pain, death seems the only way to remove it. The person may not really want to die but desperately wants the pain to stop.

Why do so many teenagers think about taking their own lives? One of the factors unique to teens is the stress experienced as a result of going through puberty and making the transition to adulthood.

did you know that...?

Suicide statistics may be significantly underreported. Parents of a teenage suicide victim may try to avoid having the death classified as a suicide because they are ashamed, embarrassed, or want to protect their family's privacy. Some medical examiners will classify a death as a suicide only if a suicide note is found, but notes are found in fewer than a third of all cases. Even law enforcement officers may classify a suicide that occurs as a result of an automobile crash as an accident. According to Tom Shires, a trauma surgeon with the Suicide Prevention Research Center in Las Vegas, doctors have even created a word for these single-car "accidents," including those showing no skid marks on the pavement: autocide. Unintentional injuries, primarily from automobile accidents, are the leading cause of death for 15- to 19-year-olds in the United States. At least some of these accidents are probably suicides. When you combine all the opportunities for faulty reporting of suicides, it seems clear that confirmed suicides are only the tip of a large iceberg.

Adolescence can be a very challenging time, physically, emotionally, socially, and mentally. Physically, your body is undergoing rapid hormonal changes. Hormonal changes, in turn, affect the emotions and make them less stable. This is one reason your moods can suddenly change for no apparent reason. Socially, you are moving from depending mostly on relationships with your family to building relationships with your peers. Mentally, you are faced with increased academic pressures and the need to solve more of your problems on your own.

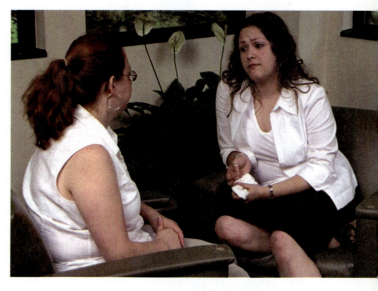

CONTRIBUTING FACTORS

There is no single factor that explains why people attempt suicide. Even in a single suicide attempt, there is likely to be more than one factor contributing to the person's decision. One single factor is probably not enough to cause a suicide attempt. But when many problems pile up, they may seem overwhelming. The person can't see any way of dealing with his or her problems. It is this sense of hopelessness and utter despair that can lead to a suicide attempt.

Certain factors have been identified that increase the likelihood an individual will attempt suicide. It is true, however, that many people have one or more of these contributing factors and yet are not suicidal. Just because a person experiences one of the contributing factors, this does not mean he or she is likely to attempt suicide. But the factors discussed in the following sections do occur often in those individuals who attempt suicide.

Mental Disorders and Substance Abuse

Ninety percent of adolescent suicide victims have at least one mental disorder, most commonly depression or substance abuse. According to statistics from the National Alliance for the Mentally Ill, almost half of the teenagers who completed suicide had had previous contact with a mental health professional. Only 15% of them, however, were being treated by a mental health professional at the time of death.

Substance abuse can occur as an attempt to medicate the emotional pain. Alcohol depresses the central nervous system. Depession of the central nervous system can lower inhibitions and impair judgment, making it more likely that an individual will act impulsively to end his or her life. Autopsy reports of adolescent suicide victims show that between one-third and one-half of the victims were under the influence of alcohol or other drugs during the time shortly before they killed themselves.

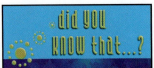

Situational Stressors

Situational stressors such as family, school, and relationship problems are often associated with suicide. These stressors are not the cause of the suicide, but rather they are triggers that make it likely the person will attempt suicide. Sometimes, teens who are in trouble at home, at school, or with law enforcement authorities see suicide as the only way out.

Many teens feel tremendous pressure to succeed academically, athletically, or socially. They may experience a major disappointment or loss, such as breaking up with a boyfriend or girlfriend or the death of someone close to them. Most teens are able to eventually resolve these difficulties, but those who have other risk factors, especially depression or substance abuse, may not have the coping skills to deal with life's problems.

Access to Lethal Methods

Almost two-thirds of completed suicides by teenagers involve a firearm. A study reported in the *New England Journal of Medicine* estimated that the likelihood of completed suicide is five times higher when a firearm is available in the home than when one is not. The reason is that gunshots are more likely to cause death than are other methods used to attempt suicide. Guns are chosen as a suicide method more frequently by teenage males than by females.

Previous Suicide Attempts

A previously attempted suicide increases the likelihood that a future attempt will result in a completed suicide. About a third of adolescent suicide victims have made a previous suicide attempt. According to the National Youth Violence Prevention Resource Center, a male teen who has already attempted suicide is more than 30 times more likely to complete suicide than is one who has made no previous attempts. A female teen who has previously attempted suicide is about three times more likely to complete suicide than is one who has made no previous attempts.

Exposure to Suicide of Others

The risk of completed suicide increases for an individual who has a family member or close friend who has attempted or completed suicide. Even a news report about a suicide or a movie that shows a fictional suicide can increase the probability of a suicide attempt for individuals who already have other risk factors. Seeing or hearing about other people who choose suicide makes it seem like a reasonable solution for problems. What the victims don't realize at the time is that there are *always* options for solving problems other than suicide, even if they are not readily apparent.

✵ teen forum ✵

Are Guns the Problem?

There are more suicides than homicides in the United States. Suicides and homicides share something in common; both are most often accomplished with a gun. Guns are easily accessible in this country, and gunshot wounds are extremely lethal. The use of a gun, in either a suicide or a homicide, dramatically increases the likelihood a death will occur. Both suicide and homicide rates are higher in western states, where guns are more readily available, than in eastern states. States with stricter gun control laws have lower rates of suicide. Some people maintain that "guns don't kill people; people kill people." Others argue that without easy access to guns, many more people would be alive today.

- Should the purchase, sale, and possession of guns be more closely regulated?
- Do guns kill people, or do people kill people? What do you think? Provide support for your answer.

"Clusters," or groups, of suicides sometimes occur among high school students. A cluster of suicides occurs when a completed suicide by one teen is followed by others, even among students who didn't know the first person who completed the suicide but heard reports about it.

PROTECTIVE FACTORS

Just as there are factors that make it more likely a person will attempt or complete suicide, there are also factors that act as protection against suicide attempts. Some of these protective factors may be genetic and unchangeable. But nongenetic factors, such as attitudes, behaviors, and

What's News?

There is no evidence that the tendency to commit suicide is inherited. However, according to the National Institute of Mental Health, there is increasing evidence that major psychiatric illnesses, which can have an inherited component, increase the risk for suicide. Depression, bipolar disorder, schizophrenia, alcoholism, and substance abuse all tend to occur more frequently in some families than in others. Researchers have linked both depression and suicidal behavior to decreased levels of serotonin, a brain neurotransmitter. Low serotonin levels have also been linked to increased impulsive behavior. Studies are currently under way to determine whether medications such as selective serotonin reuptake inhibitors (SSRIs), commonly used to treat depression, might be useful in reducing suicidal tendencies as well. Understanding more about the biology of suicidal persons can help improve treatment and save lives.

environmental characteristics, can be changed. Learning how to solve problems, control impulses, and resolve conflicts can help reduce family, school, and relationship problems before they reach the crisis point. Building resiliency skills can help children and teenagers respond more effectively to difficult life circumstances. Families and communities can provide support by ensuring that teens have access to mental health professionals when they become depressed or distressed. Teens themselves can be part of the solution by knowing where to get help and keeping this information easily available in case they or their friends need it. The restriction of easy access to the means used for attempting suicide, such as guns and pills that can be used for an overdose, can prevent impulsive deadly actions. Family, cultural, community, and religious beliefs that stress the value of life can influence teen attitudes about suicide. Recognizing and treating depression, substance abuse, and aggressive behavior can also help reduce the likelihood a teen will consider suicide.

WARNING SIGNS

There is no such thing as a typical suicide victim. Certain factors make people more vulnerable to suicide, and certain factors tend to protect against suicide. Even so, people of all ages, ethnic backgrounds, geographical locations, and socioeconomic status are represented in suicide statistics. There are some common warning signs given by people who are going to attempt suicide. It is unusual for a person to attempt suicide without ever exhibiting any of the warning signs. It is important to understand that a person who exhibits one of the warning signs is not necessarily suicidal. He or she may just be experiencing a high level of temporary stress. But, because the warning signs *can* be indications of a planned suicide attempt, you should learn to recognize them. They may be calls for help from someone who is suffering overwhelming emotional pain. Being aware of these signs can make the difference between life and death. Figure 15-1 outlines these warning signs, and they are discussed in detail in the following section.

Talking about Suicide

There is a common misconception that people who talk about suicide don't really do it. In fact, talking about suicide before actually attempting it is quite common. Talking about suicide may occur either directly or indirectly. An example of a direct comment is, "I wish I were dead." An example of an indirect comment is, "Things would be better if I just wasn't around anymore." Whether the comments are direct or indirect, anyone who talks about suicide should be taken seriously. Talk about the specific method to be used indicates a need for immediate help. Later in this chapter, we'll discuss what you should do if someone begins to talk about suicide.

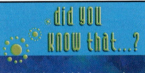

did you know that...?

Although suicide is a major problem among teens, the highest rates of suicide actually occur among the elderly, particularly older white males. In 1999, 84% of suicides in persons 65 and older were committed by males. White males 85 and older have a suicide rate six times the overall national rate.

Talking about suicide

- **Direct comments**
- **Indirect comments**

Behavioral changes

- **Trouble eating and sleeping**
- **Withdrawing from friends or becoming unusually social**
- **Preoccupation with death and dying**
- **Losing interest in hobbies and activities**
- **Giving away cherished possessions**

Emotional stressors

- **Depression**
- **Rejection, loss, or humiliation**
- **Hopelessness**

Figure 15-1
Warning signs of suicide

Behavioral Changes

Individuals who are thinking of attempting suicide may have trouble eating or sleeping. Their normal behavior may change. If they are usually outgoing, they may withdraw from friends and social occasions. On the other hand, if they are normally a loner, they may become more social. They may lose interest in hobbies, work, school, or relationships. They may seem preoccupied with death and dying. Giving away possessions that are important to them can also be an indicator they are thinking about suicide.

Emotional Stressors

Depression is one of the most common warning signs of suicide. When people are depressed, it's hard for them to see that they'll ever feel any better. Severe loss, humiliation, or rejection can increase the risk for a

What's News?

In 1999, 90% of all reported suicides occurred among white males and females. But other ethnic groups have seen substantial increases in their rates of suicide in recent years. In 1999, the suicide rate for young Native American males was twice as high as the overall national rate for males. The suicide rate of young African American males doubled between 1981 and 1998. In 1999, Hispanic females attempted suicide at a rate almost three times that of the national average for females.

suicide attempt, especially if the person is already emotionally distressed. If a loved one has recently died or the person has been rejected by a friend or romantic partner, feelings of hopelessness may trigger thoughts of suicide as a way to escape the emotional pain.

PREVENTING SUICIDE

Most people who attempt suicide are desperately crying out for help. It is common for them to give many clues and exhibit warning signs that they are considering suicide. They may not fully realize it, but they want help; they want someone to save them from themselves. Understanding the factors that can lead to suicide and being aware of the warning signs are the first steps to preventing it. Each of us can learn ways to help people we know who may be at risk. Some actions you can take yourself to give help directly. You can also connect potential victims to a mental health professional who is trained to deal with suicide or to other crisis resources. You can make the difference between life and death for someone who is having thoughts of suicide. The following sections describe some actions to take to help a person who is threatening to attempt suicide.

What You Can Do

Communicate

Be willing to talk openly and nonjudgmentally. If a person begins to talk about suicide or wanting to die, we often feel uncomfortable, embarrassed, or awkward. Sometimes we try to pretend they are only joking. We may be afraid that if we talk about suicide, the person will be more likely to actually do it. Experts recommend, however, that the best

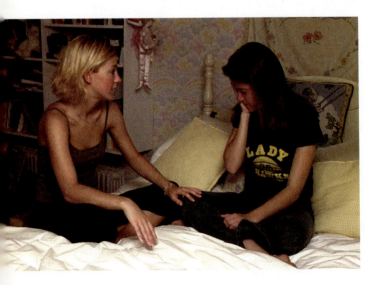

response is to talk openly about the situation. Listen carefully, and allow the person to express his or her feelings. Do not offer advice or try to convince the person he or she is wrong. It's more effective to ask direct questions to learn about the person's thoughts and intentions.

- "Are you thinking of hurting or killing yourself?"
- "Have you thought about how you would do it?"
- "Do you have the means to do it?" (For example, does the person have a gun or pills)
- "Have you decided when you will do it?"

If the answer to all of those questions is yes, the risk for a suicide attempt is extremely high, and you should take the following actions:

- Get professional help for the person immediately.
- Do not leave the person alone, even if he or she promises to get help.
- Do not agree not to tell anyone. Experts agree that many teen lives could be saved if only their friends would break the "code of silence" that exists among teenagers.

Even if you have misjudged the seriousness of the situation, it is better to be safe than sorry. A life hangs in the balance.

Suggest Alternatives

Many people who plan to commit suicide believe they have no other option for ending the pain they are experiencing. Although it is true that time has a way of healing emotional pain, when the pain is intense it can be very difficult to believe that things will get better.

Help the person identify other options for dealing with the situation. Ask the person to agree not to try to hurt or kill himself or herself without first talking with a professional. Delaying a decision can be very important because many suicide intentions are short lived. This tactic can buy valuable time to connect the person to skilled resources.

Connect the Person with Helping Resources

You can be a friend to someone who is hurting emotionally, but you probably don't have the skills needed to help a person who is suicidal. Encourage the person to get professional help and offer to go with him or her. People in crisis are not always capable of taking action without support from someone else.

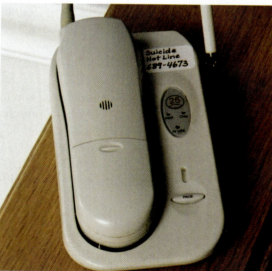

Most cities and towns have a suicide crisis hot line. The National Hopeline Network numbe is 1-800-SUICIDE. Trained telephone counselors are available at this number 24 hours a day, 7 days a week. This number can also be used to connect you with a suicide crisis center in your area. Trained mental health professionals are available to work with people in crisis who may be thinking of suicide.

There are many ways you can try to help someone who is threatening suicide, but each person ultimately has responsibility for his or her own actions. If someone you know commits suicide, it is not your fault, even if you didn't try to help. It is common to feel guilty or at fault if someone you know commits suicide. You may need to seek professional help if you are unable to accept the fact that it's not your fault.

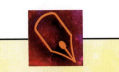

What Mental Health Professionals Can Do

Mental health professionals are trained to assess risk for suicide and to help potential victims manage the crisis until it passes. These professionals can arrange for medications such as antidepressants, if appropriate. Because antidepressant drugs take a few weeks to become fully effective, it is sometimes necessary to refer the patient for in-patient hospital treatment until the immediate danger of a suicide attempt passes. Mental health professionals also use behavioral therapy techniques to help the person resolve the crisis. If you suspect a person is thinking about taking his or her life, you should always ask that person to seek help from a mental health professional. If your friend had a broken leg, you would insist he or she seek medical treatment. If your friend has a broken spirit, that situation should not be treated any differently.

What Families Can Do

In most cases, family members know each other better than anyone else does. In today's busy society, however, many parents don't spend as much time with their children as they used to. In many families, parent–teen communication is limited to simply exchanging information. Parents may not notice signs and symptoms of distress in their children if they don't spend much time with them. Increasing family time so children have opportunities to spend time, talk, and share their feelings with family members is important for promoting good mental health. Both parents and young people should learn the warning signs for suicide so they are prepared to help family members if necessary.

What Schools Can Do

Teenagers spend a lot of their time at school. Starting at the elementary level, schools have opportunities to establish supportive atmospheres for students. Schools at all levels can play an important role in reducing early risk factors for depression and substance abuse in children and teens. They can also develop school policies against discrimination and intimidation for both teachers and students. School personnel should be aware of warning signs for depression, substance abuse, and suicide and should be able to appropriately refer students who are in crisis to the help they need.

What Communities Can Do

Communities can establish support systems to protect teens from depression and suicide. For example, they can set up programs to promote nonviolent conflict resolution and teach skills in problem solv-

✿ teen forum ✿

Suicide at School?

The tragic killings at Columbine High School in Colorado in 1999 focused attention on school violence. The media attention focused primarily on the victims of the shootings, so it was easy to forget that the two students responsible for the violence killed themselves, in addition to killing others. It appears their intent was to cause as much pain and damage as possible before killing themselves to end their own pain. In the aftermath of this shooting and other violent episodes in schools across the country, many schools have created violence prevention and crisis management plans. But a far fewer number have fully implemented suicide prevention plans. According to the U.S. Department of Education report *Indicators of School Crime and Safety, 1999*, about a quarter of deaths that occur on school grounds are actually suicides. In addition, students who commit suicide often take other victims with them as well, as evidenced at Columbine. Federal law requires schools to report suspected child abuse. Yet states currently do not require schools to notify parents if a student expresses suicidal thoughts.

- Do you think such a law should be enacted?
- What would be the pros and cons of such a law?
- Would it make students at risk for suicide less likely to ask for help?
- Provide reasons for your answers.

ing. Community members can also work to ensure that adequate help from mental health professionals is available for all teens and that teens know where they can go to get this help. Communities must let teens know they are supported. When everyone is working together to help young people who are in crisis, the risk for suicide decreases.

ARE YOU AT RISK?

This chapter discussed teen suicide in the United States, common warning signs for suicide, and ways to help a person who may be thinking about suicide. According to the CDC Youth Risk Behavior Surveillance System data for 2001, almost 20% of high school students indicated they had "seriously considered attempting suicide during the past 12 months." Are you part of that 20%? If you are, please take action to get help. Talk to someone you trust, and tell that person you need help. Many people have thought about committing suicide at some time in their lives. Fortunately, most of them didn't act on their thoughts. They eventually came to realize that the crisis was temporary, but that a choice of suicide would be permanent. Now more than ever before, help *is* available. You do not need to suffer alone. Get help *today*.

BUILDING YOUR Wellness Plan

One of the ways you can help yourself and others avoid the pain and grief associated with a completed suicide is to take action ahead of time by developing resources to be used in a crisis situation. Just as having a first aid kit can be a lifesaver in the event of an emergency, planning ahead can make the difference between life and death. Use what you learned in this chapter to create a suicide prevention plan that includes the information and resources you would want to have easily available in the event you or someone close to you had thoughts of suicide.

- A list that includes telephone numbers for community resources and suicide hot lines
- A list of warning signs
- Tips on what to do if someone threatens suicide
- Copies of the plan to keep with you and to have at home

end-of-chapter ACTIVITIES

Weblinks

Preventing Suicide

American Foundation for Suicide Prevention:
   http://www.afsp.org
The Jason Foundation:
   http://www.jasonfoundation.com
Nemours Foundation: **http://www.teenhealth.org**
   (enter the teen health site and search for suicide)
Suicide Awareness Voices of Education:
   http://www.save.org
Yellow Ribbon Suicide Prevention Program:
   http://www.yellowribbon.org

Suicide Facts

American Association of Suicidology:
   http://www.suicidology.org
Centers for Disease Control and Prevention:
   http://www.cdc.gov/ncipc/factsheets/suifacts.htm
National Institute of Mental Health:
   http://www.nimh.nih.gov/research/suifact.htm

Short-Answer Questions

1. Define the terms *suicide*, *attempted suicide*, and *completed suicide*.
2. Identify three organizations that provide information and resources related to suicide.
3. List and briefly describe the factors that may contribute to suicide.
4. List and briefly describe some of the factors that may protect against suicide.
5. List the four questions to ask someone who is talking about wanting to die.

Discussion Questions

1. Describe the relationship among mental disorders, substance abuse, and suicide.
2. Explain reasons why acts of suicide may be under-reported.
3. Discuss how the media may play a role in suicide.

4. Describe the relationship between situational stressors and suicide.

5. Discuss the relationship of guns to suicide.

☼ Chapter Vocabulary

Using a separate sheet of paper, list and define the following terms:

attempted suicide

completed suicide

suicide

☼ Application Activities

Language Arts Connection

1. Write an essay explaining your personal views regarding suicide.

2. Create a Suicide Crisis Referral pamphlet specific to the area in which you live. Include categories such as warning signs, what to do if someone you know threatens suicide, and suicide hot line numbers, along with any other information you think would be helpful.

Math Connection

Go to the Web site for the CDC Youth Risk Behavior Surveillance System, located at **http://www.cdc.gov/nccdphp/dash/yrbs/youth01online.htm.** Find the questions related to suicide (located in the section on unintentional injuries/violence). National data have been collected every two years since 1991. Find the earliest data for your state and compare them with the nation's data during the same period by creating a bar graph. Do this for each year statistics are available. Describe how teen suicide statistics in your state compare with national statistics.

Social Studies Connection

Research one of the following topics and report on your results:

1. Age-related differences in suicide attempts and completed suicides

2. Suicide attempts and completed suicides in the United States as compared with those in another country of your choosing

3. Suicide attempts and completed suicides among Native Americans, African Americans, Hispanics, or any other racial or ethnic group as compared with the national data on suicide

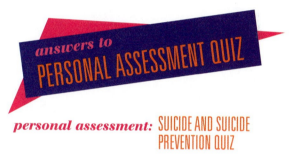

answers to **PERSONAL ASSESSMENT QUIZ**

personal assessment: SUICIDE AND SUICIDE PREVENTION QUIZ

1. False	6. True
2. True	7. False
3. False	8. True
4. False	9. False
5. True	10. True

unit 5 | Social Health

Introduction

Developing good physical and mental health habits can help you build a strong foundation for wellness. But to have an enjoyable and fulfilling life, it is also important to develop good relationships with other people. The relationships that you have with others help you learn more about others who share your world. In relationships, you learn many things about yourself as well. When you have strong, healthy relationships with others, you are likely to be both healthier and happier.

In this unit, you will have an opportunity to learn information and skills that will help you develop and maintain good relationships with others. As a child, your earliest relationships were with your family. As a teen, you now spend a lot of time with your peers as well. Perhaps you may already be involved in a romantic relationship. In all of these relationships, you will encounter conflict from time to time. The material in this unit can help you to develop good relationships with your family, friends, and romantic partners. You will also learn how to get back on track if conflict threatens your relationships.

chapter 16

Healthy Relationships at Home

Kara celebrated her thirteenth birthday just last month. Her family threw a big backyard barbecue as a surprise party. They invited a lot of her friends and relatives to celebrate "Kara becoming a teenager." Kara thinks she's pretty lucky to have such a wonderful family, but she's also feeling a little uneasy. Her brother, Todd, turned 16 about six months ago. Kara has always adored Todd and loves spending time doing things with him. Ever since he got his driver's license, however, Todd is hardly ever at home. When he is at home, it seems as if he's always arguing with someone. He showed up at her birthday party with his new girlfriend and stayed only about 30 minutes. She overheard her grandmother tell her dad, "Well, now that you have two teenagers, you'll have double the trouble." Kara wonders if her family is going to be really different than before, now that she and Todd are both teenagers.

How do you think Kara's family life will change, now that she's a teenager?

chapter OBJECTIVES

When you finish this chapter, you should be able to:

- Explain the role and purpose of a family.
- List and describe several qualities of healthy family relationships.
- Identify some of the factors contributing to changes in family structure.
- Describe the most common types of family structures.
- List and briefly describe two of the central challenges of adolescence.
- List some of the underlying stressors for families with teenagers.
- Develop a personal action plan for contributing to the development and maintenance of a healthy family.

key TERMS

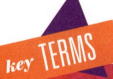

blended family
dysfunctional family
family household
healthy family
household
personal identity
traditional family

Introduction

The relationships you develop with members of your family are among the most important connections you will ever establish. These relationships provide you with many of your earliest models for establishing relationships with people outside the family. Your ideas about how families function and the qualities and skills necessary to build successful relationships are directly related to your experiences in your own family. In this chapter, we will examine what a family is, qualities of healthy families, and characteristics of family relationships, particularly during the teen years.

personal assessment: HEALTHY FAMILY RELATIONSHIPS QUIZ

Before reading this chapter, take this personal assessment to discover more about how you relate to your family members. Read the statements below and, on a separate sheet of paper, rate your answers on the basis of the way you respond most of the time. Use the following scale:
1 = Definitely True; 2 = Mostly True; 3 = Mostly False; 4 = Definitely False.
An interpretation of your results is located at the end of this chapter.

1. I treat other members of my family, including my siblings, with respect.

2. I can be trusted to keep my word and not betray a family member's confidence.

3. I am able to tell the truth when I talk to members of my family.

4. I do not have to pretend to be someone I'm not when I'm around my family.

5. I am able to express my love for my family, both physically and verbally.

6. I allow other members of my family to be themselves.

7. I am willing to help other members of my family achieve their goals and dreams.

8. If I have a problem with a member of my family, we are usually able to work it out.

9. I listen well to other members of my family, and they listen well to me.

10. In our family, we follow a structured pattern for resolving problems.

WHAT IS A FAMILY?

What are the first images that come to your mind when you hear the word *family*? Before reading any further, take a minute to construct a mental picture of your impressions when you hear the word *family*. As you read further, compare your mental picture with the following description of what it means to be a family.

Throughout history, families have formed the basic unit of society. Families provide resources and support for children as they make their journey toward adulthood. These resources include both material resources, such as food, clothing, and shelter, and emotional resources, such as love, attention, and belonging. Families try to ensure the safety and security of their members. They communicate values for decision making, model skills for social relationships, and generally help children

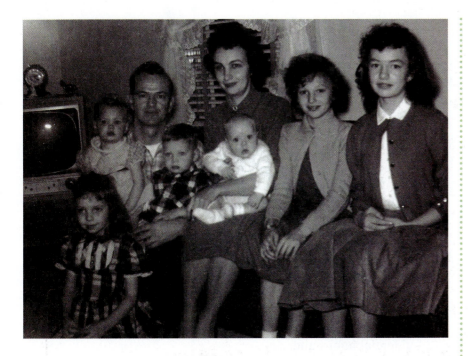

develop the skills they need to someday live successfully on their own. Although many families today may look different from families of the past, children still depend on families to provide these necessary resources and support.

Each person in a family is both an individual and a member of the family. Each family member affects and is affected by the other members. Family members share joys, sorrows, challenges, and chores. Just as in any other relationship, sometimes getting along well is easy and enjoyable, and sometimes it requires a good deal of effort. Developing and practicing skills for building healthy relationships within your family can make a big difference in the quality of your relationships with all the other people in your life.

At its best, a family provides a web of support that encourages the growth and development of each member, while also maintaining the importance of the bonds between them. A **healthy family** celebrates individual and family successes and accepts mistakes and failures as inevitable parts of growth. Healthy families are not families that never have problems. Rather, they are families that develop the qualities and skills necessary for successfully resolving problems when they occur. Despite the difficulties they experience, healthy families continue to seek positive ways to remain connected to each other.

healthy family

a family that consistently demonstrates positive qualities and skills that are characteristic of a strong, supportive family unit

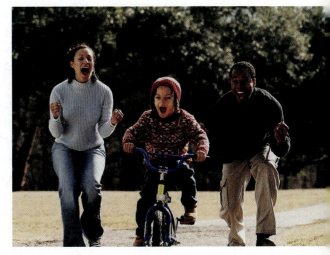

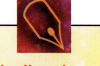

take it on home

Interview the other members of your family about how they would describe a healthy family. Listen carefully for the words they use. Are these words the same ones you would use to describe your family? In what ways could you contribute to making your family better fit the description of a healthy family? Make a note of these words, the responses of your family members, and your reactions to those responses and include them in your Health Folio.

QUALITIES OF HEALTHY FAMILY RELATIONSHIPS

For children, families provide the earliest model for all future relationships with other people. Healthy families have the same qualities that are present in healthy relationships with friends, romantic partners, and members of the extended community. Have you ever thought about what makes a healthy relationship? In all types of relationships that are healthy, you will find mutual respect, trust, honesty, and authenticity. Strong, healthy family relationships also demonstrate love, acceptance, commitment, and loyalty. Communication and problem solving are other important relationship skills that are learned and practiced within the family.

Although there will always be occasional lapses, the members of successful families practice the following 10 qualities *most* of the time:

1. *Respect.* Family members are not belittling or demeaning to each other. Both adults and children demonstrate courtesy and consideration for the other members of the family.

2. *Trust.* Family members do not intentionally hurt each other. They can be relied upon to keep promises and not to share confidential information.

3. *Honesty.* Family members tell you the truth. They do not say anything behind your back that they would not say to you personally.

4. *Authenticity.* Family members are real and genuine. They do not put on an act, pretending to be someone they really aren't.

5. *Love.* Family members are able to express their positive feelings for each other, physically and verbally. They sincerely want the best possible outcomes for other members of the family.

6. *Acceptance.* Family members allow the other family members to be themselves. They allow each other to be spontaneous and genuine, without ridicule or criticism.

7. *Commitment.* Family members are committed to the well-being of all the family members and work to ensure the best possible outcomes for each other. Families who demonstrate commitment don't give up just because there are problems or something is difficult.

8. *Communication.* Family members learn and use good communication skills, not just by talking but also by listening and reading body language.

9. *Problem solving.* Family members make the effort to acquire or develop good skills in problem solving. When they are confronted with a difficult problem, family members work together to discover new ways to solve the problem so that everyone comes out a winner.

10. *Conflict resolution.* When conflicts occur between family members, they have the necessary skills to work through the conflict

and reach a solution that is mutually acceptable to the family members involved in the conflict. Conflicts can be resolved without producing lasting bitterness and resentment, which can permanently destroy family harmony.

CHANGING FAMILY STRUCTURES

Today's families are more diverse than ever before. You may be a part of a **traditional family**, in which you share a home with your parents and brothers and sisters. Or you may be part of a **blended family** that includes a stepparent and stepsiblings. You may be an only child, or you may have several siblings. Perhaps you live with only one of your parents, with a grandparent, or in some other type of family situation. Regardless of the family situation in which you currently live, your "family" is the group of people you count on to provide the basic love, understanding, and material resources you need to make a successful transition from the dependency of childhood to the independence and self-sufficiency of adulthood.

The U.S. Census Bureau keeps statistics on the number of **households** in the United States and the individuals living in those households. The bureau conducts a census once every 10 years. The most recent census was in 2000. The U.S. Census Bureau has two broad categories of households: family households and nonfamily households. A **family household** is defined as a householder and persons who live in the same household who are related to the householder by birth, marriage, or adoption.

In the 2000 census, about 52% of all households were headed by a married couple; about 12% were headed by a single-parent female; and about 4% were headed by a single-parent male. The remaining 32% of households were considered nonfamily households, in which persons lived alone or with others who were not relatives. The 2000 census confirmed that the size of households continues to shrink, with fewer members in each household. At the same time, the percentage of single-parent households and nonfamily households continues to increase.

More children today live in single-parent households for at least part of their childhood and teenage years than they did in the past. More than half of all American children do not live in traditional two-parent families with both biological parents. According to the National Center for Health Statistics, recent data show that about 43% of first marriages end in separation or divorce within 15 years. Between two-thirds and three-fourths of persons who divorce will eventually remarry, often bringing children from the first marriage into the second marriage to form a blended family. In addition to all the challenges facing a traditional family, blended families are confronted with special challenges that occur as a result of taking two separate family units and combining them into one larger unit.

traditional family

a family that consists of two parents and their biological or adopted children

blended family

a family created when one or both of the partners who remarry bring children from a previous marriage into the new family unit

household

a person or group of persons who occupy the same housing unit

family household

a householder and persons who live in the same household who are related to the householder by birth, marriage, or adoption

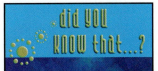

did you know that...?

More than a third of all U.S. children today are expected to live in a blended family before the age of 18.

Who's Watching the Kids?

In the past, two-parent households were much more common than they are today. In many of these families, there was a parent who did not work outside the home. It was also likely that there was a much larger extended family, such as grandparents and aunts and uncles, who lived in the same geographical area than is true for most families today. In a small town, other community members may have taken significant amounts of responsibility for children who were not their own. So there was always someone watching the kids. Today, however, circumstances have changed dramatically. There are more mothers working full time away from the home. There are more single-parent households and fewer grandparents and other family members living close by.

- Do you think these changes in family structure have resulted in positive or negative consequences for children growing up today?
- Who watched you when you were younger?
- What would you do if you were a working parent and had to find a place for your children to go after school? Give examples to explain your answer.

ADOLESCENCE: CHANGING ROLES AND RESPONSIBILITIES

Adolescence provides unique opportunities and challenges for family relationships. Even families who have previously enjoyed close, supportive relationships may find that a member reaching adolescence can create individual and family turmoil. One of the major reasons for this turmoil is that, as teenagers go through the rapid physical, emotional, and social changes of adolescence, families are also affected by these changes. If these changes combine to throw a teenager off balance, the entire family feels the effects, just like the ripple effect of a stone thrown into a pond.

One of the key functions of families is to provide physical, emotional, and social support for its members. Each person in the family has roles and responsibilities that contribute to providing this support. These roles and responsibilities are not usually created consciously. They are naturally assumed by the members without much thought or notice. Think back to the earliest time you can remember in your childhood. What were your role and responsibilities in the family? You were probably primarily a "taker" because you were too young to assume many responsibilities. Maybe some of your earliest responsibilities were to make your bed, take out the trash, or set the table for supper. As you grew older, your role changed within the family and you assumed more responsibilities.

Now, as a teenager, your role and responsibilities are changing once again and becoming more like those of the adults in the family. You may have noticed that sometimes the adult members make personal sacrifices for the good of the entire family. In the process of becoming a young adult member of the family, you may have to sometimes choose between doing what you personally want to do and what is best for your family. Making these choices will help define your new role within your family.

take it on home

Ask each of the members of your family to list their key family responsibilities. Compare responsibilities. Is the division of family responsibilities appropriate for the age, maturity, and number of nonfamily responsibilities for each member of the family? Are there any responsibilities that need to be distributed differently? Note your responses in your Health Folio.

Challenges of Adolescence

As a teenager, two of the important challenges you face on your path to self-sufficiency as an adult are establishing your individual identity separate from your role within your family and assuming primary responsibility for meeting your own physical, emotional, and social needs. We'll take a closer look at each of these challenges.

Establishing Your Personal Identity

Establishing your own **personal identity** is a key challenge of adolescence. As a child, your early identity is strongly influenced by your family. As you accumulate life experiences outside the family unit, you begin constructing your own personal identity. Early adolescence is often a time of "trying on" different identities to see what "fits" best for you—much like trying on a new hat or pair of shoes. You may rapidly discard some of these trial identities, as you would a pair of shoes you have outgrown after a rapid growth spurt. But you may keep other developing parts of your identity, as you would the old hat you've loved for years. It is likely that the adult identity you eventually establish will retain many characteristics of your childhood identity. But as you progress toward adulthood, you will be shaping and adding to your identity in ways that provide a unique fit for the person you are becoming.

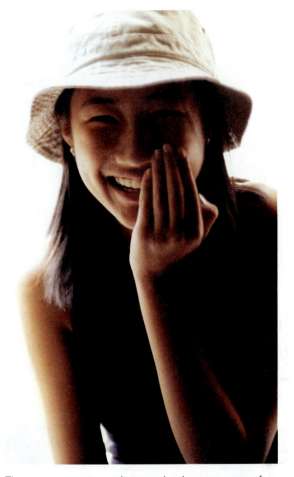

The teenage years are when you develop your sense of personal identity.

personal identity

a unified sense of self, expressing attitudes, beliefs, and actions that are uniquely characteristic of you

As they attempt to establish their own identity, teens often want to spend less time with their family and more time with their peers. This is a normal part of growing up and becoming more independent. It gives teens the opportunity to test their developing relationship skills with people they do not know as well as they know their family members. Interacting with many individuals provides important information about the relationship skills needed to be a successful adult.

Teens are often unaware of how difficult their increasing independence can be for their family members. Parents may have an especially difficult time accepting this new independence. For the past dozen years or so, you have been a part of family activities and gatherings. As you begin spending more time away, your family may feel as if you are abandoning them, although you probably are not. To ease the transition for everyone, you can make a special effort to stay connected to your family. Sometimes simple words can mean a lot, words such as: "I love you," "Thank you," and "I appreciate all the things you do for me." You can back up these words with actions, such as calling home if you have

real teens

Hi, I'm Mandy. I'm 15. I have an older brother, Trace, who is 17, and a younger brother, Mike, who is 10. We've always done a lot of things together as a family, but as soon as Trace turned 13, our family made a new rule: Tuesday night is Family Night and Family Night Rules! What I mean is that no matter what other things are going on, we are expected to spend Tuesday nights together as a family. When I was younger, I really liked Family Night because we usually got to do some- thing special and fun together, even if it was only ordering take-out pizza. Now that I'm older, there are times when I *really* wish that we had never agreed on a Family Night! Like last year, when Valentine's Day fell on a Tuesday. The drama club at school had a play for Valentine's Day, and this really cool guy asked me to meet him there. Yep, you guessed it. If I wanted to go, my whole family had to go. Actually, I guess it wasn't that bad. At least they voted to go. If anyone wants to do something "outside the family," then everyone else has to vote on whether the whole family should go or whether the person has to say no. Mostly I vote to go because we still get to do something fun. Then the next time I want a "family exception," my brothers and parents are more likely to go along. Oh yeah, one more thing I forgot: we always take pictures on Family Night. We have photo albums full of them. I have to admit that I do like looking back at all the pictures and remembering all the fun we've had together as a family. Some of my friends think we're crazy, and some of my friends wish their families were more like ours. But however they feel, they know that at our house, Family Night Rules!

a change of plans, sending a card or e-mail just to say someone is important to you, or offering to help out without being asked. These actions can help your family know they are still important to you. At the same time, these actions are also evidence that you are becoming a responsible and considerate young adult, ready for the independence you are seeking.

Meeting Your Own Needs

Independence is closely connected to responsibility. To be truly inde- pendent, you will have to assume primary responsibility for meeting your own needs. This responsibility includes providing for physical needs such as food, shelter, clothing, and financial resources. It also includes meeting your own emotional needs for love and belonging and your social needs for connection and communication.

In previous times, children and teens had to take on lots of respon- sibility at early ages. In addition to attending school, teenagers were routinely expected to be major contributors to the family. In a rural family, they might have been expected to feed and water the animals before school and to help with other chores after school. In an urban

❊ teen forum ❊

To Grandmother's House We Go?

Suppose that you and your family have always spent the last two weeks of summer vacation at your grandparents' home in another state. This summer, however, you don't want to go because you have a part-time job. Your employer would probably let you have time off, but you want to earn as much money as you can this summer. Besides, you want to spend those last two weeks before school with your friends. Your best friend says it's okay for you to stay at his house while your parents are gone. But your parents insist you have to go. Your grandparents are getting older, and, according to your parents, "they won't be around forever." They tell you that your grandparents will be very hurt and think you don't care about them if you don't come.

- What is the best way to resolve this situation?
- Should teenagers be expected to spend extended time with their family, just as they did when they were younger?
- Identify possible solutions to this dilemma. Describe in your Health Folio the possible consequences of each course of action.

family, the teens might have been expected to hold a job and contribute their earnings to the family income. Although they had large amounts of responsibility, teenagers of the past also had more opportunities for independence while still remaining connected to the family.

Today, however, teens make far fewer essential contributions to the success of the family. Even if a teenager holds a part-time job, the money earned is usually spent by the teen for things he or she wants. Few families in the United States today depend on their children to provide essential physical labor to meet their needs. Instead, most teens today are dependent members of the family structure. Because they have this role within the family, parents and other family members often view teenagers as being incapable of making healthy independent decisions.

One of the challenges that teenagers face is that, although they may feel ready to make independent choices and take certain actions without the support of their family, they still do not have the resources and skills to meet all of their own needs. For instance, you may believe you are ready for the independence of having your own car to drive yourself to and from school, work, and social activities. Yet, you are faced with the inescapable reality that you can't afford to make car and insurance payments, provide basic maintenance services for your vehicle, and pay for gas. This situation puts you, the teen, in an awkward position. You want to do something that you haven't yet acquired the skills and resources to accomplish successfully on your own. You may resent being dependent on your family and being treated like a child, but at the same time you probably feel anxious and insecure about your abilities to provide for yourself and make it on your own.

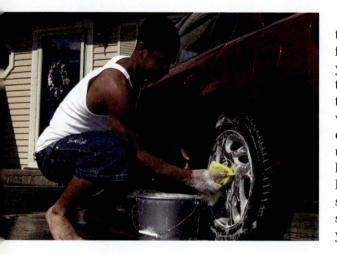

One method of working through these difficulties is to learn to negotiate as a family unit. You still need help from your parents, but you also have contributions that you can make to them. For instance, in the example about the car, you and your parents could negotiate your use of the family car. You could offer to take responsibility for washing the car and taking it to the shop for regular oil changes. In return, your parents could agree to let you use the car for a specified amount of time. Negotiations like this help everyone in the family get their needs met. In time, just as you learned to successfully tie your own shoes when you were a young child, you will gradually succeed at being independent and able to provide for your own needs.

COMMON STRESSORS FOR FAMILIES

As children become teenagers, families are faced with underlying stressors caused by changes and feelings that aren't as obvious as the conflicts associated with parent–teen struggles for independence. Teens are experiencing major physical and emotional changes associated with the hormonal changes of puberty. They no longer feel as safe, secure, and protected as they did when they were children. Instead, they face tremendous emotional and social pressures as they seek to develop their own unique personal identity. All of this turmoil occurs at the same time their parents may be facing significant midlife challenges of their own. As their own children are growing up and needing them less, they may have aging parents who require more attention. As their children become teenagers, parents are also confronted with daily evidence of their own aging. These underlying stressors can cause everyday stressors to assume exaggerated importance. See Figure 16-1 for some common everyday stressors that cause conflict in families.

> **For families with teenagers, some common everyday stressors that present the potential for conflict are:**
>
> - Hair, clothing, makeup
> - Curfews and driving privileges
> - Choice of friends
> - Time spent with family versus peers
> - Dating and sexuality issues
> - Self-destructive behaviors associated with tobacco, alcohol, or other drugs

Figure 16-1
Everyday family stressors

WHEN TROUBLE STRIKES

All families go through times of chaos and upheaval. Your family life, like other aspects of your life, will have ups and downs, good days and bad days. Some families, however, have many more relationship difficulties among their members than average. Sometimes you hear these families referred to as **"dysfunctional" families**. What does it mean to be a dysfunctional family? Experiencing occasional problems in family relationships, even if those problems are serious, doesn't make a family dysfunctional. A dysfunctional family is one in which family interactions continually negatively affect the physical, emotional, and social development of the individuals in the family. In a dysfunctional family, the sum total of all the relationship experiences in the family over time creates pain rather than pleasure.

There can be many causes of dysfunction within a family. Sometimes alcohol or drug abuse by a family member is the problem. Physical abuse and emotional neglect are other causes of dysfunction. Sometimes family members just don't have good communication, conflict resolution, and problem-solving skills. Because of this lack of skills, it's difficult for them to get along, and they don't want to spend much time together.

At its most basic level, a functional family is one that works well; it functions effectively. A dysfunctional family, on the other hand, has one or more elements of family life that are not working well. It's important to remember that even in the healthiest families, a certain amount of dysfunction exists. For instance, in almost every way imaginable, Theresa's family has healthy relationships with each other. But Theresa's dad thinks you should never publicly express anger. Now that she's a teenager, it seems as if Theresa experiences situations that make her feel angry much more frequently than when she was younger. She finds it difficult to hide her feelings, but if she shows she's angry about something, her father punishes her by sending her to her room for several hours. Because a wide range of fluctuating emotions is normal for teenagers, refusing to allow Theresa to express those emotions might be considered a mild form of dysfunction.

Theresa's situation is very different, however, from the situation in Corey's family. Corey's mom, Angela, has a very stressful job in which she has a great deal of responsibility. Sometimes when she's feeling really stressed, Angela drinks too much. She doesn't drink every day, and there are lots of days when it's not difficult at all for Corey to get along with his mom. But when she's had too much to drink, his mom comes home and yells at Corey and his little sister for any little thing. Sometimes she even spanks his little sister really hard or tells Corey that he's a no-good loser who will never amount to anything. Corey knows that she doesn't really mean to hurt them, but her behavior hurts anyway. He never knows if it will be a good day or a bad day when his mom comes home. This is an example of a family that is experiencing greater levels of dysfunction. They may need professional assistance to get their family relationships back on track.

take it on home

Have you ever considered how difficult parenting must be? Parenting is one of the most important responsibilities a person ever assumes. Yet most parents receive no training in how to be a good parent. Parents are held responsible for their children's behavior, but during the teen years, they are expected to gradually give up control. Ask your own parents or other parents you know how they prepared to become parents and what they wish they had known about parenting before they had children. If you decide you want to become a parent someday, what knowledge and skills will you want to possess first? Make a note of your answers in your Health Folio.

dysfunctional family

a family in which family interactions negatively affect the physical, emotional, and social development and well-being of the individuals in the family

When family relationships don't seem to be working, members of a healthy family have a problem-solving process they use to try to seek a solution. If they can't resolve the problem alone, they may seek assistance from resources outside the family to try to get things back on track. They may read some books on improving family relationships, seek advice from someone they trust, or make an appointment with a professional therapist. A family is not a dysfunctional family just because they are having problems. Dysfunctional families are those in which no one acknowledges that problems exist, and no one is willing to seek solutions to help the family function more smoothly.

SUCCEEDING IN FAMILY RELATIONSHIPS

Your most personal and intimate relationship is the relationship you have with yourself. Sometimes it's easy to forget that the relationship you have with yourself affects all the relationships you have with other people. So one of the most positive actions you can take to develop successful relationships with others is to learn to value and nurture your relationship with yourself.

During the teen years, having a good relationship with yourself may be more complicated than ever before in your life because you may feel as if you're constantly changing. The person you were yesterday is not the same as the person you are today. You may not even be aware of these changes in yourself unless you make a special effort to take time to notice them. If you find yourself in a situation in which you are having difficulty with family relationships or other relationships in your life, it's a good idea to spend some time reflecting on how you feel about yourself. How you feel about yourself can color the way you feel about others. Taking care of problems in this most basic relationship can often be the key to solving problems in your relationships with others, such as family members.

Families provide the "testing ground" for all the skills you are developing to serve you in your relationships throughout your life. It is within the family that you learn what works and what doesn't in respect to relationships. You have opportunities to observe the qualities that make family relationships satisfying and enjoyable—and those that don't. Family life also provides your earliest opportunities for learning and practicing skills in communication, problem solving, and conflict resolution. Teens who are fortunate enough to have good relationship role models for these skills as they are growing up have a head start in developing their own skills for healthy relationships later in life. And teens themselves can play an important role in contributing to positive family relationships.

BUILDING YOUR Wellness Plan

In this chapter, you learned about the importance of building successful relationships within your family. The relationships you have with your family can have a significant impact on your healthy development into adulthood. Your wellness plan should include information and strategies to help you become a family member who makes a positive contribution to your family unit. These should include:

- Developing a good relationship with yourself
- Understanding how you and the other members of your family contribute to the family unit
- Describing the qualities demonstrated in healthy family relationships
- Identifying the problems and stressors your family experiences
- Learning and practicing the communication and problem-solving skills your family can use to deal with these problems and stressors

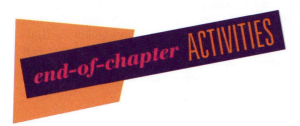

end-of-chapter ACTIVITIES

Weblink

United States Households

U.S. Census Bureau: **http://www.census.gov**

Short-Answer Questions

1. List some of the physical and emotional resources families provide for their children.
2. List and briefly describe two of the central challenges adolescents face.
3. Identify some of the everyday stressors that can cause conflict in families with teenagers.
4. List and briefly describe some of the qualities of healthy family relationships.
5. Identify five action steps you would take if you were having conflict with a parent or sibling.

Discussion Questions

1. Describe some of the societal factors that have contributed to changes in family structures.
2. Explain how your roles and responsibilities in your family have changed during the following time periods: elementary school, middle school, and high school.
3. Describe ways that a traditional family differs from a blended family.
4. Identify some of the underlying stressors that families with teenagers face.
5. Describe the process a healthy family might go through if they were experiencing a significant problem of some kind.

☀ Chapter Vocabulary

Using a separate sheet of paper, list and define the following terms:

blended family	household
dysfunctional family	personal identity
family household	traditional family
healthy family	

☀ Application Activities

Language Arts Connection

1. Using the real teen story in this chapter, write an essay describing your thoughts and feelings about Mandy's family's tradition of "Family Night Rules." How would you feel about using this tradition in your family? Give reasons for your opinion.

2. Write an essay or short story using one of your family traditions (or one you imagine) as the basis for the story.

Math Connection

Using the U.S. Census Bureau data on families (available from its Web site), construct a bar graph and a pie chart that illustrates changes in household structure over the past 50 years. Use data regarding the number of households headed by a married couple, by a single female parent, and by a single male parent and the number of households in which people live alone or with a nonrelative. In your opinion, which method of presentation (bar graph or pie chart) provides the best understanding of the data?

Social Studies Connection

1. Research and report on the historical changes in family structures from the early 1900s to now. What are some of the major effects on families today as a result of these changes?

2. Investigate various organizations in the community that provide support or resources for families. What kinds of resources are available? What must a person do to use these services?

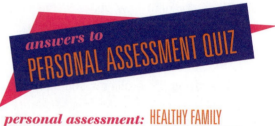

answers to
PERSONAL ASSESSMENT QUIZ

personal assessment: HEALTHY FAMILY
RELATIONSHIPS QUIZ

Answers will vary. A higher proportion of Definitely True or Mostly True responses indicates that you and your family are exhibiting the skills and qualities associated with a healthy family. It is important to note that responses to these questions will vary over time, depending on current circumstances within the family. A higher proportion of Mostly False or Definitely False responses may simply mean that your family is currently experiencing some relationship difficulties.

chapter 17

Healthy Peer Relationships

P enny has lived next door to Bradley
for the past six years. He moved
into the neighborhood when she
was in the third grade. In all those
years, they've spent a lot of time
together. They've played together,
argued and made up, and argued
and made up again. Through it all,
Penny has come to consider
Bradley a true friend. He's a year
older than she is, so he's never
been in any of her classes before. But this year
they're in the same chemistry class. Brittany, a girl Penny knows
from another class, is in their chemistry class too. Last week,
Brittany told Penny that she likes Bradley and wants Penny to help
her get a date with him. Penny has gotten Bradley dates with her
friends before, but this time is different. She doesn't know Brittany
very well, but she's heard that Brittany wants to date Bradley just
to make another boy jealous. Penny wants to be a good friend to
Bradley but isn't sure what to do.

What do you think is her role as a friend to Bradley in this situation?

chapter OBJECTIVES

When you finish this chapter, you should be able to:

- Describe the importance of social support for overall health and wellness.
- Explain the difference between social support and social networks.
- Identify some of the factors that influence the development of friendships.
- List several challenges faced in developing and maintaining teenage peer relationships.
- List and briefly describe at least five qualities of a true friend.
- Identify five skills for building healthy relationships.
- List and briefly describe five steps for dealing with peer pressure.
- Create a personal action plan to assess and develop your relationship skills.

Introduction

When you were younger, it is likely that most of your thoughts, feelings, and activities revolved around your family. Now that you're older, you're probably much more involved in social activities with your friends. You may spend a lot of time thinking about your relationships with your friends and trying to make sense of all the different feelings you have about these relationships. Just like family relationships, sometimes your peer relationships run smoothly and make life fun, interesting, and exciting. Other times, they cause you a great deal of pain and make your life very stressful. In this chapter, you will learn about the importance of social relationships and how they affect your health. You will also learn more about the qualities and skills you can acquire to help you develop strong, healthy peer relationships that are satisfying and mutually beneficial.

key TERMS

loneliness
peer pressure
reflective awareness
refusal skills
self-disclosure
social network
social support

personal assessment: HEALTHY PEER RELATIONSHIPS

Before reading this chapter, take this personal assessment to discover more about the way you currently relate to your peers. Read the statements below and, on a separate sheet of paper, rate your answers on the basis of the way you respond most *of the time. Use the following scale: 1 = Definitely True; 2 = Mostly True; 3 = Mostly False; 4 = Definitely False. An interpretation of your results is located at the end of this chapter.*

1. I treat other people with respect.
2. I can be trusted to keep my word and not betray a confidence.
3. I am able to tell the truth when I talk to my friends.
4. I am a good listener.
5. I do not have to pretend to be someone who I'm not when I'm around my friends.
6. I allow my friends to be themselves.
7. I don't pressure my friends to be like me or to do what I want them to do.
8. I am happy with the number of friends I have.
9. I am satisfied with the quality of the relationships I have.
10. If I have a problem with one of my friends, we usually are able to work it out.

WHY SOCIAL RELATIONSHIPS ARE IMPORTANT

Social relationships help to meet some of our most basic human needs: the needs for affection, love, and belonging. In Maslow's hierarchy of needs, discussed in Chapter 13, having these needs met provides the basis for becoming a self-actualized individual, which means functioning at or near your optimal level of mental and emotional health.

Developing relationships with other people also provides opportunities for you to learn more about yourself. In fact, some experts have suggested that most of what we know about ourselves comes from what we learn about ourselves from others. Our social relationships act as "mirrors" to provide feedback about how other people see us. We then use this feedback to guide our future behavior. So, in addition to making life more enjoyable, social relationships make life more meaningful.

Research indicates that social relationships also help protect your physical health. Strong social relationships help protect you against stressors that can predispose you to certain diseases. These relationships also increase your sense of well-being, stability, and control.

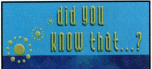

did you know that...?

From our earliest days as infants, we need social contact with other humans. According to psychologist Joan Borysenko, babies in orphanages who are fed and changed on schedule but who are neglected emotionally often develop a condition called failure to thrive. Despite having their physical needs met, these children are starved emotionally. Many of these babies die before reaching toddlerhood. Those who do survive often suffer serious psychological damage.

Numerous research studies show that people who have good relationships with other people live longer and healthier lives than do people who have negative or no social relationships.

DEVELOPING SOCIAL RELATIONSHIPS

As a child, your social relationships revolved primarily around your family. Even when you spent time with friends, those relationships were probably facilitated by an adult member of your family. You may have made friends with a particular person because that person's parent was a friend of your parent. You were also dependent on adults to make spending time with your friend possible. For example, if you played at a friend's house after school, you were probably dependent on an adult member of your family to provide transportation.

Now that you are older and becoming more independent, you want to spend more time with your friends. And, although you may still need help with transportation, you are primarily responsible for deciding with whom you spend your time and what you will do during the time you spend together.

Social Support

As you develop your own identity as a young adult, you will begin to select your own friends and develop your own social relationships with others. **Social support** is a term used to describe the degree to which a person's basic social needs are met through relationships with other people. Relationships with other people provide both **tangible** and **intangible** resources that can be used to meet our needs. Tangible resources include things such as money, transportation, or physical help of some kind. Intangible resources help to meet our emotional needs for affection, acceptance, and understanding. For example, if Kassandra is having a difficult time understanding her math homework because she missed two days of math class while she was sick, she might ask a friend in the class for her math notes from those days. This

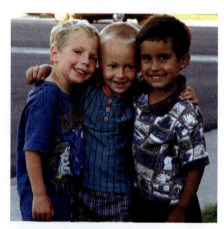

Children's friendships with other children are usually facilitated by their parents, who provide transportation and supervision and arrange times for getting together.

social support

aid and assistance exchanged through social relationships

tangible

concrete or physical; touchable

intangible

not capable of being perceived by touch, for example, emotional aid or assistance is an example of a tangible resource—class notes. Kassandra might also need some emotional support. If she talks about her difficulties in math with her dad, he might reassure her that he understands that math is hard. He might share his own difficulties in math with her or encourage her to ask the math teacher for additional help. These are examples of intangible resources—emotional support to help Kassandra resolve her problem.

Social Networks

A **social network** includes all the people with whom you have relationships. There are many kinds of relationships in your social network. Picture yourself at the center of a wheel, with the spokes in the wheel representing the various types of relationships you have. For example, your social network might include "spokes" of family, friends, classmates, and coworkers. See Figure 17-1 for an example of a social network wheel.

The **size** of your social network is the number of people in the network and may range from small (fewer than 10 people) to large

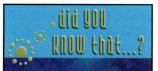

social network

a person-centered web of social relationships

size

in reference to a social network, the number of social relationships you have

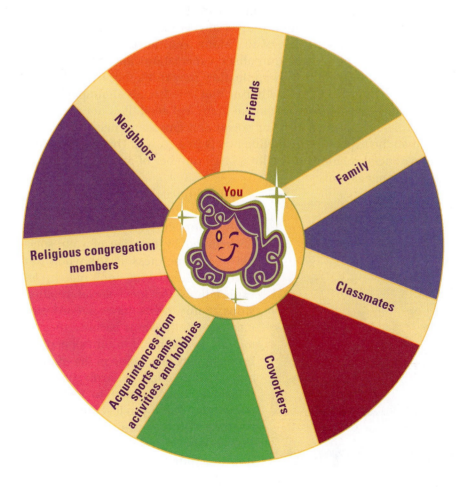

Figure 17-1
A social network is like a wheel, with you at the center and your relationships forming the spokes.

frequency

in reference to a social network, the amount of time you spend with members of your social network

intensity

in reference to a social network, the depth of interaction and intimacy you have with members of your social network

reciprocity

the "give-and-take" of a relationship; the evenness of exchange between the people involved

loneliness

an emotion that occurs when your current relationships don't match your expectations for ideal social relationships

(possibly hundreds). **Frequency** is the amount of time you spend with the members of your social network. You may spend a great deal of time with some members and relatively little time with others. **Intensity** is the depth of interaction and closeness you have with the people in your social network. You may have strong, intimate relationships with some members, such as your closest and best friends. And you may have very casual relationships with others, such as people who live in your neighborhood.

Reciprocity is another important aspect of a social network. Reciprocity is the "give-and-take" of a relationship, with this give-and-take being approximately equal among the people in the relationship. The members of your social network often provide social support, but not always. Some people in your social network may not offer any particular resources to you—tangible or intangible. That is, there is no reciprocity.

Loneliness

With all the relationships and activities that many teenagers are involved in, it might surprise you to learn that teenagers are one of the two groups of people who are most at risk for **loneliness**. (The other group is adults over the age of 80.) Many teens have a large social network, but they often have unrealistic expectations about what friendships should provide. For example, they may think that friends should always be available to each other or that true friends should always be able to meet their needs and make them feel good. It is not realistic to expect friends to meet all your social and emotional needs. Have you ever had the experience of feeling lonely in a crowd? This is how it feels to have social relationships with a large number of people without getting your needs met.

Loneliness is not the same as being alone, which means choosing to be by yourself. And loneliness is not determined by the size of your social network. Loneliness occurs when your current relationships don't match your expectations for ideal social relationships. Some teens have a hard time forming relationships because they are too shy to reach out to other people or because they lack some of the qualities and skills needed to form good relationships. It is normal to feel lonely sometimes. But if you feel lonely a lot of the time, you may want to rethink your expectations of relationships or try to improve your relationship skills.

Teens are at high risk for experiencing loneliness.

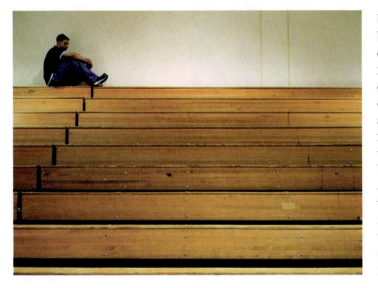

Even when you're not feeling lonely, it's good to remember that people around you might be lonely or might want to make new friends. You can help make others around you feel more comfortable by including them in your conversation or activities. By being aware of others around you who might want to develop a friendship, you have the opportunity to meet new people and make new friends.

Factors Influencing the Development of Relationships

Of all the billions of people in the world, throughout the years of your life, you will develop social relationships with relatively few of them. In addition to your own choices about who you want to develop relationships with, there are other factors that influence who the people in your life will be. Three important factors are geographical closeness, shared interests, and reciprocal self-disclosure.

1. *Geographical closeness.* Modern advances in transportation and communication have reduced our perceptions and the effects of distance. Today, it is easier than ever to develop and maintain long-distance relationships. It is more likely, however, that you will develop relationships with people who live, go to school, and work with you. Sharing a common physical space makes it easier for people to get to know each other and participate in the common activities that help a friendship thrive.

2. *Shared interests.* Social relationships often develop around a shared interest. For example, you may share with some of your friends an interest in a particular musical group or sport. These shared interests provide the "glue" that helps sustain the relationship through those early, awkward moments of trying to get to know someone.

3. *Reciprocal self-disclosure.* Social relationships may develop because of geographical closeness or shared interests, but they are maintained and deepened by reciprocal **self-disclosure**. Self-disclosure is a process of being increasingly open about who you really are as a person. Through self-disclosure, you gradually allow the other person to see you as you really are. If you disclose something about yourself to someone else, a sense of closeness between you and the other person develops. If that person does not reciprocate by sharing with you, however, you may begin to feel that the relationship is one-sided. You may then be less likely to continue disclosing things about yourself.

self-disclosure

revealing personal information

TYPES OF FRIENDS

Does it seem as if the friends you have now and those you have had in the past share many similar qualities? There are probably some differences among them, too. One way of describing types of friends is by the type of relationship you share with them. You may be surprised to see

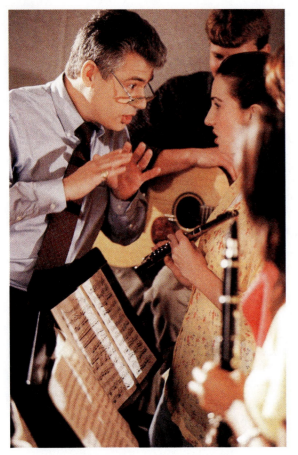

Special-interest friends are people who may not be close to you but who you see on a regular basis because of your shared interest in an activity such as band or a sport.

how many kinds of friends you have. The following are some of the most common categories:

- *Convenience friends.* Convenience friends are people with whom you are friendly and exchange small favors. You usually don't share very personal thoughts and feelings with this type of friend. An example of this type of friend is a classmate with whom you spend little time outside of class but to whom you might lend a pen or your notes for a class he or she missed.

- *Special-interest friends.* Special-interest friends are people with whom you share common interests and activities. You probably see them on a regular basis, but you may not be especially close to them. Examples of these friendships include teammates on a sports team, people with whom you work, or people who belong to the same organizations you do.

- *Historical friends.* Historical friends are friends with whom you used to spend more time but now do not see very often. If you lived in one town when you were in elementary school but moved away during middle school, one of your elementary school friends might be a historical friend.

- *Crossroads friends.* Crossroads friends are friends who were significant to you at one time in your life. You might have little contact with them now. But if you have an opportunity to

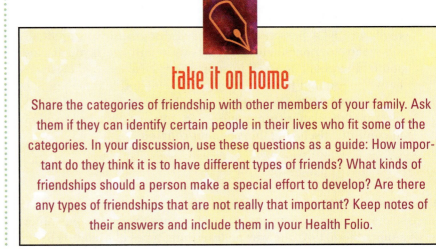

take it on home

Share the categories of friendship with other members of your family. Ask them if they can identify certain people in their lives who fit some of the categories. In your discussion, use these questions as a guide: How important do they think it is to have different types of friends? What kinds of friendships should a person make a special effort to develop? Are there any types of friendships that are not really that important? Keep notes of their answers and include them in your Health Folio.

spend time together, your closeness can be rekindled. Someone you ate lunch with every day when you used to have the same lunch period might be an example of a crossroads friend.

- *Cross-generational friends.* Cross-generational friends are friends who are younger or older than you are. You might have a friend-ship with an older neighbor or with younger children who look up to you as a role model.

- *Close friends.* Close friends are people you trust enough to share your deepest thoughts and feelings with. These are people who make you feel accepted and valued just the way you are. Close friends can remain your friends throughout your lifetime, but it is also possible that your close friends will change over time.

QUALITIES OF A TRUE FRIEND

There is a wise saying that if you have three true friends in your life, you are a rich person indeed. We usually think of true friends as those friends who are close to us and who have been our friends over a long period of time. But we might find the qualities of a true friend in any of the types of friends on the list.

True friends play many important roles in our lives. They laugh with us, cry with us, play with us, and try to understand us when we don't even understand ourselves. Many qualities have been identified to describe true friends and true friendships. Here are some of the most frequently mentioned:

- *Companionship.* True friends feel comfortable around each other. They usually spend a lot of time together and enjoy just hanging out together. They also have common activities they enjoy sharing.

- *Trust.* Trust is one of the qualities that is always mentioned when people are asked about the qualities of a true friend. It is impossible to maintain a friendship without trust. Many relation-ships are broken because one person betrays the trust of the other. Being a

real teens

Arielle Silverman is a normal American teenager who just happens to be blind. She also happens to be a very articu-late and gifted writer. Arielle won a first-place award from Arizona Press Women for her monthly essays that are pub-lished in an Arizona magazine, *Carefree Enterprise*. In one of her essays, Arielle says that, although there are times when she longs for the ability to see, she also believes that being blind has made her a better person "because I can see every human being for who he [she] is on the inside. If no one could see at all, the great barrier between the races of the world would instantly disappear. We could also for-get about perfecting our own appearance and focus more on perfecting our own character." In another one of her essays, Arielle discusses the advantages of good friend-ships and the pain that results when friendships break up. In her informal interviews with other teens, the qualities that were most consistently cited as essential for friend-ship were trust, loyalty, and honesty. Arielle describes friends as "the people who share our joy, lift us from our pain, and gently lead us in the right direction when we are confused." She concludes that, "while there are many rea-sons why some friendships end while others persist, all friends leave a mark on our hearts."

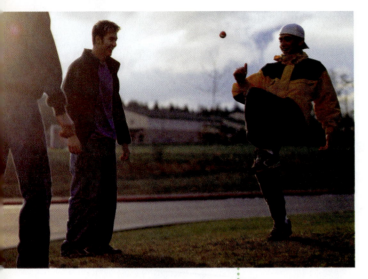

trustworthy person is one of the most important qualities you can develop if you want to have true friends in your life.

- *Mutual respect.* As with trust, friendships rarely survive if people do not have mutual respect for each other. Mutual respect involves more than just common courtesy. It is a sincere belief that the thoughts and feelings of the other person are important and valuable.

- *Acceptance.* When we allow someone to begin to know us better, we need the person to be accepting of us—warts and all. Regardless of how it appears from the outside, no one is perfect. The better we know someone, the more likely we are to discover his or her imperfections—and the more likely he or she is to discover our imperfections. True friends realize that human perfection doesn't exist. They accept you as you are, instead of always trying to change you.

- *Loyalty.* True friends are loyal. They are able to count on each other for emotional and physical help. If you have a loyal friend, you know the person won't "trade you in" when something or someone who seems better comes along. True friends value you enough to stick with you, even in difficult times.

- *Reciprocity.* True friendships have a give-and-take that is relatively equal. At certain times, one person may give more than another, but over time, the contributions the two people make to the relationship tend to even out.

COMMON STRESSORS IN TEEN RELATIONSHIPS

Although relationships can bring exceptional joy and pleasure, they can also bring a substantial amount of pain and heartache. The relationships you have as a teen can be stable, but there is a good chance they will be dynamic and changing. The person who is your "very best friend" may be the same friend you have had since elementary school. But it is just as likely to be someone you met fairly recently. It is common for teen friendships to develop quickly and fall apart almost as rapidly. Such a breakup often leaves one or both of the teens feeling hurt and confused. Let's take a look at some of the common stressors in teen relationships.

Everyone Is Changing

As we've said, adolescence is a period of great change: physically, emotionally, and socially. In relationships, not only are you changing rapidly, but so are your peers. Each of us has our own pace of growth and development. When your pace of growth and development is different from that of some of your friends, relationship difficulties can occur.

As you progress through adolescence, you may discover that your values, attitudes, beliefs, and goals change. You may find that, over time, your friends no longer see things the same way you do. This is a normal part of growing up, but it can leave you feeling lonely and isolated.

Another change may be in the activities that were once really important to you. Perhaps you have developed new interests. For example, suppose you've played on a soccer team for several years. But this year, you don't want to play. You'd rather spend your free time with the drama club instead. As a result, you may not see your old "soccer friends" as much anymore.

Unrealistic Expectations

To avoid being disappointed, you have to have realistic expectations about what a particular relationship can and cannot provide. It is unrealistic to think that any one relationship will meet all of your needs. Teens who find themselves upset and disappointed when their expectations in a relationship are not met may have had unrealistic expectations.

Insecurity

During adolescence, many teens feel awkward and insecure about every aspect of their identity. To cope with this insecurity, they try to find a group to fit into that provides a ready-made identity and where they know they will fit in and be accepted. John Powell, a gifted author, notes that many people play games with other people and are not true to who they really are. He believes people play games because they think, "I am afraid to tell you who I am, because if I tell you who I am, you may not like who I am, and it's all that I have."

Different Levels of Commitment

During your teen years, the level of commitment you want to give to relationships varies a lot. These are the years to explore various relationship options. Mature teens may be able to sustain a strong level of commitment to a particular relationship, but others are not ready to make such commitments. Or they may make a commitment and later break it. When two people in a relationship have different levels of commitment, the disparity can cause pain and confusion.

Sometimes when teens meet a new person they are interested in romantically, they begin spending time with that person exclusively, abandoning their other friends. If the romantic relationship breaks up, the person may have lost touch with his or her old friends.

Another potential source of pain is when a relationship ends. Not all relationships will last forever, whether it's a friendship or a romantic

---

✿ teen forum ✿

Best Friends?

Some teens have one special person who is their best friend. Other teens have social relationships with several people, but there isn't anyone they would describe as their best friend. Still other teens have best friends who change with the circumstances—and sometimes change as often as the weather!

- What is your opinion of best friends?

- What are the advantages and disadvantages of having a best friend?

- What do you think is the best thing to do when best friends grow in different directions and one of them no longer wants to be best friends?

- Write your responses in your Health Folio.

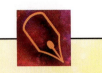

take it on home

Ask your parents or other members of your family what skills they think are most important in developing healthy relationships with others. Find out if they have ever had any type of help or training to improve their skills for building healthy relationships. If you have the opportunity, ask these questions of a grandparent or someone over the age of 65 as well. Make a note of these responses in your Health Folio.

relationship. Many relationships are temporary and exist only to fulfill a certain need or desire. Once that need or desire no longer exists, the commitment to maintain the relationship is no longer there. Even though it may be painful at first, telling the truth and being honest about your feelings about wanting to end a relationship or wanting to spend less time together is usually the least painful course of action in the long run.

SKILLS FOR RELATIONSHIP SUCCESS

Developing and maintaining good relationships can be challenging, but the rewards are worth it. Relationship skills are acquired over a lifetime, but they can be improved each day with practice. If you continually work on improving your relationship skills, you will increase your chances of having enjoyable and satisfying relationships. Let's take a look at some of the basic skills that contribute to relationship success.

Communication Skills

One of the most important skills you need to develop in order to build successful relationships is good communication. Communication was discussed in Chapter 4. You might want to go back and review some of the characteristics of good communication. As you recall, communication means much more than just talking. In fact, there are three major components to consider: the sender, the receiver, and nonverbal body language.

The Sender

The sender is the speaker. You want others to understand you, so when you send a message, state it clearly and take responsibility for your own feelings and thoughts. It's a good idea to use "I" statements—for example, "I want to go to the early movie"—so that others know where you stand and what you want. They shouldn't have to guess. It is also the responsibility of the sender to check for understanding and feedback from the listener by asking questions such as, "Does what I said make sense to you?"

The Receiver

The receiver is the listener who receives the message. Did you know the human brain can process thoughts much faster than a person can speak? Maybe you've noticed how your mind wanders when you are listening to someone, such as when the teacher lectures in class. As the listener, you

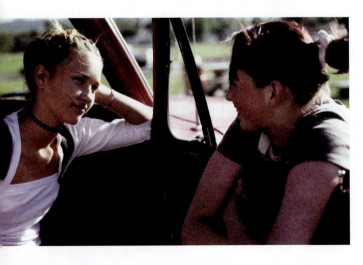

have a lot of "free" brain power. It's tempting to use this extra time and brain power to evaluate the message and think about what you might say next, but this is a poor habit that can interfere with truly effective communication. Instead, a good listener will use this opportunity to pay close attention to the speaker and understand what he or she is trying to say.

Other characteristics of a good listener include not interrupting, not giving advice, providing nonverbal feedback, and asking for clarification of anything you don't understand. An easy way to remember your responsibility as a listener is to think of the word *understand* as being "under-where-you-stand." If you can imagine what it would be like to be in the same place as the speaker, you have a good chance of being able to communicate effectively.

Nonverbal Body Language

Much of our communication comes from our nonverbal body language. You may have had an experience when you wrote a letter or sent an e-mail to someone and your message was misunderstood. Misunderstanding can happen in these circumstances because these forms of communication don't provide us with nonverbal cues from body language. When you can't see the receiver, you need to pay special attention to making sure you really understand the intended message before responding. And when you are face to face, keep in mind how much your body language is saying for you!

Reflective Awareness

Reflective awareness is your ability to identify to yourself what you are thinking and feeling at any given moment in time. To communicate well with another person and participate in a relationship, you have to know what you are bringing to the relationship. Reflective awareness means being able to identify your true thoughts and feelings about a particular situation. Knowing yourself allows you to establish an honest relationship with another person.

reflective awareness
the ability to identify to yourself what you are thinking or feeling at any given moment in time

Self-Disclosure

Self-disclosure means revealing information about yourself to friends you wish to be close to. This involves taking a risk, but it is part of establishing intimacy, a necessary part of a close friendship. Intimacy can be remembered as "into-me-see." This means letting another person see you as you really are. As trust and respect develop in a friendship, you begin to feel more comfortable letting the other person know more about you. In each relationship you have, you will face a choice of whether to reveal or conceal yourself. Which you choose will have a great influence on the final outcome of the relationship.

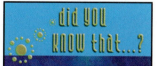

...did you know that...?

Positive mental health is characterized by high disclosure to a few significant others. Poorly adjusted persons tend to overdisclose or underdisclose to almost everyone.

Making Friends

You have probably experienced times when you wanted to get to know someone better, but the person didn't seem interested in knowing you any better. You have probably also experienced times when someone was very interested in getting to know you better, but you just wanted the person to "bug off." In both cases, you probably felt awkward and uncomfortable. Maybe you were unsure of how you should handle the situation.

- Is it best to be friends with everyone, or is it okay to just be friends with selected people?

- Brainstorm some of the different ways these issues might be resolved. What are the advantages and disadvantages of each of your solutions?

- Which option would you choose personally, and why?

- Place your answers in your Health Folio.

peer pressure

occurs when someone your own age tries to talk you into doing something you would not normally do

Decision-Making Skills

Decision-making skills help us to stay on course so that our outer lives, or actions, are consistent with our inner thoughts, feelings, and desires. As you make friends with a variety of people, you will have to make decisions such as how much time you want to spend with each person and how much you want to share with each one. Each decision represents a choice *and* has a consequence. Learning to make decisions that have positive consequences for your life is an important part of your progress toward responsible and satisfying adulthood.

Problem-Solving Skills

Even the best relationships encounter problems. People who lack maturity may walk away from a relationship at the first sign of problems. People who are more mature will try to work through problems to find a solution that works for both. Problem-solving skills were discussed in Chapter 3. You may want to review that chapter and think about how you can use those skills when you encounter a problem in one of your relationships.

PEER PRESSURE

During the teen years, a common feeling is to want to fit into a group. Being in a group helps teens feel as if they belong and have a special place. A lot of teens feel that it is more important to be a part of a group than to display their own sense of uniqueness and individuality. You may have noticed that some people want others to be like them or to do the same things they are doing. They may ridicule or otherwise mistreat people who are different or try to persuade them to join the group. This behavior is known as peer pressure, and it is not unusual among teens. **Peer pressure** occurs when someone your own age tries to talk you into doing something you would not normally do.

Peer pressure can be positive or negative. For example, if you are a member of a sports team, you might feel peer pressure from your teammates to show up for practice and work hard even when you don't feel like it. You might feel peer pressure to exercise or to do some kind of volunteer work. These are examples of positive peer pressure—the kind of pressure that encourages you to do something that will have good consequences for you.

There is also negative peer pressure. Negative peer pressure occurs when you feel as if you are being forced to engage in some type of activity that has the potential to be harmful to you. Maybe someone tries to pressure you into riding in a car, even though you know the driver has been drinking. Your peers may try to get you to disobey your parents, cheat on a test, or steal something from a local store. Peer pressure can be about something minor, such as the clothes you wear or the music you listen to. It can also be about something major, such as taking drugs or breaking the law.

Peer pressure does not always have to be verbal pressure to do something. Sometimes you may feel peer pressure to look or act a certain way or do something just because you think everyone else is doing it. Even if no one says anything specific to you, you may feel that there is an "unwritten rule" that your peers value a particular type of appearance or behavior more highly than they do another. Your perceptions about what other people think or believe may be accurate some of the time, but at other times you may be mistaken. Drawing conclusions on the basis of outward appearances can be deceiving. It's always a good idea to ask questions to find out the true situation. For example, you might ask your friends, "I know that you all seem to like to listen to hip-hop music. But I don't really like it that much. Is that a problem that would affect our friendship?" By asking questions, you get the information from your friends directly rather than drawing inaccurate conclusions.

Handling Peer Pressure

When you are faced with peer pressure, your first task is to determine what it is *you* want to do. Every choice has a consequence. Mature teens think through their options and consider the possible consequences of each of the choices. Your final decision will be a reflection of your values, your beliefs, and your ability to be true to yourself instead of being swayed by the values, beliefs, and opinions of others.

Refusal Skills

If you want to resist peer pressure, you can use **refusal skills**. Refusal skills enable you to resist giving in to peer pressure. Refusal skills allow you to be assertive about what you think and feel, instead of being passive and giving in or being aggressive and acting out. For refusal skills to work, you have to truly want to avoid the situation or action you are being pressured to participate in.

Developing good refusal skills can help you get out of uncomfortable situations without losing your friends. There are a lot of ways to refuse to do something. When you feel you are being pressured to do something you don't want to do, try practicing the following steps:

1. *Ask questions.* "What is it you want me to do?" "How will that benefit me?"
2. *Name the problem.* "You want me to steal makeup from the drugstore." "You want me to ride with you even though you have been drinking."

Many states have laws that protect teens who are pressured into sex by someone who is four or five years older. For example, in New York, a person 21 or older who has sex with a 17-year-old can be charged with 3rd degree rape—even if consent is involved! These laws protect the younger person because they:

- Reduce the likelihood of teen pregnancy
- Reduce the likelihood of sexually transmitted disease
- Take away the emotional effects of unwanted sexual behavior
- Discourage young adults from taking advantage of teens

Practicing abstinence from sexual activity as a teen is the best way to avoid these legal implications. It is also the best way to protect oneself against the emotional stress and confusion that can accompany sexual activity.

refusal skills

strategies to help you avoid situations in which you don't want to be involved

3. *Identify the consequences.* "That is against the law, and I don't want a police record!" "If I do that, I could get hurt." "I would be grounded forever if I did that!"

4. *Suggest alternatives.* "My mom has a lot of makeup she said I could experiment with." "Let's call my older brother to come pick us up." "We could go to the movies instead."

5. *Leave.* If the person still persists, leave. "I have to go now anyway." "No way, dude. I'm outta here."

As with any other skill, your ability to refuse gets better with practice. Each time you are asked to do something you really don't want to do, you have an opportunity to practice your refusal skills. Most of the time, you will be able to avoid the situation by using these steps. If you feel threatened or feel the present situation is dangerous, though, you should skip the first steps and just leave the situation as quickly as possible. Someone who is really your friend won't continue to pressure you to do something you clearly do not want to do. True friends look out for one another and try to support one another.

BUILDING YOUR Wellness Plan

In this chapter, you learned about the importance of building successful relationships throughout your life. You recognize the challenges involved in building healthy relationships, especially during the teen years. Consider the following key points when you add this important part of successful living to your wellness plan:

- Recognize that you may have a variety of types of friends, and each of those relationships can be rewarding and fulfilling.

- Understand the different stressors that can affect your relationships with others and develop ways you can cope with these stressors.

- You can develop certain qualities and skills that will help you establish and maintain successful relationships. Work on developing good communication skills, including becoming a good listener.

- Think about how you handle self-disclosure in your current relationships and how you would like to handle it in future ones.

- The next time you experience peer pressure, try using the refusal skills covered in this chapter. Think about how they worked for you and use them whenever you feel pressured to do something you do not want to do.

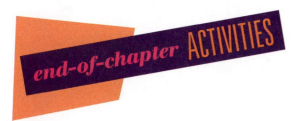

Weblink

Friendship

Arielle Silverman's essay on friendship:
http://www.carefreeenterprise.com (click on table of contents, then February 2002 link for Favorites from Months Past, and choose number 20, "A Teen's Point of View")

Short-Answer Questions

1. List three reasons why social relationships are important to health.
2. Give three examples of tangible resources for social support and three examples of intangible resources for social support that are provided by friendships.
3. Identify and briefly describe three factors that influence the development of relationships.
4. Identify at least five of the common stressors that cause conflict in peer relationships.
5. List and briefly describe three components of most communication.

Discussion Questions

1. Explain how social networks differ from social support.
2. Discuss two of the research studies mentioned in your text that illustrate the importance of social relationships.
3. Describe at least four types (categories) of friendship and give examples of each.
4. Discuss the five skills that enhance the likelihood of successful relationships.
5. Identify five steps you could take to resist peer pressure.

Chapter Vocabulary

Using a separate sheet of paper, list and define the following terms:

loneliness	self-disclosure
peer pressure	social network
reflective awareness	social support
refusal skills	

Application Activities

Language Arts Connection

1. Select a friend in one of the relationship categories discussed in this chapter. Write a letter to your friend, describing the person's importance to you.
2. Write an essay or a short story about an experience you shared with one of your friends that made a difference in your life.
3. Write an essay describing how you handled a situation in which you felt you were being pressured by a peer to do something that you didn't want to do.

Social Studies Connection

1. Research social connectedness in the United States versus that in other countries. Describe your findings.
2. Research the role of friendships as "protectors" of physical health. Suggest ways in which your community could make it easier for people to establish friendships.

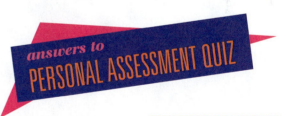

personal assessment: HEALTHY PEER RELATIONSHIPS

Answers will vary. A higher proportion of Definitely True or Mostly True responses indicates that you have skills and qualities that will enable you to develop and maintain healthy relationships. It is important to note that responses to these questions will vary over time, depending on circumstances and moods. A higher proportion of Mostly False or Definitely False responses indicates that you are currently experiencing some relationship difficulties.

chapter 18

Resolving Conflict

What a crummy day! Before he was even fully awake this morning, Ryan and his mom were arguing again. His mom said she was tired of being late to work because Ryan wouldn't get up on time to get ready for school. When he wasn't ready on time, his mom left without him, and Ryan had to ride his bike to school, making him even later than usual. His first-period teacher marked him tardy for the sixth time and reminded him that each tardy counted against his grade. At lunchtime, Ryan complained to his friend Toby about his day. To his surprise and annoyance, Toby said, "Well, man, it sounds like you're getting what you deserve." Later that day when Ryan's girlfriend, Janna, asked him if he could help her with a problem with her car, Ryan snapped at her, "It's your car. It's your problem. You deal with it." Ryan's day has gone steadily downhill, and now even Janna is mad at him.

chapter OBJECTIVES

When you finish this chapter, you should be able to:

- Describe why conflict can be considered either positive or negative.
- Explain the difference between intrapersonal and interpersonal conflicts.
- List and briefly describe several potential causes of conflict.
- Identify four broad sets of skills that support conflict resolution.
- Explain the difference between negotiation, compromise, and mediation.
- List and briefly describe the six general steps for resolving conflict.
- Create a personal action plan to assess and develop your conflict management skills.

key TERMS

bullying
coercion
conflict
conflict resolution skills
interpersonal conflict
intrapersonal conflict
mediation
negotiation
tolerance

Introduction

Experiencing conflict is a normal part of life. It is impossible to go through life without experiencing conflict on a regular basis. Sometimes the conflict is with parents or other adults. Sometimes it is with your friends or in a romantic relationship. More serious conflict can occur with legal authorities. You can even have conflict within yourself, such as when you feel confused about how you want to act in a particular situation. By developing an awareness of situations that are likely to cause conflict for you, you can prevent trouble. If you learn and practice good conflict resolution skills, you will be prepared to handle major conflicts with people around you. In this chapter, we will discuss what conflict is, how to recognize situations that might cause conflict, and what you can do to make sure you stay in control, instead of letting your emotions or other people control you.

personal assessment: RESOLVING CONFLICT

Before reading this chapter, take this personal assessment to discover more about the way you currently handle conflict. On a separate sheet of paper, respond to the statements below on the basis of the way you respond most of the time. Rate your answers using the following scale: 1 = Definitely True; 2 = Mostly True; 3 = Mostly False; 4 = Definitely False. An interpretation of your results is located at the end of the chapter.

1. I avoid conflict whenever possible.
2. I think I'm pretty good at handling conflict with adults.
3. I don't think I'm very good at handling conflict with my peers.
4. If I have a conflict with someone, I can usually resolve it by talking with the person about it.
5. I often give in to someone else rather than face an argument or disagreement.
6. I stand up for what I believe in, even if doing so might cause an argument or disagreement.
7. There are very few things I believe are worth an argument or disagreement.
8. If I can't resolve a problem with someone by myself, I ask others for help.
9. I often respond to a confrontation with someone by getting angry.
10. If I get angry with someone, I give myself time to cool down before approaching the person.

UNDERSTANDING CONFLICT

conflict

a struggle caused by incompatible or opposing interests, values, needs, or desires

Conflict is a struggle that results from incompatible or opposing interests, values, needs, or desires. Conflict can occur whenever two or more people or groups view a situation differently. Conflict is a normal part of growing up, as well as a normal part of adult life. In the Chinese language, the same symbol is used for the words *crisis* and *opportunity*. Some Chinese people believe that a crisis also presents an opportunity for growth. The same is true for conflict. Situations that cause conflict present opportunities to expand your knowledge and see multiple sides of issues. A certain amount of conflict is necessary for us to learn and develop emotionally and socially. The problem is not that a conflict occurs. Rather, the problem results when the parties involved are not able to resolve the conflict in a mutually satisfying way. The way conflict is handled is the key to whether it has a positive or a negative outcome.

Levels of Conflict

Conflict can occur at many levels. Have you ever felt as if you were in conflict with yourself? This is called **intrapersonal conflict**. It can happen when you have contradictory feelings about a particular situation or issue. An intrapersonal conflict might occur if you really want to accept an invitation to a party but you have already agreed to go to a movie with your friend Todd. You want to go to the party, but you don't want to hurt Todd's feelings. The other people involved might not even be aware of your conflict, but it exists for you. If you decide to accept the invitation to the party and back out of your commitment to go to the movie, Todd might get angry with you. At this point, you might find yourself involved in an **interpersonal conflict**, a conflict with another person or group. Interpersonal conflicts can occur with family members, your peers, or people you are acquainted with through school or work.

Conflict doesn't just occur between two people who know each other and can't agree on something they both care about. Conflicts can occur between organizations, communities, religious groups, political groups, and even entire nations. Sometimes we feel as if we are in conflict with people we don't even know. Racial tensions, religious violence, and nations at war with one another are all examples of conflict among groups.

intrapersonal conflict
confusion or struggle within yourself

interpersonal conflict
disagreement or argument between persons or groups

What's News?

One person who has been extremely effective at helping opposing groups to resolve serious conflict is former U.S. President Jimmy Carter. After leaving the presidency in 1981, he founded the Carter Center, based in Atlanta, Georgia. The organization is devoted to global peace and social justice. Carter was awarded the 2002 Nobel Peace Prize for his decades of work in seeking peaceful solutions to international conflicts and promoting social and economic justice. In awarding him the Nobel Prize, the Nobel Committee said, "Carter has stood by the principle that conflicts must as far as possible be resolved through mediation and international cooperation based on international law, respect for human rights, and economic development."

coercion

the use of physical or psychological threat or force to get what you want

bullying

the use of threats or force by one person or group to intimidate another person or group

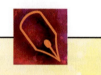

take it on home

We all occasionally try to resolve conflict in ways that aren't very positive—or effective. We may get angry; we may try to avoid the situation; or we may become aggressive and controlling. Ask members of your family how they perceive your usual responses to conflict. Ask your parents or other adults if this is the way you've always responded. Have they noticed any changes in your conflict management style over the past few years? What can you learn about yourself from their answers? Record your responses in your Health Folio.

Coercion

Conflict usually occurs because you are not getting your needs or wants met in a way that satisfies you. When you were an infant and your diaper was wet, you probably cried until someone changed it. And thus your conflict was resolved! When you were a toddler, if your playmate took a toy you wanted, you may have hit or bit or kicked to get the toy back.

Crying and hitting might work for infants and toddlers, but as you grew older, you probably learned that these tactics aren't very effective and definitely aren't socially acceptable! You learned there are better, more effective methods of getting your needs met. Unfortunately, some people never advance past the toddler stage in learning to resolve conflict. They still use some sort of **coercion** to get what they want. Sometimes coercion is psychological manipulation, and sometimes it is direct physical force. But "winning" in this manner is likely to feel like an empty victory because no one feels truly satisfied with the outcome.

Bullying

A particular type of coercion, which happens more frequently among children and teens than among adults, is bullying. **Bullying** is the use of threats or force by one person or group to intimidate another person or group. Bullying can be something as simple as pushing a student in the hallway or making fun of someone. Bullying often occurs when there is an imbalance of strength, power, or prestige.

If ignored, bullying can lead to violent acts that result in physical injury or serious emotional damage. Many elementary schools now have programs to work with children who bully other children, in hopes of stopping bullying early. Although bullying is most common in childhood and adolescence, even whole countries have been accused of bullying behavior. The use of threat or force by a large, powerful nation to intimidate a smaller, less powerful nation is an example of bullying on a large scale.

RECOGNIZING POTENTIAL CONFLICTS

Many types of issues have the potential for conflict. In general, the likelihood of conflict is highest when people feel strongly about an issue. When an issue isn't very important to you, you are likely to give in or work toward a solution, even if it means you don't get everything you want. But if the issue involves something very important to you, you are likely to have strong emotions about it. These emotions can interfere with your ability to see points of view that are different from your own. You may be blind to certain solutions because you can see the situation only from your own point of view. This narrow perspective makes it very hard to find ways to resolve the conflict.

Conflicts often arise when your feelings have been hurt or when you feel there's no way you can accept the way another person feels or thinks. In these situations, you may feel overwhelmed by anger, sadness, loneliness, or rejection. Using creative ways to express your emotions—such as writing in a journal, drawing sketches, painting pictures, dancing, or listening to music—can help you release your emotions and help you see and think more clearly. Then you can reframe the situation and see it in more neutral, less emotional terms.

Strong feelings you are unwilling to change are one cause of conflict. Some other common causes are unequal levels of power and status, different points of view, and miscommunication.

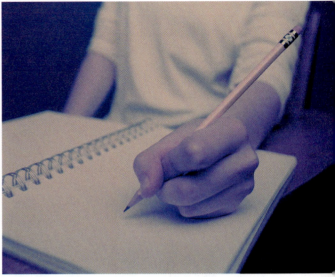

Writing in a journal is one way to express emotions and to gain a new perspective on your problems.

Power and Status

Often, the desire to establish power or gain status is a source of conflict. Feeling in control of your life and circumstances is a very important component of mental and emotional health. Sometimes your need to be in control is so strong that you resort to negative behaviors to establish power and dominance. Have you ever wanted to do something just so other people would look up to you? Status gives you a positive reputation among your peers and results in feelings of importance. It is especially important for teens to have their needs for power and status met. Any threat to the satisfaction of those needs can be a cause for conflict. The first step to resolving conflicts is to be aware of the underlying, unmet needs of the people involved, including yourself. In fact, after thinking it over, you may decide that your needs for power and control in a particular situation are hurting you rather than helping you.

did you know that...?

The Resolving Conflict Creatively Program (RCCP) is one of the largest and longest-running school-based violence-prevention programs in the United States. Designed for grades K–12, the program focuses on constructive conflict resolution and positive social relationships. It is built around a set of core skills: communicating clearly and listening carefully, expressing feelings and dealing with anger, resolving conflicts, fostering cooperation, appreciating diversity, and countering bias. A two-year study of 5,000 children in elementary schools who used the program revealed that students who participated in the program showed an increase in positive social behaviors and emotional control. Two out of three schools now use some form of ongoing violence-prevention program.

Perception and Point of View

Even people who are very much like you don't always share your perceptions of certain issues. Or they may disagree with you about what action to take in a particular situation. When you consider the vast diversity of our world today, it isn't surprising that people and groups have different perceptions and points of view.

Tolerance means promoting respect for differences and appreciating diversity. Tolerance doesn't mean you give up your own views. It simply means you understand and respect the fact that other people have views that are different from your own. Tolerance means being open minded enough to try to find common ground between yourself and persons with whom you disagree instead of insisting that everyone agree with you.

Miscommunication

Despite your best efforts to clearly communicate your thoughts and feelings, misunderstandings do occur. You can decrease the likelihood of communication misunderstandings by learning and practicing the speaking and listening skills discussed in Chapter 4. You can also become aware of your own personal emotional triggers. These are words, behaviors, and attitudes that "push your buttons" and cause responses out of proportion to the incident. If you can recognize these "buttons," you can take deliberate steps to be especially calm and careful with your communication when they are pushed.

EXPERIENCING CONFLICT AS A TEEN

You may experience more conflict during the adolescent years than during other times in your life because you are changing so quickly, physically, emotionally, and socially. Your body has changing levels of hormones during the teen years, which may make you feel more emotional than you did as a child. You are becoming more independent from your family and making more choices on your own. Independence and decision making can be sources of both interpersonal and intrapersonal conflict. You may be getting into arguments with your parents about your choices even when you're not sure yourself what choices you want to make. Your social relationships can also cause you both interpersonal and intrapersonal conflict. And your own changing viewpoints and values may result in conflict both with other people and within yourself.

You may experience more conflict when you're not feeling well, physically, emotionally, or socially. When you're feeling bad, it's tempting to take it out on those around you. Of course, lashing out doesn't solve the problem. It usually ends up making you feel worse instead of better. When you're not feeling well, you may also have less patience and tolerance than normal. Things that usually wouldn't bother you

---

tolerance

respect for people whose beliefs and practices differ from yours

take it on home

The teen years often bring increased conflicts with parents and other family members. There are many reasons for this increase in conflict. Since you have become a teenager, has the amount of conflict in your family increased, decreased, or remained about the same? Ask the other members of your family how they would answer that question. If your family feels there is too much conflict, discuss ways you might work together to decrease it. Record your family's responses in your Health Folio.

become annoying. During these times, other people may accuse you of "blowing things out of proportion" or "making mountains out of mole-hills." Later, when you're feeling better, you may even come to the conclusion that they were right!

APPROACHES TO CONFLICT

When you find yourself in a situation in which conflict is likely to occur, there are three possible approaches you can take to resolve it. These are often called "win-win," "win-lose," and "lose-lose." Let's consider a typical teen conflict using each of these three approaches. Suppose Robert and Juan have been assigned to work together on a project in history. They really didn't know each other very well before beginning the project. They have gotten along okay so far, but Juan feels as if he has been doing most of the work. He decides to tell Robert how he feels.

Win-Win

In a win-win (both parties win) approach, Juan wants to accomplish his purpose—to get Robert to do more of the work—but he doesn't want to make Robert angry or hurt him. Juan wants Robert to contribute more to the project, and he wants to get a good grade on the project. He might say, "Hey, Robert. I've been working really hard on this project because I want to get a good grade. But I need your help. We have to work on this together so that when we present our project, our presentation will go well. That way we'll both get a good grade. When can we get together to plan our presentation?"

Win-Lose

In a win-lose (one party wins; the other loses) approach, Juan wants to accomplish his purpose, and he doesn't care if Robert gets angry or hurt in the process. In a win-lose approach, Juan might tell the teacher that Robert hasn't done any work on the project and doesn't deserve credit for the project. Maybe the teacher will agree, and Juan will get a good grade without Robert's input. But Juan's denying Robert a chance to contribute more before Juan approaches the teacher can lead to an ugly confrontation between Juan and Robert and almost certainly would hurt Robert.

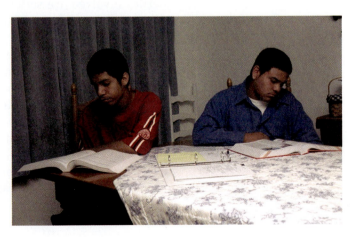

Lose-Lose

People don't approach a conflict situation intending to lose. A lose-lose outcome (both parties lose) is evidence that neither person had the skills to find a good solution to the

✴ teen forum ✴

Preventing School Violence

Although fewer than 1% of violent deaths of children and adolescents occur on school grounds, recent violent episodes in schools have attracted a great deal of media attention. In addition, many students report confrontations with other students at school. Some of those confrontations involved students who have a weapon. Schools have responded in different ways to the demands from parents and students for safer schools. Many schools have chosen to increase security personnel and increase monitoring of student behavior. School districts all over the country have decided to install metal detectors at school entrances. According to some experts, however, "an ounce of prevention is worth a pound of metal detectors." Linda Lantieri of Educators for Social Responsibility believes that relying on metal detectors and security devices to make schools safer doesn't really solve the problem of violence. Speaking about a student accused of shooting two other students to death, she noted that "the daily taunts he received would never be picked up by the metal detector his school might resort to installing."

- In your opinion, what are the most effective ways of preventing school violence? Give reasons for your responses and include them in your Health Folio.

problem. Suppose Juan tells Robert that he had better do his part of the project "or else." Robert gets mad and tells Juan that he can't make him do anything. This remark makes Juan angry, and he pushes Robert against a locker. A teacher sees the incident and Robert and Juan both get in trouble. Not only has more trouble been created, but the original problem still hasn't been solved.

CONFLICT RESOLUTION

Some problems can be resolved rather easily; others are extremely difficult to resolve. But all problems have the potential for resolution if the parties involved are seriously committed to seeking a solution instead of simply trying to win. When people are genuinely interested in solving a problem, good **conflict resolution** skills can make a big difference. Conflict resolution is a structured problem-solving process that uses reflective awareness, communication skills, problem-solving skills, and decision-making skills to prevent, manage, and peacefully resolve conflicts.

The basic skills needed to resolve conflict at the group level are the same skills needed to resolve problems between individuals. However, the more complex the conflict is, and the more people who are involved in the conflict, the more difficult it is to use these skills effectively. Practicing the use of conflict resolution skills at the individual level with daily conflicts can help you improve your skills. If you ever need to use these skills in a complex conflict that involves a lot of people, you will be better prepared.

conflict resolution

a structured problem-solving process that uses reflective awareness, communication skills, problem-solving skills, and decision-making skills to prevent, manage, and peacefully resolve conflicts

In a conflict, one party who isn't committed to resolving the problem may label the other party as the enemy. But identifying the other party as an enemy eliminates many possible options for resolving the conflict. It is likely to end in either a win-lose or lose-lose result because the "enemy" becomes someone to be beaten at all costs. This attitude can cause even minor problems to escalate into major ones. Sometimes, people or groups resort to violence to get rid of the enemy. Although it's tempting to think this will solve the problem, violence is never the best solution to a problem. Learning to resolve conflict peacefully and effectively is one of the most important skills you can acquire on your journey toward adulthood.

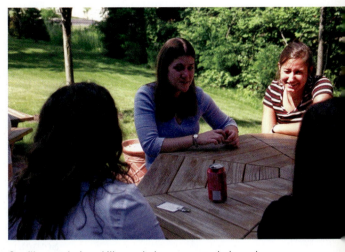

Conflict resolution skills can help groups work through complicated problems in an organized, effective way.

Conflict Resolution Skills

Good conflict resolution skills build on the other important life and wellness skills discussed in this book. Some of the skills we have already looked at include:

- Reflective awareness to help you to identify what you are feeling before you react (Chapter 17)
- Communication skills to help you present your thoughts and feelings clearly and effectively (Chapter 4)
- Problem-solving skills to help you identify possible solutions to problems that cause conflict for you (Chapter 3)
- Decision-making skills to enable you to work through possible options and select a course of action that is right for you in a given situation (Chapter 3)

You might want to review what you have learned about those topics.

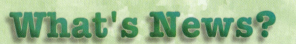

What's News?

Seeds of Peace is a not-for-profit, nonpolitical organization that helps teenagers from regions that have a lot of conflict learn the skills for making peace. The organization was founded by author and journalist John Wallach in 1993. The organization's first project was bringing together Arab and Israeli teenagers to train them in conflict resolution and help them to discover the human face behind "the enemy." In 1998, the project expanded to include other regions experiencing conflict. Since 1993, more than 2,000 teens from 22 nations have graduated from the Seeds of Peace program and returned to their home countries. They leave the program having made friends among "the enemy." It is hoped that these bright young teens will become the leaders of tomorrow and eventually bring about peace in their own countries.

Practical Steps for Resolving Conflict

There are many strategies for resolving conflict. The following six steps (see Figure 18-1) provide some general guidelines for resolving conflict. The first three steps involve preparing the ingredients for a successful outcome, just as you would do if you were following a recipe. Successful completion of the first three steps provides a good basis for resolving the conflict. The last three steps focus on actively resolving the conflict and reaching an agreement acceptable to all parties.

1. *Set the stage to meet and establish ground rules.* It will be impossible to solve a problem unless the parties involved are willing to talk about it and agree to work together to find a solution. The first step, then, to resolving a conflict is to agree to meet peacefully to establish the ground rules for your discussions. Sometimes this is a simple process, but other times it is very difficult. In situations of serious conflict, this first step can be a very large step indeed.

2. *Gather perspectives of the parties involved.* In this step, the focus is *not* on solving the problem. It is on each party's making an effort to *hear and understand* what the other one thinks and feels about the problem. It is very important to try to be nonjudgmental. At the end of this step, there should be a clear understanding of the perspectives of the people involved and exactly why this issue is important to them.

3. *Identify interests, needs, wants, and desires.* During this step, the parties are given the opportunity to clearly state what their interests are and what they feel they need to resolve the conflict. They also have a chance to state what they want to see happen and describe how the situation would look if their desires were met. It is important to separate the demands people make—what they say they want—from their underlying needs, which are often left unexpressed. For example, a teenage girl may want to stay out late for a party. That is her demand. Her *need*, however, is to feel a part of the group. There may be a solution that meets

1. **Set the stage to meet and establish ground rules.**

2. **Gather perspectives of the parties involved.**

3. **Identify interests, needs, wants, and desires.**

4. **Generate creative options.**

5. **Evaluate options.**

6. **Create a formal agreement.**

Figure 18-1
The six steps for resolving conflict

the underlying need and resolves the problem without meeting the demand.

4. ***Generate creative options.*** With the first three steps completed, the stage is set to begin actively working to resolve the conflict. At this stage in the process, it's important to think "outside the box." This means the parties don't just rely on what may seem to be the obvious solutions. One way to think of a problem is as a jigsaw puzzle to be solved. It's important to have all the pieces of the puzzle on the table for it to be put together properly. If potential pieces are left out of the problem-solving process, the parties may miss opportunities to find win-win solutions. It's important to stay focused on this step until several options have been identified that seem to have a potential for success.

5. ***Evaluate options.*** Once the parties have brainstormed as many potential options as possible, it's time to evaluate them to see which have the most likelihood for success. The parties should be willing to try a lot of different puzzle pieces to find the solution that fits best. If none of the options seems to be workable, it may be necessary to start over and go through the steps again. The goal is to create a win-win agreement for everyone involved.

6. ***Create a formal agreement.*** Once an agreement has been reached, it's a good idea to formalize the agreement by a specific action. This may be an action as simple as shaking hands. Or it may be a written document that contains the agreement and lists the consequences if the agreement is violated. Formalizing the agreement acts as a reminder to the parties, in case of future conflict, that there was agreement on this issue's resolution.

In efforts to resolve a conflict, the steps we have just discussed may be used in a **negotiation**. In negotiation, people work out their problems by talking them through. The parties reach a resolution without help from anyone else. Many problems can be resolved through negotiation.

did YOU KNOW that...?

History contains many examples of people who have used peaceful, non-violent means to address social issues about which they felt strongly. One of the most famous of these is Martin Luther King Jr. He focused on using nonviolent means to help increase civil rights for African Americans and decrease racial discrimination against them. His efforts laid the groundwork for progress toward equality for African Americans.

negotiation

a process in which two disputing parties work out their problems by talking through them without the assistance of an outside party

did YOU KNOW that...?

Throughout history, many countries have developed proverbs that are related to conflict resolution. A proverb is a saying that paints a vivid picture to help people understand a complex idea. Give some thought to how the following proverbs apply to conflict resolution:

- "Without retaliation, evils would one day become extinct from the world." (Proverb of Nigeria, West Africa)

- "To engage in conflict, one does not bring a knife that cuts but a needle that sews." (Adapted from a Bahumbu proverb of Zambia, East Africa)

- "A frog in the well does not know the ocean." (Proverb of Japan)

- "Lions believe that everyone shares their state of mind." (Proverb of Mexico)

mediation

a process in which two disputing parties work out their problems by talking through them with an outside person who facilitates the discussion

compromise

a conflict resolution in which both parties give up something

If, after trying negotiation, the parties are still unable to resolve their conflict, they may request **mediation**. In mediation, a third party steps in to help facilitate the discussion so that the two disputing parties can reach an agreement. Mediation is used in conflict resolution with individuals, groups, and nations.

It is usually impossible for both parties to get everything they want and need. If they could both get everything they want, there probably wouldn't have been a conflict in the first place. Consequently, a common outcome of negotiation and mediation is **compromise**. Compromise involves giving up some of the things that each party wants in order to reach a solution that satisfies both parties. Compromise does *not* mean giving in and accepting a solution that doesn't satisfy you. Rather, it means recognizing that there are things you are willing to give up in order to get something else you want more. Through compromise, you can create a win-win situation for both parties and a peaceful resolution to the problem.

The only way to become really effective at resolving conflict is to practice conflict resolution skills at every opportunity. Each time you practice your conflict resolution skills, you will gain insights about what works and what doesn't work for certain conflicts in particular situations. Over time, you will increase your confidence in your ability to reach positive solutions to conflict.

Creating Peace without Giving In

One of the most difficult aspects of conflict resolution is learning how to reach a peaceful solution without giving in and surrendering your values and principles. When a conflict is resolved successfully, all the people involved feel that their interests, needs, and desires have

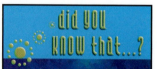

.did you know that...?

Many schools use "peer mediators" to resolve problems between students. Peer mediators are students trained in conflict resolution skills who work with other students to help them successfully work out problems. Several studies show that student peer mediation programs reduce the incidence of school suspensions. They also indicate that student violence and other hurtful behaviors have decreased when effective peer mediation programs have been implemented.

take it on home

Ask your family members to help you recall the conflicts members of your family have had with one another in the past week. Identify whether the conflicts were resolved by negotiation or mediation or are still unresolved. For any conflicts that are still unresolved, practice the six steps of conflict resolution to see if you can resolve the conflict. Practicing these skills with your family is a great way to improve your skills so you'll be ready when conflicts come up in situations outside your home.

been respected. It may not be possible to get everything you want in a solution, but you should not feel as if you had to give up everything that's important to you just to end the conflict. Giving up everything is not really a resolution. It is a passive acceptance of defeat and may ignore what you believe, need, and want. Giving in can have a negative impact in the long term because people who give in easily often find themselves feeling resentful and angry. The immediate conflict may *appear* to have been resolved, but it simply resurfaces later in another form.

Personal Boundaries

Healthy people have appropriate physical, emotional, and social **boundaries**. Boundaries are imaginary lines that indicate a limit beyond which you will not go. Boundaries help keep you safe. They help you maintain your basic values and priorities. When you are faced with a conflict, take some time to identify what your current boundaries are for this situation. You can then determine what you can compromise on and what you cannot. When you decide your boundary cannot or should not be compromised, you can clearly explain your position to the other person.

During the teen years, your peers may try to pressure you to change your boundaries. They might encourage you to cheat on a test, lie to another person, or give in to sexual pressure. There are many good reasons why you might choose to be flexible in your personal boundaries, but pressure from someone else is *not* one of them. By identifying your boundaries *before* you are faced with a difficult decision, you ensure that you are making your own choices about your life, rather than being controlled by others.

When All Else Fails

Most conflicts can be resolved using the skills and techniques we have discussed. But sometimes, despite your best efforts, you just can't seem to reach an agreement with another person or group. These instances require you to reach deep within yourself for the patience and commitment to step back and give yourself some time to consider new approaches or to develop new skills to help you resolve the conflict. Agreeing to a "cooling off period" is one way to allow the parties more time to look for solutions they may have missed. When you're in the heat of the moment, it's hard to see solutions, even when they do exist. Not all conflicts can be resolved in ways that please everyone. However, with patience and commitment to peaceful solutions, conflicts can be resolved without resorting to violence. Acting violently, whether the violence is physical or verbal, is not a real solution but only creates new problems and conflicts. Violence should be avoided at all costs.

boundaries
imaginary lines that indicate a limit beyond which you will not go

BUILDING YOUR Wellness Plan

As teenagers, you and your peers represent the future of our nation. You have the opportunity to learn skills and make choices for peaceful resolution of conflict now that can make important changes in your family, community, and world. These skills are important parts of your wellness plan because they affect so many parts of your life and the lives of those around you. After reading this chapter you should:

- Take a hard look at how you currently handle conflict when it arises. Are there areas in which you could improve your skills? What goals would you set for yourself in those areas?

- Understand that conflict is a natural part of life and can be either positive or negative.

- Recognize conflict when it occurs.

- Develop and use effective conflict resolution skills, including the six steps to conflict resolution.

- Apply other important life skills, such as communication, to conflict resolution.

- Identify the first three action steps you want to take toward improving your conflict resolution skills and write them in your wellness plan. From time to time, look back at your wellness plan to measure your progress. When you are successful most of the time in practicing those three steps, add additional action steps.

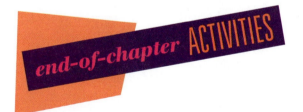

end-of-chapter ACTIVITIES

Weblinks

Peace

Seeds of Peace: **http://www.seedsofpeace.org**

Stopping Bullying

Bullying.org: **http://www.bullying.org**
Operation Respect: **http://www.dontlaugh.org**

Tolerance

Southern Poverty Law Center:
  http://www.tolerance.org

Short-Answer Questions

1. List three examples of intrapersonal conflict.
2. List three examples of interpersonal conflict.

3. Identify and briefly describe four things that make conflict likely.

4. List the primary focus of three peace-related organizations discussed in your text or in the Weblinks.

5. List the six general steps for resolving conflict.

☀ Discussion Questions

1. Explain why conflict can be either positive or negative.

2. Discuss why time can be an important factor in resolving conflict.

3. Explain why the four broad sets of skills supporting conflict resolution that are discussed in your text are important in resolving conflicts.

4. Use the six steps to resolving conflict to create and describe a solution for Keandra and Josie, two teens who are arguing about cleaning chores at the restaurant where they both work.

5. Create an example of a conflict situation and describe how it is resolved by negotiation or mediation.

☀ Chapter Vocabulary

Using a separate sheet of paper, list and define the following terms:

bullying	intrapersonal conflict
coercion	mediation
conflict	negotiation
conflict resolution skills	tolerance
interpersonal conflict	

☀ Application Activities

Language Arts Connection

1. Write an essay or short story about one of the proverbs mentioned on page 339.

2. Write an essay describing how you handled an intrapersonal conflict that you experienced.

3. Write a poem about an interpersonal conflict you faced recently.

Math Connection

Some studies suggest that an effective conflict resolution program can be successfully implemented by schools at a cost of $100 per child. Assume that this is true. The program is successful for 75% of the children. For each child for whom the program is successful, the school district saves $200 by decreased problems with conflict. How much money could a school district save (after paying for the program) if 2,000 students went through the conflict resolution program?

Social Studies Connection

1. Using your local daily newspaper, research and report on a recent conflict that affected your community. Include in your report what the source of conflict was and suggest how the conflict might be resolved.

2. Using your local daily newspaper, research and report on a recent national or international conflict. Include in your report the sources of the conflict and suggest how the conflict might have been avoided.

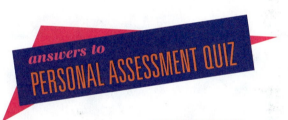

answers to **PERSONAL ASSESSMENT QUIZ**

personal assessment: **RESOLVING CONFLICT**

Answers will vary. A higher proportion of Definitely True or Mostly True responses to questions 2, 4, 6, 8, and 10 and Definitely False or Mostly False answers to questions 1, 3, 5, 7, and 9 indicates that you have skills and qualities that make it likely that you will be able to cope with conflict effectively. It is important to note that responses to these questions will vary over time, depending on circumstances and moods. A pattern of Definitely True or Mostly True responses to questions 1, 3, 5, 7, and 9 and Definitely False or Mostly False responses to questions 2, 4, 6, 8, and 10 indicates that you are currently experiencing some difficulties in resolving conflict effectively.

chapter 19

Healthy Romantic Relationships

Maggie met Nikolas last semester when he sat in front of her in geometry class. After a few weeks, they started eating lunch together a couple of times a week when they had the same lunch period. Eventually they started dating. By the middle of the semester, they were a "couple," and neither one of them wanted to date anyone else. Maggie stopped going places with her other friends and spent almost all of her free time with Nikolas. But now this semester, they don't have any of the same classes or lunch periods. Maggie and Nikolas don't have as much in common anymore, and Maggie feels bored whenever they go out. She wants to start dating other people, and she misses doing things with her friends. But she doesn't want to hurt Nikolas's feelings by breaking up with him. He's a really nice guy, and Maggie still wants them to be friends.

If Maggie came to you for advice, what would you tell her?

chapter OBJECTIVES

When you finish this chapter, you should be able to:

- Briefly explain Sternberg's three components of love.
- Describe the similarities and differences between friendships and romantic relationships.
- Explain some of the purposes of dating.
- Identify several advantages and disadvantages of various types of dating relationships.
- List and briefly describe several factors that can cause problems in a teen romantic relationship.
- Give several reasons why a teen romantic relationship might break up.
- Identify several characteristics of addictive and abusive romantic relationships.
- Create a personal action plan to guide your involvement in romantic relationships.

Introduction

Countless books, poems, and songs have been written about romantic love. Countless more plays, movies, and television episodes have used love as their central theme. Almost everyone searches for it. Some people claim to have found it, only to have it disappear later. Despite searching, some people never find it. Others find it when they're least expecting it and remain in love with the same person throughout their lives. As a teenager, you may find that a lot of your thoughts and actions revolve around romantic relationships. Or you may not be at all interested in having a romantic relationship. Both of these circumstances are normal. Over the course of an adult life, however, most people are involved in a romantic relationship at one time or another. Dating is one of the ways adolescents (and adults) gain experience in romantic relationships. This chapter will discuss romantic relationships and the pleasures and pitfalls of being romantically involved with another person.

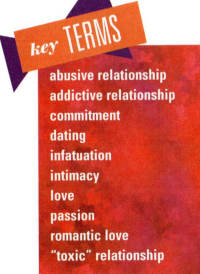

key TERMS

abusive relationship
addictive relationship
commitment
dating
infatuation
intimacy
love
passion
romantic love
"toxic" relationship

personal assessment: ROMANTIC RELATIONSHIPS

Before reading this chapter, take this personal assessment to discover more about your interest in and readiness for having a romantic relationship. On a separate sheet of paper, respond to the statements below on the basis of the way you feel most *of the time. Rate your answers using the following scale: 1 = Definitely True; 2 = Mostly True; 3 = Mostly False; 4 = Definitely False. An evaluation of your score is located at the end of the chapter.*

1. I have talked to my parents or family members about dating.

2. I have both male and female friends with whom I get along well.

3. I am comfortable with myself and who I am.

4. I am interested in dating someone.

5. I am ready and willing to assume the responsibilities of being a respectful dating partner.

6. I am able to stand up for myself and not "lose" myself in a relationship with another person.

7. I am able to accept other people as they are and not want them to change to meet my expectations.

8. My actions demonstrate respect for myself as well as for others.

9. I can communicate my needs, desires, and feelings accurately and appropriately.

10. If I became uncomfortable about any aspect of a dating relationship, I know where I could go to get advice or help.

TYPES OF LOVE

Our society uses the word **love** to describe our feelings for everything from candy and sports to marriages that last more than half a century.

- "I *love* chocolate."

- "I *love* playing soccer."

- "My grandparents have been married for more than 50 years, and you can tell that they still *love* each other."

We often use the word *love* when we're trying to describe a strong positive feeling for something or someone. There are many types of love. Some examples are love between members of a family and love between close friends. In this chapter, however, we will be discussing **romantic love** and the process that often leads to romantic love, **dating**.

---

love

a feeling of strong affection and devotion, characterized by unselfish and loyal concern for the well-being of another

romantic love

a type of love that includes an attraction to another person based on affection and sexual interest

dating

going out with another person in whom you have a romantic interest

CHARACTERISTICS OF ROMANTIC RELATIONSHIPS

Many of the characteristics that describe healthy romantic relationships are the same characteristics that describe good friendships. In fact, probably the most often cited recommendation for having a good romantic relationship is to "be friends first." Although this recommendation is often ignored, it is still excellent advice. Dating partners who take the time to be friends first give themselves time to get to know each other without being swept up in a rush of emotion. The same traits and qualities that are important to you in a friendship are the traits and qualities you should look for in a romantic relationship. For instance, if you expect your friends to be loyal and trustworthy, you will want those same qualities to be present in your romantic partner. It's a good idea to make a list of the qualities you want your romantic partner to have. You might also include a list of qualities you want to be sure to avoid.

STERNBERG'S THREE COMPONENTS OF LOVE

Objects that have at least three points of contact have a better chance of withstanding force than do those that have only one or two points of contact. A stool with fewer than three legs will tip over. But a three-legged stool can not only stand on its own, it can support additional weight as well. A psychologist named Robert Sternberg has described romantic love as having three main components: passion, intimacy,

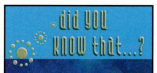

did you know that...?

Humans are fascinated with the topic of love. For example, the word *love* has more entries in *Bartlett's Familiar Quotations* than any other word except *man*. *Bartlett's Familiar Quotations* contains more than 8,000 quotations and is one of the best known references for quotations from ancient to modern literature.

Qualities I Want in a Romantic Partner

Qualities to Avoid in a Romantic Partner

What qualities do you want in a romantic partner?

and commitment. Like a three-legged stool, romantic love that is supported by these three components is more likely to stand strong than is love that has only one or two of the components (see Figure 19-1).

Passion

Passion is a romantic attraction to another person. Passion is both physiological and psychological. We are actually physically attracted to specific people because of hormones and certain brain chemicals. Passion also involves emotional feelings. The physical and emotional feelings combine to create nervousness, excitement, and anticipation about the "newness" of a relationship. Suppose you had never dived off a high board. High diving is something you really want to do, and you're kind of scared and excited at the same time. You climb the ladder and take the leap. If the dive is successful (and you don't land in a big belly flop!), you feel exhilarated and rush to do it again and again. Eventually, how-

passion

a strong liking for, desire for, or romantic attraction to another person

❤ HEALTHY PASSION ❤

Passion is a natural and important part of a romantic relationship, but it is important to understand that a relationship can contain passion without being sexual. Having strong feelings for someone does not mean that sex must be the reason for or part of the relationship. Teens will find that including sexual abstinence in a relationship takes away the risks of emotional trauma linked to unexpected pregnancy or sexually transmitted infection. Abstinence is the only behavior that is 100% effective in preventing pregnancy, sexually transmitted infections, and the emotional harm caused by either of the two.

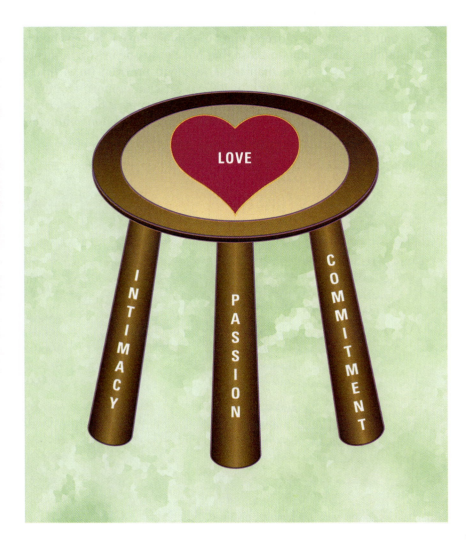

Figure 19-1

According to psychologist Robert Sternberg, romantic love is composed of passion, intimacy, and commitment.

What's News?

Research studies show that feelings of passion and infatuation are fueled by a natural brain chemical called phenylethylamine, which produces an amphetamine-like reaction within the body. Phenylethylamine is commonly called "the love drug" because it is thought to be responsible for many of the physiological reactions of the body at the beginning of a romance. Studies of the effects of this brain chemical reveal that it is impossible to maintain the passionate "high" that is experienced initially in a relationship. Over time (about 18 to 30 months) the body develops a tolerance to the effects of the chemical, and the intensity of the physiological effects diminishes and rarely returns during a relationship. This exciting period of time, however, gives a couple an opportunity to find out if there is more than passion to hold the relationship together.

ever, the excitement wears off, and it becomes "old hat." The same is true for the passion of new relationships. Passion does not have to disappear from long-term relationships, but it often feels less intense as time goes on than it did in the beginning.

Intimacy

Intimacy is a close, personal knowledge of another person. Intimacy can be physical, emotional, or both. Many teens think that intimacy is purely physical. They think of intimacy as hugging, kissing, and other sexual activities. Those are certainly intimate behaviors, but intimacy is much more than physical acts. People in an intimate relationship feel very comfortable with one another. They know each other well and reveal to each other many things about themselves that they would never reveal to people outside the relationship. Intimacy is a characteristic of both friendships and romantic relationships. As passion decreases in a romantic relationship, the amount of intimacy that has been established often determines whether the relationship will survive.

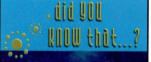

did you know that...?

An interesting fact is that the "love chemical," phenylethylamine, is one of the key ingredients in chocolate. It has been theorized that this substance is responsible for our "love affair" with chocolate!

intimacy

a close personal knowledge of another person, characterized by feelings of warmth and closeness

did you know that...?

Many studies report that males and females have differing viewpoints regarding the relationship among passion, intimacy, and commitment. Females are most comfortable with passion and intimacy in the context of a committed relationship. Males, on the other hand, seem to be more able to keep feelings of passion separate from intimacy and commitment. These findings can have important consequences for male-female romantic relationships.

take it on home

Share the information you have learned about Sternberg's three components of love with adult members of your family: parents, grandparents, aunts, uncles, or other trusted adult family members. Ask whether they agree, on the basis of their own experiences, with Sternberg's formula of love. Note your findings in your Health Folio.

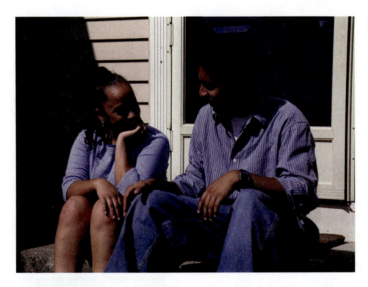

Commitment

Commitment is necessary for a relationship to endure both the good and the bad times that are a part of every relationship. Commitment in a romantic relationship is just as important as commitment in families and in friendships. Commitment ensures that the partners will not walk out at the first sign of trouble. It means being willing and able to work through problems and to stand strong in the face of difficulties. Commitment is the "glue" that holds a relationship together. It is what enables people to remain faithful to a single romantic partner.

commitment

the determination to continue in a relationship, often accompanied by an agreement or a pledge

infatuation

an idealizing, obsessive attraction to another person, characterized by a high degree of physiological arousal

INFATUATION

Infatuation, sometimes referred to as a crush, is an idealizing, obsessive attraction to another person, usually highly physical in nature. Some romantic relationships start with infatuation, but it is possible to experience infatuation without even being in a relationship. In fact, a person can be infatuated with another person without the other person's being involved at all. You or your friends may have been infatuated with a movie or sports star or with a classmate you don't even know.

If you become infatuated with someone, your infatuation could lead to a romantic relationship. But it is just as possible—maybe even more so—that you will never have a relationship with the person or you will quickly lose interest when you discover that the other person isn't really the way you imagined.

THE PROCESS OF DATING

There are many reasons why people choose to date or not to date at a particular time. Some people do not date during the teen years because of personal choice, parental disapproval of teen dating, lack of interest or acceptable partners, or involvement in other activities. It is entirely normal not to date until later in life. However, many teens do begin dating during high school. Determining when to begin dating is an issue that is usually of concern to teens. Deciding what type of dating relationships you are most comfortable with and what you will do on dates are other concerns. The following sections will examine the process of dating.

Reasons for Dating

Although the number of people who choose to remain single is growing, about 95% of adults will marry at some point in their life. Almost all married people went through a process of dating before getting married. Even people who have decided to remain single probably dated at some time. Have you ever thought about dating as having a purpose other than going out and having a good time? Some of the purposes are listed here:

- *Establishing a connection.* One of our most basic human needs is to establish meaningful connections with other humans. Dating provides a way for people to get to know each other better. Learning more about someone helps you decide whether you want to be more intimately connected to the person or to have a more casual relationship.

- *Self-discovery.* The process of dating allows you to discover more about yourself as you relate to others. Through dating, you can experiment with different roles and different types of relationships to discover the ones that most satisfying to you.

- *Finding someone special.* Dating can be simply an opportunity to spend enjoyable time with someone else. But many people date with the hopes of finding someone special–someone with whom they can have a lasting and intimate relationship. During the teen years, this "someone special" may just be someone you want to date more than once or twice. Later, you may seek a relationship that lasts much longer and might even lead to marriage.

There are many reasons to start dating. Have you thought about how you feel about dating?

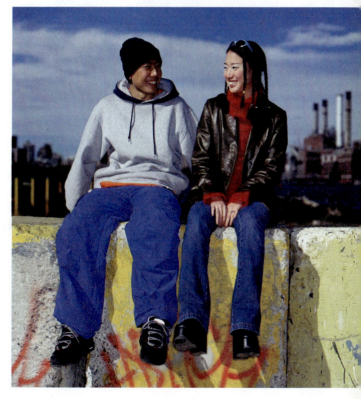

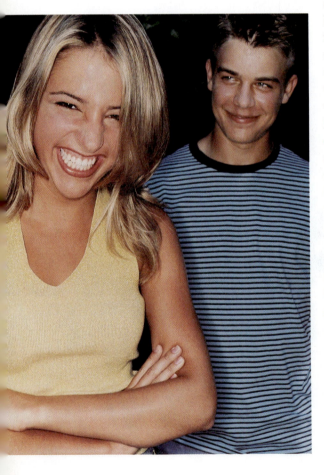

Deciding When to Date

Most people start dating when they are teenagers, usually sometime while they are in high school. Some people don't begin dating until after they graduate from high school. The age at which a person begins dating depends on a number of factors. Let's look at the examples of two students, Tamara and Gregory, to describe some of those factors.

- *Interest in dating.* Tamara is a sophomore in high school this year. Until now, she hasn't been interested in dating anyone. Because she's on the cross-country track team, she trains with other runners (both male and female) all the time. Sometimes they all get together and go somewhere after practice. She has been satisfied with her social life and has never been interested in dating anyone special. Gregory, on the other hand, always seems to be interested in some girl. He hasn't actually started dating yet, but he's definitely interested!

- *Available time and resources.* Between school, cross-country practice, and the time she spends with her family, Tamara doesn't have a lot of free time for dating anyway. Her family often depends on Tamara to watch her younger brothers and sisters because her parents have shifting work schedules. Gregory is busy too. He works at a part-time job every day after school and on the weekends. His parents helped him buy a car to get to and from school and work. Unlike some of his other friends, though, Gregory is expected to pay for some of his own expenses; he has to make his car payments and pay for entertainment and eating out.

- *Parental opinions of dating.* Tamara hasn't ever talked to her parents about dating, but she has a pretty good idea they aren't going to be thrilled with the idea. Because of their busy schedules, they already don't have as much time together as a family as they would like. When everyone is available, they like to do things together as a family. Gregory's parents agreed he could start dating after he had had his driver's license for six months. They also reminded him that he would have to pay for his dates with the money he earned from his part-time job.

- *Availability of a person you want to date.* Gregory noticed Tamara the first week of school, when he saw her out running with the cross-country team. He managed to get one of his friends to introduce them. Gregory didn't waste any time in asking Tamara to go to a movie with him. Tamara was surprised to be asked, and, even more to her surprise, she discovered she really wanted to go. But before she can say yes, she has to talk to her parents and get their permission.

Types of Teen Dating Relationships

When you are ready to begin dating, you may have many choices of people to date. You will also have a variety of options for types of dating relationships. Depending on the circumstances, your feelings, and the feelings of the other person, you may engage in one of the following types of dating:

- *Group dating.* Group dating has increased in popularity in recent years. Instead of involving just two people, group dating includes many males and females all doing something together. In this type of relationship, it isn't necessary to have an even number of males and females, and you are not necessarily paired with another person. Instead, the entire group does something together. You may "float" among people in the group, spending time with first one person and then another. You may be romantically interested in one of the other people in the group, or you may just enjoy being friends with everyone. A lot of teens like this option because it allows them to get to know many people. It also reduces the pressure many teens feel in a paired dating relationship. In group dating, financial pressure is also reduced, because everyone pays his or her own way. Parents tend to like this option best, especially for younger teens.

- *"Playing the field."* Playing the field, or "dating around," is another popular option. In this type of dating relationship, you are paired with someone for a date, but you date several people, not just one person. You might have a date with one person this weekend and another person next weekend. You may go out with the same person several times, but you don't make a commitment to date one person exclusively. Playing the field gives you a chance to get to know different people and to learn more about yourself and what qualities in a dating partner are important to you. Although this type of dating relationship doesn't provide much security, it allows for a great deal of learning, flexibility, and freedom.

- *"Going steady."* Two people who decide to go steady usually establish formal or informal expectations for maintaining the relationship. The main expectation is that the two will not date anyone else. This form of dating provides the most security of all the types of dating relationships. It also provides the opportunity to establish more intimacy with another person. However, this type of relationship requires more responsibility. Going steady does not mean a sexual relationship is necessary. Teens in a "steady" relationship who remain abstinent avoid the possible physical and emotional risks of having sex. Because of the emotional intimacy that often exists between teens who are going steady, ending this type of relationship can be more emotionally painful than with other dating relationships.

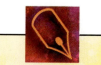

take it on home

Have a discussion with your parents or other adults in your family about what their expectations are for you in a dating relationship. Even if you will not be dating any time soon, discussing these matters ahead of time can help you understand their expectations of you. Make a note of these expectations in your Health Folio.

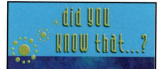

did you know that...?

Dating, as we know it today, was "invented" in America. Only the industrialized nations have a dating custom.

take it on home

Talk to the adult members of your family about the lessons they learned from their dating experiences. What things would they do differently? Is there a particular type of dating they would recommend or avoid? Being willing to learn from the experiences of others is a mark of maturity and good judgment. Note their responses in your Health Folio.

Dating Ethics

Regardless of the type of dating you choose to do, it is important to show respect, caring, and consideration for the person you are dating. Dating partners should demonstrate their care for each other by being honest and by never trying to take advantage of the other person. Neither person should try to dominate the other or always insist on having his or her way. Learning to treat romantic partners well is an important sign of maturity.

What to Do on a Date

When you are ready to begin dating, common questions are, "What should we do?" "Where can we go?" Some common date activities are high school extracurricular events and movies. Fortunately, there are many other options, even for teens who live in a small town or remote area. Finding something to do may require a bit of creativity, but you might discover something that can make a date more fun and interesting than a movie or school event. For example, picnicking in the park might help you get to know the other person better because you have more time to talk than if you were watching a movie or a sporting event. Creative dates also give you an opportunity to learn more about each other's interests and to experience new things.

Tough Teen Dating Issues

Dating can be awkward for people of all ages. Even adults with lots of experience in dating sometimes feel awkward and uncomfortable, especially when dating someone new. Because most teens are new to dating, they often feel nervous about it. Let's discuss some of the most common concerns.

Fear of Rejection

Fear of rejection may be the worry most often mentioned by teens when they are asked about dating-related problems. Fear of rejection can be a paralyzing force that stops you from moving forward toward something you really want. It takes a lot of courage to invite someone to get to know you better, and that's what dating is all about. If things don't go well, your self-esteem may be threatened. Remember that everyone faces the possibility of rejection at some time or another and that learning to handle rejection is part of the growth experience from adolescence to adulthood. Make a conscious decision to take a chance and not to let your fear of rejection keep you from enjoying potential new relationships.

Communication

Good communication skills you have learned with your family and peers are especially important in a romantic relationship. To maintain a relationship with a romantic partner, you need to be able to express yourself clearly and honestly and to be able to listen well. Romantic relationships can also provide an important opportunity to test your conflict resolution skills.

Passion

The rapid hormonal changes of adolescence can result in sexual urges that may be difficult to handle appropriately and responsibly. A healthy, ethical romantic relationship includes respect for yourself *and* for the other person. It also includes being willing and able to take responsibility for your actions. Thinking carefully about the possible long-term effects of your actions and making your decisions on the basis of these long-term effects rather than what you want at the moment is a mature and responsible way to respond to your feelings of passion.

Jealousy

Because many teens feel insecure about themselves and their ability to be accepted and valued, they often try to control others. Jealousy is motivated by insecurity and demonstrated by possessiveness. You may think that your romantic partner's jealousy shows that he or she cares about you. In reality, however, jealousy is usually a sign of insecurity and the need to control the partner's contact with other people.

Unrealistic Expectations

It is common for teens to have unrealistic expectations of a romantic relationship. They "put all their eggs in one basket," expecting one person to meet all of their social and emotional needs. This is an impossible task and can put a lot of strain on a romantic relationship. You may find, after you have been in a relationship for a while, that you want the other person to change and be more like you. But a necessary part of a healthy romantic relationship is respecting and honoring the differences between you and your partner. Another unrealistic expectation during the teen years is that the relationship will be permanent. Although some relationships do last, the vast majority of them end within a few weeks or months. Recognizing this fact allows partners in a relationship to make decisions based on reality rather than on fantasy.

Lack of Maturity

Lack of maturity is a factor that makes all of the other problems in teen relationships more difficult. Just as it is unrealistic to expect a five-year-old child to sit quietly for hours at a time, so is it unrealistic to expect teens to make mature decisions 100% of the time. But in romantic relationships, it is especially important to have the maturity to think about the consequences of your actions and to think about the interests and

Pressure to engage in sexual activity does not contribute to a healthy relationship. Among the problems associated with teens having sex is that the experience may leave them with emotional scars following the event. It is true that many states have laws protecting teens from having sex with older partners. Teens can protect themselves as well by remembering that abstinence is the only 100% effective method of avoiding problems associated with sexual encounters.

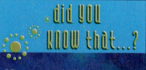

did you know that...?

Many teens believe that jealousy shows that their romantic partner likes them a lot. Sometimes people even try to make their partner jealous, to prove that he or she cares. In reality, jealousy can be a danger sign in a romantic relationship. Jealousy can even be a predictor of dating violence, especially if the jealousy continues, and the person becomes even more controlling. Jealousy in a partner should always be a warning sign that you may be in a potentially abusive situation.

safety of the other person. As much as possible, you want to keep from hurting both yourself and the other person by your actions and choices.

Breaking Up Is Hard to Do

Regardless of how wonderful your first romantic relationship seems at the time, it is extremely rare for first romantic relationships to result in

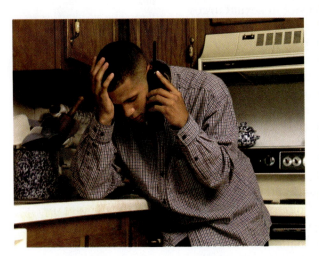

"living happily ever after." This is much more likely to be the stuff of fairy tales, rather than the real world. Although you occasionally hear of long-term successful relationships with the first person someone ever kissed, this is definitely the exception rather than the rule.

There are many reasons why relationships that seem so right in the beginning fall apart. A high percentage of breakups happen because the two people have different expectations about the three components that support relationships: passion, intimacy, and commitment. If a couple is unable to resolve these differences successfully, the relationship is likely to end. Let's look at some of the problems that can occur.

Problems with Passion

At the beginning of a romantic relationship, passion is high. Indeed, it is often the driving force for the relationship. When passion is "in the driver's seat" of the relationship, one of the persons may be more interested in romantic or sexual activities than the other person is. Negotiating when and how passion is expressed is part of the development of a relationship. Moving too fast or pushing another person into action before he or she is ready can cause stress in the relationship.

Problems with Intimacy

Dating partners often have different ideas about intimacy – both physical and emotional intimacy. One partner may want a lot of physical intimacy but not be willing to be emotionally intimate. Teens often find it much easier to establish physical intimacy than emotional intimacy. Because emotional intimacy requires the core of a person's identity to be exposed and vulnerable, it can seem very scary and risky. There are risks in both emotional and physical intimacy, especially if you don't feel you can fully trust your partner. To safeguard against taking risks you may later regret, moving slowly toward intimacy is the wisest course of action.

Problems with Commitment

One of the most difficult things for teens to deal with when they are dating is the area of commitment. It's unrealistic for a teen to make a

BENEFITS OF SEXUAL ABSTINENCE

- No worry about unexpected pregnancy. Remember, there is no such thing as "partially pregnant."
- It allows a relationship to mature and a couple to develop romantic intimacy without the complication of sex.
- No worry about sexually transmitted infections.
- No feelings of guilt or regret.

long-term commitment to another person. You have just begun to explore the world of potential partners, and it's unfair to both you and the other person to make promises of long-term commitment that you aren't likely to keep.

Even so, a certain level of commitment is necessary to sustain a dating relationship. When the time comes that you or the other person wants to leave the relationship, the breakup can be very difficult for both of you. It's not a healthy choice to stay in a relationship you no longer want to be in or to try to force another person to stay when he or she is ready to leave the relationship. It takes a great deal of maturity and honesty to leave a relationship—or to allow the other person to leave—with grace and dignity. Even in the best of circumstances, there are likely to be some hurt feelings for a while.

UNHEALTHY RELATIONSHIPS

"Toxic" relationships are romantic involvements that result in negative consequences for one or both partners. In toxic relationships, people become so focused on their partners that they don't take good care of themselves. As with alcohol and other drugs, relationships can be addictive. In an **addictive relationship**, one partner becomes the center of the world for the other person. In effect, the partner becomes the "drug of choice," someone the person depends on in an unhealthy way. Sometimes addictive relationships can also become abusive relationships. In an **abusive relationship**, one of the partners uses power and control over the other in order to get what he or she wants. Let's take a closer look at these types of relationships and what you can do to avoid them.

Addictive Relationships

Patterns of addictive relationships are quite common in teen dating relationships. The initial fascination and attraction of a new relationship can cause teens to give up other interests and friendships in order to spend more time with a particular person. In their desire to achieve closeness and belonging, teens are often willing to give up important elements of their identity to be accepted by another person. A person who is addicted to a relationship allows the other person to control his or her life, just as addicts allow alcohol or drugs to control their lives.

For example, suppose Tabitha begins dating Robert, who loves playing video games. Tabitha loves the outdoors and has always spent a lot of time with both male and female friends in outdoor activities. She never had any interest in being inside, playing video games. But now, she rarely spends any time with her friends. She stays at home to wait for Robert to call. When she and Robert are together, they play video games for hours at a time. Tabitha's friends are concerned and annoyed, but Tabitha insists that it's none of their business. She says she'd rather spend time with Robert, no matter what they're doing.

"toxic" relationship

romantic involvement that results in negative consequences for one or both partners

addictive relationship

relationship in which the object of your affection is the center around which your world revolves, or your "drug of choice"

abusive relationship

relationship in which one of the partners uses power and control over the other in order to get what he or she wants

Tabitha is exhibiting the patterns of an addictive relationship. If she and Robert break up, Tabitha may have difficulty returning to the friends and lifestyle she once knew and loved.

Abusive Relationships

In an abusive relationship, one person controls the behavior of the other person. A person can be abused physically, emotionally, or sexually. Hitting, pushing, throwing things, and using a weapon are some examples of physical abuse. Emotional abuse can be just as devastating as physical abuse. Emotional abuse includes verbal insults and threats. It can also include blaming or trying to manipulate the other person. Sexual abuse is any type of force to get a person to do a sexual activity that he or she does not want to do.

The Cycle of Abuse

The use of alcohol and other types of drug use are frequently present in abusive relationships. The abuse may worsen when the abuser is under the influence of alcohol or a drug. Abuse often involves a predictable cycle of violence. Tension in a relationship increases, and the abuse gradually intensifies, until an explosion of some type occurs. After the explosive incident, the abuser promises never to do it again and is especially nice to the partner. The abused partner tries to prevent another abusive incident by trying to control situations so that the partner doesn't get angry again. The abused partner is always "walking on eggshells" to prevent another conflict. Despite his or her best efforts, however, another episode of violence is sure to break out.

Dealing with Abuse

An abusive relationship can be changed or stopped through the efforts of either the abuser or the abused or both. People who are abusive need outside help to change their behavior. They are rarely able to change on their own, and often don't admit the need for help or simply refuse to get it. Therefore, it is often up to the abused person to stop the abuse. Often, however, it is very hard for someone who is being abused to get out of the relationship and get help. Abused partners may love their partner, may believe that he or she will change, or may be afraid of what the partner will do if abandoned. At the first signs of abuse, even emotional abuse, it is extremely important for the abused person to demand that the abuse stop immediately and permanently. If the abuse continues or is repeated, the abused person must leave the relationship. Failure to leave may result in long-term emotional or physical injury or even death. The best time for both the abuser and the abused person to get help is while they aren't involved in the relationship. This may be after the relationship ends or just a "time-out" period. This allows both parties to work on the issues that contributed to the abusive relationship.

They can then consider beginning another relationship, either with someone new or with the same partner. In most cases, professional assistance is necessary. In some cases, legal assistance may also be required to protect one's physical safety.

BUILDING YOUR Wellness Plan

In this chapter, you learned about romantic relationships. It is likely that romantic relationships will play an important role in your life. Your wellness plan should include information about how to increase your chances of success when you begin dating and how to have a respectful, healthy romantic relationship when you date another person. Key aspects of your personal wellness plan should include:

- Practicing mutual respect in your relationships
- Understanding the three components of romantic relationships: passion, intimacy, and commitment
- Being familiar with the different types of dating and appropriate activities for teens to do on dates
- Recognizing the warning signs of unhealthy relationships and knowing strategies to avoid or leave them
- Knowing the consequences of sexual behavior and understanding that abstinence enhances emotional health and is 100% effective in preventing pregnancy and sexually transmitted infections.

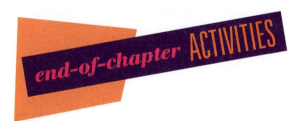

end-of-chapter ACTIVITIES

Weblinks

Dating

Slickditty: **http://www.leisureideas.com** (click on "Other Fun Things" and then on "Some Fun Things to Do on a Date")

Teenager's Guide to the Real World: **http://www.bygpub.com** (click on "Free Online Resources" and then on "Great Dating Ideas for Teenagers")

Toxic Relationships

Teen Relationships: **http://www.teenrelationships.org** (click on links to "What's Respect?", "What's Abuse?", and "How's Your Relationship?")

Short-Answer Questions

1. Briefly explain Sternberg's three components of love.
2. List the similarities and differences between friendship and romantic love.

3. List and briefly explain three purposes of dating.

4. Identify several of the tough teen issues in dating.

5. Identify some of the danger signals of a toxic relationship.

☀ Discussion Questions

1. Discuss the differences between romantic love and other types of love.

2. Explain what infatuation is.

3. Describe the advantages and disadvantages of various types of dating relationships.

4. Describe several reasons why teen relationships break up.

5. Discuss some of the reasons it is difficult to get out of an abusive relationship.

☀ Chapter Vocabulary

Using a separate sheet of paper, list and define the following terms:

abusive relationship	intimacy
addictive relationship	love
commitment	passion
dating	romantic love
infatuation	"toxic" relationship

☀ Application Activities

Language Arts Connection

1. Write a fictional or nonfictional essay or short story about two adults who exhibit Sternberg's three components of love in their relationship.

2. Write an essay describing the advantages and disadvantages of different types of dating relationships.

3. Write a poem that describes your feelings about love or romantic love.

Social Studies Connection

1. Collect evidence from television programs of different examples of dating relationships. What conclusions can you draw from your findings?

2. Research and report on community resources for places where teens can get help if they are in an abusive relationship and want to get out.

3. Research dating patterns in another country (such as England, Mexico, Saudi Arabia, or China) and compare them with dating patterns in the United States. What are the similarities and differences?

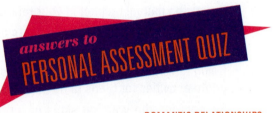

answers to PERSONAL ASSESSMENT QUIZ

personal assessment: ROMANTIC RELATIONSHIPS

Answers will vary. A higher proportion of Definitely True or Mostly True responses to questions indicates that you have an interest in dating and the skills and qualities necessary for a healthy dating relationship. A higher proportion of Definitely False or Mostly False responses indicates that you may not be interested in dating or ready to date at this time. It is important to note that responses to these questions will vary over time, depending on circumstances.

The Greatest Risks to Health and Wellness

Introduction

In earlier units, you learned about the leading causes of death in the United States and the meaning of risk factors as they relate to health and wellness. You may recall from those discussions that we no longer face major death threats from germs and other microscopic organisms. The disease threats to health come from conditions that are not caused by germs. Our current major health threats are heart disease, stroke, and cancer.

But there are other conditions that threaten your well-being, such as abuse of alcohol, tobacco, and drugs. These conditions can have negative effects on a person's health status, now and in the future. It is well known that these behaviors do not add to a person's health status, and that poor personal behavior choices can put a person at risk. In this unit, you will find information to help organize your wellness plan to avoid or reduce threats from these risks. We hope you will develop attitudes and behaviors that protect you for your lifetime.

chapter 20

Tobacco

Mel and her friends are not smokers. When they see some of the other kids around town who do smoke, they have a hard time understanding why people would want to intentionally breathe smoke into their lungs. Mel thinks that smoking cigarettes is like standing in front of a campfire and letting the smoke blow in your face. Her friends wonder why anyone would want to do something that is so harmful to health and that, once started, is so hard to quit. The group is not interested in smoking, nor have they even considered trying it. Besides, in their state, it's against the law for kids their age to buy or possess cigarettes. Mel and her friends feel very good about the fact that they can protect their health and not engage in a behavior that is against the law.

chapter OBJECTIVES

When you finish this chapter, you should be able to:
- Describe the structure and function of the respiratory system.
- Explain how tobacco products harm the body.
- List and explain the diseases associated with tobacco use.
- Explain why it is hard for teens who smoke to quit.
- List ways you can help someone quit smoking.
- Explain why there is no such thing as a safe cigarette.

key TERMS

bronchiectasis
carbon monoxide
carcinogen
cartilage
chronic bronchitis
cilia
diaphragm
emphysema
leukoplakia
periodontal tissue

Introduction

Cigarette smoking is not only harmful to health, it is also *the* number one most preventable cause of illness and death in the United States. If you have chosen not to smoke, you have made a decision that will help you live a longer and better-quality life. Making this decision as a teen is especially important because the vast majority of smokers begin smoking as teens—young teens. Beyond ninth grade, fewer and fewer young people start smoking because, as teens become young adults, the peer pressure to begin smoking cigarettes decreases and interest in practicing wellness increases.

This chapter contains information to reinforce your motives not to smoke. If you have thought about starting to smoke, the information and activities presented in this chapter should help you strengthen your commitment to wellness by not smoking.

personal assessment: TEEN SMOKING

Copy these statements on a separate piece of paper. Indicate which of the items you think are true, and which of the items you believe to be false. You can check your answers against the correct answers at the end of the chapter.

1. More than 5 million smokers under the age of 18 who are currently alive will die from a smoking-related disease.

2. The younger a person is when he or she starts smoking, the greater the risk of lung cancer.

3. Most of the adolescent smokers who buy their own cigarettes prefer the most heavily advertised brands.

4. Teen smoking is often a warning sign of future health problems such as drug use or social troubles such as violence.

5. Research indicates that nicotine is addictive to teens in ways similar to those of heroin, cocaine, and alcohol.

6. Studies have shown that early signs of the blood vessel damage that could cause heart attack or stroke can be found in adolescents who smoke.

7. Teenage smokers suffer from shortness of breath almost three times as much as teens who do not smoke.

THE RESPIRATORY SYSTEM

The respiratory system is directly affected by tobacco smoke because most smokers inhale smoke directly into the lungs. It makes sense, then, that much of the harm inflicted by cigarette smoke occurs in the mouth, throat, and lungs. Before you learn how smoking cigarettes harms the respiratory system, it may be helpful to review the parts of the respiratory system and how breathing occurs. Refer to Figure 20-1 as you read about this important body system.

The **trachea** is the main airway that extends from the throat to the lungs. The trachea is made of **cartilage**, a firm material that keeps the

trachea

the airway that extends from the throat to the lungs

cartilage

a firm but elastic material that keeps the trachea open for the passage of air

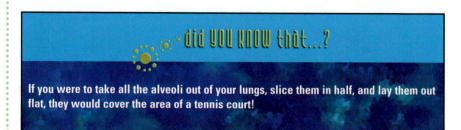

did you know that...?

If you were to take all the alveoli out of your lungs, slice them in half, and lay them out flat, they would cover the area of a tennis court!

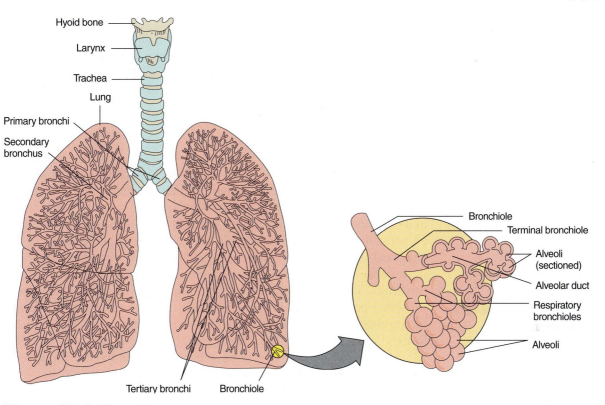

Figure 20-1 The respiratory system

airway open for the passage of air from outside the body. The trachea branches off into two main sections that enter into each lung. These branches are known as **bronchi**. As the bronchi enter the lungs, they divide into smaller and smaller branches. The smallest of these branches are known as **bronchioles**, and at the end of the smallest bronchioles are the **alveoli**. The alveoli have the appearance of microscopic grape clusters. Like tiny balloons, they fill with air when we inhale. The bronchioles consist of thin layers of tissue that are wrapped with **capillaries**, and it is here that oxygen and carbon dioxide are exchanged in the lungs.

Breathing

The purpose of breathing, also called respiration, is to allow air to enter the lungs so the blood circulating in the capillaries of the alveoli can dump carbon dioxide and pick up oxygen. Breathing is controlled by the **diaphragm**, a large muscle that sits just above the abdomen at the base of the chest. Although breathing seems automatic and continuous to most of us, it is actually a complex process that is controlled by a detection system in the nervous system. When the amount of carbon dioxide reaches a certain level in the bloodstream, the nervous system triggers the breathing mechanism. This starts with the diaphragm's contracting and lowering toward the stomach. This movement increases the volume in the chest cavity, and, as the volume increases,

bronchi
the branches of the airway that enter the lungs

bronchiole
the very ends of the bronchial tree

alveoli
structures at the ends of the bronchioles that inflate with air when we breathe

capillaries
the smallest of blood vessels, where oxygen and nutrients are exchanged for carbon dioxide and waste at the cell level

diaphragm
a muscle just above the abdomen that causes breathing

the pressure in the lungs decreases, creating a situation in which the air pressure inside the lungs is lower than the air pressure outside the body. This difference in pressure causes air to rush into the lungs. If the airways are clear, the air travels all the way to the alveoli, which then expand. When the diaphragm relaxes, the volume in the chest cavity decreases, and air is forced out of the lungs.

Defenses of the Lungs

Have you ever noticed how many tiny particles are floating in the air? They are easy to see when a stream of natural light enters through a window. The air we breathe contains a variety of particles, organisms, and chemicals that are continually inhaled into the lungs. The body has amazing defense mechanisms that work together to prevent germs and chemicals from harming the lungs and airways. For example, the hairs in the nose filter particles in the air and prevent them from going into the lungs. The trachea and airways in the lungs are lined with special cells that contain **cilia**, microscopic hairlike structures that move and sweep dust, chemical residue, and debris up from the lungs to the throat. Coughing and clearing the throat then remove this debris. When we get throat or airway infections, our bodies produce more mucus to capture infectious materials so they can be removed from the body before reaching the lungs.

WHY PEOPLE SMOKE

Why do you think people start to smoke? And continue to smoke? After all, just about everyone knows that smoking is a harmful, expensive, unpleasant-smelling habit. These facts make it hard to imagine why anyone would want to smoke in the first place. There are actually many reasons why people use tobacco products, and the reasons can be complex. Try answering the two questions below on a separate piece of scrap paper, using only a few words.

1. Why do young people start smoking?

2. Why do adults smoke?

Typical teen answers to the first question include "to be cool," "because my friends smoke," "because I'll appear older," and "because I want to." Teens are *not* likely to include "for good health," or "because I'm addicted" as reasons to smoke. On the other hand, common answers to the second question include "it's a habit," "I'm addicted," "I can't stop," or "to calm my nerves." Why do teens and adults have different reasons for smoking? Why don't adults smoke to be cool? The answers lie in the needs that are satisfied by smoking. Teens want to be recognized and are concerned about their image among their peers. Some use smoking as a way to satisfy their need for recognition.

The motivation for teens to fit in is very strong, and this may explain why 90% of all smokers start smoking before age 19. Once they have started, the addictive nature of tobacco takes over and becomes the

cilia

microscopic hairlike projections on certain cells that line the airways and sweep mucus and debris up the airway to the throat

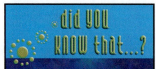

did you know that...?

In 1900, tobacco consumption averaged only 54 cigarettes per person per year. Consumption rose to about 4,345 cigarettes per adult in 1963. This number, by the way, was just before the U.S. Surgeon General disclosed the link between cigarette smoking and lung cancer. In the years that followed the Surgeon General's report, cigarette smoking among adults began to decline.

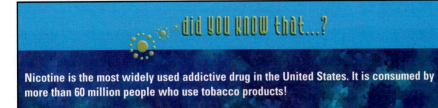

did you know that...?

Nicotine is the most widely used addictive drug in the United States. It is consumed by more than 60 million people who use tobacco products!

main reason for adult smoking. Tobacco contains an addictive chemical called **nicotine**. Addiction means the body has developed a physical need for a substance that makes quitting physically uncomfortable. The addictive nature of tobacco is what makes cigarette smoking a high-risk behavior. Teens who think they can smoke now and quit later are likely to regret their decision to start smoking because they may find themselves as adults with an expensive, unhealthy habit that is tough to give up.

Teen Smoking

Although most teens don't smoke, there is still a large number who do. Consider the following figures:

- Approximately 4.5 million U.S. teens are cigarette smokers.
- Each day, nearly 4,800 adolescents smoke their first cigarette.
- Nearly 43% of students in grades 9–12 have used tobacco.

These numbers are of concern because of the many harmful effects of tobacco. Some teens believe they can smoke while they are young and quit later before diseases such as lung cancer, emphysema, and heart disease occur. It's easy to believe that the harm to health associated with smoking happens only to adults – and older adults at that. But there are several things wrong with this reasoning. For instance, the nicotine in cigarette smoke is an addicting drug, and the addictive effects of the drug are **dose related**. This means that the more tobacco smoke consumed, the greater the exposure to nicotine, and the higher the level of addiction. This addiction can become a difficult barrier to the smoker's desire and ability to quit smoking. One-third of the people who started smoking as teenagers and were unable to quit as adults will die prematurely from tobacco-related illnesses.

Teen smokers may experience a number of harmful effects to their health. Research indicates that:

- Teen smokers suffer from shortness of breath almost three times as much as teens who don't smoke.
- Smoking by young people has been shown to interfere with both the function and growth of the lungs.
- Secondhand smoke is a major cause of respiratory problems for everyone who breathes it, especially infants and children.
- Early signs of heart disease and stroke are already present in some teenage smokers.

nicotine

an addictive chemical substance in tobacco

dose related

referring to the effects of a substance that are related to how much of the substance is consumed over time

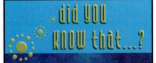

did you know that...?

The rate of cigarette smoking among teenagers is lower now than it was in 1990. The U.S. Centers for Disease Control and Prevention surveys high school students in all 50 states every two years. The information reported in 2001 indicated that only about 14% of the teens surveyed were regular smokers, compared with almost 17% in 1999.

EFFECTS OF TOBACCO SMOKE

The first time a person tries to smoke a cigarette, he or she is likely to cough a lot because the body is trying to eliminate the irritating foreign substance that is entering the airway and lungs. In fact, smokers have to train and discipline themselves to tolerate smoke in the throat and lungs! If beginning smokers paid attention to the reaction of their body to the cigarette smoke and quit smoking before they got addicted, they could prevent a lot of health problems.

Without question, the greatest threat to the respiratory system is cigarette smoke. This smoke is not simply gray air, but a vapor that contains almost 2,000 known chemical substances. Particulate matter (solids and liquids) makes up about 21% of the smoke, and gases make up the rest. Some of these substances are poisonous or otherwise harmful to the cells in the lungs. Other substances in smoke are addictive or cause birth defects and cancer. Some of the more common substances in cigarette smoke are listed in Table 20-1.

As the smoke is inhaled, the chemicals it contains are deposited on the tissues of the mouth, throat, and airways. Over time, the constant assault of these chemicals harms these tissues. Because the damage caused by cigarette smoking is dose related, that is, the earlier a person begins smoking and the more cigarettes smoked and the deeper the smoke is inhaled, the greater the harmful effects will be.

Harm to the Respiratory System

Because tobacco smoke is inhaled through the mouth and makes its way to the lungs, it stands to reason that the primary effects of smoking are on the structures of the respiratory system. Some of the effects, such as bronchitis, can occur within a relatively short period of time; other conditions, such as lung cancer, appear after many years of smoking.

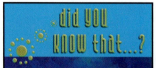

.did you know that...?

Research reported by the American Cancer Society indicates that cigarette smoke is 40% tobacco and 60% poison. Why doesn't smoking one cigarette kill a person? Because the total amount of poisonous substances in each cigarette is not enough to immediately poison an individual; the poisons have their effect over years of exposure.

Table 20-1 Examples of Harmful Chemicals Found in Cigarette Smoke

Chemical	Commonly Found	Poison	Cancer	Birth Defects
Acetone	Nail polish remover			X
Arsenic	Poison	X	X	X
Benzene	Paint, plastic, pesticides		X	X
Cadmium	Rechargeable batteries		X	X
Carbon monoxide	Engine exhaust	X		
Formaldehyde	Preservative for body tissue		X	X
Hydrogen cyanide	Gas chamber poison	X		
Toluene	Industrial solvent			X
Vinyl chloride	Plastic pipes		X	X

Bronchitis

Bronchitis is a condition in which the airways of the lungs (bronchi) become inflamed. Inflammation can come from a variety of sources, including the chemicals in tobacco smoke. Symptoms of bronchitis are a persistent cough and fever. The condition can become chronic, meaning that it continues for a long time. Have you ever heard the term *smoker's cough*? This is a cough that often occurs in the morning and is characteristic of **chronic bronchitis**.

Bronchiectasis

The constant irritation from chronic bronchitis can lead to a condition called **bronchiectasis**, in which the airways become scarred, swollen, and filled with mucus. The result is that even though the smoker can inhale air as the chest expands, exhaling is difficult because the airways close quickly and trap air and chemical irritants in the air sacs of the lungs. The chemicals eventually create a destructive effect on the air sacs, paving the way for emphysema.

Emphysema

Bronchiectasis can lead to **emphysema**, a word that comes from the Greek word *emphysan*, which means "to inflate." The irritants and air trapped as a result of bronchiectasis cause the tiny alveoli to overinflate. The increased pressure from overinflation and trapped chemicals from the smoke eventually cause the alveoli to tear. Once they are torn, the alveoli cannot be repaired and no longer function properly in the exchange of oxygen and carbon dioxide. This condition, known as emphysema, is almost exclusively a smoker's disease. If the individual with emphysema continues to smoke, the alveoli will continue to tear, eventually causing death when the lungs can no longer transfer needed oxygen into the body. Interestingly, the person with emphysema has no trouble inhaling but experiences a great deal of difficulty completely *exhaling*. Figure 20-2 shows photographs of both a normal lung and a lung with emphysema.

> **bronchitis**
> inflammation of the bronchi (airways)

> **chronic bronchitis**
> bronchitis that continues for a long time

> **bronchiectasis**
> a condition in which the airways of the lungs become scarred, swollen, and filled with mucus

> **emphysema**
> a condition in which the alveoli tear because of overinflation

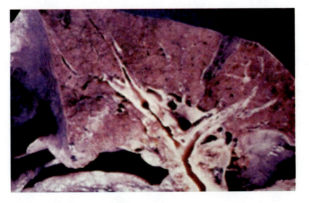

Normal lung   Emphysema

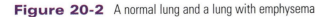

Figure 20-2 A normal lung and a lung with emphysema

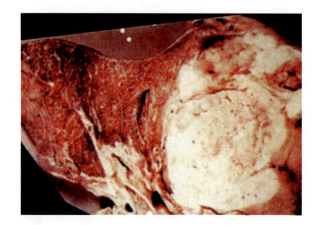

Cancer

Figure 20-3
A cancerous lung

Lung Cancer

The tar in cigarette smoke is actually the solid matter that contains about 63 chemical substances that are known to cause cancer. Tar is what gives smoke its gray color and what makes tobacco a **carcinogen**, a cancer-causing substance. Five cigarettes contain about a half-teaspoon of tar. It is a sticky, brown smelly liquid that clings to hair, skin, clothes, and lung and throat tissue. The manner in which tobacco smoke contributes to lung cancer is now well known. Over time, the smoke that enters the lungs delivers so much tar that the cilia become paralyzed and can no longer sweep out the smoke materials, chemicals, and mucus. The chemicals, especially tar, remain trapped on the lung tissue and cause alterations in the cells so that they become cancerous. Figure 20-3 shows a picture of a cancerous lung.

Lung cancer is very serious. By the time symptoms develop, the cancer is likely to have spread to other parts of the body. For this reason, most lung cancer victims do not survive the disease. Approximately 90% of lung cancer patients are smokers, and only 1 out of every 10 lung cancer patients lives more than five years after diagnosis.

carcinogen

a substance that causes cancer

What's News?

According to the National Center for Health Statistics, lung cancer is now the number one cause of cancer death among women! In fact, the lung cancer rates for women have steadily increased since 1950, when such cancer statistics were first reported. As more and more women have become smokers, the lung cancer death rate for women has risen from approximately 5 per 100,000 women in 1950 to 40 per 100,000 in 2000. Currently, the percentage of the population who smoke is getting lower. This may mean that the lung cancer death rate will be lower in years to come.

Harm to the Circulatory System

Tobacco smoke not only harms the respiratory system, it also causes considerable harm to the circulatory system. The chemicals in cigarette smoke that pass through the alveoli into the bloodstream negatively affect the circulatory system. (See Figure 20-4 to view the major structures of the circulatory system.)

We know that nicotine is the substance in cigarette smoke that makes cigarettes addicting, but it also causes the heart to beat more rapidly than normal. At the same time, other chemicals in smoke cause

take it on home

Talk with adults in your home or neighborhood about their smoking habits. Find out:

• If they ever smoked

• How old they were when they started

• How old they were when they quit (if they have quit) and what made them decide to quit smoking

• Why they started smoking (or why they chose not to start)

Write a summary report of your findings and place it in your Health Folio.

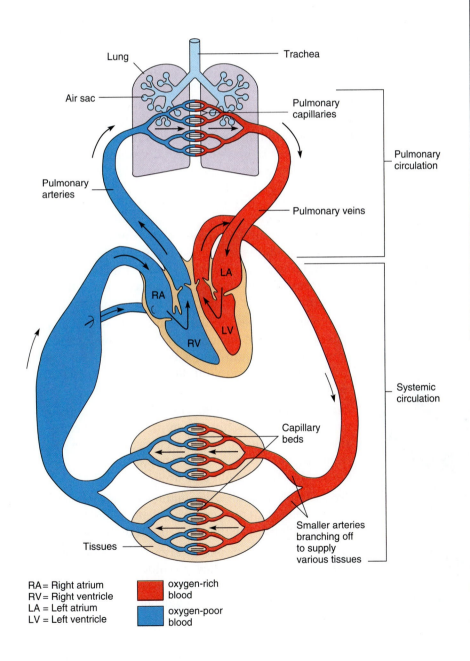

RA = Right atrium
RV = Right ventricle
LA = Left atrium
LV = Left ventricle

oxygen-rich blood
oxygen-poor blood

Figure 20-4
Schematic drawing of the circulatory system and lungs

the capillaries to constrict (get smaller). The combination of rapid heartbeat and narrowed blood vessels causes the heart to work harder. The result is often high blood pressure.

Nicotine also increases the likelihood that cholesterol will build up in the blood vessels, a leading factor for developing heart disease. The more cigarettes a person smokes, the greater the possibility that circulatory problems and premature death will occur. In fact, a smoker has three times the risk of having a heart attack than a nonsmoker.

Cigarette smoke contains **carbon monoxide**, a colorless, odorless gas that enters the bloodstream through the lungs. This poisonous gas is also a major ingredient of automobile exhaust. If enough carbon monoxide enters the bloodstream, it can cause death because it interferes with the blood's ability to transport oxygen to the body's cells. Here is what happens: When red blood cells pass through the capillaries in the alveoli, **hemoglobin** normally acts as an oxygen magnet, picking it up and carrying it throughout the body. But if carbon monoxide and oxygen molecules are both present, hemoglobin is more likely to attract the carbon monoxide. Smokers are unable to transport a full load of oxygen because so much of their hemoglobin is tied up with carbon monoxide. This process helps explain why smokers get winded so quickly and tire more easily than nonsmokers.

Harm to Appearance

Most teens are concerned about their appearance. Unfortunately, cigarette smoking can quickly affect someone's appearance in a very negative way. Many nonsmoking teens find smokers unattractive because of tobacco's effect on a person's appearance. Here are some of the negative effects that smoking can have on both appearance and health:

- *Breath.* Cigarette smoke dries out the mouth and throat. This drying encourages the growth of bacteria that cause odors. Smoke also clings to the mouth and airways and causes smelly tobacco breath. Mint gum does not mask it well, especially if a person has smoked for a long time.

- *Hair and clothes.* Smoke clings to the hair and clothes because it has a positive chemical charge whereas hair and clothing have a negative charge. The two charges create an attraction, and the smoke stays on long after the smoker has put out a cigarette.

- *Teeth.* Smoking causes the enamel of the teeth to yellow. The chemicals in the smoke also contribute to gum disease, which can eventually result in tooth loss.

- *Skin.* Teens who smoke cigarettes may not notice the wrinkle effects until they get older, but studies show that cigarette smokers have more wrinkles in their skin than nonsmokers. The skin ages because nicotine prevents a good blood flow to the skin cells.

carbon monoxide

a colorless, odorless poisonous gas

hemoglobin

an iron-rich compound in blood that carries oxygen

Choosing not to smoke can be good for your appearance.

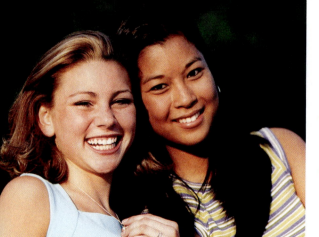

Harm to Others

There is little doubt that cigarette smoking harms the smoker. Evidence is accumulating now that cigarette smoking also is harmful to the environment, to nonsmoking individuals who spend time around smokers, and to developing fetuses.

Environmental Damage

Cigarette smoking can do great harm to the environment. Most of this damage results from fires caused by mishandling cigarettes. The tobacco in cigarettes is designed to smolder as it burns, so when a cigarette is carelessly discarded or accidentally dropped into a cushion, it can smolder, unnoticed, until the smoker has left the area. When it does erupt into a blaze, there may be no one available to put it out. Even worse, people may be sleeping and not able to escape the fire in time. According to the American Cancer Society, more people die from cigarette-caused fires (about three people every day) than from fires started by any other single cause.

Smoking also contributes to litter in the environment. Take a look at the areas outside of nonsmoking buildings or at the pavement and gutters near a bus stop. Most likely, they are littered with cigarette butts. Not only is this litter unsightly, the cellulose filters on the cigarettes present health problems to animals or small children who may eat them.

Environmental Tobacco Smoke

Did you know that it's possible to have your health negatively affected by smoke even if you never light a cigarette yourself? There is considerable evidence that both exhaled smoke and smoke from the burning end of a cigarette are harmful to the health of nonsmokers who are in the area. When smokers take a drag on a cigarette, they inhale **mainstream smoke**. Mainstream smoke is filtered by the tobacco and the filter on the cigarette. Once exhaled, it is called **exhaled mainstream smoke** and contributes to **environmental tobacco smoke**. Commonly referred to as secondhand smoke, environmental tobacco smoke is

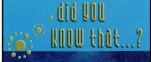

The worst industrial disaster in U.S. history took place in April 1947 at a ship loading dock in Texas City, Texas. A careless smoker cast a cigarette butt into the hold of a ship fully loaded with ammonium nitrate. The ammonium nitrate exploded, and the explosion damaged 90% of the buildings in the nearby city, killed almost 600 people, and hospitalized more than 4,000 people. The cost of the disaster was more than $4 billion.

mainstream smoke
smoke that comes directly to the smoker from the cigarette

exhaled mainstream smoke
smoke that is exhaled by the smoker

environmental tobacco smoke
smoke that people breathe when they are in a smoky environment; also called secondhand smoke

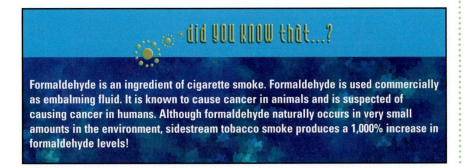

Formaldehyde is an ingredient of cigarette smoke. Formaldehyde is used commercially as embalming fluid. It is known to cause cancer in animals and is suspected of causing cancer in humans. Although formaldehyde naturally occurs in very small amounts in the environment, sidestream tobacco smoke produces a 1,000% increase in formaldehyde levels!

✿ teen forum ✿

Nonsmoking Areas

Clean-indoor-air laws and policies that restrict smoking to designated areas have been enacted in 49 states and the District of Columbia. These laws vary from restricting smoking to certain sections of restaurants and civic buildings to banning smoking in all public places such as government buildings, schools, elevators, and retail stores. The purpose of the laws is to protect nonsmokers from the harmful effects of secondhand smoke. Some people think that such laws take away from the freedom of smokers.

- How do you feel about this kind of restriction?
- Should smokers be forced to give up something they want to do so that nonsmokers can have a smoke-free environment?

inhaled by anyone who is near a smoker or in a smoky environment. The smoke that comes from the burning end of a cigarette between puffs or from a cigarette sitting in an ashtray is known as **sidestream smoke**. Another source of harm are the contaminants that diffuse through cigarette paper into the environment and contribute to the chemical composition of secondhand smoke.

Environmental tobacco smoke (ETS) contributes to a variety of ear, nose, and throat infections among nonsmokers. Children exposed to ETS have higher rates of bronchitis and asthma than do children not exposed to ETS. More important, ETS ranks third as a major preventable cause of death. Only direct smoking and alcohol abuse rank higher as preventable causes of death. It is estimated that ETS is responsible for approximately 3,000 lung cancer deaths among nonsmokers each year. In June 2002, a group of scientists in the World Health Organization reviewed 50 research studies and concluded that secondhand smoke is linked to cancer. Information on the harmful effects of ETS has prompted many local and state governments to pass laws to ensure smoke-free environments for nonsmokers.

Smoking during Pregnancy

Smoking during pregnancy is not a good idea. Remember that cigarette smoke contains thousands of chemicals that enter the bloodstream of the smoker. A woman who smokes during pregnancy will deliver these chemicals through her bloodstream to the bloodstream of her fetus. These chemicals can produce harmful effects both before and after birth.

1. Smoking women are likely to deliver before their scheduled due date.

2. Fetuses born to smoking mothers are likely to be low-birthweight babies (those who weigh less than 5.5 pounds at birth). Low-birthweight babies are at risk of dying before their first birthday.

3. Children born to smoking mothers are at greater risk for birth defects than are children of nonsmokers.

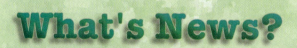

What's News?

Even if a woman does not smoke during her pregnancy, her fetus can still be harmed by the smoking of others. Secondhand smoke is an environmental hazard and can adversely affect fetal development and elevate the risk for low birthweight. Low birthweight can cause many other problems for an infant. In addition to not smoking themselves, pregnant women should avoid exposure to ETS.

COST OF SMOKING

Smoking costs money. The costs built into every pack of cigarettes include the cost of manufacturing and distributing the cigarettes, profit for the seller, and taxes paid by the consumer. The federal government imposes a tax of about $.40 on each pack of cigarettes. Each state has the capacity to collect a tax on each pack of cigarettes according to its own desires. New York's tax on a pack of cigarettes is $1.50; Illinois collects $.98 per pack; California collects about $.90 per pack; Virginia and Kentucky collect about $.03 per pack. The taxes on cigarettes serve to bring revenues to the state and federal government, but they also have an effect on tobacco use. As taxes go up, cigarette sales drop, and the people who quit smoking or smoke less don't require as much health care and miss fewer days of work. It is estimated that for every $.10 increase in cigarette tax, we save $7 on health care and loss of work time because the increase causes many people to quit smoking.

The amount of money spent on tobacco products is large and provides huge profits for the tobacco companies. For example, Philip Morris, one of the largest tobacco corporations in the United States, records profits in excess of $5 billion a year. Did you ever stop and think about what goes on behind the scenes to encourage people to purchase cigarettes? An advertising agency is a group of people who are paid money to create advertising campaigns that motivate people to buy certain products or services. Ad agencies are responsible for most of the commercials we see on television. Imagine that you own an advertising agency and a customer asks you to develop an advertising program to help sell a product. When you ask the customer to provide you with information about the product, you learn that:

- It is taken by mouth but has no nutritional value whatsoever.
- Once it gets into the body, it robs it of oxygen.
- It is addictive.
- People who use it die sooner than people who don't.
- It kills almost 450,000 people a year.
- The product costs about $12 a pound.

As the owner of the ad agency, how would you feel about accepting money to promote such a product? Do you think you could create an advertising message to motivate someone to buy this product? Clearly, advertising this product would not be an easy task. It is difficult to "sell" tobacco products using health-promoting messages. What messages have you seen in tobacco ads that try to make tobacco use appealing?

LOW-TAR, LOW-NICOTINE CIGARETTES

There are companies that advertise low-tar and low-nicotine cigarettes. Are these cigarettes safe for the user? The answer is no. It seems as if low-nicotine cigarettes would be less addictive than high-nicotine cigarettes, but they aren't. Research shows that smokers who are addicted require certain levels of nicotine. When using low-nicotine cigarettes, they inhale more deeply, smoke faster, and actually consume more cigarettes than when they smoke regular cigarettes.

Research on cigarette smoking now shows that people who smoke the so-called low-tar cigarettes often inhale the same level of cancer-causing tar as people who smoke regular cigarettes and are just as likely to suffer the negative health effects of smoking as those who smoke regular cigarettes. Even low-tar cigarettes contain tar and other chemicals. If the companies were to eliminate all tar, they would be eliminating the smoke and then cigarettes would not be pleasing to smokers. The truth is, there just isn't any level of tar that is safe.

BIDI CIGARETTES

Bidis are hand-rolled cigarettes from India that have no filter. They are made with tobacco from the Southeast Asia region. The cigarettes have been used by young people because they are sweetly flavored with strawberry, chocolate, cherry, and mango (because the tobacco is harsh), and they are less expensive than American cigarettes. The cigarettes should not be viewed as a natural substitute for cigarettes that is safe and trendy. Despite their sweet flavor and colorful packaging, bidis represent a greater health risk than American cigarettes.

1. Research on bidis indicates that, ounce for ounce, bidis contain much higher levels of the toxic substances in standard cigarettes.

real teens

Frank used to smoke cigarettes. When he was 14 years old, he tried a cigarette a friend offered him, just to see what it was like. He never really intended to be a smoker. He knew cigarettes were bad for his health, but he got caught up trying to be liked by his friend. When the friend moved away, Frank regretted that he had started smoking, so he decided he would try to quit. He didn't want to ask his parents for help because he didn't want them to know he was smoking. He surfed the Web to find sites that offered suggestions for quitting. Sure enough, he found some good ones, even some containing personal stories from people who had quit. The information Frank gathered, along with his sincere desire to not smoke, has motivated him to stay tobacco free for almost two years.

2. The tobacco in bidis contains 8% nicotine (compared with 1% in regular cigarettes), making them more addicting and more harmful to the circulatory system.

3. Bidis contain no filter, so the burning product releases three to five times more tar and nicotine than regular cigarettes.

4. The tobacco does not burn well, and the user has to "drag" more strongly to keep the bidi lit. In the process, pieces of tobacco and paper are inhaled into the throat and lungs.

HELPING SOMEONE QUIT SMOKING

Do you know someone who wants to quit smoking—maybe a parent, relative, neighbor, or friend? There are things you can do to help, but first you must understand that smoking plays a significant role in the life of the smoker. It is a strong habit, both physically and psychologically, and can be very difficult to give up. It takes courage to first decide to quit smoking. Quitting successfully also requires *continual motivation* to not smoke. This is where you can help by acting as a member of the ex-smoker's **social support network** and helping him or her keep focused on success and on what triggered the desire to quit smoking. This trigger may have been a doctor's order, the desire for wellness, the need to set an example for children, or the high monetary costs of smoking. The closer your relationship to the ex-smoker, the greater the opportunity you have to reinforce his or her motives for not smoking.

When someone you care about announces the intention to quit smoking, you can do more than just say, "That's nice" or "Congratulations!" You can help reinforce the person's motives, strengthen his or her resolve, and even strengthen your relationship with the person by doing some of the following:

1. Ask the person to tell you how he or she feels after not smoking. Talking about feelings helps the quitter develop nonsmoking attitudes and strengthens their motivation to stay off tobacco.

2. If the person complains about how difficult it is to give up smoking, tell the person how proud you are of him or her and that you are confident he or she can succeed.

3. Don't let the person get away with saying he or she is going to start up again. There are several things you can say to help the person over the hump:

   • Let the person know he or she seems healthier since they have quit smoking.

   • Remind the person that every day makes a difference.

   • Tell the person you know how much better off he or she will be after working through it.

   • Ask the person to retell you the things that motivated him or her to quit in the first place.

> **social support network**
>
> a network of family, friends, and acquaintances who encourage, support, and provide positive feedback

- Encourage the person to talk about the sense of pride and accomplishment he or she will feel after completely quitting.
- Remind the person of the money that will be saved, and encourage him or her to put the money into a savings account to save for something special.

Perhaps you can think of other ideas. The key is that you remain involved with the ex-smoker and do all you can to help keep the focus on the positive reasons for not using tobacco.

Ex-smokers need new behaviors to occupy the time formerly occupied by smoking. You can help by inviting them to exercise with you, share a hobby, listen to music, do homework, play video games, or even just hang out and talk. Watching television is not a good idea because it lets them sit too quietly and be in a situation that may leave them feeling the urge to light up.

SMOKELESS TOBACCO

smokeless tobacco

tobacco that is not smoked but is used orally, such as snuff or chewing tobacco

Only about 8% of young people use **smokeless tobacco**, and its use has declined since the early 1990s. The Monitoring the Future Study in 2001 found that almost three-fourths of tenth and twelfth graders surveyed disapproved of smokeless tobacco use. The decline in smokeless tobacco use and high level of disapproval indicates that there is little support among our young adults to use smokeless tobacco. This is good news because smokeless tobacco is not a safe alternative to cigarettes. Smokeless tobacco contains chemicals that are highly addictive and some materials that can lead to cancer and heart disease. Other serious health conditions associated with the use of smokeless tobacco are:

- *Tooth abrasion.* Grit and sand particles in smokeless tobacco can scratch teeth and wear away the tooth enamel.
- *Gum recession.* The tobacco is typically held in the same spot in the mouth. This habit can result in permanent damage to **periodontal tissue** (the supporting tissue around the tooth root). The injured gum can pull away from the tooth and eventually cause loss of the affected teeth.

periodontal tissue

supporting tissue around the tooth root

- *Increased tooth decay.* Sugar is added to smokeless tobacco during the curing and processing to improve its taste. This sugar reacts with the naturally occurring bacteria in the mouth and leads to tooth decay.
- *Oral cancer.* Tobacco and its irritating juices are left in contact with gums, cheeks, and lips for long periods of time. This long-term contact can eventually result in a condition called **leukoplakia**. Leukoplakia appears either as a smooth white patch or as leathery-looking wrinkled skin around the gum line. It results in cancer in 3%–5% of all cases. Oral cancer treatments can disfigure patients because a lot of bone and tissue must be removed from the patient's face. Oral cancer is especially dangerous because it can spread quickly to the brain.

leukoplakia

a precancerous sore that develops after prolonged exposure to tobacco

BUILDING YOUR Wellness Plan

Your wellness plan related to tobacco is very simple: Don't use tobacco products! Cigarette smoking is the number one most *preventable* cause of death in the United States because it is a *voluntary* behavior with very high risk to health. Teens may not believe they are being harmed by smoking, but those who smoke are setting themselves up for a life of addiction and many future health problems. Develop your wellness plan to include a goal related to tobacco use. You might want to select from the list below or create your own.

- Define and clarify your wellness goals to include abstaining from tobacco use as a wellness practice.

- Sharpen your refusal skills so you can resist pressure from others who try to convince you that smoking is cool.

- Use your health literacy skills to learn more about the dangers of tobacco use.

- Support someone you know who is trying to quit.

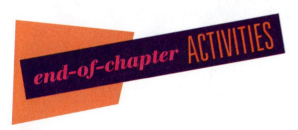

end-of-chapter ACTIVITIES

Weblinks

Help with the Process of Quitting Tobacco

QuitNet.com, Inc.: **http://www.quitnet.com**

Tobacco-Related Laws and Policies of Every U.S. State

American Lung Association:
http://www.virtualsql.com/abcqxyz/dev/lungusa

Up-to-Date Reports about Smoking and Its Effects on the Body

National Library of Medicine:
http://www.nlm.nih.gov/medlineplus/smoking.html
Patient Education Institute:
http://www.nlm.nih.gov/medlineplus/tutorials/smokingthefacts.html

Short-Answer Questions

1. Name the structures in the lungs where oxygen and carbon dioxide are exchanged between the lungs and the bloodstream.

2. How would someone know he or she has bronchitis and not just a cold?

3. List three chemicals in cigarette smoke that harm the body.

4. What is the substance in cigarette smoke that causes one's cholesterol level to get higher?

5. Name the precancerous condition in the mouth that occurs before oral cancer develops.

☀ Discussion Questions

1. Describe what happens during the breathing process.
2. List and discuss the major health risks associated with smokeless tobacco.
3. Explain why there is no such thing as a safe cigarette.
4. Discuss why cigarette smoking is harmful to the circulatory system.
5. Describe some ways you can help someone quit smoking.

☀ Chapter Vocabulary

Using a separate sheet of paper, list and define the following terms:

bronchiectasis	cilia
carbon monoxide	diaphragm
carcinogen	emphysema
cartilage	leukoplakia
chronic bronchitis	periodontal tissue

☀ Application Activities

Language Arts Connection

Write a letter to one of your local city council members or commissioners explaining why it would be healthy to pass policies to prevent smoking in public places. Include in your letter the issues related to secondhand smoke and the unappealing nature of cigarette smoke to nonsmokers. You can include the letter in your Health Folio. If you are in favor of such a policy, consider sending a copy to the council or commissioners.

Math Connection

Find out approximately how much cigarettes cost in your community. Suppose someone you know smokes one package of cigarettes per day. How much will the person spend on cigarettes over 1 year? Over 10 years? Over 20 years? Now suppose this person has to be treated for chronic bronchitis six times during that 20-year period. Research the cost of treatment with a local health care provider or on the Web and add it to the 20-year total. If you had the money spent on smoking and illnesses related to smoking, what would you do with it?

Science Connection

Find a cigarette butt (handle it carefully with rubber gloves or tweezers to avoid germs) and remove the paper and tobacco from the filter. Write a report of your observations: What color is the filter just behind the tobacco? What does it smell like? What do you think is trapped in the filter? Do you think the filter traps all harmful materials? Prepare a summary of your findings and include it in your Health Folio.

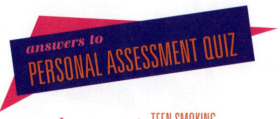

answers to
PERSONAL ASSESSMENT QUIZ

personal assessment: TEEN SMOKING

Each of the statements is true!

chapter 21

Alcohol

As are many of her friends and classmates, Clarissa is struggling with the news of a tragedy. Brent, one of the most popular kids in school, was seriously injured at a party over the weekend. He was at the gathering after the basketball game, and some older kids brought liquor to the party. Brent, who was not a drinker, decided that he would try some alcohol this time to celebrate the team's victory. After a few drinks, he started acting silly. People were laughing at his antics, especially when he was dancing with a lamp. The fun turned horrible in an instant. Brent, a gifted athlete who was on the gymnastics squad, tried to do a handstand on a dining room chair. The alcohol interfered with his ability to do the trick. He lost his balance and fell, striking his back on another chair. He was taken by ambulance to the hospital, where doctors confirmed that Brent had broken his back and damaged his spinal cord. They are concerned that he may never walk again.

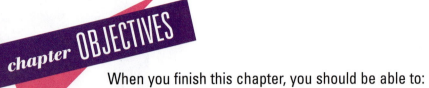

chapter OBJECTIVES

When you finish this chapter, you should be able to:

- Explain how alcoholic beverages are made.
- Explain why ethyl alcohol is considered a drug.
- Give reasons why teens should avoid alcohol consumption.
- Explain the meaning of binge drinking and why it is harmful.
- Describe both the negative and positive effects on the health of adults who engage in moderate alcohol consumption.
- Explain how alcohol is metabolized in the body.
- Summarize the effects of alcohol on selected body structures.
- Discuss personal and social factors related to alcohol abuse and alcoholism.
- Discuss trends in teen alcohol consumption.

key TERMS

alcohol dehydrogenase
alcohol poisoning
binge drinking
blood alcohol concentration
cardiomyopathy
fermentation
fetal alcohol syndrome
hypothermia
proof
withdrawal

Introduction

Humans have consumed alcoholic beverages for almost as long as there have been civilizations. Archeological digs indicate that alcohol has been used by human beings for more than 8,000 years. For example, earthenware pitchers used by Neolithic tribes in 6400 B.C. were found to contain berry wine residue. It is no wonder, then, that alcohol is part of the social fabric of the United States. Although alcoholic beverages are consumed by most adults in this country, people tend to overlook the fact that alcohol presents many personal and social problems if it is not used properly. It is important to understand that alcohol is a powerful drug that can cause death if consumed in sufficient quantities. It is also a product that has no nutritional value.

A young adult's decision to drink alcoholic beverages is a personal one that should be made carefully and should be based on information about the risks associated with alcohol use. In this chapter, you will gain information about alcohol to help you make an informed choice about whether to drink alcohol as an adult.

personal assessment: FACTS ABOUT ALCOHOL

Read each of the statements below and mark on a separate piece of paper whether you think each one is true or false. You can find all the answers at the end of the chapter.

1. There are no calories in alcoholic beverages.
2. Liquor that is consumed with soda will affect the body more quickly than liquor consumed by itself.
3. Eating while consuming alcoholic beverages will slow the absorption of alcohol.
4. Coffee and a cold shower will sober up a drunk.
5. Before the days of modern medicine, alcohol was used as a sedative for surgical procedures.
6. A person cannot become an alcoholic by drinking only wine.
7. Most alcohol consumed is absorbed into the body through the stomach.
8. Given the same amount of alcohol and the same body weight, a woman will be more affected by alcohol than a man.

THE NATURE OF ALCOHOL

Beverage alcohol is known as ethanol or ethyl alcohol. It is the only form of alcohol that is fit for human consumption. Ethyl alcohol contains calories but has no nutritional value. When alcohol is consumed, the human body metabolizes the alcohol first and uses the calories for body processes. Food calories are metabolized after the alcohol. If the energy needs of the body are met by the alcohol, the unused food calories are stored as fat in the body.

Alcohol Production

Alcohol is a by-product of **fermentation**, a process in which sugars from fruits or grains are allowed to sit without oxygen in the presence of yeast. The yeast uses the sugar as a food source and produces ethyl alcohol as a by-product. The fermentation process varies depending on whether the manufacturer intends to produce wine, beer, or liquor. Alcoholic beverages contain different levels of alcohol. In general, 12 ounces of beer, 5 ounces of wine, and 1.5 ounces of liquor each contain about the same amount of alcohol (approximately one-half ounce). Beer is usually 4%–6% alcohol. The percentage of alcohol in wine varies and is given on the label. Alcohol in liquor comes from a process known as distillation, in which the alcohol is removed from fermented

fermentation

the process of converting sugars into ethyl alcohol and carbon dioxide

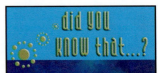

You may be using *denatured* ethyl alcohol in the alcohol burners in your science class. This is the same alcohol that comes from the sugar fermentation process—but don't try to drink it! This kind of alcohol has specific materials mixed with it that make it unfit for human consumption.

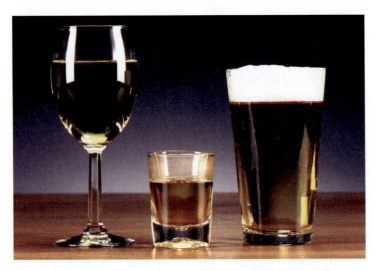

Each of these drinks contains approximately the same level of alcohol.

proof

the measure of the amount of alcohol in a liquor; a 90-proof liquor is 45% alcohol

products such as barley, corn, or potatoes. Liquor expresses the amount of alcohol as "**proof**." Proof is stated on the label and is twice the amount of alcohol. For example, 86-proof bourbon is 43% alcohol.

Alcohol the Drug

Alcohol is a depressant drug. It causes central nervous system impulses to travel more slowly and has a sedating effect by causing body functions to slow down. More than 100 years ago, doctors used alcohol as anesthesia for surgical procedures. This practice was risky because the amount of alcohol needed to mask pain is extremely close to the amount that leads to death. If enough alcohol is consumed, it depresses the brain centers that control respiration and heart rate and causes them to shut down. This danger is why medical scientists have developed safer anesthetics.

The body protects itself from overconsumption of alcohol by triggering a vomiting response that removes alcohol from the stomach before it can fully enter the bloodstream and depress brain function. Some people believe that vomiting during a drinking episode is a result of drinkers "mixing their liquors," but this is not the case. Vomiting is a clear sign that the amount of alcohol consumed is reaching a dangerous level.

tolerance

physical change in the body that causes one to adapt to the effects of a drug, causing the person to use more of the drug to get the same effect

The most common reason people drink alcohol is to achieve a "drug effect." The problem is, as with other depressant drugs, the body builds up a **tolerance** to the effects of alcohol. To continue to achieve the desired drug effect, a person has to consume larger and larger amounts of alcohol. The stronger the effect desired, the more the alcohol that must be consumed. It is common for heavy drinkers to feel a sense of discomfort, including nausea, when they do not have alcohol in their bloodstream. This discomfort is a condition called **withdrawal**.

withdrawal

feelings of discomfort that occur when the body is deprived of a drug to which it is addicted

DRINKING BEHAVIORS

Each person has to decide what role alcohol will play in his or her life. Many people choose not to drink any alcohol; some choose to drink occasionally; others choose to drink more than is good for them. All behaviors related to alcohol consumption can be viewed as being part of a continuum that ranges from abstinence to alcoholism. Definitions of consumption should be used with caution, however, because there are factors other than the amount of alcohol, such as how people respond to alcohol, the length of time over which consumption takes place, the type of drink consumed, and the body size of the drinker.

Responsible Drinking Behaviors

Abstinence and light and moderate consumption represent responsible adult drinking behaviors. There are other factors that contribute to responsible drinking behaviors, including:

- *Decision-making skills.* When young adults turn 21, they should know how to make responsible decisions about whether to drink alcohol. They should also have developed the communication skills needed to express their values and turn down invitations to drink if they have decided doing so is best for them.

- *The ability to say no.* Resisting pressure from others to engage in behaviors you have decided not to do is responsible, adult behavior.

- *Acceptance of abstainers.* Adults who make the decision to drink alcohol should never pressure those who choose not to. The decisions others make for themselves should be respected.

Abstinence

Not everyone feels a need to consume alcohol, and no one should be made to feel they must consume alcohol. Data show that most people in the United States who are age 12 and older do not drink alcohol. The 2001 National Household Survey on drug abuse reported that 51.7% in this age group had not consumed alcohol at any time in the 30 days prior to the survey. The Centers for Disease Control and Prevention reported in 2001 that less than half of the high school students surveyed had consumed alcohol in the 30 days prior to the survey. People who abstain from alcohol consumption do so for a variety of reasons:

- They are concerned about their *health and well-being* and recognize that alcohol is a chemical irritant and carcinogen estimated to contribute to about 4% of cancer cases. Some people have been advised by their doctors to stop drinking. The National Institute on Alcohol Abuse and Alcoholism recommends that certain people should not drink alcohol at all. These include women who are pregnant or trying to conceive; people who plan to drive or engage in other activities that require attention or skill, such as airline

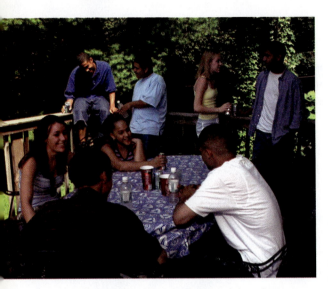

Choosing to abstain from alcohol doesn't mean having less fun!

pilots and surgeons; people taking medication, including over-the-counter medications; recovering alcoholics; and persons under the age of 21.

- They hold *religious beliefs* that advocate abstinence as a way of keeping the body pure and healthy.
- They have decided that the *cost* of alcohol, a nonfood substance, is more than the product is worth.
- They want to be a *positive role model* and set a good example of healthy habits for friends and younger children and teens.

Light Consumption

There are people who do not abstain from alcohol use but drink very lightly. They may have a glass of wine with a meal, for example, or one drink at a social event where alcohol is being served. Light consumption is no more than one drink a day three or fewer times a week.

Moderate Consumption

The moderate drinker consumes no more than one or two drinks a day—one drink for a woman, two drinks for a man. Three drinks on any

---

There will come a time in your life when you will have to make a decision about consuming alcohol. When that time comes, the following points may help you with your decision.

- Drink only if it is *your* choice. *You* have responsibility for your own health, and you don't have to drink alcohol.

- If you choose to drink, drink moderately; *never* have more than three drinks in one drinking episode.

- Don't drink more than one alcoholic beverage per hour.

- Don't engage in "drinking games" or drinking challenges.

- Consider drinking nonalcoholic "look-alikes." It helps keep "alcohol pushers" away.

- Be aware of drinking roles. If you go to a party and choose to be the designated driver, remember you have the responsibility to be the designated nondrinker. Remember that not being the designated driver does not mean you should be the designated drunk.

- Always drink responsibly.

Tips for responsible drinking

single occasion represent the upper limit of moderate alcohol consumption. It is important to remember that both the number of drinks and their distribution over time are important in defining moderate consumption. For example, people who do not drink all week so they can have more than three drinks per episode would *not* qualify as moderate drinkers.

Alcohol Abuse

Alcohol abuse occurs if the upper limit of moderate consumption is exceeded during any single drinking episode. Drinking beyond this limit on a continual basis can lead to medical (liver damage and accidents) and social (drinking-and-driving offenses, public intoxication, abuse) problems.

Binge Drinking

A significant drinking problem is the practice of **binge drinking**. Binge drinkers consume five or more drinks in any single drinking episode. Although these drinkers don't drink every day, when they do drink, they drink to excess. Approximately 5 million teens engage in binge drinking each year in the United States. Many binge drinkers start at about age 13. Binge drinking behavior increases during the teen years and then begins to decrease toward the mid-twenties.

The most serious consequence of binge drinking is **alcohol poisoning**. Alcohol poisoning is a severe and potentially fatal overdose of alcohol. If too much alcohol is consumed over a short period of time, the depressing nature of alcohol deprives the brain of oxygen. Signs of alcohol poisoning include:

- Vomiting
- Unconsciousness
- Breathing slowly (fewer than eight breaths a minute or 10 or more seconds between two breaths)
- Pale, cold, clammy skin

A person showing any of these signs needs immediate medical help because these are indications that a dangerous level of alcohol is in the bloodstream. A common misconception is that vomiting means the body has rid itself of alcohol. Vomiting is actually a sign that an overdose of alcohol has entered the bloodstream. Anyone vomiting or showing any of the other symptoms of alcohol poisoning should not be left to "sleep it off." Nor should other attempts, such as giving the person coffee or a cold shower, be made to help the person sober up. Call 911 and request medical attention.

Binge drinking leads to other problems in addition to poisoning the body. Possible consequences of binge drinking include causing automobile accidents, physically or sexually assaulting other people, and damaging property.

binge drinking

drinking that consists of five or more alcoholic drinks in a row for males and four or more for females

alcohol poisoning

overdose of alcohol that can lead to death

What's News?

Research is beginning to suggest that heavy alcohol use by teenagers contributes to brain damage. Three studies indicate that binge drinking may contribute to impaired memory, sluggish recall, and poor verbal skills. These problems were magnified in subjects who also consumed illegal drugs.

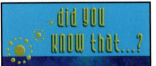

did you know that...?

There are many types of alcoholics. A common belief is that alcoholics are people who are drunk all the time or who physically abuse family members. But there are alcoholics who hold a steady job and others who don't drink often but occasionally drink themselves into unconsciousness. These individuals are known as **functional alcoholics**.

functional alcoholic

a person who frequently consumes alcohol to the point of drunkenness but who is able to carry out responsibilities of daily life

in-patient

referring to treatment programs that take place while the patient stays in a hospital or other health care setting

out-patient

referring to treatment programs given to patients who do not stay in a health care setting

Alcoholism

If you were asked to define the word *alcoholism*, what would you say? If you have trouble answering, you aren't alone. In fact, health professionals have many definitions for alcoholism. Simply put, alcoholism is a level of alcohol consumption marked by continued alcohol abuse. At exactly what point abuse turns to alcoholism is not easy to explain, but the National Institute on Alcohol and Alcoholism describes alcoholism as a disease with four main characteristics:

- A craving to drink alcohol
- The inability to control drinking behavior once it begins
- Withdrawal symptoms (nausea, anxiety) after drinking stops
- Tolerance, which means have having to drink more and more in order to get "high"

Currently, about 1 of every 14 adults, or about 14 million Americans, is an alcohol abuser or an alcoholic.

Causes of Alcoholism. It appears that personality, social, and genetic factors all contribute to the development of alcoholism, with estimates that almost 60% of the risk for developing alcoholism is genetic. This does not mean that alcoholism is inherited; it means that genes play a role in how an individual responds to alcohol. Anyone who has a family member who is an alcoholic would be well advised to avoid alcohol use altogether.

Treatment of Alcoholism. Almost 700,000 people in the United States receive treatment for alcoholism. Just as there are various forms of alcoholism and causes of alcoholism, there are various ways that alcoholism can be treated. The first step in all treatment programs is to separate the patient from alcohol and rid the system of the physical need for it. In a hospital treatment, this step can be done on either an **in-patient** or an **out-patient** basis. Counseling is another aspect of treatment. Alcoholics Anonymous is a support program that helps alcoholics remain abstinent.

Prevention of Alcoholism. The best way to prevent alcoholism is to avoid using alcohol. After all, individuals cannot get addicted to a drug

real teens

Mya is worried about her friend Dana. Mya suspects that Dana has developed a dependence on alcohol. She certainly has a greater interest in drinking than all the other friends Mya has. Mya has observed Dana's change over the past four months. Dana never had a lot of interest in drinking alcohol until last summer, when she visited her cousin in another state. Now she seems more interested in drinking than sharing time with her friends. Mya made a list of the drinking behaviors she sees in Dana:

1. She drinks a lot and very often—not just at parties on the weekend.
2. She does not tell the truth about how much she drinks.
3. She will hide liquor in her room and drink by herself when she listens to music.
4. She often chooses to stay home and "listen to her music" instead of going out with her friends.

Mya has decided to search the Web to find out if these behaviors are related to a teen drinking problem. Mya believes they are, but she wants to learn more, and she wants to find out what she can do to help her friend.

they don't use. Abstinence is especially important for teens who have relatives with drinking problems. Someday, there may be a simple blood test to identify genetic predisposition for alcoholism. This type of screening could be done on infants and the information used to counsel the child to avoid alcohol as an adult. The second best preventive measure is to provide information about alcohol-related problems so that abstinence or responsible-use patterns can be incorporated into personal wellness plans.

EFFECTS OF ALCOHOL CONSUMPTION ON HEALTH

As a chemical compound and a drug, alcohol has an effect on body tissues, especially the brain and the rest of the central nervous system. The immediate effects of alcohol are dose related, meaning that the effects are greater at higher doses and lesser at lower doses.

Alcohol Metabolism

Metabolism is the process of converting food substances into energy for use by the body. Alcohol absorption begins as soon as it reaches the stomach, although most of the absorption actually takes place in the small intestine. It is here that alcohol enters the bloodstream and

metabolism

the process of converting food substances into energy for the body

What's News?

Scientists continue to study biological conditions in individuals that can predict a predisposition for alcoholism. In one study of adolescent boys, a particular brain wave exhibited by sons of alcoholics as a response to a stimulus predicted alcoholism and drug addiction.

enzyme

a complex protein substance in the body that helps create chemical reactions

alcohol dehydrogenase

an enzyme in the liver responsible for alcohol metabolism

passes through the liver, where it is metabolized by an **enzyme**, **alcohol dehydrogenase** (ADH). The process of metabolism produces carbon dioxide and water as end products as alcohol is metabolically removed from the body. If it were not removed, it would create a toxic environment for the body's tissues and organs, and as the alcohol level builds up, it can lead to death.

Individuals respond differently in the way they metabolize alcohol. The rate of metabolism is fixed, according to the drinker's genetic makeup, at about one alcoholic beverage per hour. Because alcohol is absorbed in the stomach and small intestine at a rate much faster than the rate of metabolism, some alcohol will circulate in the blood and affect the nervous system. This effect is what gives the drinker a sedated feeling. If a drinker consumes more than one drink per hour, the amount of alcohol that is not metabolized raises the level of alcohol in the blood and also the magnitude of the sedating effect. Too much alcohol consumed in a short period of time can lead to alcohol poisoning.

Nothing can increase the rate of alcohol metabolism and reduce drunkenness. Some people believe that exercising ("Let them walk it off"), drinking lots of coffee, or taking a cold shower will sober up a drunk. None of these techniques work. The best way to avoid drunkenness is to not drink too much in the first place.

Body Structures Affected by Alcohol

Alcohol circulating in the bloodstream affects a number of body structures. It slows down the brain and nerve activity. Muscular coordination is affected; reaction time is increased; speech is slurred; and concentration and decision making are impaired. People under the influence of alcohol tend to do unreasonable things they probably wouldn't do otherwise.

Alcohol's effects on the circulatory system are reportedly both good and bad. The type of effect seems to be related to the amount of alcohol consumed. Alcohol causes the blood vessels in the circulatory system to dilate (widen), resulting in the skin's feeling warm. A common belief is that alcohol is good for warming you up in cold weather. Actually, just the opposite is true. Dilation of the blood vessels causes

❧ teen forum ❧

Should Physicians Encourage Their Patients to Consume Alcohol to Protect Their Health?

Medical evidence appears to support the notion that light to moderate alcohol consumption can be good for one's health. On the other hand, it is also clear that people who consume alcohol beyond moderate levels may experience negative health effects.

- What is your view on this practice?
- If you were a physician, would you counsel patients to consume alcohol? Explain the reasons for your opinion.

the body to *lose* heat, so drinking alcohol in cold weather increases the risk of **hypothermia**, a condition that can be life threatening.

One of alcohol's beneficial effects on the circulatory system is its influence on fat deposits in the bloodstream. Evidence indicates that *light* to *moderate* alcohol use can reduce these fat deposits, thus decreasing the risk of heart disease. (More information about heart disease is presented in Chapter 24.) On the other hand, high doses of alcohol negatively affect the circulatory system by contributing to an enlarged and weakened heart muscle. This condition is known as **cardiomyopathy**. Consistently high alcohol consumption also contributes to high blood pressure, a risk for cardiovascular disease.

Alcohol has no beneficial effects on the digestive system. In the short term, it disrupts the absorption of nutrients. In the long term, heavy alcohol use can contribute to the formation of ulcers in the stomach and cancers of the mouth, esophagus, stomach, and liver. Individuals who both drink and smoke increase their risk for mouth and throat cancers.

hypothermia

loss of body heat due to exposure to extreme cold

cardiomyopathy

damage to the heart muscle caused by long-term alcohol abuse

did you know that...?

Women are more susceptible to alcohol-caused cardiomyopathy than men. In fact, it appears that women's susceptibility occurs with less alcohol consumption than men's.

What's News?

A 12-year study of 38,077 male health professionals found that men who drank approximately one alcoholic drink three or more days a week had a reduced risk of heart attack compared with men who drank less frequently.

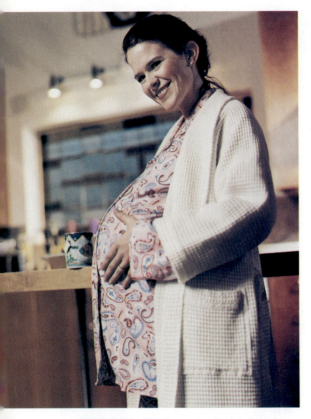

A good mother begins caring for her baby long before it is born.

FETAL ALCOHOL SYNDROME

Fetal alcohol syndrome (FAS) is a condition that can cause birth defects in babies born to women who drink alcohol during their pregnancy. It is estimated that each year there are as many as 12,000 cases of FAS and as many as 48,000 cases of a milder form of the syndrome. The effects on the child are dose related, meaning that the more the mother drinks, the more serious the effects. Of all forms of birth defects, FAS is the easiest to prevent. In fact, it is 100% preventable because the syndrome never appears in babies born to women who do not drink during their pregnancy.

The birth defects associated with FAS can affect the baby in three ways:

- *How a child looks.* Examples of FAS characteristics include low weight at birth, small head circumference, and abnormalities of the face such as flattened cheekbones and small eye openings.
- *How a child's brain and nervous system develop.* The child may have learning difficulties or epilepsy, a disease characterized by abnormal electrical activity in the brain.
- *How a child grows and develops.* The child doesn't develop at the same rate as other children. There may be social withdrawal, poor coordination, lack of imagination, and poor social skills.

ALCOHOL AND THE LAW

Alcohol use is controlled by laws and regulations because of its potential to harm both the individual who drinks and others in the community. It is a drug with drug-related problems, such as the potential for addiction, overdose, and automobile accidents.

Legal Drinking Ages

At one time, alcohol use by children was not controlled. When the medical and legal community determined that many young people could not handle alcohol responsibly, they passed laws regulating the age at which a person can drink legally. In most states it was age 21, but in the 1970s, many states lowered the legal drinking age to 18. Many problems with teen drinking developed after this change, so in 1984, states were encouraged to return the legal drinking age to 21. Taking this action has saved many lives: in 1987, there were 1,017 fewer alcohol-related highway deaths among those in the 18–20 age group. A large amount of research data supports having the legal drinking age set at 21. Here are some facts:

- In states with the higher drinking age, 16–21 year olds drink less frequently than those in the states with a lower drinking age.

- The *1978 National Study of Adolescent Drinking Behavior* reported that tenth to twelfth graders in states with lower drinking ages drank significantly more, were less likely to abstain from alcohol, and were drunk more often than tenth to twelfth graders in states with a drinking age of 21.

- Young people who begin drinking before age 15 are four times more likely to develop dependence on alcohol than those who begin drinking at age 21.

Blood Alcohol Concentration

When alcohol enters the body, it is quickly absorbed into the bloodstream. The resulting level of alcohol in the blood is known as the **blood alcohol concentration** (BAC). Sometimes the BAC is expressed as BAL (blood alcohol level) or blood alcohol percentage. The level of BAC reached depends on four conditions:

1. *Body size.* A large person has a greater volume of blood and water in which to disperse the alcohol.

2. *Amount of body fat.* Alcohol does not penetrate fat tissue well.

3. *Amount of food in the stomach.* Food in the stomach, especially fats and starches, slows alcohol absorption.

4. *Amount of alcohol consumed in a particular time frame.* The longer it takes an individual to consume the alcohol, the less likely the BAC level will rise because the body will have time to metabolize the alcohol.

As BAC increases, so does alcohol's sedating effect on the body. The same number of drinks will result in different BAC levels for men and women, but the same BAC level will produce the same types of effects on the nervous systems of both sexes. For example:

- At a BAC of 0.02, light to moderate drinkers begin to feel some effects.

- At a BAC of 0.08, there is definite impairment of muscle coordination and driving skills; this is the level at which intoxication is legally defined. The person may have difficulty balancing and will probably have slurred speech.

- At a BAC of 0.12, vomiting usually occurs.

- At a BAC of 0.40, most people lose consciousness; some die.

- At a BAC of 0.50 (that's one-half of 1%!), death usually occurs.

Tables 21-1 and 21-2 show the effects and legal implications of various alcohol levels on men and women.

Because of all the research on the effects of BAC on behavior, judgment, and driving skill, by 2002, 33 states had enacted laws that established the legal limit for alcohol intoxication at 0.08. The BAC level is even lower (0.02 or less) for *teens* in 38 states. Teenage drivers exhibiting that level of intoxication may lose their driver's license for a year. Teens not possessing a driver's license who are caught using alcohol while driving have their application for a driver's license suspended for a year.

blood alcohol concentration
the percent of ethyl alcohol present in the bloodstream after drinking alcoholic beverages

Table 21-1   Blood Alcohol Levels for Men

Number of Drinks*	Approximate Blood Alcohol Concentration (Percent)								Effect
Body weight (pounds)	100	120	140	160	180	200	220	240	
1	0.04	0.03	0.03	0.02	0.02	0.02	0.02	0.02	Alcohol effect
2	0.08	0.06	0.05	0.05	0.04	0.04	0.03	0.03	Driving skills affected
3	0.11	0.09	0.08	0.07	0.06	0.06	0.05	0.05	
4	0.15	0.12	0.11	0.09	0.08	0.08	0.07	0.06	
5	0.19	0.16	0.13	0.12	0.11	0.09	0.09	0.08	Legally intoxicated
6	0.23	0.19	0.16	0.14	0.13	0.11	0.10	0.09	
7	0.26	0.22	0.19	0.16	0.15	0.13	0.12	0.11	
8	0.30	0.25	0.21	0.19	0.17	0.15	0.14	0.13	
9	0.34	0.28	0.24	0.21	0.19	0.17	0.15	0.14	Criminal penalties
10	0.38	0.31	0.27	0.23	0.21	0.19	0.17	0.16	

*One drink = 1.25 oz. of 80-proof liquor, 12 oz. of beer, 5 oz. of wine.
Note: Subtract 0.01% for each 45 minutes of drinking.

Table 21-2   Blood Alcohol Levels for Women

Number of Drinks*	Approximate Blood Alcohol Concentration (Percent)								Effect
Body weight (pounds)	90	100	120	140	160	180	200	220	
1	0.05	0.05	0.04	0.03	0.03	0.02	0.02	0.02	Alcohol effect
2	0.10	0.09	0.08	0.07	0.06	0.05	0.05	0.04	Driving skills affected
3	0.15	0.14	0.11	0.10	0.09	0.08	0.07	0.06	
4	0.20	0.18	0.15	0.13	0.11	0.10	0.09	0.08	
5	0.25	0.23	0.19	0.16	0.14	0.13	0.11	0.10	
6	0.30	0.27	0.23	0.19	0.17	0.15	0.14	0.12	Legally intoxicated
7	0.35	0.32	0.27	0.23	0.20	0.18	0.16	0.14	
8	0.40	0.36	0.30	0.26	0.23	0.20	0.18	0.17	
9	0.45	0.41	0.34	0.29	0.26	0.23	0.20	0.19	Criminal penalties
10	0.51	0.45	0.38	0.32	0.28	0.25	0.23	0.21	

*One drink = 1.25 oz. of 80-proof liquor, 12 oz. of beer, 5 oz. of wine.
Note: Subtract 0.01% for each 45 minutes of drinking.

Teen Drinking

Teen drinking can result in actions that will negatively affect teens and their families for the rest of their lives. The following facts illustrate some of these problems:

- For the three leading causes of death for teenagers—motor vehicle accidents, homicides, and suicides—alcohol use is strongly implicated.
- In 1999, 21% of drivers in the 15- to 20-year-old age group who were killed in vehicle crashes were intoxicated.
- Researchers report that alcohol use is implicated in one-third to two-thirds of the sexual assault and acquaintance or "date rape" cases reported by teens and college students.

Despite the fact that it is illegal for teenagers in the United States to purchase or consume alcohol, some teens continue to report using alcohol. There are a number of national studies of adolescent alcohol use. The three major studies are listed below with the findings related to alcohol use.

1. *2002 Monitoring the Future Study*
   - Between 2001 and 2002, alcohol consumption declined significantly for the eighth and tenth graders studied.
   - The rate of binge drinking among tenth graders declined between 2001 and 2002.

2. *2001 National Household Survey on Drug Abuse*
   - Among teens surveyed, ages 12–17, an estimated 17.3% used alcohol in the month prior to the survey interview.
   - The highest prevalence of both binge and heavy drinking was for young adults aged 18–25, with the peak rate occurring at age 21.
   - Twenty-nine percent of persons age 12–20 reported drinking alcohol in the month prior to the survey interview.
   - Underage alcohol use rates were relatively similar for all areas surveyed—cities, towns, and rural areas (about 28%).

3. *Youth Risk Behavior Surveillance–2001*
   - Forty-seven percent of the students surveyed indicated they had had at least one alcoholic beverage within 30 days of taking the survey.
   - Twenty-nine percent of the students reported consuming at least five alcoholic drinks at least one time within 30 days prior to taking this survey.
   - Nationwide, 13.3% of the high school students surveyed reported that they had driven an automobile after consuming alcohol.

The good news from these reports is that a decreasing number of students are drinking alcohol and that they are, as a whole, drinking

take it on home

Have a conversation with your family about drinking alcohol. Find out if the adult members of your family drink alcohol. If they do, ask what it is about drinking that appeals to them. If they don't drink, ask about their reasons for not doing so. Express your views on alcohol. What kind of response do you get? Do your family's views and attitudes match yours? Write up your findings and include them in your Health Folio.

less. The bad news is that there are high school students in the United States who drink alcohol, even though it is illegal for them to do so. Even more serious, some teens operate automobiles after drinking. And almost one-third of high school students have participated in binge drinking behaviors, despite the extreme risks involved.

BUILDING YOUR Wellness Plan

Alcohol consumption is a behavior for adults and a matter of personal preference. Not everyone needs to consume alcohol. Adults who choose to consume alcohol should drink responsibly. Your own health and the well-being of others are important considerations in making choices about drinking. Now is the time for you to begin making your decisions about alcohol's role in your life. The wellness plan you develop now will serve you in the future. Consider the following suggestions to include as part of your wellness plan.

- Develop a list of strategies you might use to guide your drinking (or nondrinking) behavior.
- Create a plan that would limit alcohol consumption during pregnancy.
- Develop a set of resources to help someone who has a drinking problem.

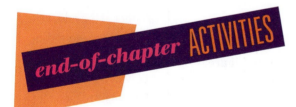

end-of-chapter ACTIVITIES

Weblinks

Facts for Teens about Drinking

Alcoholics Anonymous: **http://www.alcoholics-anonymous.org** (find "message to teenagers")

American Academy of Family Physicians: **http://familydoctor.org/handouts/273.html**

Help for Teens Affected by Someone's Alcohol Problem

Alateen: **http://www.al-anon.alateen.org** (click the Alateen link)

Short-Answer Questions

1. Name the chemical process that produces alcohol.
2. What kind of drug is alcohol?
3. Name the controlling factor in alcohol metabolism.
4. How many drinks would be the upper limit of moderate alcohol consumption for males and females?
5. What is the legal limit of alcohol intoxication?

Discussion Questions

1. Discuss why alcohol consumption is not a good idea for teenagers.
2. List and explain the circumstances that affect the blood alcohol concentration while consuming alcohol.
3. Describe behaviors that are examples of responsible alcohol use.
4. Discuss the significance of binge drinking among teenage drinkers.
5. Summarize the research related to teen drinking patterns.

Chapter Vocabulary

Using a separate sheet of paper, list and define the following terms:

alcohol dehydrogenase

alcohol poisoning

binge drinking

blood alcohol concentration

cardiomyopathy

fermentation

fetal alcohol syndrome

hypothermia

proof

withdrawal

Application Activities

Language Arts Connection

Advice columnists are people who write responses to letters from people asking for help with their problems. Imagine you are an advice columnist. Write replies to the following.

1. My friend went to a party last weekend. Some kids brought alcohol and offered her some, and she tried it. I told her it was a bad idea. Should I leave her alone or try to convince her not to do it again? What can I say to her?
2. I went to the beach with friends last week. One guy brought beer, and everyone was drinking except me. The ride home scared me because the driver was feeling the beer. I am 15 and can't drive. What should I do the next time this happens?

Math Connection

An average high school male has 5 quarts of blood in his body; an average high school female has 4 quarts. Calculate the blood alcohol levels if they each had 6 ounces of alcohol in their bloodstream. Do the same for 9 ounces and 12 ounces.

Social Studies Connection

Search the Web for your state's traffic safety Web site. Find out what your state laws are for underage drinking and driving. Prepare a report of your findings.

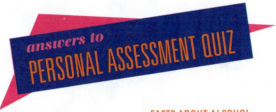

answers to
PERSONAL ASSESSMENT QUIZ

personal assessment: FACTS ABOUT ALCOHOL

1. False. Alcohol itself is a source of calories. Other calories come from the products that are mixed with the alcohol.
2. True
3. True
4. False. Nothing can cause a person to sober up faster than the person's own body processes.
5. True
6. False. Any alcoholic beverage can contribute to alcoholism.
7. False. Ninety percent of the alcohol is absorbed through the small intestine.
8. True

chapter 22

Drug Abuse

All the kids at school liked Mark. He had the good looks of a pop star, was on the high school baseball team, and had a great girlfriend, Jane. But trouble began at the end of his sophomore year, when he got addicted to drugs. It started when he tried alcohol, then marijuana, and he eventually experimented with acid. At first, his drug use was experimental, but soon he was doing drugs all the time and lost interest in many other things that really mattered in his life. Mark's grades started to slip; he lost his starting position on the baseball team; Jane broke off their relationship; and kids at school began to avoid him. His mother didn't notice the changes that were taking place because she was working long hours to support him and his younger sister. Mark finally ended up in jail for a traffic violation. His former baseball coach, Mr. Novak, helped him get out of jail and offered to help him get cleaned up. The coach organized a group of Mark's friends to help and encouraged him to start meeting with the school counselor. This team approach has worked for Mark. He is now surrounded by people who really care about him; his grades are coming back; and he will be graduating this year. Although Mark feels as if he lost a year of his life while he was on drugs, he is rebuilding his life and is enthusiastic about the future.

chapter OBJECTIVES

When you finish this chapter, you should be able to:

- Identify the risks and dangers associated with drug abuse.
- Discuss current trends of teen drug abuse.
- Explain the difference between over-the-counter, prescription, and illicit drugs.
- State common reasons why young people abuse drugs.
- List and describe classifications of abused drugs.

key TERMS

amphetamines
anabolic steroids
drug abuse
drug dependence
flashback
medicine
opium
over-the-counter medications
tolerance
withdrawal

Introduction

Drug abuse is a significant social problem in the United States. Drug abuse has been around since the late 1800s. In 1875, the government outlawed opium dens, where people gathered to smoke opium. In 1937, marijuana was declared illegal. The problem became magnified when drugs moved from dark alleys and crime-ridden areas into ordinary homes throughout the country. Increasing numbers of otherwise good kids turned to drugs "for fun" and found themselves in a downward spiral of dependency. Parents, teachers, politicians, religious leaders, law enforcement personnel, and the health care community became concerned about this growing problem when it began to hit middle-class families in the 1960s. In 1981, President Reagan declared the war on drugs, and his wife, Nancy, popularized the phrase "Just say no." The United States launched its "war against drugs" to dissuade teens and young adults from engaging in drug abuse. It was not that adults didn't want teens to have fun; they were concerned about teens engaging in behaviors that had serious consequences.

Many teens realize the dangers associated with drug use. In fact, 71% of teens believe that alcohol and drug use is the most serious issue facing them today, and most don't use illegal drugs. This chapter provides information to support the decision not to try drugs. It explains the dangers of "just experimenting" and how to avoid being vulnerable when drugs are offered by "friends."

personal assessment: DRUG FACTS

Use a separate sheet of paper to record your responses to the following statements. Decide whether each is true or false. Keep the sheet with your wellness plan. Check your responses at the end of the chapter.

1. Most teens do not use drugs.

2. Teens who learn about the risks of drugs from their parents are half as likely to use drugs as are teens who hear nothing from their parents.

3. The average age for starting drug use in the United States is 18.

4. A person cannot get addicted to marijuana.

5. Most prison inmates in the United States have used drugs.

6. Drug use among U.S. teens is on the decline.

THE IMPORTANCE OF MEDICINES

A **medicine** is any substance used to treat an ailment or illness. Medicines have been used by people for centuries. The ancient Greek physician Hippocrates prescribed a form of aspirin to control the pain of childbirth. More than 30% of all medicines used today come from natural products.

Medicines of all types are available in one of two forms. **Prescription medicines**, also called drugs, must be prescribed by a trained physician to ensure they fit the medical condition for which they are being taken. **Over-the-counter medications** do not require a doctor's prescription but should always be used according to the directions on the label.

Medical Uses of Drugs

Scientists have developed and tested drugs and medicines to determine the most effective dose and means of getting them to the troubled area of your body as quickly and safely as possible. Drugs are formulated to be effective and safe for children, adults, and the elderly. Each of these three age groups will require a different amount of a drug to produce a safe effect. Drugs come in different forms, depending on the purpose of the medication. Have you ever wondered why some drugs come in tablets and others in capsules? The following list explains different forms in which medications are available:

- *Tablet.* Tablets are designed to dissolve in the stomach so the medicine can be absorbed into the bloodstream. Aspirin is an example.

- *Capsule.* Medicines in capsule form are designed to be absorbed in the small intestine rather than in the stomach, where the medicine would be made ineffective by the stomach's strong acids.

---

medicine

a chemical substance used to treat an ailment or illness

prescription medicines

medicines that must be prescribed by a trained physician to ensure they fit the medical condition for which they are being taken

over-the-counter medications

medicines that do not require a doctor's prescription

Removing medicine from a capsule before taking it can decrease its effectiveness. Some cold medications come in capsule form.

- *Ointment or cream.* Creams and ointments are used to treat skin conditions on which they can be directly applied. Anti-itch and some antibiotic medications are available in this form.

- *Aerosol.* Aerosol sprays are used to administer medication into the nose or throat. Nasal sprays are often used to relieve the congestion of a cold.

- *Injection.* Some medicines are injected just under the skin to be absorbed by the bloodstream; others are injected directly into a vein so they can act very quickly; still others are injected into muscle tissue. Some diabetics take a daily injection of insulin.

It is extremely important to read label directions carefully, especially with over-the-counter medications, to make sure the medicine is used correctly. When medicines are prescribed, patients should discuss their proper use with their pharmacist or doctor. Although medicines are safe and effective if used correctly, there can be harmful consequences if they are misused. For example, not taking the entire prescription of antibiotic medication for an infection can result in a return of the infection. People's failure to take the entire prescription of antibiotic is also one reason for the development of bacteria that are resistant to antibiotics, making it very difficult to treat future infections. Patients should also be aware of the possible side effects of medications they are taking and which ones are serious and require contacting the physician. Doctors will also monitor all drugs a patient uses in order to avoid problems caused by medication interactions.

Misuses of Medicines

Drugs and medicines should be used only according to directions or as prescribed. They should be destroyed when they are no longer needed or if they have passed their expiration date. All drugs, including over-the-counter drugs, should be kept away from children and discarded when they expire. Occasionally, someone may misuse prescription drugs. A prescription drug is considered to be *misused* if it is taken in any of the following ways:

- Taking more of a drug than has been prescribed or continuing to use it when a qualified health care provider indicates it is no longer needed

- Using a drug for a medical condition other than that for which it was intended

- Using a medication that is prescribed for someone else

Prescription drug abuse occurs when a prescription medicine is used for something other than the drug's intended purpose. The most commonly abused forms of prescription drugs are painkillers and mood suppressants.

prescription drug abuse

the use of a medical drug product for nonmedical reasons

DRUG ABUSE

Drug abuse is the use of chemical substances to achieve an abnormal mental state. These chemical substances can be drugs that have legitimate medical value (amphetamines, sedatives, morphine), substances that have no or limited medical value (alcohol, LSD, heroin, PCP), or chemicals designed for other purposes (aerosol paint). Misusing substances in this way is also called illicit drug use because it is against the law.

Social Costs of Drug Abuse

There are many costs and harmful consequences associated with drug abuse. The total economic cost of alcohol and drug abuse in the United States in 1992 was estimated at $102 billion. In 1998, the figure rose to $142 billion. Almost $90 million of this amount was crime-related costs, including crime-victim health care expenses, work productivity loss, and costs associated with the criminal justice system. Other costs include medical costs of abusers themselves and the repair of damaged property.

Drug abuse also contributes to poverty, dysfunctional neighborhoods, homelessness, gang activities, drug trafficking, and the disruption of family systems. Drug users are often involved in domestic violence and divorce.

Human Costs of Drug Abuse

Drug abusers have a shorter life expectancy than do people who don't abuse drugs. Approximately 20,000 people die every year from causes related to illicit drug use. Drug abusers expose themselves to the risks of overdose, poisoning, liver damage, and accidental death. Nonphysical consequences include job loss, ended friendships, and legal punishment such as imprisonment.

The risks and consequences of various drugs are presented in the following sections. Although there are many physical and psychological problems related to drug abuse, the real tragedy lies in the users' loss of personal control and failure to achieve life goals. The preoccupation with drug use takes young people away from the really important task of preparing for their adult life. Most drug abusers end up in one of three ways:

1. They outgrow or overcome their need for drugs and get on with their lives.
2. They are sent to jail.
3. They die while using drugs (overdose, accidents, homicide).

Drug Abuse among Teens

Drug use among our nation's youth is of great concern to parents and educators because these adults care about teens and don't want to see

teen forum

Drug Testing

Drug abuse is of such concern that some employers use drug testing to ensure that their employees are not drug users. Organizations such as airlines, hospitals, and law enforcement agencies, where drug use by employees puts the public at risk, have adopted this strategy. Other companies may choose to conduct drug testing to avoid having employees with drug problems. Imagine that you are applying for a job, and the employer asks you to submit to a drug test.

- How would you feel about being asked to take such a test in order to get the job?
- Should companies be permitted to make drug screening a condition for employment?

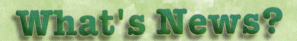

A 22-year study tracked almost 750 randomly selected young people from adolescence through their late twenties. Findings from the study reveal that when the subjects reached their late twenties, 8.3% had developed a major depressive disorder, 5.2% were dependent on alcohol, and 6% had a substance abuse disorder.

them negatively affecting their growth and development. Researchers have been studying teen drug use for almost 30 years. The current trend shows that drug use among young people is holding steady or declining slightly, depending on the type of drug.

The *Monitoring the Future* study began in 1975 to research drug use trends among teens in the United States. In 2002, more than 43,000 students in grades 8, 10, and 12 were surveyed. Researchers asked questions about drug use during the 30 days prior to the survey, the past year, and the entire lifetime. This is what the *2002 Monitoring the Future* study found about teen drug use:

- For the sixth straight year, drug use stayed the same or went down.
- Teens overwhelmingly disapprove of people who use drugs.
- Teens believe that people who use drugs, alcohol, and tobacco on a regular basis are at risk for harming themselves.
- Teens strongly disapproved of the drug ecstasy. This trend was significant for eighth, tenth, and twelfth graders.

It appears that, although most teens don't approve of drug use, some young people do use illicit drugs, including alcohol and tobacco.

Reasons Why People Abuse Drugs

People start using drugs for a variety of reasons, which vary from drug to drug. Our culture places heavy emphasis on the use of drugs to cure all sorts of problems, both physical and mental. Have you noticed the number of television advertisements for prescription drugs? Illicit drug use is influenced by our cultural belief that all physical ailments can be corrected with medicinal drugs. As a result, some young people see drug use as a type of "medication" for the normal growth and development "pains" they have to go through.

Here are some other reasons for drug use uncovered by researchers:

- *Curiosity.* People hear a lot about drugs. Some want to try them just to see what they are like. This type of experiment involves a great deal of risk, however, because all addicts began by "just trying" drugs. There is no way to know in advance if you are highly susceptible to drug addiction. In one case, a parent reported that her son tried alcohol for the first time on his sixteenth birthday and immediately became an alcoholic. It wasn't until the young man reached age 24 that he was able to free himself of the addiction. What do you think he might have accomplished during all those lost years?

- *Emotional pressures.* Some people use drugs in an attempt to ease emotional problems. Anger, stress, depression, rejection, and boredom are some of the feelings that people seek to relieve with a drug effect. This is a bad strategy because when the drugs are gone, the feelings are still there. Even worse, drug use just creates another set of problems.

- *Social pressures.* Many people who use drugs want to get others to use drugs with them. Every young person wants companionship. Those who choose to use drugs want others to be like them and may push drug use on other young people. Drug users who sell drugs also have an interest in getting others to use with them because new users can become customers and a source of more income.

- *Perception.* Some young people believe that "everyone else" is using drugs and they don't want to be left out. The truth is, most teens *don't* use drugs, as you saw in the statistics given earlier in this chapter.

- *Peer selection.* The Center for Substance Abuse Prevention has reported that lonely people sometimes begin drug use when approached by drug users who take advantage of them by offering friendship. Rather than being true friends, users most often are simply looking for others who will share their habit and, if they are also selling drugs, become their customers.

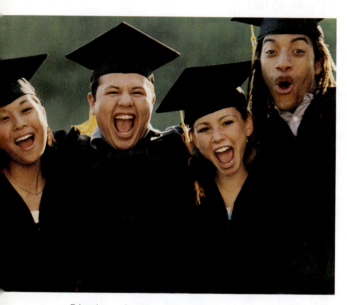

Friends are important to you and good for your life.

Drug Dependence

Drug dependence is the need for a drug because of mental or physical changes that make it difficult for users to control or stop their drug use. There are two types of drug dependence:

1. *Psychological dependence.* A drug is constantly on the user's mind, and he or she feels an overwhelming need to use the drug often. The drug becomes an important part of the user's daily activities.

drug dependence

a need for a drug that results in continuous use of the drug

2. *Physical dependence.* The user's body needs the drug in order to avoid the discomfort of withdrawal. Not all drugs produce physical dependence, but they may still be abused because of their perceived effects or as a result of psychological dependence.

Withdrawal

When individuals stop using drugs on which they have become dependent, they go through a process of withdrawal. **Withdrawal** involves feelings of discomfort that can be both mental and physical and range from mild to severe. The amount of discomfort varies according to the type of drug, the amount being used, and the length of time the drug has been used. Many long-term drug users are no longer seeking a high but are using drugs to avoid the discomfort of withdrawal. Withdrawal symptoms are listed in Figure 22-1. Severe cases of withdrawal require medical attention.

Tolerance

Tolerance is the physical adjustment of the body to a drug. It develops over time with regular drug use and results in the user needing increased doses of the drug to get the same effect. Eventually, the dosage becomes more than the body can handle, and the user becomes ill or dies. Not all drugs contribute to the tolerance effect. Table 22-1 lists drugs of abuse and the degree to which each drug produces dependence or tolerance.

Drugs That Are Abused

Most young people in the United States are not drug abusers. Research studies of teens who have used drugs give us a clear picture of the

> **withdrawal**
> feelings of discomfort that occur when the body is deprived of a drug to which it is addicted

> **tolerance**
> the physical adjustment to a drug that causes the user to require increased doses to feel the same effect

- Cold sweats
- Headaches
- Delusions
- Tremors
- Extreme restlessness and agitation
- Hallucinations
- Convulsions
- Nausea and vomiting
- Anxiety

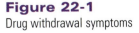

Figure 22-1
Drug withdrawal symptoms

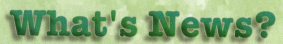

What's News?

Research is now pointing to the fact that drug tolerance may be a learned response. Scientists believe that if tolerance to a drug is something that is learned, addicts may be able to "unlearn" their tolerance and reduce their addiction.

Table 22-1 Dependence Potential of Abused Drugs

Drug	Psychological Dependence	Physical Dependence	Tolerance
Heroin	High	High	High
Barbiturates	Moderate	High	Moderate
Alcohol	Moderate	Moderate	Low
Amphetamines	Moderate	Maybe	High
Cocaine	High	Maybe	Low
LSD	Low	None	None
Marijuana	Low	None	Very low

kinds of drugs they used. The drugs discussed in this section include the ones reportedly used by teens who do use drugs. They appear in descending order, with the most widely used drug listed first. Figure 22-2 illustrates the degree of drug use among teens and adults studied in the National Household Study on Drug Abuse. Alcohol, the drug most abused by young adults, is not included here. It is discussed in Chapter 21.

Marijuana

Although no more than one-third of the students surveyed in the *2002 Monitoring the Future* study had used marijuana, it is the illegal drug most likely to be abused by teens. Marijuana has many names, including pot, grass, reefer, weed, herb, and Mary Jane. It is a mixture of the dried, shredded leaves, stems, seeds, and flowers of a variety of hemp plant, *Cannabis sativa*. The major active ingredient in marijuana is known chemically as delta-9-tetrahydrocannabinol (THC). It is THC that provides the mind-altering effect produced by the burnt marijuana.

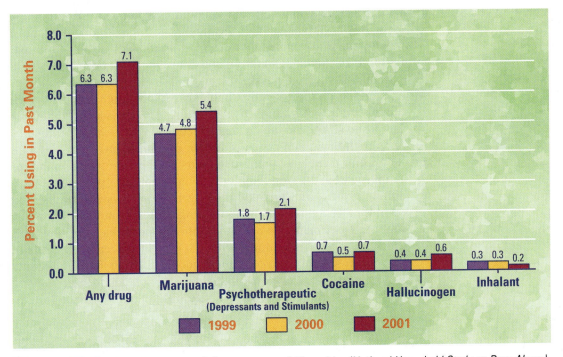

Figure 22-2 Illicit drug use trends by persons aged 12 or older *(National Household Study on Drug Abuse)*

When marijuana is smoked, it is inhaled into the lungs. From there, THC passes rapidly into the bloodstream, which carries the chemical to organs throughout the body, including the brain. The effects of marijuana on the brain can last for days or weeks after the immediate mind-altering effect wears off.

Scientists have researched the effects of marijuana use for more than 30 years. Their findings indicate there are both short-term and long-term problems associated with marijuana use.

Over the short term, marijuana can produce changes in the nervous system. These changes cause distorted perceptions, poor judgment, problems with memory and learning, difficulty thinking and problem solving, and loss of coordination. Marijuana also produces an increased heart rate.

Over the long term, marijuana smoke, just like smoke from cigarettes, harms the lungs. In fact, it is more harmful than tobacco smoke, for several reasons:

1. Marijuana is not grown under the same controls as tobacco. Growers may use pesticides that are not approved for normal agricultural use.

2. Marijuana smoke contains 50% to 70% more cancer-causing chemicals than tobacco smoke. The smoke causes production of an enzyme that accelerates cancer growth.

3. Marijuana smoke is generally inhaled more deeply into the lungs than tobacco smoke.

did you know that...?

An average marijuana cigarette today may contain 150 milligrams of THC. This is 10 times the amount of THC in the marijuana smoked in the 1960s. The amount of THC has increased because growers constantly attempt to "improve" their product, with genetic combinations and good farming techniques so it will sell better.

There is evidence that the chemicals found in marijuana smoke (specifically THC) weaken the body's ability to fight disease. In fact, marijuana smokers are ill more often than nonsmokers. Because THC is stored in the fat cells of the body, a person who uses marijuana will have a difficult time passing a required drug test.

Research indicates that babies born to women who use marijuana during their pregnancy display altered responses to visual stimuli, increased shakiness, and a high-pitched cry, which may indicate problems with brain and nervous system development.

Long-term marijuana use leads to dependence for many people. Withdrawal symptoms include cravings for the drug, irritability, difficulty sleeping, and anxiety. Long-term, heavy users are also likely to exhibit more aggression on psychological tests than are nonusers, with the worst performance occurring about one week after they last used the drug. These individuals will also exhibit a decreased motivation to do well in school or to look for a good job. High school students who smoke marijuana are less likely to graduate than their nonsmoking peers. They are also less likely to do well on standardized tests.

Hallucinogens

Hallucinogens, sometimes called psychodelics, are chemicals that alter how the brain perceives time, reality, and the environment. Users may believe they are hearing voices, seeing images, and feeling things that don't exist. Or they may think they are doing something for five minutes when it has actually been an hour.

Hallucinogenic drugs include LSD, PCP, mescaline, and psilocybin (a hallucinogenic mushroom). In the United States, it is illegal to use, possess, or manufacture hallucinogens.

When hallucinogenic drugs cause distortions, users sometimes engage in unusual, unexpected, or dangerous behaviors. There are tragic reports about the harm suffered. For example, a teen using LSD reportedly thought he could fly, jumped out a second-story window, and pierced his leg on an iron fence below. You may have heard about people having **flashbacks** after using drugs. This is one of the most profound side effects of hallucinogens. Flashbacks have been known to occur days, weeks, or even months after the user's original "trip." You can imagine what would happen if this were to occur while the user was driving a car or involved in some other activity that requires full attention.

The power and purity of hallucinogens vary because they have no standard dosage and are manufactured in uncontrolled and often unsanitary laboratories. As a result, users have no way of predicting what effects might occur, effects that can be as serious as causing the user to go into a coma.

The use of hallucinogens can change the emotions and cause confusion, disorientation, and feelings of suspicion. Evidence indicates that PCP use may also interfere with the hormones related to normal growth and with the learning process.

flashback

an unexpected hallucinogenic experience that occurs long after the effects of the drug have worn off

Depressants

Depressants are drugs that slow the function of the central nervous system. They have some medical value and are often used to induce sleep and relieve stress and anxiety. Examples of depressants include barbiturates such as Seconal, Nebutal, or Ambytal and tranquilizers such as Valium or Librium. The effects of depressants are similar to those of alcohol, and these drugs are referred to among drug users as "downers." Most misused depressants are stolen from medical supply sources. Very few are manufactured in home laboratories.

Small amounts of depressants can relax muscles and produce a state of calmness; larger doses can cause slurred speech, staggering, and altered perception. Very large doses can lead to respiratory depression, coma, and death. When depressants and alcohol are combined, there is a multiplying effect that increases the health risks.

The regular use of depressants over time can result in physical and psychological dependence. Withdrawal symptoms range from mild anxiety to death. Babies born to mothers who abuse depressants can be physically dependent on the drugs and experience withdrawal symptoms after birth. Prolonged depressant use has a tendency to cause mental health problems and is often associated with suicide.

Stimulants

Stimulants comprise several groups of drugs that affect the nervous system by increasing alertness and physical activity. Their use results in rapid heart rate, high blood pressure, dilated pupils, and decreased appetite. The main groups of stimulants are amphetamines (pharmaceutical stimulants), street drugs such as MDMA (ecstasy), and cocaine. Stimulants act on the body just the opposite as depressants.

Amphetamines. **Amphetamines** are powerful stimulant drugs such as Desoxyn, Dexidrine, and Ritalin that increase activity in the central nervous system. Their effect is similar to that of the body's adrenaline. Although amphetamines mimic the effects of adrenaline, they affect the body for a much longer period of time. Some people use amphetamines to counter the effects of sleeping pills, thus creating an unhealthy "roller coaster effect."

Amphetamine users may feel a temporary boost in self-confidence and power, but abuse of the drug can cause delusions, hallucinations, and feelings of paranoia. These feelings, in turn, can then lead to bizarre and even violent behavior. Amphetamines, more than any other illegal drug, are associated with violence and antisocial behavior. The negative feelings associated with amphetamine abuse often disappear when the drug is no longer taken.

Amphetamines have the potential to be psychologically addictive because users want to avoid the depressed feeling often experienced when the drug's effect wears off. This dependence can cause the user

take it on home

Talk with your family about drug use. Ask the adults in your family about the extent of drug use around them when they were teens. See if they think things are different now. Compare and discuss the differences between then and what you observe now. Write a report of your discussion and keep it in your Health Folio.

amphetamines

powerful stimulant medications that are sometimes abused to create an energetic euphoria (exaggerated feelings of well-being)

What's News?

A dangerous drug known as PMA (para-methoxyamphetamine) is being sold on the streets as MDMA (ecstasy), and dosages of ecstasy that contain PMA are also being sold.

The danger of PMA is that it is about 20 times stronger than Ecstacy. PMA can cause cardiac arrest, breathing problems, coma, and death.

to turn to stronger stimulants, such as cocaine, or to larger doses of amphetamines to maintain a "high."

Ecstasy. Ecstasy is the street name for a drug with the chemical name of 3, 4-methylenedioxymethamphetamine (MDMA). MDMA is a synthetic (human-made), psychoactive drug that has amphetamine-like and LSD-like properties. It is another drug that is manufactured in non-medical labs, so purity is always suspect.

Brain-imaging research in humans indicates that MDMA injures the brain by affecting neurons. The National Institute on Drug Abuse reports that ecstasy users can expect:

- Psychological difficulties, including confusion, depression, sleep problems, drug craving, severe anxiety, and paranoia. These can occur immediately and sometimes weeks after taking ecstasy.
- Physical symptoms such as muscle tension, involuntary teeth clenching, nausea, blurred vision, rapid eye movement, faintness, chills, and sweating
- Increases in heart rate and blood pressure

Cocaine. Cocaine is a product of the South American coca plant. It comes in the form of a white powder that the user sniffs (snorts) into the nose. Cocaine is so psychologically addicting that some users become addicted the first time they use it.

Perhaps the most harmful effect of cocaine use lies in the user's response to the effect of the drug. The high is intense but lasts for only a short period of time (35–40 minutes), leading users to continually seek the high. This search results in larger and larger doses. The amount of money needed to buy the drug continues to increase as the user rides an ongoing roller coaster of being high, crashing, and getting high again. Many cocaine users turn to illegal means of funding the habit, and their lives spin out of control. Physical problems associated with cocaine use include:

- Damage to nasal passages; diminished sense of smell
- Convulsions, heart problems, and even death
- Malnutrition due to the appetite-suppressing effect of the drug
- Risks of stillborn infants and birth defects if cocaine is used during pregnancy

Drug	Form	Street Names	Effects	Potential for Dependence	Health Risks
Marijuana	Smoked, oral	Butter flower, cannabis, tea, duby, joint, MJ	Euphoria, relaxation, loss of coordination, heightened senses	Physical: unknown Psychological: low	Disoriented sense of time, loss of coordination, lung irritation, possible birth defects (if used during pregnancy)
Hallucinogens	Liquid, tablets, mushrooms	Acid, blotter, boomers, buttons, Mesc	Unpredictable behavior, increased blood pressure, distortion of time, hallucinations	Physical: uncertain Psychological: low; except for PCP (high)	Irregular breathing, elevated blood pressure, changes in senses, unexpected flashbacks, coma, death
Depressants	Capsules, tablets	Backwards, bambs, bluebirds, yellow bullets, tranq	Calmness similar to alcohol, sensory alterations	Physical: high Psychological: moderate to high	Shallow respiration, coma, death possible from failed respiration
Amphetamines	Tablets, injection	Dexies, jolly bean, road dope, sweets	Increased heart rate, high blood pressure, decreased appetite, possible loss of coordination	Physical: possible Psychological: moderate	Agitation, hallucinations, convulsions, death
Cocaine	Snorted, smoked, injected	Angie, base, beam, esnortiar (Spanish), heaven	Increased heart rate, irregular heartbeat, high blood pressure, anxiety	Physical: possible Psychological: high	Agitation, hallucinations, convulsions, death (especially if mixed with heroin)
Inhalants	Inhaled chemicals	Air blast, amys, highball, oz, spray	Dizziness, slurred speech, sleepiness	Physical: some Psychological: mild	Nausea, vomiting, memory loss, lung damage, brain damage, death
Steroids	Oral, injected	Gym candy, pumpers, therobolin	ncreased body weight, increased aggressiveness	Physical: possible Psychological: possible	Skin rash, impotence, shrunken testicles (males), irreversible masculine traits (females)

Effects of abused drugs

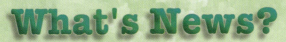

When users mix cocaine and alcohol, they are performing a complex chemical experiment in their body and compounding the danger each drug poses. Researchers are finding that the human liver combines cocaine and alcohol and manufactures a third substance, cocaethylene. This substance intensifies cocaine's effects and may increase the risk of sudden death.

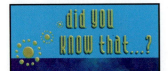

A crack cocaine high lasts only 5–20 minutes.

Crack cocaine is cocaine that is processed in a form that can be smoked. The high from crack cocaine is more intense than the high from the powder, but it does not last long. Consequently, users take more doses, thereby increasing the likelihood of addiction. When the high from cocaine wears off, a rapid "down" is experienced that leaves users feeling lower than before they used the drug. Many cocaine addicts turn to other drugs to help them deal with the discomfort.

Inhalants

Inhalants are volatile (evaporate quickly) substances, normally found in household cleaning products. The vapors in these products are rapidly absorbed into the bloodstream and carried throughout the body. Once in the brain, the chemicals quickly cause users to experience dizziness and slurred speech. Depending on the type of material inhaled and the level of inhalation, users may even experience hallucinations, convulsions, and death. Research indicates that inhalant abuse reaches a peak among young teens in eighth grade, with about 4% of teens using inhalants regularly.

A number of short- and long-term conditions affect inhalant users. The effects are related to the type of product inhaled and the length of time the user inhales. Short-term effects include:

- The replacement of oxygen in the bloodstream by inhalant chemicals, which reduces the supply of oxygen to brain tissue and reduces brain functioning

- Nausea, vomiting, and loss of appetite

- Poor motor skill and a lack of attentiveness that can result in accidents

Long-term effects include:

- Compulsive use and mild withdrawal symptoms when inhaling is discontinued

- Physical effects such as weight loss; muscle weakness; damage to the nose, throat, and lung tissues; damage to the liver and kidneys; and lack of coordination

- Mental effects such as inattentiveness, irritability, disorientation, and depression

Narcotics

Narcotics are pain-killing drugs made from **opium**, opium derivatives, and their semisynthetic or totally synthetic substitutes. Medical morphine, codeine, and heroin are all made from opium. Opium comes from the opium poppy, which grows in Afghanistan, the country that supplies most of the world's opium.

Drug abusers choose narcotics because they produce a sense of well-being and calmness. If doses are too high, however, narcotics can cause coma and death. Narcotics are particularly dangerous drugs because regular users quickly

opium

a narcotic drug derived from the sap of the opium poppy

real teens

Eric is a young adult, just out of his teen years. He grew up in a nice family in Southern California. After high school, he needed to earn money to support himself while he was trying to break into show business. A guy he met at a party offered him an opportunity to travel overseas and pick up "leather samples" in Pakistan. He would be paid $800 plus all expenses for each trip. What Eric didn't know was that the suitcases containing the "samples" actually contained raw opium sewn into the suitcase linings. The opium came from the Afghanistan poppy fields, where 94% of the world's opium is grown. Eric was caught with the opium when he tried to leave the airport in Pakistan. Normally, his punishment would have been death by hanging, but because he gave information to the Pakistani authorities, implicating others in the plot, he was spared. He is now serving a seven-year sentence in a Pakistani prison.

develop physical and psychological dependence. As tolerance increases, the amounts necessary to achieve the desired results increase, and dosage levels can lead to overdose and death. You may have read about celebrities who died as a result of drug overdoses.

Tolerance can also be a problem for people who are given narcotics for pain. They become addicted and continue to use the drugs when they are no longer medically necessary. Some users continue taking the drug to keep from experiencing the discomfort of withdrawal.

did you know that...?

Morphine has been used by doctors as a pain killer for more than a century. In 1895, heroin was developed as a substitute for morphine because it was believed to have fewer side effects. It turned out to be more addicting than morphine, and its use was suspended. Unfortunately, stopping the medicinal use of heroin didn't prevent it from becoming an illegal street drug.

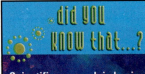

anabolic steroids

a class of synthetic drugs
designed to build muscle

did you know that...?

Scientific research is beginning to show that anabolic steroid abuse contributes to aggression and has other psychiatric side effects.

Steroids

Have you heard about young athletes taking "roids," or steroids? Some young people believe that using **anabolic steroids**, drugs designed to build muscle, enhances athletic performance. Steroids have legitimate medical purposes. Some of these purposes include correcting delayed onset of puberty or other medical conditions related to low levels of male hormones and counteracting the body wasting among AIDS patients. But using them without a prescription can result in serious health problems. And, although they can build muscle, anabolic steroids cannot increase skill or speed.

Although the *Monitoring the Future* survey indicates that fewer than 5% of adolescents use anabolic steroids, some teens do use them. Steroids are particularly bad for young people because, although muscle growth is enhanced, growth in general is interrupted. This means that teens who use steroids may develop muscle but may never reach their full potential height. Other problems include:

- Increased cholesterol levels
- Liver tumors and cancer
- Shrinking of the testicles and low sperm count
- Baldness
- Increased risk of prostate cancer
- Facial hair, alterations of the menstrual cycle, baldness, and a deepened voice in women who use steroids

PREVENTING DRUG ABUSE

As a teen, you can contribute to the important work of preventing drug abuse. There are many actions you can take as an individual, as a student, and as a member of your community. It is essential that you first take care of yourself. This means resisting any temptation to try drugs. Keep in mind your values – what you believe in – and what you want from life. Then consider the harmful consequences of drug abuse and the problems that can start when kids just want to "see what it's like." Stand up for your beliefs and say no to drugs, alcohol, and tobacco. Remember, the people who offer you drugs don't really care about you. They have selfish motives; they either want you to be like them or want you to buy drugs from them.

If you find yourself in a place where drugs are being abused, leave immediately. But don't simply ignore behaviors you know are wrong. If you see or know of someone using or selling drugs, tell a trusted adult. He or she can give you guidance for handling the situation. And your actions may save a life.

Take a look at the antidrug programs at your school. Is there a group you can join to help make a difference? It takes a lot of effort and cooperation to tackle tough problems, and everyone can contribute in some way.

Just like your school environment, healthy communities need people who care about the welfare of everyone. Drug dealers and criminals have no place in these communities, and there are programs, such as Neighborhood Watch, that encourage neighbors to look out for each other. If your community does not have such a program, see if there is interest in starting one. If there are existing service groups, consider joining one and doing your part to promote social wellness.

BUILDING YOUR Wellness Plan

Drugs do not create value in one's life. Teens who get involved in drug use generally find themselves dropping out of school or getting low-paying jobs. Although some young people claim they are able to use drugs only occasionally, the reality is that many people whose lives have been ruined started drug use out of curiosity. They never planned to become drug abusers. Here are some specific things to consider adding to your wellness plan:

- Look for constructive activities to keep you busy. Examples include developing a hobby, participating in school activities, and doing volunteer work. People sometimes use drugs because they are bored. People are bored only if they want to be.

- Call on your communication skills and create a set of refusal skills. Practice saying no confidently and comfortably.

- Find a trusted adult or family member to talk with about problems and feelings that seem unsolvable. We all need help from time to time. There are safe solutions for all problems.

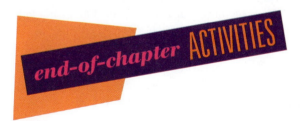

end-of-chapter ACTIVITIES

Weblinks

Effects of Alcohol and Drugs

South Coast Drug Information:
http://www.jeweldesigns.com/scdi/teens.htm

Effects of Marijuana

National Institute on Drug Abuse:
http://www.nida.nih.gov/MarijBroch/Marijteens.html

Substance Abuse and Alcohol Self-Assessment

Health Central: **http://www.healthcentral.com** (click on the topic center that interests you)

Short-Answer Questions

1. Name two kinds of over-the-counter medicines.
2. Name the five main forms of drugs and medicines.
3. List four illegal drugs that are abused.

4. Name the active ingredient in marijuana smoke.

5. State what anabolic steroids are used for.

☀ Discussion Questions

1. List and discuss the personal, social, and economic consequences of drug abuse.

2. Describe the differences among drug use, drug misuse, and drug abuse.

3. Discuss why some young people choose to abuse drugs.

4. Explain the addictive nature of cocaine.

5. Identify the three drugs most likely to be abused by adolescents and describe their health effects.

☀ Chapter Vocabulary

Using a separate sheet of paper, list and define the following terms:

amphetamines	medicine
anabolic steroids	opium
drug abuse	over-the-counter medications
drug dependence	tolerance
flashback	withdrawal

☀ Application Activities

Language Arts Connection

Pretend you are creating a communitywide antidrug campaign. In a letter to your mayor, explain why you think the campaign is necessary and explain in detail your plan for carrying out the campaign.

Math Connection

Visit the National Institute on Drug Abuse Web site at **http://www.nida.nih.gov** and find out how much the United States spends each year attempting to stop drug abuse. Then use the Web to find out how many people live in the United States at this time. Imagine that drug use stopped today and all the money spent on ending its use was divided equally among the U.S. population. How much would each person get?

Social Studies Connection

1. Search the Web to learn about state-funded programs in your state that provide rehabilitation for drug users. Prepare a report about these programs.

2. A number of famous people have died as a result of drug use. Research one of those famous people and prepare a report on his or her life, use of drugs, and cause of death. In your report, describe what the person or his or her friends might have done to prevent the death.

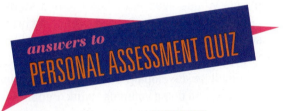

answers to PERSONAL ASSESSMENT QUIZ

personal assessment: DRUG FACTS

1. False. The answer would be true if alcohol were excluded. Remember that alcohol is a drug.

2. True.

3. False. The average age is 13!

4. False. Recent evidence indicates that physical addiction can be demonstrated in laboratory animals.

5. True. In fact, more than 75% of prison inmates used drugs before they went to prison.

6. True. The rates of drug use declined after 1979 but showed a slight increase in 2001.

chapter 23

Infectious Diseases

Eliot has always been interested in science. It was his favorite subject in elementary school, and he also learned a lot about life sciences in middle school. He has now taken a special interest in microbiology, the study of microscopic organisms and how they affect the environments in which they live. In addition to his high school classes, Eliot is taking a microbiology course at the local community college. He likes the lab sessions best because he can work with the organisms under experimental conditions. Eliot is quite sure he wants to study microbiology when he goes to college, and he is even considering a career in medicine.

chapter OBJECTIVES

When you finish this chapter, you should be able to:

- Define *infectious disease*.
- Explain why most infectious diseases are not as dangerous as they once were.
- State the causes of infectious diseases.
- Describe the chain of infection.
- Discuss ways of preventing infectious diseases.
- Describe the five stages of disease.
- List the most common infectious diseases in adolescents, their causes, and specific ways to prevent them.
- Explain the meaning of *bioterrorism*.

key TERMS

bioterrorism
carrier
chain of infection
fomite
infectious disease
modes of transmission
opportunistic infection
pathogenic organisms
secondary infection

infectious diseases

diseases that are caused by some form of pathogenic organism

pathogenic organism

also called a pathogen; a living organism that can cause disease by invading the body's tissues and multiplying; commonly referred to as germs

Introduction

If you are like most teenagers, you stay pretty healthy. It would be nice if we always stayed healthy and well, but everyone gets sick with an infectious disease at one time or another. **Infectious diseases** are caused by **pathogenic organisms**, living organisms that invade the body's tissues and multiply. These diseases can be spread from one person to another or in other ways, such as through contaminated food. Not all germs cause serious illnesses because the body has a well-developed set of defense mechanisms. Some infectious diseases are easily cured, with the body healing naturally, but others need medical attention and can last a lifetime. Still others can result in death. This chapter is about infectious diseases, how they affect your health, and how you can prevent illnesses that are caused by infectious organisms.

personal assessment: PERSONAL HABITS

Read each of the statements below and record your answers on a separate sheet of paper. Briefly explain your reasons for doing or not doing each of the behaviors. An interpretation of your answers is located at the end of the chapter.

Do you:

1. Know which immunizations you have had and when you had them? List the immunizations and the dates they were given.

2. Wash your hands often and especially before you eat?

3. Share grooming products (razor, makeup, hairbrush, comb, etc.) with others?

4. Cover your nose and mouth when you sneeze and cough?

5. Share food, eating utensils, straws, or drinks with others?

6. Wear clean socks and clothes?

7. Get regular medical checkups? Give the date of your last checkup.

8. Avoid coming into contact with the blood or body fluids of another person without wearing protection?

9. Know how to safely handle and store food?

10. Take care of your body by eating a balanced diet, getting lots of exercise, and getting plenty of rest?

HISTORY OF INFECTIOUS DISEASES

Infectious diseases were the number one cause of death throughout history until the early 1900s. Few children in the past lived to see adulthood, and most adults died by the time they were 35 years old. It is hard to believe now that during the Spanish-American War in 1898, only 968 U.S. soldiers died of battle injuries. The other 5,438 deaths were the result of infectious diseases. In 1900, the major causes of death were tuberculosis, pneumonia, diarrhea, and intestinal and stomach diseases.

Research has contributed much to our knowledge of infectious diseases. The good health practices, such as handwashing and bathing, that you know about as a teen were unknown in the past. These practices, combined with improved medications, have greatly reduced deaths caused by bacterial and viral infections. By the mid-1940s, chronic diseases replaced infectious diseases as the number one cause of death, and the human life span was greatly increased. Do infectious diseases still kill people? Yes, but far fewer than 100 years ago.

In the late 1800s, fear of infection and epidemics led to mandatory physical examinations of immigrants while at Ellis Island to prevent the spread of infection between countries.

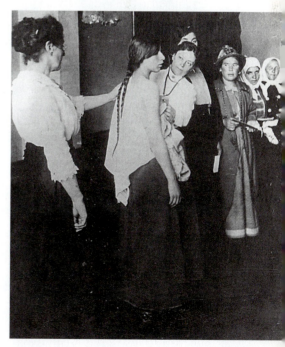

CAUSES OF INFECTIOUS DISEASES

The organisms that cause infectious diseases come in a variety of forms and sizes. You have probably heard about bacteria or viruses, but you may not know that fungi and parasites can also cause disease. Each specific pathogenic organism causes a specific disease. Table 23-1 lists the types of pathogens, and they are discussed in more detail in the next section.

Viruses

Viruses are the smallest of all life forms, so small that they can be seen only with very powerful microscopes. Viruses need host cells in order to reproduce. When a virus enters your body, it will seek out a specific type of cell and attach itself to that host cell. For example, the cold virus will affect only the nasal passages and airway. Here's how it works:

1. A virus particle enters your body because you touched a contaminated surface and brought your fingers to your mouth or inhaled droplets with viruses from the air.

2. The virus attaches to cells lining your nose or throat.

3. The virus quickly produces new viruses using the genetic material from the host cells.

4. The host cells break, sending new viruses into your bloodstream and into your lungs. Because you have lost some cells that line

Table 23-1 Types of Pathogens

Pathogen	Description	Common Diseases	Treatment
Viruses	Smallest unit of living material; requires host cells to reproduce	Common cold, measles, mumps, chicken pox, influenza, herpes, AIDS	No cure; drugs and medications to relieve symptoms
Bacteria	One-celled microorganisms; some beneficial, some harmful	Tetanus, strep throat, food poisoning, tuberculosis, pneumonia, syphilis, gonorrhea	Antibiotics. There are about 150 antibiotics available; certain antibiotics are cures for specific bacterial infections.
Fungi	Plantlike pathogens such as molds and yeasts	Athlete's foot, vaginal yeast infection, athletic itch, ringworm	Various antifungal medications
Protozoa	One-celled microscopic animal-like organisms	Dysentery, giardiasis, malaria, vaginal infection	Various medications designed to kill the organism
Multicellular parasites	Organisms composed of numerous cells that use humans or animals as hosts	Scabies, tapeworm, hookworm	Various medications designed to kill the organism

What's News?

A virus usually found in the Middle East appeared in New York City in 1999. Known as the West Nile virus, this organism is transmitted by mosquitoes that feed off infected birds. The disease has moved from the New York area to the central United States, down the east coast and west toward Texas. Although the virus is not life threatening to everyone, it is a special problem for young children and elderly adults.

your throat and sinuses, fluid is able to flow into your nasal passages, giving you a runny nose.

5. Viruses in the fluid that drips down the back of your throat also attack cells lining your throat, causing your throat to feel sore.

6. Viruses in your bloodstream can attack muscle cells and may cause you to have muscle aches.

Diseases can be caused by different forms of the same virus. For example, there are many types of influenza virus. Figure 23-1 illustrates how one type of virus can be more prevalent than another during the same time period in different parts of the country.

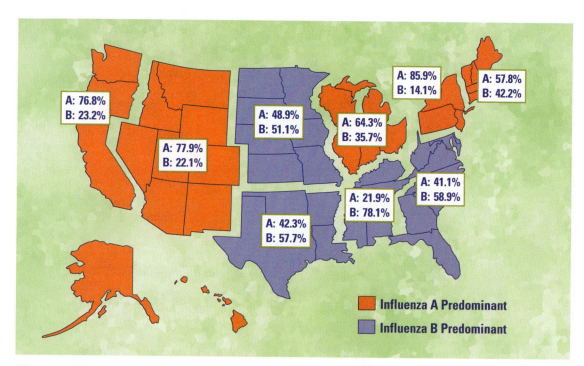

Figure 23-1 Distribution of influenza forms, September 2002 to May 2003

Bacteria

Bacteria are larger and more complex than viruses. They come in many forms. Figure 23-2 shows some of the common bacteria types. Some bacteria can survive temperatures hot enough to boil water and cold enough to freeze your blood. Some bacteria are "friendly," living in

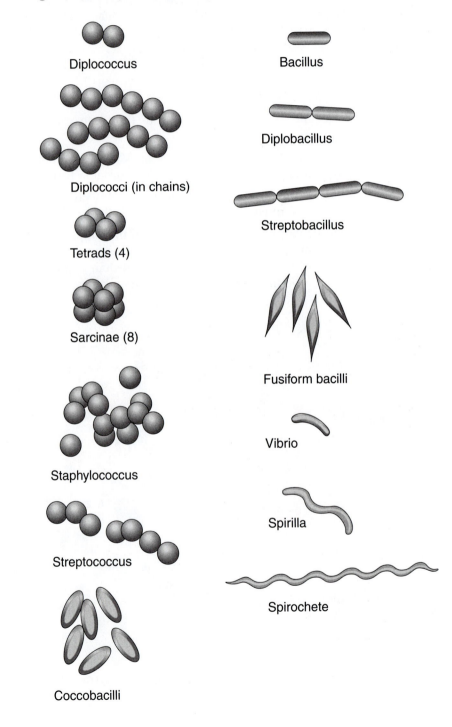

Diplococcus

Diplococci (in chains)

Tetrads (4)

Sarcinae (8)

Staphylococcus

Streptococcus

Coccobacilli

Bacillus

Diplobacillus

Streptobacillus

Fusiform bacilli

Vibrio

Spirilla

Spirochete

Figure 23-2
Basic forms of bacteria

your intestines, where they help digest food, or putting the "sour" in sourdough bread. But other bacteria contribute to diseases in humans, causing conditions such as strep throat, food poisoning, wound infections, tuberculosis, gonorrhea, and tetanus.

Bacteria do their damage in the body through one of two mechanisms. Some forms of pathogenic bacteria produce **exotoxins**, which are poisons that are produced by the bacteria. These toxins are harmful to the living body cells, producing such health effects as food poisoning, whooping cough, or diphtheria. Other bacteria may produce **endotoxins**, which are poisons manufactured in the cell wall of the bacteria. Diseases such as **botulism** and **tetanus** are caused by endotoxins. Most often the poisons are released to the body when the bacteria die. In other instances, the bacteria may transmit the toxin simply by coming into contact with the healthy cells.

Bacterial diseases can be prevented with **immunizations** and can be cured with the use of **antibiotics**. There are more than 150 antibiotics that can treat bacterial infections. Each disease has to be matched with the antibiotic that will cure that particular infection. Only medical professionals know which antibiotic will work on which disease.

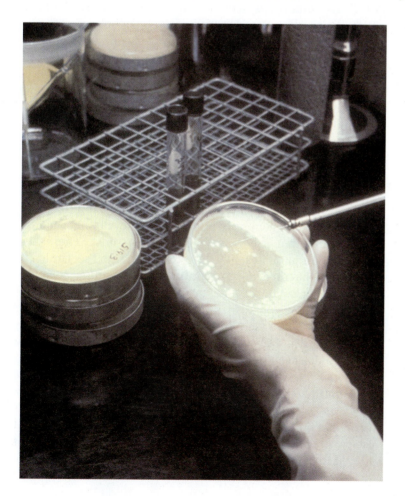

A microbiologist is studying a culture of botulism bacteria.

exotoxin

poison produced by and released from certain bacteria

endotoxins

poisons that come from the cell wall of certain bacteria when they die

botulism

a strong toxin that affects muscles in the body that can result in death if not treated quickly and properly; most often due to improperly canned foods

tetanus

a bacterial disease that affects the nervous system, commonly known as lockjaw; results in death about 10% of the time

immunization

a process that enables the body to become immune to specific infectious diseases

antibiotics

a class of medications that kill bacteria and clear up infection

Fungi

Fungi are plantlike organisms such as molds, yeasts, and mushrooms. More than 70,000 forms of fungi have been identified. Fungi range from single-celled microscopic organisms to what might be one of the largest organisms on the earth. (In 1992, scientists discovered an underground fungus in Michigan that was almost 40 acres large and weighed more than 100 tons!) Not all fungi cause disease. For example, certain yeasts can be used to make bread; one form of mold, *Penicillium chrysogenum*, is used to make penicillin; other yeasts can be used to ferment fruits or grains to produce carbonated or alcoholic beverages. Pathogenic fungi can be the cause of ringworm, athlete's foot, or yeast infections, and certain species of mushroom are poisonous.

Protozoa

parasite

an organism that relies on a host organism for survival; usually the host organism is harmed in some way

Protozoa are one-celled, animal-like microscopic organisms. Some protozoa are harmful to humans because they are **parasites**, although there are fewer than a dozen such parasites in the United States. One of them is *Giardia intestinalis*, which can be picked up by drinking untreated water. Have you heard commercials advertising "fresh mountain water"? The truth is, some mountain streams are contaminated, and hikers who drink the water can become very ill after a few days, with abdominal cramps, nausea, vomiting, and diarrhea. The condition is not life threatening, but it is very uncomfortable. Giardia can be avoided by boiling water or treating it with appropriate chemicals. If the source of drinking water is not a treatment plant, an approved well, or at the site of a melting glacier, it must be treated before it is safe for drinking.

Multicellular Parasites

The largest of the pathogenic organisms are the multicellular parasites. These organisms generally undergo a life cycle that includes stages of development that are outside the human host. There are very few multicellular parasites that affect humans in the United States, and those cases that do occur are confined to the southeastern United States. Some multicellular parasites are very small; others are up to 20 feet long. Some of these parasites are small mites (0.3–0.5 mm), such as those that cause **scabies** (see Figure 23-3). Scabies is not a life-threatening disease, but it is uncomfortable because it itches a lot. The mites that cause the disease do not multiply on the human host. The condition is cured with the correct type of prescription lotion.

scabies

infection caused by a small mite

Another example of a multicellular parasite is a roundworm known as *Ascaris lumbricoides*. This roundworm is the most common worm infection in humans and can be found in rural areas of the southeastern United States. It is transmitted as an egg through contaminated soil that may be accidentally swallowed. Once it enters the host's body,

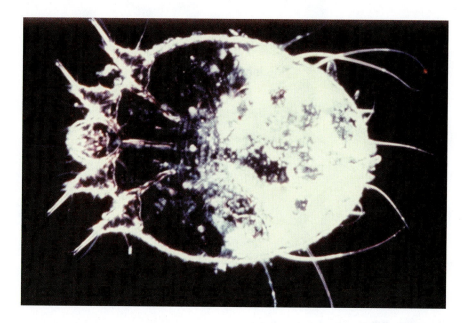

Figure 23-3
Scabies mite

it lives in the small intestine, where it feeds off the host. The organism may live one or two years and generally produces no discomfort unless there are several worms present.

THE CHAIN OF INFECTION

Infectious diseases are spread in a variety of ways. Some diseases are communicable, which means they are spread from one person to another. Because some pathogens can be transmitted in the air or by touch, it's important to cover your mouth when you sneeze and wash your hands before handling food. Other ways of transmitting infectious diseases include contact with infected food and animals.

A model that illustrates the infection process is called the chain of infection. In Figure 23-4, each link of the chain represents an element that must be present for infection to spread. Infectious diseases are controlled by breaking one of the links through preventive practices such as ensuring clean water supplies and careful handwashing. There are six links in the chain of infection:

1. *Infectious agent:* A pathogenic organism such as a virus or bacterium is present
2. *Reservoir host:* A place where the organism can grow and reproduce. This may be inside a human or an animal or in a substance such as water or food.
3. *Portal of exit:* A way for the pathogenic organism to leave the reservoir. Portals of exit vary, depending on the organism. For example, the cold virus exits from the nose or mouth, and some infections can exit through sores on the surface of the skin.

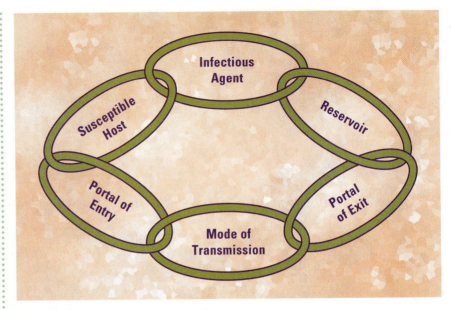

Figure 23-4 The chain of infection

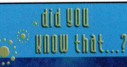

4. *Mode of transmission:* A way for the organism to move from the reservoir into another host, which may be a human. Modes of transmission may involve direct contact, such as kissing, sneezing, coughing, consuming or handling contaminated food or water, and insect or animal bites. Some organisms are transmitted by way of **fomites**. A desktop in your classroom is an example of a fomite. You are actually more likely to catch the cold virus from a germy desktop than from breathing the same air as another student who has a cold.

5. *Portal of entry:* The location and means by which the pathogen enters the body. Examples are eyes, nose, mouth, skin, and urogenital openings. Cold and flu viruses enter through the mouth and nose. Bacteria that produce food poisoning enter through the mouth and then move down the esophagus to the stomach.

6. *Susceptible host:* An individual who has no immunity against the pathogen and so is likely to "catch" the illness. This can be a person who is not immunized against the disease, who has a weak immune system, or whose behavior puts him or her at risk for a disease. Not everyone who is exposed to a pathogen becomes ill. Some people have a very good immune system that keeps them healthy. Depending on the disease, a susceptible host can become a new reservoir.

PREVENTING INFECTIOUS DISEASES

Our best weapon against infectious organisms is using our understanding of the chain of infection. Applying our knowledge about how these organisms are transmitted gives us the ability to manage them and prevent disease. Another weapon against infectious organisms is immunization.

Breaking the Chain of Infection

It's only necessary to break one link in the chain of infection to stop infectious organisms in their tracks. Let's take a look at ways to break each of the links.

1. *Infectious agents.* These can be killed with chemicals that destroy organisms or prevent their reproduction. Water is chlorinated in the United States because chlorine kills harmful bacteria and other germs. When you are camping, you can make your drinking water safe by boiling it. Other things you can do to kill infectious agents are to thoroughly cook foods that require cooking and to keep your environment clean of waste materials and trash.

2. *Reservoir host.* Steps can be taken to prevent bacteria and other harmful pathogens from multiplying. Refrigerate leftover foods as soon as you finish eating. Wash your hands after handling raw meat. Keep cold foods cold and hot foods hot. Stay home when you are ill.

3. *Portal of exit.* Cover your mouth when you cough or sneeze. Throw away infected tissues and bandages, disposing of them in a covered trash can. If you have a communicable disease, stay away from other people. This method is called **self-imposed quarantine**.

4. *Mode of transmission.* One of the most effective ways of stopping the mode of transmission, according to the Centers for Disease Control and Prevention, is to wash your hands often. Sexually transmitted infections can be avoided by practicing abstinence or postponing sexual activity until you know the person very well and are comfortable discussing these infections and ways to prevent them. Medical personnel never touch the body fluids of another person without protective gloves.

5. *Portal of entry.* Avoid touching your face, especially during the cold and flu season. *Stay away* from injected drug use unless prescribed by a doctor. Don't share eating utensils, straws, or drinks. Never share toothbrushes or razors.

self-imposed quarantine
voluntarily staying away from other people when you are ill so as not to spread disease

did you know that...?

One major study showed that children with asthma were more likely to have upper respiratory infections if they lived where there was a high cockroach population.

✳ teen forum ✳

A Position on Immunization

Although immunization has saved countless lives, it is not without controversy. There are arguments against requiring vaccines. Some people say, for example, that the diseases have been eliminated, that some people get sicker from the immunization, and that immunizations are costly. Those in favor, however, argue that everyone should get immunized to protect themselves and society.

- If your local health department announced it had a new vaccine that prevented HIV infections, would you be willing to get the vaccine, or would you hold off and see how it affected other people? Give the reasons for your answer.

human immunodeficiency virus (HIV)

a virus that can multiply and destroy a portion of the immune system

6. *Susceptible host.* Keep your body healthy with plenty of rest, exercise, and a balanced diet. Don't put yourself at risk of getting diseases. Have regular checkups to detect signs of disease. Get all necessary immunizations and keep them up to date.

Immunizations

Immunity means being resistant to catching diseases. Immunization (sometimes called vaccination) is a process that enables the body to become immune to specific infectious diseases. There are two ways to immunize against a disease caused by a virus. The first is natural exposure, which occurs when you become infected with a disease. For instance, a person who got chicken pox would build up immunity and would not be likely to have that disease again. The second way to immunize is artificial exposure, in which parts of the viral agent are put into your body by injection, by mouth, or by other means. This exposure causes your body to make weapons (antibodies) against the infectious agent. If you are exposed to the disease later, your body is prepared to fight it.

Most of the important immunizations we have today were developed at the beginning of the twentieth century. Since the process of immunizing began, billions of people have been protected from devastating diseases such as diphtheria, whooping cough, tetanus, and yellow fever. Perhaps you never heard of some of those diseases. Your not having heard about them demonstrates the miracle of immunizations because in the past these were common diseases that affected every neighborhood. Smallpox, once a major concern and life threatening, is now virtually extinct, and polio and measles have been eliminated from the United States. Polio and measles are still found in some countries that do not have aggressive immunization programs.

STAGES OF DISEASE

Infectious diseases progress through five separate stages (see Figure 23-5).

1. *Infection.* Infectious diseases begin when a susceptible host becomes infected with a pathogenic organism. The organism enters the body and "sets up housekeeping" where it can grow and multiply.

2. *Incubation stage.* During this stage, the pathogenic organism starts to multiply. The incubation period varies with each disease and ends when symptoms appear. Incubation may last hours (food poisoning), or a couple of days (common cold), or even years (**human immunodeficiency virus**). At the end of the incubation stage, a disease is usually highly contagious.

3. *Prodromal stage.* Infected people in this stage will begin to feel sick, although they won't have all the symptoms of the disease.

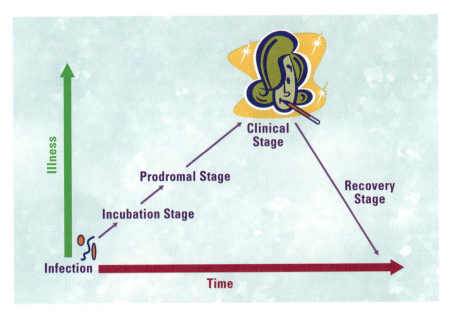

Figure 23-5
Stages of infectious diseases

They may start running a fever or feel achy and tired. Although the person is not really ill, he or she can still pass the disease on to someone else.

4. *Clinical or illness stage.* It is during this stage that symptoms appear. For example, a person who is clinically ill with the common cold will sneeze, cough, and have a runny nose.

5. *Recovery stage.* Recovery begins when the body's immune system starts to overcome the pathogenic organisms and symptoms begin disappearing. This may take a few hours or a few weeks, depending on the disease. Many bacterial illnesses can be treated with antibiotics. Specific antibiotics cure specific diseases; there is no one antibiotic for all diseases. An important fact about antibiotics is that they can't kill viruses, which is why there isn't a cure for the common cold. It is important when taking antibiotics to take the entire prescription, even if you begin to feel better before you use all the medication. If you stop taking the antibiotic just because you think you are cured, the few bacteria that remain can reproduce, but they become capable of altering their genetic core to create a resistance to the antibiotic. One form of the bacterium that causes gonorrhea has mutated to the point where the bacteria actually use antibiotic penicillin as a food source! During the recovery stage, disease-causing organisms are still in the body. It is possible in some instances for a person suffer a **relapse**. A relapse is a condition in which someone gets sick with the same illness before fully recovering. It is important to take care of yourself during the recovery stage so that relapse does not occur.

relapse

a condition in which a person experiences an illness a second time before completely recovering from the first occurrence

MAJOR INFECTIOUS DISEASES

Many kinds of infectious diseases affect humans, however, we are more likely to be infected with certain pathogens than with others. Knowing which diseases are most likely to infect teens and young adults, along with knowing the pathogens that cause them, how they are spread, and how they can be prevented, will help you avoid the pathogens and stay well.

The Common Cold

The most frequently occurring infectious disease is the common cold. More than 200 viruses are known to cause colds. Contrary to popular belief, colds are *not* caused by cold temperatures or cool drafts. The "cold season," the time of year when the majority of colds occur, is usually between early September and late April. The reason has to do with how colds are transmitted, which is from person to person. During the cooler months, people spend more time indoors together, thus increasing the chance of being exposed to cold viruses.

There are several ways that colds can be spread from one person to another. The most common is by touching an infected surface (fomite) and then touching the eyes, nose, or mouth. You can see how effective frequent handwashing is for preventing illness during the cold season. Inhaling the virus when someone sneezes or coughs is another way of becoming infected. The least likely way a person can become infected with a cold is by inhaling virus particles that have been suspended in the air because the virus particles are widely dispersed in the air.

Colds are usually most contagious from the second to the fourth day of infection, when the greatest number of viruses is present in nasal fluids. Colds usually last 7 to 14 days, and symptoms include sneezing, nasal discharge, obstruction of nasal breathing, swelling of the sinus membranes, sore throat, cough, and headache.

Because most colds are caused by viruses and usually go away on their own, seeing a doctor for antibiotics won't help; it's actually a waste of money. The only effective way to treat a cold is to get rest and drink lots of fluids. You may need to see a doctor, however, if you develop a **secondary infection**, one of the harmful side effects of colds. Secondary infections occur when the cold turns into another type of infection such as bronchitis, ear infection, or pneumonia. If you have a cold that worsens rather than improves after a week or two, you should see your doctor to find out if you have a secondary infection that is treatable.

Influenza

Another common infectious disease is influenza, or "flu." There are three main types of flu virus: A, B, and C. Viruses A and B are most likely to cause flu in humans, and there many variations of the A and B types. Flu is caused by one of these virus subtypes and is spread when an infected person coughs and the virus is transmitted into the air,

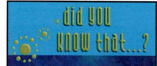

The National Institute of Allergy and Infectious Diseases estimates that there are more than 1 billion common colds in the United States within a one-year time span!

secondary infection

an infection that arises at a location other than the original site; usually involves a second pathogen or irritant

Table 23-2   Symptoms of Colds and Flu

Symptom	Cold	Flu
Fever	Rare	Yes: 102–104 degrees Fahrenheit
Cough	Yes	Yes
Stuffy nose	Yes	Sometimes
Sneezing	Yes	Sometimes
Sore throat	Yes	Sometimes
Aches and pains	Slight, if at all	Yes
Headache	Rare	Yes
Chills	Rare	Yes
Tiredness	Slight	Yes

where it can be breathed in by others. The flu, like the common cold, can also spread through fomites, so it's important to avoid touching your face and mouth, especially during the flu season.

The incubation period for the flu is one to four days, and a person is considered contagious between the day before symptoms appear and three to five days after they begin. These symptoms include headache, chills, dry cough, body aches, fever, stuffy nose, and sore throat and may last for one or two weeks before they start to improve. (See Table 23-2 for a comparison of cold and flu symptoms.) Although the flu may cause teenagers to feel miserable for only a week or two, it can be deadly in the elderly and young children. Scientists have recently developed medications to help treat the flu. Known as antiviral medications, they must be started very soon after the symptoms begin in order to be effective.

Food Poisoning

Food poisoning is another type of infectious disease, usually caused by food that is contaminated with certain types of bacteria. Some foods, such as toadstools, are toxic themselves.

Salmonella, probably the most common form of food poisoning, is caused by *Salmonella* bacteria. Poultry, meat, or fish can be contaminated with the bacteria, which can multiply if the food is allowed to sit at room temperature. In the United States, it is estimated there are between 1 and 2 million cases of salmonella each year. Mild cases of salmonella are often undiagnosed, so the exact number of actual cases is difficult to determine. Symptoms of salmonella usually develop within 12 to 72 hours after infection and may include diarrhea, fever,

salmonella

food poisoning caused by *Salmonella* bacteria that are found in food sources, especially chicken and other meat products

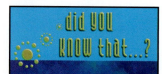

Scientists have isolated at least 250 diseases that are caused by spoiled and contaminated food.

and abdominal cramps. Salmonella food poisoning usually lasts from four to seven days, and most people recover without treatment. In some cases, however, the diarrhea is so severe that the infected person must be hospitalized. Without prompt treatment, the infection can spread from the intestines to the bloodstream and result in death.

An estimated 55% of all food poisoning cases are caused by improper cooking and storage of foods; 24% are caused by poor hygiene, such as not washing the hands before handling food and using unclean preparation surfaces. Only 3% of food poisoning cases are caused by an unsafe food source. You can prevent food poisoning by practicing the following safe food-handling behaviors, which are also mentioned in Chapter 8.

- Keep your hands clean while working with or eating food. This is the *single most important thing* you can do to prevent food poisoning.

- Refrigerate leftover food as soon as possible. If food of any kind smells bad, do *not* attempt to eat it. It should be discarded.

- Never eat vegetables, such as beans, asparagus, or greens, that come from a can that has a bulge in it. The bulge is caused by gases produced by *Clostridium botulinum*, a potentially deadly bacteria. This type of food poisoning is called botulism.

- Always cook ground meat thoroughly. The less the meat is cooked, the greater the likelihood of food poisoning.

- Never defrost poultry at room temperature; thawing should be done in the refrigerator.

- Avoid cross-contamination. This means not allowing raw meat, poultry, or fish or any surface touched by these raw foods to come into contact with other foods.

- Don't use a wooden cutting board because organisms breed in the grooves made by knives. It is safer to use a ceramic or acrylic cutting board if the board is cleaned after each use. If you do choose to use a wooden board, be sure to periodically disinfect it with bleach.

Mononucleosis

Infectious mononucleosis is an extremely common disease among high school and college students. It is caused by a common virus called the Epstein-Barr virus. Often referred to as "mono," infectious mononucleosis is nicknamed "the kissing disease" because it spreads primarily through intimate contact with infected saliva. The incubation period for mono is from four to six weeks. Symptoms, which usually last about four weeks, include swollen glands in the neck, white patches in the back of the throat, fever, sore throat, headaches, tiredness, and lack of appetite. Although mono goes away without treatment, individuals with the disease should get plenty of rest and drink lots of fluids. In some cases, the tonsils and adenoids become so enlarged they make it difficult to breathe. This condition requires a doctor's care and may be treated with steroids to reduce the swelling.

Conjunctivitis

Conjunctivitis, also known as pinkeye, is another common infectious disease. Conjunctivitis is caused by several viruses and bacteria and is spread by contact with either respiratory fluids or eye discharges from infected individuals. It can also be spread by sharing articles of clothing, towels, makeup, and grooming supplies that touch the face or eyes, so it's important for teens not to share these items.

Symptoms of conjunctivitis include a white or yellowish discharge from under the eyelid, matted eyelids during sleep, reddening and swelling of the eyelids, tearing, and pain. The incubation period is 1 to 3 days for bacterial conjunctivitis and 5 to 21 days for viral conjunctivitis. Most cases are mild and go away on their own. If you have conjunctivitis in which the symptoms are very painful or last for more than 5 days, you should see a doctor.

Strep Throat

Strep throat is a serious throat infection caused by bacteria called streptococci. Strep throat is transmitted by sneezing and coughing or from items that touch the mouth, such as a straw, fork, or glass. The incubation period for strep throat is about five days. Some people, known as **carriers**, can be infected with strep throat and have no symptoms. Although they are not sick themselves, they can infect others. Animals, including pets, can also be carriers of strep throat.

The symptoms of strep throat include fever, stomachache, headache, and a throat that hurts so badly it is hard to swallow. Strep throat is usually easy to treat with antibiotics, but it is important to take the medicine exactly as it is prescribed. Not taking all of the medicine or not taking it in the manner prescribed can result in a relapse. Strep throat that has relapsed can be harder to treat because the streptococci can develop resistance to the original antibiotic, making it ineffective in killing them.

Strep throat can be very serious. If left untreated, it can even result in death. If you develop a sore throat and know you have been around someone who has been diagnosed with strep throat, you should see a doctor as soon as possible to be tested for the bacteria. The doctor will take a swab of your throat and have it tested for the presence of the bacteria.

Tuberculosis

Tuberculosis (TB) was the number one cause of death in the early 1900s. For many years, the number of cases greatly declined, but, unfortunately, TB is making a comeback. This infection is caused by bacteria that travel through the air. It is spread when an infected person coughs

carrier
an infected person who does not show symptoms of a disease but who can spread it to others

acquired immunodeficiency syndrome (AIDS)

a condition caused by HIV infection whereby a portion of the immune system is destroyed, making it easy for the infected person to get life-threatening diseases

opportunistic infections

specific infectious diseases that occur when part of the body's immune system is damaged

or sneezes, propelling the bacteria into the air, where they can be inhaled by other people. Because the bacteria are inhaled, TB usually infects the lungs, but it can also infect other organs such as the brain, kidneys, and liver. Left untreated, it can be fatal. Some types of TB are easily cured with antibiotics, but there is a new type of the disease that is resistant to many antibiotics and can be deadly.

Symptoms of TB include weight loss, night sweats, feeling sick or weak, and fever. When it has infected the lungs, the symptoms include coughing, chest pain, and coughing up blood. If you think you have been exposed to TB, you should see your doctor as soon as possible because exposure can be determined by a simple skin test. People who test positive for TB exposure may have medications prescribed to kill the bacteria before they develop the illness.

Sexually Transmitted Infections

Sexually transmitted infections (STIs; sometimes called sexually transmitted diseases, or STDs) are other examples of infectious diseases. As their name suggests, they are spread by sexual contact.

Chlamydia

The most common STI in the United States is chlamydia, caused by a bacterium called *Chlamydia trachomatis.* The Centers for Disease Control and Prevention estimates that about 1 in every 10 adolescent girls has been infected with *Chlamydia.* Most people infected with *Chlamydia* don't have symptoms. If symptoms do develop, they usually appear within one or two weeks after exposure. Symptoms of chlamydia include a burning sensation when urinating, eye inflammation, minor discharge from the vagina, or pus discharge from the penis, and pain or swelling of the testicles. More advanced cases may cause lower back and abdominal pain and fever. If chlamydia is left untreated, it can result in many serious complications, such as sterility, in both men and women.

Human Immunodeficiency Virus

Although chlamydia is the most common form of STI, the most life threatening is human immunodeficiency virus, commonly referred to as HIV. This virus was first diagnosed in the United States in 1981, but it probably existed here before that. When HIV gets into the body and multiplies in sufficient numbers, it causes a breakdown of the T4 cells, an important part of the body's immune system. This is the condition known as AIDS, **acquired immunodeficiency syndrome**. When the immune system cannot function properly, the body is susceptible to infections caused by organisms that usually do not cause disease in healthy individuals. These infections are called **opportunistic infections** because they would not occur if the immune system were working normally. But they can be fatal to someone with AIDS.

What's News?

The major cause of death among HIV patients has been a form of pneumonia caused by *Pneumocystis carinii*. The illness is commonly referred to as PCP (*Pneumocystis carinii* pneumonia). Until 1988, the organism that causes PCP was thought to be a protozoan. Although the organism was renamed *Pneumocystis jiroveci* in 2002 because it had the characteristics of a fungus, the scientific and medical literature still refers to AIDS cases as PCP (using *Pneumocystis jiroveci* pneumonia).

Tests for the presence of HIV in the body can be performed using either the blood or saliva. The virus can be detected four weeks after infection. The incubation period for HIV to become AIDS varies. It usually ranges from 7 to 10 years, but shorter and longer time periods have been reported. HIV is not transmitted through casual contact with a person infected with HIV or by insect bites or stings. For example, you cannot get it from shaking hands with an infected person or from a toilet seat. HIV is spread through contact with body fluids, such as blood. Sexual contact and sharing infected needles while injecting drugs are two common ways to contract

WHY CONDOMS FAIL

Latex condoms are theoretically effective in preventing STIs and pregnancy. They lose their effectiveness if they are:

- Stored someplace where the temperature is very high
- Damaged by fingernails or jewelry during application
- Not removed properly right after sexual intercourse

real teens

Many famous people have died as a result of AIDS. Perhaps the most famous is Ryan White, a young man who died in 1990 at the age of 18 after living with AIDS for five years. Ryan contracted HIV from a blood transfusion. He had a disease called hemophilia, in which the blood cannot form blood clots and patients bleed excessively from even minor wounds. Hemophilia is a genetic disorder, not an infectious disease. Ryan was barred from his school in 1985 when officials there learned he had AIDS, which he developed when he received a contaminated blood product that was to help him with his hemophilia. Little was known about HIV, and school officials were afraid the other students could get the disease from Ryan. Ryan's parents fought the ruling, and he was allowed to go back to school. He was later banned once more. When Ryan returned to school, he faced very difficult conditions. He was required to use his own private bathroom and use disposable eating utensils. Many kids treated him very badly. In May 1987, Ryan's family moved to another town. The school officials at the new school were ready for Ryan's arrival. They had learned as much as they could about HIV and had educated the parents and children. Ryan was treated with dignity and respect and allowed to live as a normal teenager. Congress passed a law called the Ryan White Comprehensive AIDS Resources Emergency Act of 1990 (Ryan White CARE Act) that provides medical support for AIDS patients. Ryan's bravery contributed to better understanding and more humane treatment of people with AIDS.

HIV. Anyone who has been involved in any unprotected sexual activity or has injected drugs should be tested for HIV.

Preventing Sexually Transmitted Infection

There are some things a person can do to decrease his or her chances of getting any STI, including HIV:

- Practicing abstinence. Sexual abstinence is the only way of preventing any sexually transmitted infection. The absence of close sexual contact prevents any pathogen from moving from one reservoir to a new host.

- Using a latex condom or female condom creates a barrier between the two partners which may help prevent the spread of a pathogen from one partner to another. A condom does not cover all areas of the genitals so the exposure to a pathogen still exists; therefore, a pathogen may still be transmitted. Abstinence is the only 100% effective method of preventing the spread of a STD.

- Avoiding illegal drugs, especially injected drugs.

- Not using anyone else's razors or toothbrushes. HIV can spread through fresh blood on these items.

- Not touching the body fluids of another person without wearing latex gloves. This is especially important if there is any chance that those fluids will come in contact with any break in the skin. As with the condom, latex gloves offer barrier protection from HIV transmission.

BIOTERRORISM

You may be familiar with terrorism as a behavior used by some political groups to gain control, inflict damage to communities, or raise awareness of their political causes. Terrorism can occur in many forms, such as suicide bombings. **Bioterrorism** is terrorism through the use of biological weapons such as the spread of deadly anthrax spores into a community. The threat of bioterrorism is monitored by the U.S. Department of Homeland Security, created in response to terrorist attacks in New York City and Washington, D.C. in 2001. In addition to developing plans to address threats by all types of terrorism, the department developed categories to classify biological weapons in order of their potential threat. Category A agents pose the greatest threat to the American public, are easily transmitted, and have high mortality rates. Anthrax and smallpox are examples of Category A threats. The government is doing the most to address threats from this category. Category B and Category C threats are not easily transmitted and are less life threatening.

bioterrorism

a form of terrorism in which biological agents (pathogens) are used to infect large segments of a population

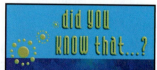

did you know that...?

No one has ever died from AIDS. People with AIDS die from diseases that arise because of a weakened immune system.

Anthrax

Anthrax is a Category A agent we heard a lot about in October 2001. Several citizens and government employees received letters in the mail that included a fine white powder, which, when analyzed, turned out to be anthrax. Anthrax is a bacterial infection that can be transmitted in a number of ways, but it cannot be spread from person to person.

1. ***Inhalation.*** This is the most serious form of anthrax and causes death in 99% of the cases if not treated quickly. This is what happened to some of the people who opened the contaminated mail. Inhaled anthrax infection usually starts with symptoms that are the same as severe colds and flu, but breathing soon becomes difficult. The general public does not come into contact with this form of anthrax unless it is introduced to the environment by criminals or terrorists. Farmworkers can be exposed when they deal with materials from infected animals.

2. ***Skin contact.*** Anthrax can cause infections if it comes into contact with cuts or scratches. This is the least serious form, causing painless blisters that break and develop black scabs.

3. ***Oral consumption.*** This is the least common method of spreading anthrax to humans. It can be caused by eating undercooked meat from an infected animal.

Our bodies have some natural defenses to anthrax so that not everyone who is exposed to the bacteria gets the disease. All three types of anthrax are treatable with antibiotics, so it is important see a doctor quickly if exposure is suspected. Although there is a vaccine available for anthrax, it may have serious side effects.

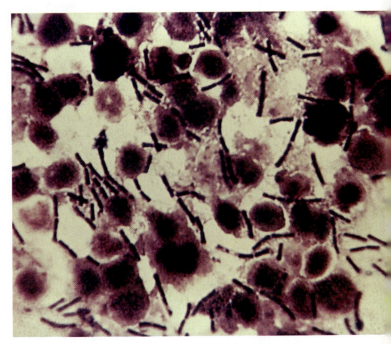

Photomicrograph of *Bacillus anthracis* (anthrax bacteria)

Smallpox

Another Category A agent is smallpox. Smallpox is a serious, contagious, and sometimes fatal infectious disease that is caused by a virus. There is no treatment or cure for smallpox, but there is a vaccine. Because of this very effective vaccine, the last case of naturally occurring smallpox in the United States was in 1949, and the last case in the world was in 1977 in Somalia. The symptoms of smallpox are high fever, headaches and body aches, nausea, and scabs that crust over and leave scars. Smallpox is usually spread by person-to-person contact, body fluids, or touching clothing or other contaminated items. Smallpox is rarely spread through the air because it is a fragile virus.

BUILDING YOUR Wellness Plan

Infectious disease is a significant health problem, but it is something that can be easily prevented by including certain behaviors discussed in this chapter in your wellness plan.

- Keep your hands clean, especially after using the toilet and before eating.
- Be sure you and your family members are fully immunized according to medical recommendations.
- Understand the chain of infection and practice the behaviors that prevent transmission of infectious diseases.
- Understand that barrier contraception, such as condoms, is only partially effective in preventing the transmission of STIs, while abstinence is 100% effective.
- Learn all you can about infectious diseases and keep up to date with prevention practices and treatments.

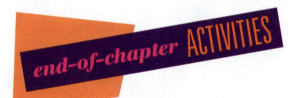

end-of-chapter ACTIVITIES

Weblinks

Bioterrorism

Centers for Disease Control and Prevention:
http://www.bt.cdc.gov

Food Handling

Center for Food Safety and Applied Nutrition:
http://www.cfsan.fda.gov

Fungi

Tree of Life: **http://tolweb.org/tree** (search for fungi)

HIV and AIDS

Body Health Resources: **http://www.thebody.com**

Centers for Disease Control and Prevention:
http://www.cdc.gov/hiv/dhap.htm

Infectious and Parasitic Diseases

Centers for Disease Control and Prevention:
http://www.cdc.gov/ncidod/dpd

West Nile Virus

Centers for Disease Control and Prevention:
http://www.cdc.gov/ncidod/dvbid/westnile

Short-Answer Questions

1. What do you think is the most important way you can prevent the spread of the common cold and flu?
2. Name three common infectious diseases that spread easily from person to person.
3. List six types of pathogenic organisms.
4. What is the portal of entry for the common cold?
5. Name the most deadly form of anthrax.

Discussion Questions

1. Describe the importance of the chain of infection and explain each link.
2. List and explain the stages of disease.
3. Explain how personal behaviors can contribute to food poisoning.

4. Discuss two ways you can prevent food poisoning.

5. Explain the concept of bioterrorism and why it is currently such an important issue.

☀ Chapter Vocabulary

Using a separate sheet of paper, list and define the following terms:

bioterrorism	modes of transmission
carrier	opportunistic infection
chain of infection	pathogenic organisms
fomite	secondary infection
infectious disease	

☀ Application Activities

Language Arts Connection

Visit the Centers for Disease Control and Prevention (CDC) Web site and locate information on bioterrorism. Write a report about how communities can prepare to handle biological threats.

Math Connection

Choose an infectious disease and gather information about the distribution of disease cases in the United States by all races. Prepare a graph that compares the number of cases of the disease for each race over the past three years.

Social Studies Connection

Using the same disease you chose in the Math application activity, visit the CDC's or your state health department's Web site and locate statistics about it. Create a chart that shows the trend of disease cases over the past 10 years, and prepare a report that explains what can be done to reduce the number of cases.

answers to PERSONAL ASSESSMENT QUIZ

personal assessment: PERSONAL HABITS

1. You want to make sure you have all the immunizations you need for your age group. Some immunizations require booster injections at certain time periods.

2. The germs that make you sick, such as the common cold virus, are most likely to get into your body because of dirty hands.

3. Some diseases, such as head lice or ringworm, can be transmitted by hair-care devices. Blood-borne diseases can be transmitted by razors.

4. If you don't, you may be contaminating surfaces and spreading disease to others.

5. If they have a cold or flu, you can become infected (and you can't wipe the germs off the bottle, can, or straw).

6. Clean footwear can reduce the possibility of foot odor and athlete's foot.

7. Your teen years are pretty healthy, but a checkup can find disease problems before they get too advanced.

8. HIV infection is incurable. It is transmitted by blood-to-blood contact.

9. Everyone should know how to handle food products to reduce the possibility of food poisoning.

10. Each of these activities is a good wellness practice.

chapter 24

Chronic Diseases

When her grandmother was diagnosed with cancer of the thyroid, Leena was really upset. She is very close to her grandmother, and it was scary knowing that she had a serious disease. Leena didn't know much about cancer but had heard it could be fatal. Her mom didn't know much either, so Leena decided to put her health literacy skills to work and get some information. She went on the Web and, after looking for "cancer," narrowed her search to "thyroid cancer." She learned that this type isn't usually a deadly form of the disease. In fact, most women who get thyroid cancer can be cured. Leena is still concerned, but she feels better knowing her grandmother's condition is not as serious as she first thought. She's also glad that the cancer was found early, an important factor in successful treatment.

chapter OBJECTIVES

When you finish this chapter, you should be able to:

- Explain the difference between infectious disease and chronic disease.
- State the known risk factors for heart disease.
- List the common causes of heart attacks and strokes.
- List the signs and symptoms of heart attacks and strokes.
- Explain what cancer is.
- List the risk factors for some cancers.
- Describe the following conditions: asthma, diabetes, and migraine headaches.

key TERMS

atherosclerosis
benign tumor
biopsy
cholesterol
coronary artery disease
diabetes
hypertension
insulin
metastasis
migraine

chronic disease

a disease condition that continues for a long time

Introduction

For centuries, infectious diseases were the major killers of people of all ages. With the introduction of better health practices and the development of antibiotics, infectious diseases are no longer the threat they once were. **Chronic diseases** are currently the leading causes of death among Americans. Chronic diseases are conditions that are not caused by pathogens and tend to last for a long period of time. With the control of infectious diseases, people live much longer, and, as they age, the risks increase for conditions such as heart disease and cancer. There are many chronic conditions that are not life threatening, but they can reduce the quality of life for people who have them.

Most teens don't worry too much about chronic diseases, believing them to be problems of older adults. But the teen years are actually the best time to develop the habits that help prevent chronic conditions from occurring later. And there are chronic conditions, such as migraine headaches or arthritis, that can affect teens. This chapter discusses chronic diseases, what they are, and what you can do to reduce your risks of getting many of them.

personal assessment: HEART DISEASE

What do you already know about heart disease? Read each of the statements below and record on a separate sheet of paper whether you think each is true or false. The answers appear at the end of the chapter.

1. High blood cholesterol is a risk factor for heart disease that you can control.
2. A blood cholesterol level up to 240 is okay for adults.
3. Fish oil supplements are good for lowering blood cholesterol.
4. Vegetable oils are good for lowering cholesterol.
5. The number one cause of death in the United States is heart disease.
6. All children should have their cholesterol level checked.
7. All types of vegetable oils help lower blood cholesterol levels.

THE NATURE OF CHRONIC DISEASES

Chronic diseases affect the majority of people in this country at some point in their lives. To see just how widespread they are, take a look around your classroom and count the students. Divide the total by four. Now multiply your answer by three. This is how many of your fellow students are likely to die of a chronic disease later in life. That's right; about 70% of all deaths in this country are caused by some form of chronic disease.

Because chronic diseases are related to lifestyle habits and not usually caused by bacteria, antibiotics cannot cure them. Among the diseases that cannot be cured with antibiotics are the three leading causes of death in the United States: heart attack, cancer, and stroke. The good news is that the health behaviors under your control are your best defense against chronic diseases. Applying what you learn in this chapter can positively influence both how well and how long you live.

CARDIOVASCULAR DISEASE

The most common chronic disease, responsible for more than 40% of the deaths in the United States, is **cardiovascular disease**, which is any disease of the heart and blood vessels. The most common cardiovascular diseases are **hypertension**, **heart attack**, and **stroke**.

Hypertension

Hypertension means blood pressure that is always higher than normal. Blood pressure is the force exerted by the blood as it travels through the

cardiovascular disease

a disease condition that affects the heart or circulatory system

hypertension

increased pressure in the arteries against which the heart must pump the blood

heart attack

the death of heart muscle cells due to an inadequate supply of oxygen

stroke

an event in the brain that cuts off the blood supply to a section of brain tissue

arteries. Normal blood pressure is about 120/80 mm Hg. Blood pressure is measured in millimeters of mercury (mm Hg). The higher number in this ratio is the measure of pressure when the heart contracts and squeezes blood out into the arteries. This is known as **systolic pressure**. The lower number (**diastolic pressure**) is the pressure of blood in the arteries as the heart relaxes between beats. Hypertension can strain the heart, causing it to enlarge and weaken. It can also cause the arteries to harden, or lose their elasticity.

In the United States, one out of five Americans (one in four adults) has hypertension. About one third of these people don't know they have it, which is why it's called "the silent killer." Left untreated, hypertension can lead to stroke or damage the heart, kidneys, and other organs. The cause of hypertension in 90%–95% of cases is unknown, although the risk factors for cardiovascular disease, discussed later in this chapter, contribute to hypertension.

Because there are no symptoms, the only way to diagnose hypertension is by having the blood pressure checked with an instrument called a **sphygmomanometer** (see Figure 24-1). This is a special cuff that is put around the upper arm and inflated with air to cut off the blood flow through the arm. The air is then let out of the cuff to allow the blood flow to return to the arm. With a manual sphygmomanometer, a trained person listens to the sounds in the blood vessels with a stethoscope. With an electronic sphygmomanometer, the sounds in the blood vessels are detected with a machine.

Blood pressure readings above 140/90 are considered to be high. Individuals with high blood pressure may be advised to change one or more of their lifestyle habits. Depending on the person, these changes might include increasing physical exercise, quitting smoking, reducing alcohol consumption, losing weight, using less salt, or managing diabetes. If following these recommendations doesn't lower the blood pressure to within a normal range, medication may be prescribed.

There is a medical condition known as low blood pressure, but the condition is generally not life threatening the way high blood pressure is. Low blood pressure does not cause a strain on the heart; rather, it can produce feelings of light-headedness or dizziness. It is important to see your health care provider if you experience symptoms such as shortness of breath, fainting spells, headaches, or fever over 101 degrees Fahrenheit.

Heart Attack

The heart is a muscular organ that needs its own blood supply to function properly. Special arteries, different from those that supply the rest of the body, ensure that the heart receives the nutrients it needs to continue pumping. Called coronary arteries, their insides are normally smooth, much like a nonstick cooking surface. This surface can become very uneven because of the gradual buildup and hardening of

systolic pressure

pressure measured in the arteries as the heart is pumping blood into the arteries

diastolic pressure

pressure measured in the arteries as the heart relaxes to fill with blood

sphygmomanometer

a device used to measure blood pressure

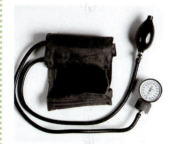

Figure 24-1
A sphygmomanometer

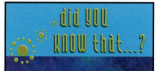

The average person's heart beats 72 times a minute, or 103,680 times a day! A good aerobic exercise program will make the heart muscle more efficient so that when the body is at rest, the heart can beat at a slower rate to move the same amount of blood.

atherosclerosis

a buildup of firm fatty deposits along the inner lining of the arteries, which causes the opening inside the artery to narrow and lose elasticity

coronary artery disease

atherosclerosis in the coronary arteries

material known as plaque. This process is known as **atherosclerosis** and can be the result of both hereditary factors and lifestyle habits. If there is too much atherosclerotic plaque, the coronary arteries can become partially blocked and unable to supply the heart muscle with the blood and nutrients it needs (see Figure 24-2). This condition is called **coronary artery disease**. As the arteries become more and more clogged, the heart will actually start to hurt, a condition called angina. This is the heart's way of saying it needs more oxygen. If the condition continues to worsen, it can result in what we call a heart attack. Heart attacks vary in the amount of damage involved. In some cases, the heart continues to pump, but some of the muscle cells die for lack of sufficient oxygen. In other cases, a coronary artery becomes so restricted that the heart stops working altogether. These differences explain why some people have a heart attack and don't even know it, whereas others die before they fall to the floor.

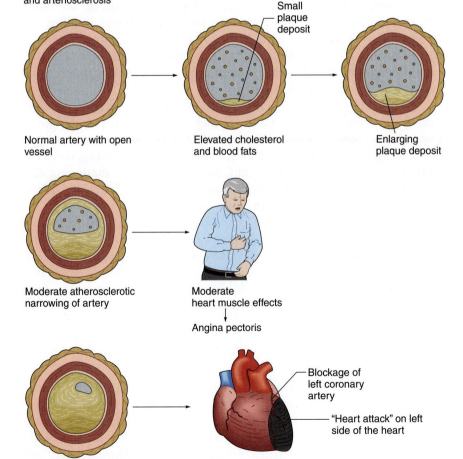

Cross sections through a coronary artery undergoing progressive atherosclerosis and arteriosclerosis

Small plaque deposit

Normal artery with open vessel

Elevated cholesterol and blood fats

Enlarging plaque deposit

Moderate atherosclerotic narrowing of artery

Moderate heart muscle effects

Angina pectoris

Blockage of left coronary artery

"Heart attack" on left side of the heart

Complete/almost complete blockage, with hardening due to calcium deposits

Severe acute heart damage

Figure 24-2

Atherosclerosis: narrowing of the artery

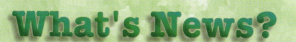

What's News?

Research by Robert J. Genco, D.D.S., Ph.D., at the University of Buffalo School of Dental Medicine, has uncovered a possible link between gum disease and heart disease. It appears that the bacteria that contribute to gum disease may also play a role in causing plaque buildup in coronary blood vessels. One more reason to take good care of the teeth and gums!

Symptoms of a heart attack vary from person to person, ranging from no symptoms at all to any of the following:

- *Chest pain.* The pain is not usually sharp. Victims of heart attacks describe it as a crushing, squeezing pain or a tight constriction. This pain usually starts in the center of the chest and then spreads or moves around, going to either shoulder, down the arms, or into the jaw.

- *Heavy sweating.* Most heart attack victims sweat very heavily, even if they are not doing any physical activity.

- *Nausea.* Nausea is a common heart attack symptom, especially in women.

- *Shortness of breath.* Many heart attack victims report it is hard for them to "catch their breath."

- *Fainting.*

Most heart attack victims, when experiencing symptoms, deny the possibility they are having a heart attack. This attitude prevents them from getting needed help. Most deaths from heart attacks occur within two hours after symptoms begin, with the victim never reaching the hospital. Permanent damage to the heart and death can often be prevented if the victim gets help and treatment without delay. If you are

✢ teen forum ✢

Should Tobacco Companies Pay?

Cigarette smoking has been linked to both heart disease and cancer. Several states have sued the tobacco industry for billions of dollars to recover some of the money they spent caring for people with tobacco-related illnesses. The states believe the tobacco companies have been dishonest about their products and don't care if cigarettes make people sick. Talk with your family and friends about the responsibility for tobacco-related illnesses.

- Should the tobacco companies bear some responsibility for illness, or are the people who use tobacco products at fault?
- Should smokers be required to pay for their own health care?

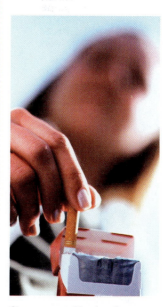

Cigarette smoking has been found to cause both heart disease and cancer.

with someone who is experiencing any of the symptoms of a heart attack, have the person stop whatever he or she is doing and rest. If the symptoms last for more than a couple of minutes, contact the emergency medical services. Heart attack is a true medical emergency.

Treating Heart Disease

Medical advances have resulted in a variety of treatments for heart disease, ranging from cholesterol-lowering medications to heart transplants. One commonly used procedure to enlarge clogged arteries is called **angioplasty**, in which a small balloon is inserted into a clogged artery. The balloon is then inflated to press the plaque against the wall of the artery and increase the size of the opening allowing better blood flow. If the blockage is too great, coronary bypass surgery is performed. In this procedure, the surgeon removes a small section of vein from the patient's leg and attaches it to the heart to create a "bypass" around the damaged artery (see Figure 24-3). Have you heard the term *triple bypass*? This is the procedure performed when three arteries are blocked and they are replaced by three veins.

Stroke

A stroke occurs when the blood supply to the brain is cut off. Stroke can be caused by a blockage in the arteries (atherosclerosis) that supply oxygen to the brain, or it can be caused by a ruptured blood vessel. Because a stroke usually occurs on only one side of the brain, symptoms

angioplasty

medical procedure in which a small balloon is inserted into a clogged coronary artery and inflated to reduce an obstruction

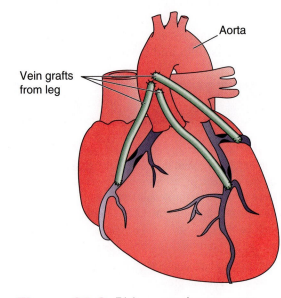

Figure 24-3 Triple coronary bypass surgery

usually occur on only one side of the body. Possible symptoms of stroke include:

- Sudden weakness, numbness, or paralysis in an arm, a hand, leg, foot, or the face
- Sudden loss of speech, slurred speech, or incoherent speech, and/or trouble understanding the speech of others
- Sudden loss of vision or experience of dimness (usually happens in only one eye)
- Sudden unexplained dizziness, unsteadiness, or falling
- Loss of consciousness

Because stroke affects the brain, it is important to contact emergency medical services immediately, even if symptoms are slight or only temporary. Symptoms that last for less than 24 hours may be a ministroke. Ministrokes tend to occur just before a full stroke. The sooner a stroke victim gets medical attention, the less brain damage will occur. Stroke is another true medical emergency.

Risk Factors for Cardiovascular Disease

Years of research have revealed that certain characteristics put people at risk for cardiovascular disease. Two types of risk factors have been identified:

1. Risk factors you cannot change or control (nonmodifiable risk factors)
2. Risk factors you can change or control (modifiable risk factors)

The three major nonmodifiable cardiovascular risk factors are heredity, age, and gender.

1. *Heredity.* Having close family members who have heart disease is a significant risk factor for the disease. Certain racial groups are at a higher risk than others. For example, approximately 30% more African Americans will die from heart disease than will white Americans.

2. *Age.* The older a person is, the more likely he or she will develop heart disease. One reason is that as a person ages, the arteries lose some of their ability to expand and relax easily as the blood is pumped through them. But heart disease can start very early in life. Deposits of plaque have been found in the arteries of children and teenagers, so it is clear that preventive behaviors are important to young people.

3. *Gender.* During their childbearing years, women have less heart disease than men of the same age because of a protective effect from estrogen. Once women go through menopause and estrogen levels decrease, they are just as likely to develop heart disease as men.

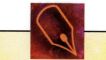

take it on home

Talk to as many of your family members as you can to find out if there is a history of heart disease among your relatives. If there is, collect information about members who have heart disease, or had heart disease but did not die from it, or had heart disease and died from it. What risk factors did they have? Prepare a short report for your Health Folio that summarizes what your risks might be, based on what you learned. Identify what your wellness plan should include to reduce any risks you might have.

Smoking, inactivity, high cholesterol, obesity and overweight, and hypertension are five of the most important modifiable risk factors—factors that are under *your* control.

Smoking

Smokers have a much higher risk of heart disease than nonsmokers because smoking raises the level of carbon monoxide in the blood, which can damage the walls of veins and arteries. Smoking also makes the heart beat faster, narrows the blood vessels, raises blood pressure, and causes the blood to become sticky so it clings to the walls of arteries more easily.

Inactivity

Lack of exercise is a major risk factor for cardiovascular disease. Exercise, especially aerobic exercise, makes the heart stronger and more efficient, helps the body manufacture the good kind of cholesterol known as **high-density lipoprotein** (HDL), and improves circulation.

High Cholesterol

Cholesterol is a type of fatty substance found in the body and circulates in the bloodstream. There are different types of cholesterol, each with a different effect on the body. The "bad" cholesterols are LDLs (low-density lipoproteins) and VLDLs (very low-density lipoproteins). Lipoproteins are protein molecules that carry fat. High-density lipoprotein (HDL) is considered "good" cholesterol because HDL molecules act as "cholesterol sponges," picking up and carrying off large amounts of fat from the bloodstream. When large amounts of bad cholesterol are present in the bloodstream, they can accumulate in the arteries and make them narrower. Therefore, as blood cholesterol rises, so does the risk of coronary artery disease. Table 24-1 lists the levels of cholesterol and their degree of risk.

Whereas smoking and eating a high-fat diet cause the body to produce bad cholesterol, exercise helps it produce good cholesterol.

high-density lipoprotein

fatty protein in the blood that helps carry cholesterol

cholesterol

a soft, waxy type of fat that circulates in the bloodstream

Table 24-1 Cholesterol Levels and Risk

Total Cholesterol (mg/dL)		LDL Cholesterol (mg/dL)		HDL Cholesterol (mg/dL)	
<200	Desirable	<100	Optimal	<40	Low
200–239	Borderline high	100–129	Near optimal/above optimal	≥60	High
≥240	High	130–159	Borderline high		
		160–189	High		
		≥190	Very high		

What's News?

A new blood test is now available that detects heart attack risk. The test detects levels of C-reactive protein (CRP), an indicator of inflamed blood vessel walls, which are associated with heart attack risk.

Cholesterol level is also affected by age, sex, and heredity. Have you heard the term *hardening of the arteries*? Atherosclerosis is the medical term for this condition, and it is one of the consequences of high cholesterol levels, especially LDLs. As fat deposits and calcium build up along the walls of the arteries, they form a substance called plaque. Atherosclerosis can start early in childhood. In fact, scientists have found evidence of the beginning of fat streaks in the arteries of children as young as three years old.

Obesity and Overweight

People who have excess body fat are more likely to develop cardiovascular disease, even if they have no other risk factors. Excess weight raises blood pressure, which in turn causes a strain on the heart and also raises LDL cholesterol and triglycerides (fats that are converted from foods we eat). Overweight also causes lower levels of HDLs.

Hypertension

Hypertension is a risk factor for heart disease. It is normal for blood pressure to vary from moment to moment, and it is highly influenced by factors such as activity level, eating, and stress. But blood pressure that consistently measures over 140/90 is considered hypertension.

Understanding your risk factors not only helps you know if you are at risk for cardiovascular disease, it also lets you know the specific modifiable risk factors you can change. Although there are risk factors you can't change or control, it is important to identify and work on those risk factors that you can change. Doing things to eliminate risk factors is a wise decision even as a teen or young adult.

CANCER

Cancer, the uncontrolled growth and spread of abnormal body cells, is a very significant chronic condition. The American Cancer Society reports that one out of every two men and one out of every three women will have some form of cancer sometime during their lifetime. Hardly anyone escapes either getting cancer or having someone close to them develop the disease. Although 77% of all cancers occur in people over age 55, it can occur at any time during the life span.

cancer

the uncontrolled growth and spread of abnormal cells in the body

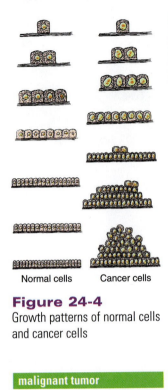

Figure 24-4
Growth patterns of normal cells and cancer cells

malignant tumor
abnormal growth of cells forming a cancerous tumor

metastasis
the spread of cancer from one site to another location in the body

benign tumors
abnormal growth of cells that form a noncancerous tumor

biopsy
the removal of a tiny piece of a tumor for examination under a microscope

Can you see the difference between the cancerous and normal cells in Figure 24-4? Normal cells reproduce and grow at a certain set, controlled rate. For example, one cell divides into two cells; two cells become four; and so on. Cancer cells grow at a faster, abnormal rate. They develop into bundles of cells called **malignant tumors**, which can interfere with the body's normal functions. When cancer cells first begin to grow, they usually stay in one area of the body. If they are not treated, they can eventually detach from the original tumor and spread to other sites in the body. This process is called **metastasis** and often results in death. Lung cancer, for example, often spreads to the brain.

Not all tumors are cancerous. Some tumors are known as **benign tumors** because they don't spread wildly or threaten life. Table 24-2 compares the characteristics of normal and cancer cells. If a doctor suspects that a person has cancer, a **biopsy** is performed. This is a surgical procedure that involves removing a tiny piece of the tumor and examining it under a microscope to see if the tissue is cancerous. Malignant tumor cells are irregular in shape, size, and growth patterns and usually invade the surrounding tissue.

Factors That Contribute to Cancer

Certain types of cancer are related to personal behaviors. For example, smoking causes lung cancer and contributes to other types, such as cancer of the bladder, esophagus, and breast. In fact, one-third of all cancer deaths are caused by smoking. Smokeless tobacco causes oral cancers such as cancer of the tongue and mouth.

Many years of scientific research have revealed a number of other factors, in addition to smoking, that are related to cancer formation. Notice how many of these are under your control. Think about how

Table 24-2 Cell Growth

Characteristic	Normal Cells	Cancer Cells
Genetic makeup	Identical	Varied
Cell structure	Identical	Varied
Cell function	Serve a purpose	Loss of identity so they fail to function as normal cells do
Location	Stay where they originated	Loose, can easily spread to other areas of the body
Cell life	Fixed and finite	Longer than normal cells
Cell reproduction	Regulated	No regulation

having this information gives you the power to effectively fight one of the top killers of our time.

1. ***Diet.*** There appears to be a strong relationship between diet and certain cancers, both positive and negative. Some foods, especially fruits and vegetables that supply antioxidants, beta carotene, and fiber, protect against cancer. On the other hand, some foods, especially those that contain large amounts of sugar and dietary fat, can contribute to cancer formation. Excessive amounts of alcohol also contribute to the formation of certain cancers.

2. ***Occupational and environmental factors.*** Exposure to certain chemicals may cause brain, lung, and other cancers. Perhaps the most common environmental factor is sun exposure, which is strongly related to skin cancer. Most cancers from sun exposure develop years after the exposure takes place. Every year in the United States, there are about a million new cases of skin cancer, more than the number of all of other cancers combined. Individuals exposed to the sun for more than a half-hour are advised to use sun protection.

3. ***Infectious Agents.*** Certain viruses are related to some types of cancer. For example, the same virus that causes mononucleosis is responsible for Burkitt lymphoma, a type of cancer found in African children. Many cases of liver cancer have been connected to hepatitis A and B viruses. And some cases of cervical cancer have been linked to the human papilloma virus, the same virus that causes genital warts and is transmitted through sexual contact.

4. ***Obesity.*** Obese individuals will not necessarily get cancer, but evidence does suggest that obesity may be a risk factor.

5. ***Inactivity.*** Scientists believe that about one-third of all cancer deaths are related to diet and lack of exercise. The latest guidelines suggest that exercising for at least 30 minutes a day, five times a week can protect against cancer. Forty-five minutes is recommended for preventing breast and colon cancers.

6. ***Genetics.*** Some types of cancer tend to run in families. These include breast cancer, colon cancer, ovarian cancer, and uterine cancer.

Cancer Treatments

The sooner cancer is detected, the more likely it is to be cured. One of the best things you can do to protect yourself against this disease is to know and watch for the warning signs of cancer, listed in Figure 24-5. In addition, self-examinations should be performed monthly: breast exams for women and testicular exams for men.

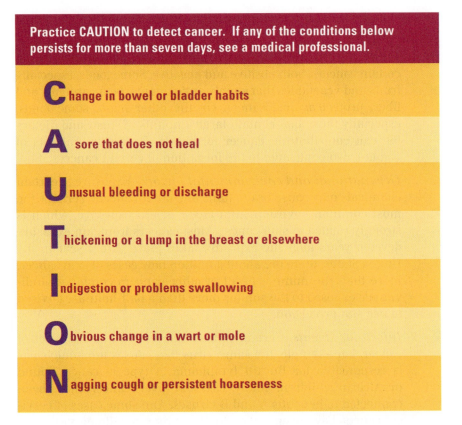

Practice **CAUTION** to detect cancer. If any of the conditions below persists for more than seven days, see a medical professional.

Change in bowel or bladder habits

A sore that does not heal

Unusual bleeding or discharge

Thickening or a lump in the breast or elsewhere

Indigestion or problems swallowing

Obvious change in a wart or mole

Nagging cough or persistent hoarseness

Figure 24-5
The seven warning signs of cancer

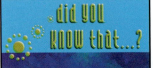

did you know that...?

Chemotherapy causes hair loss because the treatment is designed to stop fast-growing cells, such as cancer cells, from reproducing and growing. The problem is that hair follicles are also fast-growing cells, so hair growth stops until chemotherapy treatment has been completed.

There are several kinds of treatment for cancer; the kind used depends on the type of cancer and the stage at which it is detected. The most common treatment is surgery, in which the malignant tumor and a large area of normal tissue around it are removed. Nearby lymph nodes are often removed to ensure that cancer cells do not travel through the lymph system and metastasize. A patient is considered cured if the cancer has not metastasized into nearby lymph nodes or the bloodstream and if the surgeon is able to remove all the cancerous cells. Cancers that are treated with surgery include cancers of the head and neck, lung, breast, colon, ovaries, prostate, uterus, and thyroid.

The second most common type of treatment is radiation, received by almost half of all cancer patients. Radiation beams do not kill cancer cells but destroy their ability to reproduce. Radiation is used for treating Hodgkin's disease and cancers of the brain, throat, bone, testicles, and cervix. Unfortunately, radiation has some unpleasant side effects, which include diarrhea, fatigue, difficulty swallowing, intense itching, and lack of taste and smell.

Chemotherapy, another type of cancer treatment, involves giving drugs or hormones, or both, to treat cancer that has spread from its original site. As does radiation, chemotherapy often has unpleasant side effects, which can be quite serious and may include nausea, vomiting, diarrhea, anemia, hair loss, and lowered immunity.

OTHER CHRONIC CONDITIONS

In addition to the life-threatening chronic conditions, there are less serious chronic ailments that are troublesome to good health and can require continual medical attention. These conditions can affect teens as well as adults.

Asthma

Asthma is a chronic disease in which the airways (bronchial tubes) swell, spasm, and produce larger than normal amounts of mucus. During an asthma flare, sometimes called an asthma attack, breathing is difficult. A flare may be brought on by a variety of triggers such as allergens, tobacco smoke, exercise, changes in weather, viral infections, and smog. Because the triggers vary from person to person, treatment also varies. Some people can control their asthma by avoiding their triggers; others need medication.

Asthma is the number one reason for school absences among children. In fact, about 14 million days of school are missed each year by kids who have asthma. Asthma can be a serious condition, so if you sometimes have difficulty breathing, it is best to see your doctor.

asthma

a condition of the lungs characterized by periodic episodes of airway spasms, causing shortness of breath

Diabetes

Most of the food we eat is turned into sugar to be used as energy by our body cells. **Insulin** is a hormone produced in the pancreas that enables sugar molecules to enter the body cells. When the body either does not produce enough insulin or cannot correctly use the insulin that is produced, a condition known as diabetes develops. **Diabetes** is characterized by high levels of sugar in the bloodstream. Excessively high blood sugar levels can result in many serious complications, including death. In the United States, diabetes is the seventh leading cause of death.

There are three major types of diabetes:

1. Type I diabetes: must be controlled with a daily insulin injection (shot)
2. Type II diabetes: less severe form that can be managed without insulin injections
3. Gestational diabetes: affects only pregnant women

About 85% to 90% of American diabetics have type II diabetes, and most of these people are mature adults. Diabetes is becoming more prevalent, and, with the rising level of obesity in children, physicians are now seeing many teens with type II diabetes. Most type II diabetics can control their diabetes with diet, exercise, and weight control. In some cases, drugs are also used to bring the disease under control.

Type I diabetes is most often found in children and young adults. Gestational diabetes is usually temporary and goes away after the woman gives birth. Women who have had gestational diabetes are,

insulin

a hormone produced in the pancreas that is used by the body to turn sugar into energy

diabetes

a disease characterized by high levels of sugar in the bloodstream caused by the body's either not producing enough insulin or not correctly using the insulin that is produced

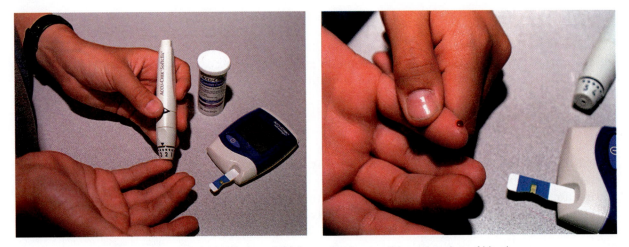

Blood glucose monitoring is now a relatively simple and painless procedure requiring only a drop of blood.

however, at higher risk of getting diabetes in the future than are women who do not experience gestational diabetes.

We don't know what causes diabetes, but heredity, obesity, and lack of exercise play an important role in the development of the disease. Diabetes is diagnosed with blood tests, and its symptoms include frequent urination, excessive thirst, unexplained weight loss, fatigue, and sores that heal slowly.

Diabetes can be very dangerous if it is not treated because it can lead to cardiovascular disease, kidney disease and failure, blindness, severe damage to the hands and feet that can require amputation, and damage to the nervous system. Diabetics must monitor their blood sugar to make sure it is under control. There now are simple test kits that require only one drop of blood, and the National Aeronautics and Space Administration (NASA) is working on a painless technique that can monitor blood sugar through the skin.

Migraine Headaches

Headaches are one of the most common reasons for doctors' office visits in the United States. There are many types of headaches, some more painful than others. One of the most debilitating is the **migraine** headache. This is a brain and nervous system disorder that is characterized by recurrent attacks of severe headache accompanied by various combinations of symptoms that include nausea, vomiting, and sensitivity to light and sound. The headache lasts from 3 to 72 hours, with the pain usually occurring on only one side of the head. Some migraine sufferers see flashing lights and bright spots or experience other changes in their vision just before the onset of the headache.

There is no known cause of migraine. The most widely accepted theory is that migraines have a hereditary component. People prone to migraine seem to have a nervous system that is very sensitive to

migraine

brain and nervous system disorder characterized by recurring attacks of severe headache

What's News?

Terrell Davis was not a teen when he played in Super Bowl XXXII for the Denver Broncos, but his story is a good example of someone who lives successfully despite suffering migraine headaches. During the first quarter of the game, Terrell was hit hard and developed the symptoms of a migraine. The bright sunlight, for example, made him feel worse, so he left the field to take his medication. He was able to return to the game in the second half, scored the winning touchdown, and earned the Most Valuable Player award for Super Bowl XXXII.

sudden changes in the body or the environment. Scientists believe that abnormal cells in the brain play a role in migraine and that certain factors, called migraine triggers, cause these abnormal cells to produce a headache. Here are some common triggers reported by migraine patients:

- Lack of food
- Lack of rest or sleep
- Exposure to light
- Hormonal disturbance, especially in women
- Stress
- Alcoholic drinks
- Chocolate
- Foods, such as cheese, sour cream, and yogurt, that contain a chemical called tyramine
- Citrus fruit, such as oranges and grapefruits
- Certain food additives, such as nitrites, MSG, and aspartame (Nutra-Sweet and Equal sweetener)

There are different types of treatments for migraines. In the past, doctors gave migraine sufferers pain medication and told them to go home and sleep. Now doctors can treat the migraine itself instead of just the pain because scientists have developed a prescription family of drugs, known as ergot alkaloids, that are effective in treating severe migraines. These drugs halt a migraine attack by preventing dilation of the blood vessels in the brain. Some migraine sufferers help themselves with relaxation exercises, stress management strategies, and biofeedback. These techniques can also be used to prevent migraine headaches from occurring in the first place.

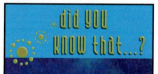

did you KNOW that...?

Women are three times more likely to suffer from migraine headaches than men. There is no clear reason why, but scientists suspect it is related to female hormones and the reproductive system.

Osteoporosis

Osteo means "bone," and *porosis* means "porous." Thus, osteoporosis is a condition in which the bones are porous and brittle. The condition can affect men and women, but of the approximately 44 million Americans at

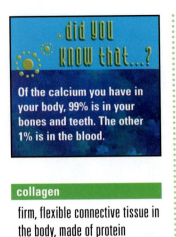

collagen

firm, flexible connective tissue in the body, made of protein

risk for this disease, 68% are women. Although osteoporosis is more likely to occur in the older adult, young people can have the condition. More important, osteoporosis begins to develop during the teen years.

Your bones are living tissue. They are made primarily of calcium and **collagen**, a protein substance that gives structural flexibility in bones and other tissues such as your nose and ears. During your lifetime, calcium is constantly removed from bone and replaced. During your childhood and teen years, calcium is replaced faster than it is removed, causing the bones to become stronger. In your later years, the calcium tends to be removed faster than it is replaced.

This imbalance results in the bones becoming more brittle as you age. For some people, this brittling is severe. The bones become very porous and fragile (osteoporosis), and they are easily broken, especially at places where breaks normally do not occur.

A number of risk factors are associated with the development of osteoporosis. Some of these factors are not within your personal control, such as your gender, your genetic makeup, and your age. But there are things you can include in your wellness lifestyle that reduce your chances of getting osteoporosis: exercise, calcium intake, and avoiding tobacco use. The more of the controllable risk factors you manage, the more you can offset uncontrollable risk factors. Table 24-3 lists some of the risk factors for osteoporosis.

Table 24-3   Osteoporosis Risk Factors

Uncontrollable Risk Factors	
Gender	Your chances of developing osteoporosis are greater if you are a woman. Women generally have less bone tissue and lose bone more rapidly than men because of estrogen loss during menopause.
Body size	Small-framed women are at greater risk than large-framed women.
Race	Anglo and Asian women are at greater risk than Hispanic and African American women, though their risk is still significant.
Family history	People who come from a family in which someone has osteoporosis are at greater risk for the condition than are people whose family has no history of osteoporosis.
Age	The older a person is, the greater the risk.
Controllable Risk Factors	
Hormones	Abnormal absence of menstrual periods, low estrogen level (menopause), and low testosterone level in men increase the risk.
Diet	A lifetime diet low in calcium and vitamin D increases the risk.
Exercise	An inactive lifestyle, especially the absence of weight-bearing exercise, increases the risk.
Cigarette smoking	Women who smoke have lower levels of estrogen than do nonsmokers.
Alcohol	Two or 3 ounces of alcohol daily can have a harmful effect on the skeleton.

BUILDING YOUR Wellness Plan

The causes of many chronic diseases are under your control, developing habits to reduce your risks is a very important part of your wellness plan. The behaviors you practice as a teen set the stage for the condition of your body in adulthood.

Prevent cardiovascular disease by following these recommendations:

- Don't smoke.
- Get plenty of exercise.
- Eat fruits and vegetables and avoid high-fat foods.
- Keep your weight within a normal range.

Some cancers can be prevented. Here are some things you can do now to decrease your chances of getting cancer in the future:

- Don't smoke.
- Protect yourself from the sun's harmful rays.
- Eat a low-fat diet rich in fruit and vegetables.
- Get regular exercise.
- Protect yourself from things in your environment that may cause cancer.
- Get regular medical checkups.
- Perform self-examinations such as breast exams and testicular exams.
- Learn and remember the early warning signs of cancer.

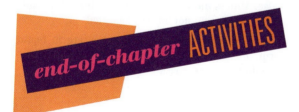

end-of-chapter ACTIVITIES

Weblinks

Circulatory System, Heart Disease, and Stroke
American Heart Association:
  http://www.americanheart.org

Lung Health
American Lung Association: **http://www.lungusa.org**

Nutrition and Cancer
American Cancer Society: **http://www.cancer.org**

Short-Answer Questions

1. Name the leading cause of death in the United States.
2. List the heart disease risk factors you can change or control.
3. Describe the symptoms of a heart attack.
4. List the symptoms of a stroke.
5. List the symptoms of a migraine headache.

Discussion Questions

1. Discuss the reasons why chronic disease has replaced infectious disease as the leading cause of death in the United States.

2. Describe what takes place when a surgeon performs "triple bypass" surgery.

3. Using two chronic diseases as examples, explain why it is important to pay attention to risk factors related to chronic diseases.

4. List the seven warning signs of cancer and explain what should be done if a person has one of these signs for more than seven days.

5. List and explain the various types of cancer treatment.

Chapter Vocabulary

Using a separate sheet of paper, list and define the following terms:

atherosclerosis	diabetes
benign tumor	hypertension
biopsy	insulin
cholesterol	metastasis
coronary artery disease	migraine

Application Activities

Math Connection

Research on the Web to find the costs for some important cardiovascular tests and procedures such as blood tests, electrocardiograms, angioplasty, and bypass surgery. Prepare a table that lists the procedures and the cost, and then prepare a report that explains what you can do now to avoid having to pay those costs later in your life.

Science Connection

1. Measure your blood pressure by learning to take it yourself, asking your physician, or finding a blood pressure machine that can be used for free. Many pharmacies and supermarkets have them available. Ask adult family members what their blood pressure is. Write these numbers down. Is your blood pressure higher or lower than theirs? Do any of them have high blood pressure?

2. Take a deep breath and exhale slowly. This is probably easy to do. Now, jump up and down for two minutes without stopping. Then put a straw in your mouth and close your lips tightly around it. Breathe in and out only through the straw. This is difficult to do, isn't it? Now, fold the straw in half and continue to breathe in and out only through the straw. This is how it feels to have asthma. Write down how it feels to breathe this way.

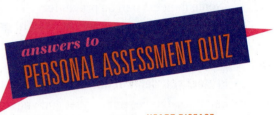

answers to
PERSONAL ASSESSMENT QUIZ

personal assessment: HEART DISEASE

1. True.

2. False. The desirable level is 200 or below.

3. False. Although fish oil supplements can have some beneficial effects, eating fish is the best way to receive the protective effect.

4. True.

5. True.

6. False. Unless there is a medical condition that calls for it, children do not have to be tested.

7. False. Vegetable oils can help if they are in liquid form. But hydrogenated oils, such as margarine, contain trans-fats, a risk for heart disease.

unit 7

Healthy Consumerism

Introduction

Throughout this book, you have learned that, through your actions, you can practice wellness and create a lot of control over your health. Wellness behaviors you develop now will affect your life as a teen and an adult. In addition to the wellness skills you have developed already, it is important for you to recognize how you may be affected by outside influences from others. Many of these outside influences will attempt to influence how you spend your money on health-related products and services.

In this unit, you will learn about the mass media and the positive and negative influences that the media may have on your health. You will also see how your critical thinking and problem-solving skills can be used to make wise choices. You will learn how to become a better consumer of information, as well as how to shop and wisely buy products and services that others want to sell you. All of these skills will be important to your wellness program as you move into adulthood.

chapter 25

Understanding the Media

Last night Chad was surfing the television channels trying to find something to watch. He passed up the dramatic shows (mostly about cops, lawyers, or doctors) and all the news talk shows. He considered a couple of comedies as possibilities but decided he really wasn't in the mood. He finally settled on an action movie with cool car crashes and people shooting at each other. After an hour or so, he got tired of watching it and turned off the television and headed for bed. He didn't think about the movie again until this morning in his health class when the teacher announced they were starting a new unit in which they would be discussing the way the media influence health. The girl who sits behind him whispered, "That means the way the media use sex to sell products and violence to solve problems." Chad thought again about the shows he had surfed last night and the movie he had watched. He wondered if watching television really had anything to do with health.

chapter OBJECTIVES

When you finish this chapter, you should be able to:

- Explain the meaning of the terms *medium*, *media*, and *mass media*.
- Define the term *media literacy*.
- Identify several ways the mass media affect health.
- List five key things to be aware of when you see, read, or hear a media message.
- List and briefly describe several ways advertisers market their products.
- Identify several questions you can ask to analyze or evaluate a media message.
- Describe some of the effects of violence and sex in the media.
- Create a personal action plan to become a wise media consumer.

Introduction

Throughout much of history, the major way to send and receive information was the spoken word. When the printing press was invented in the fifteenth century, books and newspaper "dailies" became important methods of communicating and sharing information. News could be sent over greater distances. Hundreds of years later, radio was invented and more recently television, which has become a key part of the lives of most Americans. Although television plays a role in transmitting news and information, it is used mostly for entertainment.

Now in the twenty-first century, Americans have access to more types of media than ever before. From portable radio/CD/MP3 players to films, the Internet, and DVDs, most Americans are regular consumers of media products that didn't even exist a few years ago. Various forms of the media have made important contributions to our lives and have changed the way we live, work, and play. In this chapter, we will examine media influences and their effects on our health.

key TERMS

advertising
constructed
consumers
cross-promotions
feedback
mass media
media
media literacy
media target audience
medium
product placement

Before reading this chapter, take this personal assessment about your current experiences with media products. Read the questions below and answer them as yes or no on a separate sheet of paper. Base your answers on how you feel most of the time. An interpretation of your answers is located at the end of this chapter.

1. I watch at least two hours of television almost every day.

2. I see most of the new "teen" movies at the theater.

3. I have a personal collection of movie videos.

4. I don't know how many music CDs and music videos I own.

5. I regularly talk to my friends about shows I watch on television.

6. I often buy products I see advertised on television.

7. I am among the first to know about the newest advertisements.

8. I know what products are associated with being "cool."

9. Our family has a cable connection with multiple channels.

10. Our family has an Internet connection.

DEFINING TERMS

A **medium** is any method used to communicate. **Media** is the plural form of the word *medium*. Some of the more common forms of media are books, newspapers, magazines, telephones, radios, televisions, films, and the Internet. **Mass media** are the channels for communication of messages that are produced by a few people and intended for consumption by many people, such as television programs. The intended audience for a particular form of mass media is known as the **media target audience**.

Most mass media are one-way forms of communication. **Consumers** of mass media messages have little or no opportunity to give any type of immediate **feedback** to the people who produce the messages. By contrast, in face-to-face communication, the receiver of the message may disagree, ask a question, or clarify the information received from the sender. The two parties who are communicating can discuss the message. Personal telephone calls and letters are two forms of media, or channels of communication. Both the sender and receiver can take active roles in these types of communication. Phone calls and letters are not considered to be mass media, however, because they are not intended for large numbers of people. An important characteristic of mass media is that consumers of mass media messages are mostly passive, rather than active. For example, even if you yell at the television

medium

any method used to communicate; the singular form of the word *media*

media

various methods used to communicate, such as televisions, radios, telephones, and newspapers

mass media

channels for communication of messages that are produced by a few people and intended for consumption by many people

media target audience

the group of people identified to receive a particular media message

consumers

the people who purchase a product or service

feedback

the part of the communication process in which a person can disagree, ask questions, clarify understanding, or otherwise "talk back" did you know that...?

According to a 2002 report by the Kaiser Family Foundation, on average, boys spent about a half-hour a day playing video games, whereas girls played only about 8 minutes a day. Girls, on the other hand, spent more time each day than boys listening to CDs, tapes, and the radio. Music videos were popular among both boys and girls; 49% of those interviewed said they watched these daily.

during an exciting sports event, only you and the people within hearing range are aware of your enthusiasm.

You might be surprised to learn that teenagers are one of the most common media target audiences, especially for music, television, and film products. Teenagers devote so much time and attention to these mass media products that they have been called "screenagers." Advertisers hope to shape the lifestyles and buying habits of teenagers in order to gain lifetime customers.

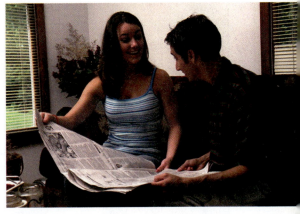

Because teenagers are such a common media target audience, it's important for you to learn to read, analyze, and evaluate the messages sent from all kinds of media. Experts believe that another important skill for modern teens is the ability to produce and communicate your own messages through many different media formats. These skills are called **media literacy**. Media literacy can contribute to developing the health literacy you learned about earlier in this text because media messages can have such a major influence on your life.

media literacy

the ability to read, analyze, evaluate, and produce communication messages in a variety of media forms

WHY ARE THE MASS MEDIA IMPORTANT TO HEALTH?

We live in a media-rich society, and Americans now spend the majority of their leisure time interacting with some form of mass media. Some experts believe that the mass media have more influence on our society than do families and schools. Children, in fact, spend twice as much time watching television as they do in school. A 1995 *Entertainment Monitor* study of 8–18 year olds found that 66% of them had a television in their bedroom. In 1997, an article in *USA Today* reported that 80% of homes in the United States had a VCR. It is estimated that more than three-quarters of homes in the United States today have cable television access. Many cable companies provide hundreds of channels. It is not surprising, then, that the mass media affect every aspect of our lives and of our health–physical, mental, social, emotional, and spiritual.

take it on home

Conduct a survey of your household and make a list of all the products that give you access to mass media messages. Interview family members about how much time they spend each day using the various types of media. How have things changed since your parents or other adult members of your family were young? What are the advantages and disadvantages of so much available media? Keep track of everyone's answers and place them in your Health Folio.

✳ teen forum ✳

Media Entertainment versus Physical Activity

As a teen, you are likely to be busy with school, extracurricular activities, work, and social activities. Most teens still manage to fit in many hours of watching television, playing video games, listening to music, and taking part in computerized entertainment. Teens who spend lots of time engaged in these activities are less likely to be physically active. This lack of physical activity is contributing to the rising rates of obesity in adolescents and may result in health problems later in life.

- In your opinion, is the time that teens spend on mass media entertainment a health problem? Give reasons for your opinion.
- What, if anything, should be done to deal with this problem (if one exists)?

When individuals spend most of their free time viewing mass media messages, they may have little time left over for other activities. It is not uncommon for teenagers to spend the majority of their leisure time watching television and videos, listening to music CDs, and playing electronic games. There is nothing wrong with those activities, but spending time with media products reduces the time available to participate in physical activities, interact with family and friends, engage in social activities, and complete schoolwork assignments.

The mass media also influence our health in more subtle ways than just consuming time. An interesting idea suggested by Bill Walsh in an article for *Media Literacy Review* is that watching large amounts of television *changes* us. It changes how we see things, what we think is important, and what we think is normal. It also influences our expectations both of ourselves and of others. Do you think watching television might have this kind of impact on you? If watching television does change us, other forms of media influence probably do too. As you read the rest of this chapter, think about how the mass media may be affecting your physical, mental, emotional, social, or spiritual health. Consider whether these effects are positive or negative.

THE MEDIA AND SOCIAL REALITY

Whether media messages are part of a television show, movie, magazine advertisement, or computer game, they all have the same purpose: to influence their audiences to think, feel, or act in a certain way. Through images, music, sound effects, special visual effects, and printed words, media messages try to spark an emotional response in the receiver of the message.

Most of us rarely try to critically analyze or evaluate what these media messages are trying to "sell" us. We are too focused on all the special effects. Let's take a look at some important facts we need to be aware of whenever we see, read, or hear a media message.

Media Messages Are Constructed

Referring to a media message as **constructed** means that producers of the message took what *really* happened and interpreted it from their particular viewpoint. Media constructions may use text, sounds, or visual effects; many use all three. The message becomes the creator's way of telling the story. Complete stories can never be told because of limited time and space. For example, all the work needed to solve a crime cannot be shown on a one-hour television police show. Only parts of the story can be represented. The same is true of news programs, magazine articles, and movies. The creators of the message choose what to put in the story and what to leave out. As the audience, we never see the parts that were left out. It's easy to make the mistake of believing we are getting the full story. But, in fact, we are getting only one small piece of the story. Informed consumers of media messages always ask themselves, "What is *not* being represented?" Thinking about this question can help you understand the intended effects of the media message.

Media Messages Use Special Language

The "language" of the media has its own rules. Think about the last scary movie you saw. Special music was probably used to heighten your sense of fear during really scary parts of the movie. This is part of the language of the media, used in this example to communicate fear. If you see a newspaper article with large headlines, you may believe that this story is more important than another story that has smaller headlines. In a movie or television show, the camera angles focus your attention on specific things. Each form of media has its own perspective and language that help determine how stories are presented and how they are received by their audience.

Media Messages Are Perceived Differently

People perceive the same media message differently, so there will be as many perceptions of a media message as there are people who experience it. As we take in a media message, we form our own impressions and conclusions. We interpret media messages on the basis of a variety of factors, including our age, level of maturity, education, and previous experiences. As an experiment, ask your friends to watch a music video with you. Then, each of you decide for yourself what you think the "message" of the video was. When you talk about your perceptions, you may find that you and your friends reached different conclusions about what you saw and heard. It is quite common for people to see the same thing and yet interpret it differently.

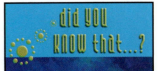

did you know that...?

It is estimated that children growing up in the United States today watch an average of 1,000 hours of television every year. It is expected that they will continue to watch at least that many hours of television throughout their lives. By the time young people graduate from high school, they will have spent more time in front of the television than they did in school.

constructed

in reference to the media, pertains to the process of taking objective reality and interpreting it according to a particular viewpoint

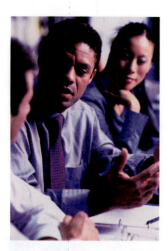

Many people come together to carefully plan media productions.

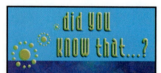

...did you know that...?

A survey of fifth graders conducted by New York University revealed that 90% of the respondents read four minutes or less each day. These same fifth graders watched an average of 130 minutes—more than two hours—of television daily.

Most Media Messages Have a Profit Motive

Some messages are clearly designed to sell a product or service. For example, commercials are called that because their intent is to sell a commercial (for-profit) product or service. It may not be as obvious, however, that even newspapers and the news programs you hear on television are driven by a profit motive. If they do not sell their product or service well, the audience may buy a different newspaper or tune in to a different television network. Because advertising sponsors pay for time and space on the basis of the number of people expected to see their commercials, media messages during television programs of all types are constructed to keep the targeted audience interested and coming back for more.

Media Messages Contain Specific Information

Media messages convey information about who and what is important to the creator or producer of the message. The age, gender, and race of characters; the environment in which the story takes place; and the actions of the plot all give us clues about the values and viewpoints of the creator of the message. Frequently, media messages tell the stories of persons with power and privilege rather than those of ordinary people. This focus can give a distorted view of the real world. For example, think about how television shows and movies traditionally portrayed the health care field. Most, if not all, the doctors were male, and the stories usually focused on them. This bias is slowly changing; more female doctors and health care providers are now portrayed, but there is still a distorted view of health care settings. For example, although the number of male nurses is increasing in the real world, few male nurses appear on television shows that take place in medical settings. Another example is the type of families that are shown in soap operas. Soap operas rarely focus their story line around working-class families. Instead, they almost always show families that are well-to-do.

What's News?

Many educators are concerned about the lack of media literacy demonstrated by their students. Although mass media are the dominant source of Americans' information about what's going on in the world, they are rarely a study subject in schools. Although mass media are often used as teaching tools, few schools have specific programs to teach students how to analyze and evaluate media messages. Some other countries, including Great Britain, Canada, Australia, and Spain, include media education in elementary schools. Some states in the United States have begun to require that their students complete a course in media literacy before high school graduation. Teacher training programs have been started so that teachers can learn to integrate media literacy into other subjects at all grade levels.

ADVERTISING IN THE MASS MEDIA

Rarely a day goes by when we do not hear or see a large number of media messages. Many of these messages are intended specifically to motivate you to purchase a product or service. Companies that want to sell a product or service use **advertising** to reach their target audiences. Advertising is usually distributed through some type of mass media, such as television, radio, magazines, or newspapers, so that many people will receive the same message. Companies frequently target teen audiences for ads featuring clothing, cosmetics, music, videos, and films because these are products they know teens are interested in and might buy.

Creating Needs

Advertising is one way that companies try to create the impression that teens "need" their products. They send the message that the products are necessary for people to be attractive and successful. It has been said that the main purpose of advertising is not simply to sell a product but to create the impression that a person who doesn't own or use the product being advertised is a "loser." One approach companies use is to create the perception that their product is a "cool" item you simply must have. This advertising trick takes advantage of teenagers' natural insecurity and anxiety about how they are perceived by others. There are even research companies that specialize in searching for the next cool teen trend. Commercial companies pay for this research information in order to market more successfully to teens. Their message is that being cool is based on what you *buy*, which is something they just happen to *sell*. To ensure continued sales, commercial companies continually change what is considered cool. Teens, therefore, become constant customers, continually buying new things to keep up with the created image of being cool.

Expert critics of the media suggest that when you see or hear an advertising message, you should ask yourself, "What dream is being sold here?" You will frequently find that companies are using our dreams for happiness, success, and acceptance to feed their need for

advertising

a form of communication that uses the mass media to sell a product or service to an intended audience

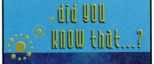

did you know that...?

Up to 40% of the cost of a product is the cost of advertising! Companies are willing to spend a lot of money on advertising because they believe advertising is necessary to get consumers to buy their product. Competition is especially fierce between producers of very similar products, such as Coke and Pepsi.

did you know that...?

A 30-second commercial for Super Bowl XXXVI (2002) cost almost $2 million. Apparently, advertisers think the cost is worth it in order to reach an estimated 140 million television viewers. An estimated 8% of the Super Bowl viewers tuned in just to see the advertisements! Interestingly, tobacco giant Philip Morris bought Super Bowl advertising minutes to air a commercial *against* smoking. Their purpose was to create the impression that they don't want teenagers to start smoking. What potential benefits could this advertisement have for a producer of cigarettes?

✴ teen forum ✴

Fast Food in School?

The United States is faced with a rising epidemic of obesity. Many studies show that lifestyle behaviors related to obesity begin early in life. These studies conclude that two of the most important factors are diet and physical activity. The fast-food industry, in particular, has been blamed for contributing to the poor eating habits of Americans. At the same time, the fast-food industry has become a major force in school cafeterias. Suppliers such as Burger King, Taco Bell, and Pizza Hut have formed partnerships with schools in which the schools receive a percentage of the profits from in-school food sales. The same is true for soft-drink, candy, and other snack-food companies. Many schools use the money from these sales to pay for educational programs. Opponents of these commercial partnerships believe that schools are endangering the health of young Americans by providing them with such easy access to unhealthy foods.

- Do you think the monetary benefits of these partnerships outweigh any potential health problems?

- Does your school participate in these partnerships? If it does, do you support or oppose its position?

- Be prepared to defend your answers. Include your answers in your Health Folio.

cold, hard cash. Think about advertisements for tobacco or alcohol. There is usually an emphasis on attractive people having a wonderful time. Viewers are left with the impression that the people's beauty and happiness are related to their use of tobacco or alcohol. Teens who are aware of this technique of manipulation can examine advertising messages closely and determine what methods advertisers are using to promote their products. They can then make informed choices about whether to purchase the products.

Product Placement

product placement

a form of advertising that takes place within entertainment, rather than as a separate commercial

Product placement is a form of advertising that takes place *within* a form of entertainment rather than as a separate commercial. It places a brand-name product within a television show or movie as a part of the setting and environment, such as the car the main character drives or the soft drink the children drink. The product appears very visibly so the audience can't miss it.

There are many advantages to product placement for both the television or movie producer and the advertiser. Product placement helps producers cut costs and makes their story seem more like real life. For instance, if a particular type of car is featured in a movie, the producer can use the car without purchasing it. At the same time, advertisers get tremendous value for their money. In contrast to a newspaper or television advertisement that is a "one-shot" event, product placements in movies and television shows live on indefinitely. Each time the television show or movie is shown, the audience sees the product again.

Cross-Promotions

Another way that commercial companies make a great deal of money is from **cross-promotions** using product placement. Consider a Disney film that becomes a blockbuster movie. Certainly, Disney makes money from the film itself. However, a great deal of money is also generated by the sale of the character dolls and toys, clothes, storybooks, games, and fast-food promotions that are associated with the movie. Next time you walk down the aisle in a toy store, notice how many of the toys are cross-promotions from a television show or movie. When you are in a fast-food restaurant, pay attention to the toys that are featured in the kids' meals. Chances are, you will find they are connected to a current movie or television show.

Controversial Advertising

One controversial form of advertising related to product placement is the portrayal of characters who smoke in movies or television series. Although a particular brand of cigarette may not be featured, this practice promotes smoking. The percentage of people who smoke in movies is much higher than the percentage in the general public. A survey conducted between 1990 and 1996 showed that 80% of male leading characters smoked. Of the top 200 television shows of 1996–1997, 89% contained smoking. Although smoking rates vary by education level, geographic location, and other factors, only about 25% of the American public smoke. But when we see such a large number of characters in movies and television shows smoking, it is easy to think that "everyone's doing it," even though that is far from the truth.

VIOLENCE IN THE MASS MEDIA

For years, adults have worried about the effects on children of violence in the mass media. The question has been repeatedly asked, "Does violence on television and in the movies make children more likely to commit a violent act?" Media violence often suggests that the use of force is the primary way to solve problems and interpersonal conflict. Concern about violence and the media increased after the school shootings at Columbine High School in Littleton, Colorado, especially after it was reported that the two teen shooters favored violent music, video games, movies, and Internet sites. You may also have heard of teens who commit a violent crime and then say they were copying something they saw in a video game, movie, or television episode.

Experts are suggesting that we may have been asking the wrong questions about violence and the media. Although it is difficult to link specific acts of real-world violence to specific television shows or films, there is

cross-promotions
the creation and advertising of products related to other products or forms of entertainment

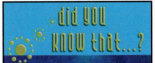

BMW reportedly paid $3 million for its Z3 roadster to be the car that James Bond drove in the 1996 film *Golden Eye*. Car industry sources estimate that the use of this car in the movie generated $240 million in advance sales alone!

Continual exposure to violence through the mass media may result in what experts call a "mean world syndrome."

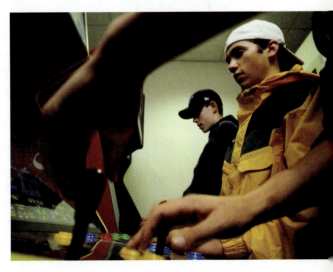

What's News?

In November 2001, the American Academy of Pediatrics issued the following Policy Statement on media violence: "The American Academy of Pediatrics recognizes exposure to violence in media, including television, movies, music, and video games, as a significant risk to the health of children and adolescents. Extensive research evidence indicates that media violence can contribute to aggressive behavior, desensitization to violence, nightmares, and fear of being harmed."

did you know that...?

Violence in movies appears to be on the increase. In the movie *Die Hard 2*, 264 people were killed. In the original *Die Hard*, only 18 people were killed.

evidence that continual exposure to violence through the mass media may result in what is called a "mean world syndrome." This means that people begin to think of the world as a mean, dangerous place where they are likely to experience violence. Thus, even as acts of violence in real life are declining, the *perception* is that they are becoming more common. As a result, people become more fearful of being victims of violence. As does smoking on television and in movies, violent acts occur much more frequently in the media than in real life. One study of television programs showed that 58% of all male major characters and 41% of all female major characters were involved in some type of violence in any given week of the series. It also reported that violence was the main theme of almost half of the television programs or movies exported from the United States. Film producer Michael Moore focused on the fear in America created by this portrayal of violence in his 2002 documentary movie *Bowling for Columbine*.

real teens

A 13-year-old Canadian teenager named Virginie Lariviere was devastated after her little sister was robbed, raped, and strangled to death in 1991. Virginie believed that there was a connection between violent television programs and the violent manner in which her sister was murdered. She began to collect signatures in a personal campaign against television violence. Two years and 1.3 million signatures later, the Canadian government announced a five-part strategy to deal with violence in television. The strategy focuses on action by broadcasters, producers, advertisers, educators, and parents. A Virginie Lariviere Television Award was created to recognize people whose contributions help decrease the amount of violence shown on television. Interestingly and sadly, much of the violence on Canadian television is from programs that are picked up from the United States. Thus, joint efforts with U.S. broadcasters are considered key to the future success of the initiative.

SEX IN THE MASS MEDIA

Just as with the portrayals of smoking and violence, portrayals of sex in the mass media bear little resemblance to real life. The mass media are often accused of showing sex as a casual, recreational activity rather than as a physically and emotionally intimate act between two loving adults. One research study examined prime-time television shows popular among young viewers. Results from the study showed that as much as 50% of the character interaction revolved around sexual references. On television and in the movies, having sex rarely results in negative consequences. In real life, however, each year about 25% of sexually active teens are diagnosed with a sexually transmitted infection. Once again, the media portrayal presents an inaccurate picture of the real world.

The mass media are also partly responsible for the negative self-esteem issues that females have regarding body image. The mass media frequently present gender stereotypes of men as the aggressors and females as the sexual objects who are valued primarily for their physical appearance. In real life, of course, it is impossible to compete with these unrealistic media images of beauty and attractiveness. Females have much more to contribute to society than just physical appearance. But the emphasis on physical appearance, in every form of mass media, creates the impression that physical appearance is the only thing that really matters.

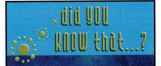

One study revealed that more than 75% of the content of MTV music videos involved sexual themes. In addition, the characters of music videos were shown in stereotypical male-female roles.

ANALYZING AND EVALUATING MEDIA MESSAGES

Most people don't spend much time, if any, analyzing and evaluating the hundreds of media messages they see and hear each day. After considering the information presented in this chapter, you may be interested in taking control of how you perceive these messages. Taking control begins with paying attention to what the creators and producers of these messages are trying to accomplish. What is their intention? What effect do they hope to have on you? Media literacy gives you the power to be in charge and ask questions about what you're seeing and hearing.

In an article in the *Media Literacy Clearinghouse*, Elizabeth Thoman suggests some questions you might ask yourself:

1. Who is the producer/storyteller of the message?
2. What is their purpose/motive/agenda? (to inform, to persuade, to educate, to call to action, to entertain, to shock)
3. What does the message say? How does it say it?
4. What format/medium does the producer use?
5. What are the advantages of the format/medium?
6. What methods/techniques does the producer use to make the message believable?
7. What lifestyle is portrayed in the message?
8. Who makes money or benefits from the message?

9. Who/what is left out of the message?

10. Whose interests are served by telling/showing the message in this particular way?

11. Do I agree with the message?

12. How might different people interpret the message differently?

13. What can I do with the information I have obtained from this message?

BUILDING YOUR Wellness Plan

Once you know how frequently you are exposed to mass media products, you might recognize that they have a greater influence on you than you first thought. Developing a planned approach to evaluating mass media can help you retain control over important aspects of your life. Paulo Freire, a well-known Brazilian educator, developed a four-step process for active learning. This process can be used as a good method for approaching media messages. The four steps are:

1. Become aware of the issue. ("How is a particular issue portrayed by the media?")

2. Learn more about the issue and how it is being represented. ("What?")

3. Think about the meaning associated with the issue. ("So what?")

4. Determine the best action. ("Now what?")

You can practice these steps to become more aware of the effects the mass media have on all aspects of your life and your health. You can then decide what response would help you develop healthy behaviors for this area of your personal wellness plan.

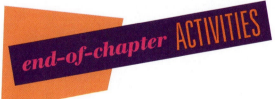

end-of-chapter ACTIVITIES

Weblinks

Influence of the Media

Media Literacy Clearinghouse:
  http://www.med.sc.edu/medialit

Sexism, Stereotyping, and Violence in the Mass Media

Media Awareness Network:
  http://www.media-awareness.ca

MediaWatch: **http://www.mediawatchyouth.ca**

Short-Answer Questions

1. List three ways in which the mass media can affect physical health.

2. List three ways in which the mass media can affect other components of health.

3. Identify five key things to be aware of when you see, read, or hear a media message.

4. Identify three examples of the use of a cross-promotion.

5. Give three examples of questions you might ask to determine the purpose of a media message.

Discussion Questions

1. Explain the difference among the following terms: *medium*, *media*, and *mass media*.

2. Discuss some of the differences between real life and the mass media construction of real life.

3. Discuss some of the possible effects of violence in the mass media.

4. Discuss some of the possible effects of sex in the mass media.

5. Give several reasons for including media literacy in schools.

Chapter Vocabulary

Using a separate sheet of paper, list and define the following terms:

advertising	media
constructed	media literacy
consumers	media target audience
cross-promotions	medium
feedback	product placement
mass media	

Application Activities

Language Arts Connection

1. Create your own print "advertisement" for a commonly advertised product. Compare your advertisement with an existing advertisement for the same product. Invite several people to analyze which advertisement they think is most truthful and which they think is most effective at selling the product.

2. Working together with a classmate or small group, create the text, sound, and visuals for a "documentary" video clip describing teens' opinions of the effects of violence or sex in media messages.

Math Connection

1. Look over the many brands and types of breakfast cereals sold at your local grocery store. Select five and compare the prices of the heavily advertised cereals with those of the generic brands that are not advertised. How much more, expressed in percentages, do the advertised brands cost? Then calculate how much more money you would pay for the heavily advertised cereal over the course of a year if you purchased cereal twice a month for 12 months. How much additional money would you spend on an advertised brand of cereal over the course of a year?

2. Select a 60-minute action show to watch on television. Count the number of violent incidents and note how many minutes each violent incident lasted. Also count the number of commercials and the number of minutes they were on the screen. Subtract the number of minutes for commercials from the total length of the show (60 minutes). Create a bar graph or pie chart to show the number of minutes of violence in the show compared to nonviolence. Create a separate bar graph or pie chart comparing the total minutes of the show and the total minutes of commercials.

Social Studies Connection

1. Watch a popular television show and analyze the way the following groups are represented: men, women, minorities, teenagers, and the elderly. How is each group portrayed? What type of role does each group have in the story line? In what ways are the groups treated differently?

2. Interview a police officer about his or her view of the way the police are represented in a particular television show or movie. How close is the representation to reality? What conclusions can you draw about how the media portray reality in a law enforcement situation?

3. Research the "mean world syndrome" and prepare a report on its possible effects on society.

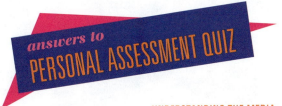

answers to PERSONAL ASSESSMENT QUIZ

personal assessment: UNDERSTANDING THE MEDIA

Answers will vary. A higher proportion of yes responses indicates that you spend a lot of time using mass media products. A higher proportion of no responses indicates that you are not a heavy consumer of mass media. Regardless of your score, it is not necessarily good or bad; it is simply an indicator of your current use of mass media. It is important to note that responses to these questions may vary over time.

chapter 26

Understanding
Health Information

As do many other teenage males, Randy wants to be stronger and more muscular. He's tall for his age and pretty quick. He thinks that if he were stronger and more muscular, he would have a better chance at a starting position on the basketball team. He works out on a regular basis, using a weight-training program designed for him by his basketball coach. A teammate told him about a nutritional supplement that is supposed to build muscle faster. He asked his coach about it, but his coach said he didn't think such a product was a substitute for hard work. Randy thinks if he uses a nutritional supplement *and* works really hard, he could have an advantage over the other guys when the basketball season starts in a couple of months. Randy's health is important to him, though, and he doesn't want to do anything that would hurt him. He also doesn't want to waste his money on things that don't work.

chapter OBJECTIVES

When you finish this chapter, you should be able to:

- ☀ Describe several sources of health information.
- ☀ Explain the difference between reliability and validity.
- ☀ Identify some of the common characteristics of health fraud or quackery.
- ☀ List several ways to practice good self-care.
- ☀ List and briefly describe the major differences between conventional and complementary, or alternative, medicine.
- ☀ Identify the major difference between prescription and nonprescription drugs.

key TERMS

complementary, or alternative, medicine
conventional, or Western, medicine
health fraud
medications
quackery
reliability
self-care
side effects
validity

Introduction

Throughout your lifetime, you will find yourself in many situations that require you to make judgments about the health information you read and hear about. You will base your actions, some of them very important, on the information you receive. Some situations that require action will be relatively minor, such as deciding what type of medicine to take when you have a bad cold. Other situations may be much more serious, such as determining the best way to recover from a serious injury or what type of treatment to seek for a life-threatening disease such as cancer. You may not realize it, but every day you are reading and hearing information that, if acted on, can affect your health either positively or negatively. How well you analyze, interpret, and use this information makes a big difference in how healthy you are, both now and later in life. In this chapter, you will learn the skills needed to acquire and understand health information to use in making decisions that contribute to good health.

personal assessment: UNDERSTANDING HEALTH INFORMATION

Before reading this chapter, take this personal assessment to discover more about the methods you currently use to acquire health information. Read the statements below and record your responses on a separate sheet of paper. Base your responses, using the following scale, on the way you feel most of the time. 1 = Definitely True; 2 = Mostly True; 3 = Mostly False; 4 = Definitely False. Interpretation of responses is located at the end of the chapter.

1. I believe I can safely rely on health information on the Internet to be accurate.

2. I know at least three places to find accurate health information.

3. When I see a physician or health care provider, I feel uncomfortable asking questions.

4. I believe that if advertising claims about a health product sound too good to be true, then the claims probably aren't true.

5. Under certain circumstances, I would take a prescription drug that was prescribed for someone else.

6. I can read and understand the labels on medications.

7. If I see an article on health information in a well-known magazine, I am confident that the information provided is accurate.

8. I know the meaning of the terms *complementary* and *alternative* medicine.

9. I depend on my physician to keep me healthy.

10. I can determine when I need to see a physician for a health problem and when I can take care of it myself.

HEALTH CARE IN THE UNITED STATES

Almost everyone needs health care services sometime during their lifetime. The United States spends billions of dollars every year trying to keep its citizens healthy. Despite efforts to keep health care costs down, however, they continue to rise rapidly. You have learned that health literacy is the ability to obtain, interpret, and understand basic health information and services. The focus of this book is to help you acquire the skills you need to become a health-literate teen. These skills will help you become more responsible for your own health. They will also enable you to help others become more responsible for their own health. As a health care consumer, you can do your part to keep health care costs down by developing and practicing your health literacy skills.

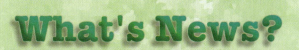

What's News?

The United States spends more money than any other nation in the world on health care. Spending on health care is 20% of the federal budget and of most state budgets as well. In 2001, the cost of health care in the United States increased more rapidly than during any year in the past decade—to $1.4 **trillion**. Health care is the single largest category of spending in the U.S. budget. The United States spends more money on health care than on defense, education, or housing, an annual average of $5,035 per person. Many people, including policy makers, are concerned about the rising cost of health care in the United States and whether these increased expenditures really result in better health for the American people.

Making good decisions about health information requires skills in communication, critical thinking, problem solving, and decision making. This chapter covers some information you might need to make a good decision and how you can find this information if you are facing health-related problems.

FINDING HEALTH INFORMATION

There are many ways to obtain health information. You probably receive health information every day that can have an effect on your health, and most of it comes with little or no effort on your part. For example, you may hear on the news something about a new genetic discovery. Or a friend may tell you about a new exercise program that is supposed to help you quickly lose weight and gain muscle. Or maybe when you're surfing the Internet you see an interesting Web site about a teenager with diabetes. Perhaps during your last visit to the doctor, she gave you a brochure on sun exposure.

The mass media provide a great deal of health information to the public. There are television specials devoted to specific health topics. News reports give updates on scientific research about health topics. Companies that produce health products and services provide information on how to use their products and services through television or magazine advertisements in an attempt to sell them for profit.

Reliability and Validity

Applying good health literacy skills includes determining whether the information received from a particular source has **reliability** and **validity**. Some sources of health information are considered to be more reliable and valid than others. For example, although a physician is not always correct, information from a physician has a higher likelihood of being accurate than information from a popular teen magazine or a television

reliability
the extent to which the information reported can be tested and confirmed by multiple trusted sources

validity
the accuracy of the information obtained

advertisement. Health-related articles that are published in professional medical or health journals have been evaluated by other experts in the health field and have met the criteria for publication. These contrast with articles in popular magazines, which may or may not have been evaluated for accuracy. Some Internet Web sites represent the opinions of highly respected health organizations. Other Web sites contain the personal opinions of individuals who are not health experts. And many Web sites are hosted by people who simply want to sell their products, such as weight-loss programs or nutritional supplements.

You can ask the following questions to help determine the reliability and validity of all types of health information:

1. Does the information come from a trusted source?
2. Is the information consistent with information from other sources?
3. Is the information based on reliable facts or on personal opinions?
4. Who produced the health information message, and what are their credentials?
5. Does the producer of the health information message have something to sell or gain?

Sources of Health Information

There are times when you need to search for health information on your own. You may not have the facts you need, or you may need additional information. You will probably be able to find the information you need from one of the following sources.

Family or Friends

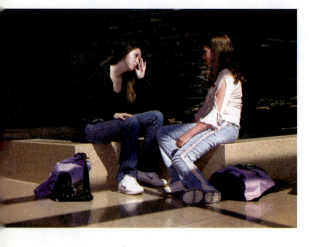

Asking friends for health advice is a good way to find out about other resources to answer your questions, but you shouldn't rely on a friend's advice alone.

When faced with a need for health information, most people turn first to family members or friends. It's always a good idea to ask people you know for health resources. But you also need to recognize that one person's experience is simply that—*one* person's experience. It is inaccurate to assume that what has worked for one person will automatically meet your needs. So when you seek health information from family or friends, be sure to consult other sources as well.

The Internet

A huge amount of health-related information is available on the Internet. You can put a search term, such as the name of a disease, into an Internet search engine, and you will usually obtain hundreds of possible sources for information. Many of these sites on the Internet provide good information, but you will need to use your media literacy skills (discussed in Chapter 25) to make sure that the information is accurate.

Books

You can visit any local bookstore or library to find books that are written on the health topic in which you are interested. When you search books for health information, you should evaluate the credentials of the person who wrote the book.

- Is the author a medical professional?

- What type of training in this specific area does the author have?

- Does the book give information, or is it trying to sell you something?

- Does the book have a reference section?

Articles in Newspapers, Magazines, and Health Journals

Other common sources for health information are articles in newspapers, magazines, and health journals. Articles in newspapers often report breaking news about a particular topic. One potential problem with these newspaper reports is that the amount of information presented is usually very limited because of space considerations. Another problem is that it is sometimes difficult to determine if the information is based on scientific research. Magazine articles about health are often written by individuals with no professional training in the health topic. Articles that are published in health journals that are reviewed by other health professionals are more likely to have accurate information. In many cases, though, this information is written very scientifically and may be difficult to understand.

Educational Brochures and Videos

Many community health agencies have educational brochures and videos about certain health problems. For instance, if you are interested in a certain type of cancer or heart disease, you might look in the phone directory to see if your community has a local American Cancer Society or American Heart Association. These agencies usually have many educational brochures available at no cost. You may also be able to check out a video about a certain topic. If your community does not have these organizations, you may be able to find educational brochures or videos at your local community health center or public library.

Your Physician or Other Health Care Professional

If you are not satisfied with the information you are able to find on your own, talk to your physician or another health care professional. Health care professionals are good sources of trusted information. If they can't help you, they can refer you to someone else with more experience with that particular issue.

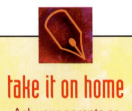

take it on home

Ask your parents or other members of your family if they have ever been the victim of health fraud. Ask if they ever purchased a product that met one of the five criteria listed in Figure 26-1. If they did, were they pleased with the product? Would they recommend it to others?

HEALTH FRAUD

The U.S. Federal Trade Commission (FTC) estimates that consumers waste billions of dollars every year on health care products and treatments that are unproven, useless, or even harmful. **Health fraud** occurs when a manufacturer claims that a product is effective for treating a particular condition when in fact it is not. For example, a manufacturer might claim that its product cures cancer, but it does not. Another commonly used term for health fraud is **quackery**.

People who have a disease for which there is no known medical cure are often desperate for a way to cure the illness. Other people just want a quick fix to treat a condition that usually takes a longer period of time to resolve in a healthy way. For example, people who want to lose weight quickly may be tempted to try a weight-loss product even though there is little or no likelihood that it will work. Elderly people are particularly susceptible to health fraud. They may hope that a medication will make them feel better or live longer. Or they may not be educated about how to carefully evaluate health information. If you have good health literacy skills, you are able to differentiate fact from fiction.

SELF-RESPONSIBILITY FOR HEALTH

As a teen, you have a great deal of control over your own health. Every day you make decisions and take actions that either help or hurt your health. Some of these actions affect you immediately, and some of them may not affect you until years later. You can use health information to manage your own care in certain situations. **Self-care** is managing a health-related situation without direction from a health care professional. You can probably handle many minor health problems on your own. For example, if you have a headache caused by stress, you may be able to relieve it by taking a walk or a nap. Or you may need to take

If you have doubt about a particular health product, ask yourself the following questions. If you answer yes to one or more of these questions, you might suspect health fraud. Investigate the product more closely before deciding whether to purchase or use it.

1. **Is the product being advertised as a quick and effective method to cure one or more health problems?**

2. **Does the manufacturer use "testimonials" claiming impressive results?**

3. **Is the product sold only by mail or Internet from a single source?**

4. **Does it require payment in advance?**

5. **Is the product described as a "scientific breakthrough" or does it contain a "secret ingredient"?**

Figure 26-1
Spotting quackery

real teens

Carey's best friend, Neisha, was recently diagnosed with diabetes. Neisha is upset that she has diabetes, and she doesn't look forward to having to exercise, control her diet, and take insulin. Neisha's doctor gave her some brochures about diabetes, but Carey and Neisha wanted to find out more. They went to the Internet and started looking for information about diabetes. They found a Web site from a person who claimed to be cured of diabetes. According to the information on the Web site, there is a new pill you can take that will cure diabetes. You must take the pill each day for one year, but then you will be cured. Best of all, you don't need to exercise, diet, or take insulin. The pill is available only from this Web site by sending $59.95 for a one-month supply. Neisha really wanted to order the pill, but Carey said that Neisha's doctor would have told her if there were really such an easy answer to diabetes. Carey also reminded Neisha that she would have to have her parents' permission to order any medicine. Because Carey knew how to spot health quackery, she saved Neisha from spending money on a product that was worthless or potentially harmful.

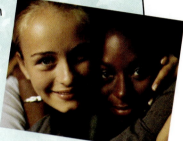

aspirin or another over-the-counter pain reliever you have on hand to stop the pain. If you get a small cut on your finger, you may be able to use a bandage to stop the bleeding. See Figure 26-2 for some tips to help you practice good self-care.

Your body is actually quite skilled at healing itself. If you treat it with a little extra care and attention, it can often heal itself without medical intervention. Here are some tips to help you practice good self-care:

- Be a good observer of your body. Pay attention to how you're feeling and be aware if there is anything about your body that seems unusual.

- Practice habits that may prevent the need to frequently use medicine. These include getting enough sleep, eating well, and exercising.

- Be well informed about different options for taking care of common health problems, such as headaches, colds, and muscle soreness.

- Know where to find information about different types of health-related problems. You can solve problems that are not serious on your own by referring to books, articles, brochures, Web sites, and other sources of health information.

- Know when to seek professional advice. Self-care is not appropriate for all health problems.

Figure 26-2
Tips for practicing good self-care

WHEN TO SEE A HEALTH CARE PROFESSIONAL

Some health problems are relatively minor. If you are well informed, you can make decisions about these problems on your own or by talking with your parents or other trusted adults. More serious problems require the attention of a physician, dentist, or other health care professional, such as an X-ray technician, dietician, or physical therapist. It is sometimes obvious that you need to see a physician or go to an emergency clinic. Other times it is not as clear.

Symptoms are signals from our bodies that something might be wrong. Pain, fever, coughs, and chills are examples of symptoms. Symptoms can be used as guidelines to help you determine if you need to seek professional advice:

- How severe are the symptoms? For example, how much pain are you experiencing?
- How long have the symptoms lasted? For example, how long have you been coughing?
- How frequently do the symptoms occur? For example, if you have a headache, do you have one every day or only once or twice a month?
- Are the symptoms unusual? For example, have you noticed a lump somewhere in your body or a change in a wart or mole?

Symptoms you may be able to treat on your own include those that are mild, don't last very long, occur infrequently, and are fairly common. If your symptoms are severe, long-lasting, frequently occurring, or unusual, however, you need to consider seeking professional advice rather than relying only on self-care. If you take time to pay attention to your body on a daily basis, it will be easier for you to notice when you are experiencing symptoms that are out of the ordinary and need medical attention.

TYPES OF HEALTH CARE

One of the decisions you will eventually face is what type of health care to seek. You can apply your skills in seeking health information to seeking appropriate health care as well. In the United States, the most common form of health care is **conventional**, or **Western**, **medicine**. This is the type of health care and medical practices taught by most U.S. medical schools and offered in most U.S. hospitals. **Complementary**, also known as **alternative**, **medicine**, is health care and medical practices that are not commonly part of conventional or Western medicine. Many complementary or alternative medical practices have been widely used in other countries since ancient times. Some of these practices have been gaining popularity in the United States. For example, Chinese medical practices, such as acupuncture and herbal medicines, are being used by a growing number of Americans. See Table 26-1 for a comparison of conventional and complementary medicine.

symptoms

signals from the body, such as fever, cough, or chills, that you have a health problem

conventional, or Western, medicine

the type of health care and medical practices taught by most U.S. medical schools and offered in most U.S. hospitals

complementary, or alternative, medicine

health care and medical practices that are not commonly part of conventional or Western medicine

Table 26-1   Conventional versus Complementary Medicine

Conventional or Western Medicine	Complementary or Alternative Medicine
Focused on the physical body and its symptoms	Focused on the relationship or balance between physical, mental, emotional, and spiritual systems of the body
Believes that disease can be traced to an identifiable physical cause or causes	Believes that disease is a disruption in the balance of body systems
Based on scientific method and research	Based on years of accumulated experience
Believes that disease is cured by drugs, surgery, and technology	Believes that the body is healed by restoring the whole person to harmony

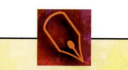

take it on home

Ask your parents or other members of your family if they have ever used a complementary or alternative health care professional. If they have, were their experiences positive or negative? Why? If they have not used a complementary or alternative health care professional, would they consider doing so? Why or why not?

SELECTING HEALTH CARE PROFESSIONALS

You want the people who take care of your medical needs to be knowledgeable and competent. One way to find a good physician is to ask for a referral from someone you trust. Another way is to find out where doctors received their medical training, how many years they have been practicing, and what experience they have had with problems like yours. You can also check with the Better Business Bureau and the local medical society in your town to see if any complaints have been filed. By searching for this information before you actually need care, you have a good chance of finding a physician with a reputation for quality care.

If you have a serious medical condition requiring surgery or extensive treatment, you may want to get a **second opinion**. This means asking one or more additional physicians for their opinions about your medical condition before making decisions about treatment options. When two or more physicians agree, you feel more confident that you are receiving the best medical care possible for your particular situation.

Establishing a Physician-Patient Partnership

Many people like to have the same person care for them every time they need medical services, and many insurance companies *require* you to have your medical care coordinated by a single physician. Your physician is an excellent source of health information. A primary care physician knows you personally and coordinates the care you receive from other health professionals. By using a primary care physician, you know there is one person who is aware of all the medical care and drug treatments you are receiving. Having one person coordinate your care

second opinion

an opinion from a physician or other health care provider about diagnoses and treatment options in addition to the one made by the original treating physician

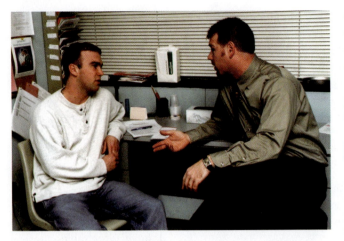

You can talk to your doctor or a health care professional for trustworthy health and wellness information.

can prevent confusion and misunderstanding among health care professionals. The primary care physician can also treat many common illnesses, diseases, or injuries. Many teens have the same primary care physician as the other adult members of their family.

Medical Specialties

In some cases, your primary care physician may recommend that you see a **specialist**. A specialist focuses on a specific area of care, such as cardiology or gynecology. Some of the more common types of specialists are listed in Table 26-2.

specialist

a health care provider who focuses on one area of care, such as cardiology or gynecology

Other Health Care Providers

In addition to physicians, there are other types of health care providers who play an important role in the diagnosis and treatment of illness and disease. Nurses, for example, outnumber physicians and all other categories of health care providers. They provide much of the direct care that patients receive. Although the demand for nurses continues to rise, there is a diminishing supply of people training to become nurses. The resulting nursing shortage is one of the most critical problems facing the U.S. health care industry today.

Nurse practitioners and physician assistants have job responsibilities that are similar to those of physicians. They can diagnose and treat illness and disease. They also conduct health assessments and can prescribe medications. They work under the supervision of a physician but are trained to make many decisions about patient care without needing to consult the physician.

Table 26-2 Types of Medical Specialists

Type of Specialist	Description of Specialty
Cardiologist	Heart and circulatory system
Gynecologist	Female reproductive system
Dermatologist	Skin disorders
Obstetrician	Pregnancy and childbirth
Orthopedist	Bones and joints
Psychiatrist	Mental health
Oncologist	Cancer

Sometimes physicians, nurse practitioners, and physician assistants refer patients to **allied health care practitioners** for a particular type of care. Allied health care practitioners support and assist the physician in providing a specialized type of patient care. Examples of allied health care practitioners include physical therapists, laboratory technicians, medical records technicians, and X-ray technologists. Paramedics and dental hygienists are also considered allied health care practitioners.

> **allied health care practitioners**
>
> health care workers with specialized technical skills who support and assist the physician in providing some types of patient care

COMMUNICATING WITH HEALTH CARE PROVIDERS

It is important to feel comfortable talking to your physician, sharing information, and asking questions about health concerns that are important to you. It is also important to feel comfortable talking to other health professionals who may be involved in your treatment, such as nurses, technicians, or physical therapists. It is easy to feel intimidated when you are in the presence of a busy health professional who has a great deal more medical knowledge than you do. However, getting the best health care and medical treatment involves a partnership between you and the health care professionals who treat you. If you can't talk honestly with your health care providers, they may not have all the information they need to help you. Communicating important information to all health care providers helps them to treat you effectively and efficiently. You have the best chance to receive good medical care if you establish a partnership with your physician or health care provider. Even as a teen, you have the right to be listened to with respect by health care professionals. After all, you know your body better than anyone. If you don't feel comfortable with your current physician, you may want to ask your parents or guardians about finding a different physician with whom you feel more comfortable.

Physicians have a limited amount of time to spend with a patient. When you go to see a physician, one way to make the best use of your time with him or her is to write a list of your symptoms and questions before your appointment. Remember, when you're not feeling well, it can be hard to remember everything the physician tells you, so take along a pencil or pen to make notes.

USING MEDICATIONS WISELY

Medications are drugs used to treat an illness or injury. The two broad categories of medications are prescription drugs and over-the-counter (OTC) drugs. Prescription drugs must be prescribed by a physician and are usually obtained at a pharmacy. Over-the-counter drugs are medications that the U.S. Food and Drug Administration (FDA) has recognized as safe for use without a prescription. More than half of all medications are sold as OTC medications. Many of these OTC drugs originally required a prescription. After these prescription medications have been used by a large number of people over a long period of time

> **medications**
>
> drugs used to treat an illness or injury

side effects

unintended results of taking a medication

generic drug

a drug not protected by a trademark granting an exclusive right to market the product

brand-name drug

a drug whose manufacturer has an exclusive right to sell it

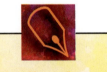

take it on home

Ask your parents for permission to survey the prescription and over-the-counter drugs that are currently in your household. What percentage of these drugs are generic, and what percentage are brand-name drugs? Discuss the advantages and disadvantages of generic versus brand-name drugs with the adults in your family. Which do they prefer and why? Write a report of your findings and keep it in your Health Folio.

without dangerous **side effects**, the FDA determines them to be safe enough to be sold over the counter to consumers.

Reading Drug Labels

Both prescription drugs and OTC drugs have labels that give the consumer information about the drug, recommended dosage, and possible side effects. In addition, purchasing many prescription drugs requires the patient to receive personal counseling from a pharmacist about the drug. You may also be given a written version of the pharmacist's verbal explanation. Over-the-counter drugs usually contain a package insert that gives more detailed information about the drug than will fit on the label. It is important to read this package insert so that you will know how to use the drug safely and effectively.

Generic versus Brand-Name Drugs

One way you may be able to save money on medications is to use a **generic** equivalent of a **brand-name drug**. When a new medication is developed by a manufacturer and approved for public use, the maker of the product has an exclusive right to market the product for a certain number of years. This right provides an incentive for pharmaceutical companies to spend time and money developing new drugs. It also allows them to recover some of the expenses of developing, testing, and marketing the drugs. After a drug has been on the market for a specified number of years, other companies may market the same medication with government approval.

In most cases, generic drugs are just as effective as brand-name drugs. Occasionally, there is a reason for using a specific brand-name drug instead of a generic equivalent. When your doctor writes you a prescription, you should always ask if it is okay to substitute a generic equivalent. Even when you are purchasing drug products over the counter, you can often save a lot of money by choosing a generic or "store brand" rather than a brand-name drug.

Medication Dangers

All medications have the potential to be dangerous, so it is very important to carefully follow the manufacturer's recommendations for OTC drugs or the physician's directions for prescription drugs. If medications are not taken correctly, they can cause dangerous (or deadly) side effects. They also may not achieve the desired results. For example, people sometimes stop taking a prescribed antibiotic as soon as they start feeling better. When they do this, the drug is not as effective. The pathogens that caused the illness can continue to reproduce, and the person can become sick again. Another consequence of stopping a medication too soon is that the pathogens left behind can become drug resistant and the medication will no longer be effective against them.

Drug Interactions

You must be careful about drug interactions between different medications. When two or more drugs are taken at the same time, they can have effects on each other within the body. Some interactions simply make the drugs less effective, but in some cases, the interaction of the drugs can produce a dangerous medical situation. When a new drug is prescribed, always let your physician and pharmacist know if you are taking any other medications. Even OTC drugs such as aspirin can affect the way other OTC or prescription drugs are processed by the body.

Guidelines for Safe Medication Use

Here are some guidelines to help you use OTC and prescription medications safely and effectively:

- Take medications, including OTC medications, only if necessary.
- Take prescription medication only if a physician has prescribed it for *you*. Never take prescription medications prescribed for someone else.
- Always read and follow label directions carefully.
- Ask your physician or pharmacist about potential drug interactions *before* combining medications.

✹ teen forum ✹

Advertising Prescription Drugs

If you watch television or read magazines, you may have noticed the many advertisements for prescription drugs. In the past, prescription drugs were marketed to physicians by the pharmaceutical companies that produced them. Physicians then determined whether the drugs were appropriate for use in specific medical situations for individual patients. In the past few years, instead of focusing all their advertising efforts on physicians, pharmaceutical companies have begun direct-to-consumer (DTC) advertising. In this type of advertising, the pharmaceutical companies encourage consumers to self-diagnose their health problems and then visit their physician to request the advertised "fix." Prescription drugs certainly offer potential solutions for some health problems. But many people believe it is the role of the physician, not of the consumer, to determine whether a certain drug should be used in a given situation. They believe that DTC advertising causes consumers to pressure their physicians to treat them with a specific prescription drug. Other people argue that DTC advertising results in better-informed consumers and increases positive health outcomes.

- In your opinion, what are the pros and cons of DTC advertising? Give a rationale for your answer.

- Do not exceed or change the recommended dosage or length of treatment without talking to your physician.
- Store medications in a cool, dry place and do not use them past the expiration date printed on the label or packaging.

BUILDING YOUR Wellness Plan

Because everyone will use health information from various sources many times in their lives, it is important that you develop and practice your health literacy skills. On the basis of what you have learned in this chapter, think about how you normally obtain health information. Are there areas in which you should improve your skills? What goals can you set for yourself in these areas? Understanding and using health information wisely includes:

- Knowing how to find reliable and valid sources of health information
- Being able to detect health fraud and quackery
- Practicing good self-care and seeing a health care provider when necessary
- Communicating well with health care providers
- Knowing how to use prescription and OTC drugs wisely

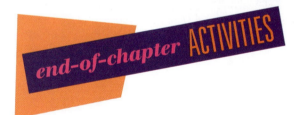

end-of-chapter ACTIVITIES

🔗 Weblinks

Be an Active Part of Your Health Care Team

U.S. Food and Drug Administration:
**http://www.fda.gov/cder/consumerinfo/
active_member.htm**

☼ Short-Answer Questions

1. List four skills needed to make good decisions about health information.
2. Identify four sources of health information.
3. Identify three types of individuals who might be vulnerable to health fraud.
4. List four questions to ask yourself about your symptoms when deciding whether you need to see a health care professional.
5. List four guidelines for using medications safely.

☼ Discussion Questions

1. List three sources of health information, and describe the advantages and disadvantages of each.
2. Explain the major differences between conventional, or Western, medicine and complementary, or alternative, medicine.
3. Discuss ways you might determine whether health information is reliable and valid.

4. Describe some of the common characteristics of health fraud or quackery.

5. Compare and contrast prescription and nonprescription drugs.

☀ Chapter Vocabulary

Using a separate sheet of paper, list and define the following terms:

complementary, or
    alternative, medicine

conventional, or Western, medicine

health fraud

medications

quackery

reliability

self-care

side effects

validity

☀ Application Activities

Language Arts Connection

1. Write an essay describing how a teenager can find out whether the claims made on a health product are accurate.

2. Design a brochure for a health problem of your choice. Be sure your information is accurate and easily understood.

Math Connection

1. Research information about the amount of money the United States spent on health care in 1980, 1990, and 2000. Create a bar graph to compare the expenditures during those years.

2. It is estimated that health care costs are approximately $5,000 per year for each man, woman, and child in America. What is the estimated annual expenditure for health care for the citizens of a city that has a population of 48,850?

Social Studies Connection

1. Compare health care costs in the United States with health care costs in three other countries. How does the U.S. system of health care differ from those of the other countries?

2. Conduct a sample survey to find out where people in your town or city are most likely to obtain the health information they need.

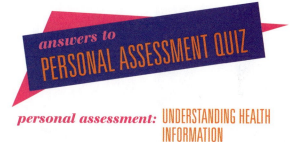

answers to
PERSONAL ASSESSMENT QUIZ

personal assessment: UNDERSTANDING HEALTH INFORMATION

Answers will vary. A higher proportion of Definitely True or Mostly True responses to questions 2, 4, 6, 8, and 10 and Definitely False or Mostly False answers to questions 1, 3, 5, 7, and 9 indicates that you have skills and qualities that enable you to find and understand health information effectively. A pattern of Definitely True or Mostly True responses to questions 1, 3, 5, 7, and 9 and Definitely False or Mostly False responses to questions 2, 4, 6, 8, and 10 indicates that you have room for improvement in your health literacy skills.

chapter 27

Shopping versus Buying

Javier's mom tripped coming down the stairs and sprained her ankle. It began to swell immediately, so she propped her foot up and put some ice on it. Javier and his girlfriend, Katrina, offered to fix dinner for the family that night. They decided to have spaghetti, salad, and bread, so they went to the grocery store for spaghetti sauce, bread, and the ingredients for the salad. His mom also asked them to pick up an ankle wrap, a cold pack, and something to help her ankle stop hurting so much.

Once at the grocery store, Javier and Katrina discovered they had some decisions to make. It was pretty easy to decide on the salad ingredients, and the family always uses a particular brand of spaghetti sauce, but there are dozens of choices of bread. After making a choice, they went on to the pharmacy. The pain reliever was easy to find, but Javier and Katrina had never purchased an ankle wrap or cold pack and weren't sure how to choose the most effective ones. They decided they would ask the pharmacy assistant for advice.

chapter OBJECTIVES

When you finish this chapter, you should be able to:

- Identify differences between shoppers and buyers.
- List and briefly describe five shopping skills of a wise consumer.
- Explain how credit cards and interest work.
- Describe what to do in case of identity theft.
- Explain several reasons teenagers are a popular target market for advertisers.
- Describe how health insurance works.

key TERMS

claims
consumer
disposable income
identity theft
insurance
out-of-pocket expense
premiums
target market
third-party payment
uninsured

Introduction

Most teens love shopping—and buying! You are probably already responsible for shopping and buying many things on your own. You may already have had to make some decisions about purchasing different types of foods, clothes, and health care products. As you get older and accept responsibility for making more of your own decisions, you will have many more opportunities to make choices among various products. Developing the knowledge and skills to purchase products that are safe, effective, and a wise use of your money is an important task of young adulthood. In this chapter, we will discuss shopping and buying, particularly as they are related to health-related products and services.

personal assessment: CONSUMER SKILLS

Before reading this chapter, take this personal assessment to discover more about your knowledge and skills as a consumer. Read the statements below and record your responses on a separate sheet of paper. Base your responses, using the following scale, on the way you feel most of the time: 1 = Definitely True; 2 = Mostly True; 3 = Mostly False; 4 = Definitely False. Interpretation of responses is located at the end of the chapter.

1. I compare prices when I shop for products and services.
2. I often buy items I did not intend to buy before I went shopping.
3. I set a budget before going shopping, and I stick to it.
4. If there is something I really want, I will borrow money or charge it in order to get it.
5. I am not easily convinced that advertising claims are really true.
6. If a product is highly advertised, I am more likely to buy it.
7. I manage my expenses so they don't exceed my income.
8. I wouldn't know what to do if I lost my purse or wallet.
9. I understand how the health care insurance system works.
10. If I get sick and the doctor's office is closed, I go to the emergency room.

BECOMING A WISE CONSUMER

consumer

a person who purchases a product or service

A **consumer** is a person who purchases a product or service. Throughout your lifetime, you will make choices as a consumer that will affect your health. When you go to the grocery store, you can choose foods that contribute to your health – or foods that don't. When you purchase over-the-counter medications, you can select products that are effective and expensive – or products that are just as effective but cost less. And when you buy fitness footwear or equipment, you have to choose among the various types and brands. Later, as an adult, you will have to make decisions about health insurance.

Becoming a wise consumer requires a number of skills. You must be able to understand the information the manufacturer or salesperson gives you about the product or service. You must know how to compare the advantages and disadvantages of the variety of products and services you want or need. Most of us have a limited amount of time to devote to researching what to buy and a limited amount of money to spend. Applying your health literacy and decision-making skills will help you to spend your time and money wisely and to purchase products and services that are safe and effective.

Are You a Shopper or a Buyer?

Some people like to shop; other people just like to buy. "What is the difference?" you may ask. **Shoppers** use their knowledge and skills to make comparisons and seek the best product or service for the best price. **Buyers** purchase products and services without making comparisons. Both shoppers and buyers are consumers, but shoppers have the characteristics of a wise consumer. They are willing to invest the necessary time and energy to research and compare options before making a buying decision.

Consider the shopping habits of Whitney and Adam, who are both looking for new running shoes. They go to their local sporting goods store, and Adam buys the first pair of shoes he tries on. He says they feel fine, and he has enough money to pay for them. Whitney tries on several brands of shoes. She finds a couple of pairs she likes and asks the salesclerk for additional information. The salesclerk recommends a couple of brands on the basis of customer satisfaction and length of wear. Whitney doesn't buy the shoes but, instead, goes home and looks up the brands on the Internet. She compares the Internet prices with the prices at the store. She decides to buy the pair at the local store, even though they are a few dollars more, because she can get them immediately and she doesn't have to pay the shipping charges. In this example, Whitney exhibits the characteristics of a shopper, but Adam is clearly a buyer.

Developing Your Shopping Skills

Not every purchase is worth the time spent shopping. Sometimes, the best use of your time and money is simply to buy, especially if the product or service is relatively inexpensive or if the quality of the product is not that important. For example, suppose you are considering buying disposable forks and spoons for one-time use at a picnic or three-ring paper folders for a school report. In these cases, it may be a better use of your time and money to simply buy something that meets your needs than to shop. But when quality is important and a lot of money is involved, as when choosing a car or a computer, it is a good idea to take the time to apply your shopping skills. Here are some ways to develop your shopping skills and become a wise consumer:

1. *Know what you're looking for.* Is this something you really need or just something you want or wish you could have? Is appearance important, or do you just care that it works well? Having a good idea of what you're looking for before you start shopping helps you narrow your options and saves you time.

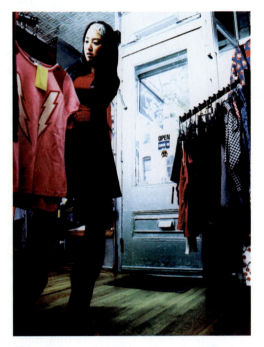

Shoppers invest time and energy to learn about a product before making a purchase.

2. *Know your budget.* Determine how much you can spend and don't waste time looking at products that cost more. It's almost always a bad idea to go into debt to purchase things, even if you think you really need them.

3. *Gather key information.* What features are important in the product or service? Read product labels or ask salesclerks for information. You can also use the Internet to visit Web sites to get technical information provided by the manufacturer or advertiser of the product. Use all this information to help you decide if a product is likely to meet your needs.

4. *Compare your options.* Once you have found two or three products that are within your budget and seem acceptable, compare the features. How do the products compare in price? How do the various features compare? If there is a particular product you prefer, identify why you prefer it over the others.

5. *Purchase your best option.* Many factors can influence a purchasing decision. Sometimes it's best to choose the product offered at the lowest price. Other times you may be willing to spend a little extra money to have the product you like best or the one that has the highest quality.

TEEN CONSUMER SPENDING

target market

the intended group of consumers for a particular product or service

disposable income

money that is left over after basic needs have been satisfied

Teenagers represent a very important **target market** for manufacturers of personal products and services because today's teens have more money to spend than ever before. Many teens have an after-school or a weekend job. Some receive additional spending money from their parents. In addition to things they need, teens may buy extras such as music CDs, magazines, and movie tickets with their **disposable income**. Money that is left over after basic needs have been satisfied is called disposable income. It makes sense for companies to target much of their advertising to teens because teens are often tempted to buy items they don't truly need. Companies also hope to win lifetime customers by building loyalty to a particular brand at a young age, generating customers for many years into the future.

did you know that...?

Today's teenagers represent a major target market for producers of goods and services. The 32 million teens in the United States are the largest group of teenagers in the nation's history. They also have the most discretionary (disposable) income of any group of teens in history. According to Teen Research Unlimited, the nation's premier market-research firm focusing on the teen market, a typical teen spends more than $5,000 a year in discretionary spending. In 2001, teen spending totaled $162 billion.

BECOMING A SAVVY SPENDER

One of the most important tasks of young adulthood is learning to manage your money well. Smart money management can make your life simpler and more enjoyable. Yet even many adults don't have good money management skills. Despite its importance, even fewer teens have developed the skills necessary to manage their money well.

Opening a Checking or Savings Account

Many teens find that they need to open a checking or savings account to manage their money. A bank account enables you to deposit money you have earned or that has been given to you in a safe place until you need it. When you want to purchase something, you can write a check or withdraw cash instead of having to carry cash. You can also request a debit card, which allows you to make purchases or withdraw money directly from your account without writing a check. Learning to manage a checking or savings account is also one of the most basic money management skills needed as an adult.

How Credit Cards Work

When you buy something on credit, someone (usually a bank or a credit card company) loans you the money to make the purchase. Then they charge you **interest** for the privilege of buying the item before you had the cash in hand. Interest is the monthly amount that companies charge you for the privilege of purchasing on credit. Some credit card companies also charge you an annual fee for the privilege of having the credit card, whether you use it or not. Credit cards provide a way for young people to buy things they want or need, even if they don't have the money to pay for them right away. Credit card companies know that if they can "hook" teens early into buying products on credit, they will make a lot of money in interest charges over the years. For example, if you buy a $499 television set and pay for it over 18 months at 18.8% interest, the final cost of the television will be about $575.

interest

the monthly amount that companies charge you for the privilege of purchasing on credit

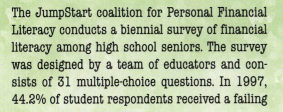

What's News?

The JumpStart coalition for Personal Financial Literacy conducts a biennial survey of financial literacy among high school seniors. The survey was designed by a team of educators and consists of 31 multiple-choice questions. In 1997, 44.2% of student respondents received a failing score. Worse yet, failing scores are on the increase! In 2000, 59.1% of students failed, and the failing percentage rose again in 2002 to a whopping 68.1%. This survey provides evidence that high school students have a lot to learn when it comes to managing money.

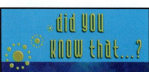

The problem is that it's easy to let charges pile up. When the bill comes due, there may not be enough money to pay it. It's a good idea to buy only those things you have the cash to pay for. Otherwise, you may be tempted to buy things you think you need, when they are really only things you want, but cannot afford. Learning now to live within your means is an important skill you will need to acquire and practice as a young adult to avoid financial problems.

Some companies offer a prepaid or stored-value card for teens. These cards work similarly to the way a prepaid phone card or a gift card from a retail store works. A certain amount of money is deposited on the card, and the person uses the card instead of cash to make the purchase. Prepaid credit cards can be handy to have when you don't want to carry cash, but they serve the same basic purpose as an ATM or debit card or a checking account. It is just another way of spending money that you already have.

Even responsible adults sometimes make unwise purchases. But as a teen, you may be especially vulnerable to marketing and advertising gimmicks. As you are developing your own identity, you may go through stages as you work toward personal independence. You may find yourself tempted to buy things as a way of expressing your changing identity. In addition, some teens are inexperienced in making purchasing decisions, have not developed good shopping skills, and have little experience knowing what is true and what is false in advertising. Remember that the purpose of advertising is to sell you something—whether you need it or not!

Identity Theft

identity theft

another person's use of your personal information to create a new identity and use your financial resources

Once you have a credit or debit card or even a driver's license, you become a target for **identity theft**. This is one of the fastest growing crimes against consumers, according to the nonprofit Institute of Consumer Financial Education. In identify theft, a thief uses your personal information to create a new identity and use your financial resources. If your wallet or purse has been lost or stolen and you have any personal financial information inside, follow these steps to protect yourself financially:

1. Call the three major credit reporting agencies (Equifax, Experian, and TransUnion). Ask them to place a Fraud Alert on your name and Social Security number.

2. Notify the Social Security national fraud hotline at 1-800-269-0271.

3. Cancel all of your credit cards immediately.

4. Contact your bank if you had checks lost or stolen.

5. File a police report the same day if at all possible.

Purchasing Health-Related Products

Companies know that personal appearance is important to teens, so they market many health-related products that involve improving one's appearance. Teens are also a natural target market for nutrition and fitness products and services. One of the techniques used by these companies is to try to make you feel insecure about how you look. Then they can sell you a product that will help you "improve" your appearance.

Think about some of the products you frequently see advertised on television. You can buy shampoos and hair care products to make your hair "bouncy and more luxurious." You can purchase toothpaste that "makes your smile whiter and brighter." You can purchase mouthwash to "keep your breath fresh and clean." All these advertisements focus on identifying some "problem" with your appearance and providing a product that claims to solve the problem. Even if there really isn't a problem to begin with, this is a way for the advertiser to sell a

did YOU KNOW that...?

Sellers of herbal supplements often claim their products can help you increase your energy or lose weight. Herbal supplements are not regulated by the Food and Drug Administration (FDA), and some of the active ingredients in herbal supplements can be harmful or can interact with other medications in a dangerous way. The FDA reports that ephedra, a popular herb that advertisers claim has benefits for bodybuilding and weight loss, appears to have been responsible for about 100 deaths among users.

What's News?

A report issued by the Federal Trade Commission (FTC) in September 2002 found that 55% of weight-loss advertisements make claims that are very likely to be false or that lack proof to support them. According to the FTC, any advertisement that uses the claims listed below should send up a "red flag," cautioning you to have doubts about the truth of their claims:

1. Consumer testimonials and before-and-after photos

2. Rapid weight loss

3. No diet or exercise required

4. Long-term/permanent weight loss

5. Clinically proven/doctor-approved

6. Natural/safe weight loss

Consumers spent about $35 billion on weight-loss products in 2000. Surgeon General Richard Carmona says that "the public must adopt a healthy skepticism about advertising that promotes miracles and scientific breakthroughs." If claims sound too good to be true, they are probably false.

real teens

Tobias tried out for his high school football team last year, but he was cut from the squad during the last trial. He plans to try out again this year. He knows he needs to get into better shape to improve his chances of making the team. He talked his parents into signing a contract at a local fitness gym that has great new weight equipment. He promised to pay the monthly fees from the money he earns from his after-school job. Tobias and his parents had a choice of signing a six-month contract with a higher monthly fee or a one-year contract with a lower monthly fee. Tobias wanted the one-year contract because he would have lower monthly payments. His parents convinced him that a six-month contract would be better. It would give him an opportunity to see if he really used the gym without committing to a whole year of payments. After working out at the gym for a couple of months, Tobias realized that it was always crowded during the only free time he had to work out. He also felt left out because all the other club members were adults. He decided that he would rather work out with his friends at the local public gym, even though their weight equipment isn't as nice. It also costs less. When he tried to get out of his contract, the managers at the gym said he had to pay the remaining four months on his contract. Now he's really glad his parents convinced him to get a six-month membership instead of a one-year membership.

---

product—one that you may not even need! As a wise consumer, you have to determine if these products really do what they claim to do before spending your money on them. Your health literacy skills and decision-making skills can help you determine whether advertising claims are true.

PAYING FOR HEALTH CARE

Almost everyone in the United States uses the health care system at one time or another. When you become independent, you will need to make a decision about health insurance. Many people have health **insurance**, but a large number of people in the United States are **uninsured**. If you are uninsured, you must pay for medical treatment yourself. This method of payment is called an **out-of-pocket expense**. Even the most routine medical care, such as visiting a doctor for a sore throat, can cost more than a hundred dollars. If your medical condition requires hospitalization or surgery, the expenses can run into thousands of dollars. Therefore, people who are uninsured often can't afford the medical care they need. As a result, they may delay or avoid treatment, allowing a minor problem to turn into a major, expensive medical problem.

---

insurance

a form of full or partial coverage for health services that is based on collecting a certain amount of money in advance from a consumer in return for payment for approved charges when they occur

uninsured

referring to people who do not have insurance

out-of-pocket expense

payment for health care made directly by the person receiving the care

How Insurance Works

When you buy insurance, you pay a certain amount, usually each month, to the insurance company. These payments are called **premiums**. In return, the insurance company promises to pay for part or all of your care if you become sick or injured. The insurance company does this by pooling all the money it collects from the people who pay monthly premiums. When individuals receive medical care, the health care providers (or sometimes the patients themselves) submit **claims** to the insurance company, requesting payment. The insurance company must be able to pay these claims from the premiums it collects. An insurance company's payment for medical services is known as a **third-party payment**. The insurance company is the "third party," who pays the "second party" (the physician or hospital) for services that the "first party" (the patient) received.

Although many people obtain health insurance through their employment, there are still many others who don't have insurance. In 2001, it was estimated that 41 million Americans did not have health insurance, or about 14.6% of the total population. Many of the people who don't have health insurance work full time, but their employers are small businesses that don't offer health insurance to their employees. Other uninsured people work part time and are not eligible for the employer's health benefits. Still others cannot afford the premiums they would be required to pay. In 2001, the average cost of insurance coverage for an individual was nearly $3,000 per year.

About four-fifths of all medical payments in the United States today are made through the third-party payment system. Not all third-party payments are made through private insurance companies, however. A large number of payments are the responsibility of the government through **Medicare** and **Medicaid** payments. Medicare is a program sponsored by the federal government to help provide medical care for citizens 65 years of age and older and those who are disabled. Medicaid is a joint federal-state program to help make medical payments for people whose income falls below a certain level.

---

premiums

monthly payments made to an insurer in exchange for the insurer's commitment to pay any covered claims received

claims

in reference to insurance, requests for payment that are made by health care providers to insurers

third-party payment

a health insurance term meaning that approved charges are paid by the insurance provider rather than by the patient

Medicare

a federal program that provides medical insurance for citizens 65 years of age and older and those who are disabled

Medicaid

a joint federal-state program that provides medical insurance for people whose income falls below a certain level

---

did you know that...?

Young adults, ages 18–24, are the least likely of all age groups to have health insurance coverage. If their parents have insurance, many young adults who attend college can remain on their parents' insurance policy. But after age 18, many young adults don't qualify for their parents' health insurance. They may work part time or at small businesses that don't offer health benefits. They may decide that insurance is too expensive during a time of their lives when they are generally healthy.

Controlling Health Care Costs

If you have insurance, it may not seem as if it costs very much to see the physician. But every time an insured person visits the doctor, has medical tests done, or receives treatment, the insurance company must pay the bill. Over time, if a lot of people who are insured have medical expenses, the cost of the claims submitted to the insurance company may be more than the amount of money the insurance company has collected. Insurance companies then must raise the rate of the monthly premiums. Because of the rising costs of health care, insurance has become quite expensive.

As a teen, you can help keep insurance premiums and health care costs down by using health care services only when you really need them. Prevention and early treatment are much less expensive than waiting until you are very ill before seeking treatment. Hospital care is extremely expensive, so waiting until a condition is very serious and requires hospitalization increases the overall cost of health care. In fact, using the emergency room at the hospital is one of the most costly ways of obtaining medical care and should be used only in a true emergency.

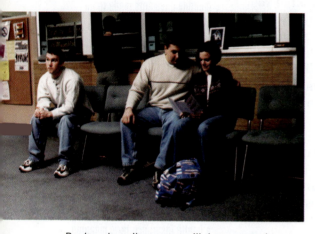

Don't wait until you are so ill that you need to go to the emergency room. Seeking prevention and early treatment services will be less expensive and better for your health.

YOUR RIGHTS AS A HEALTH CARE CONSUMER

As a health care consumer, you have the right to be treated with respect and to ask questions about things you don't understand. Remember, you are the consumer and you are paying your health care professionals for the knowledge, expertise, and care they provide. If the medical information you receive from a health care professional is confusing, it is important that you ask questions.

�֎ teen forum ✤

Paying for Health Care

The United States is the only industrialized country in the world that does not have some type of national health care plan for its citizens. Instead, we have focused on a free market approach of supply and demand for health care. At the same time, the United States spends more than any other nation in the world on health care for its citizens. Even with these large expenditures, Americans do not enjoy the best health status in the world.

- Compare the United States' spending on health care with that of several other industrialized nations. What are some possible reasons the United States spends so much more money than other countries?

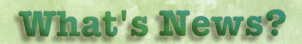

What's News?

Historically, the regulation of health care has been left to the individual states, which have laws to protect citizens who need health care services. Recently, however, consumer advocacy groups have pushed for a federal patient protection act that would apply standard patient protection regulations to all Americans. This is sometimes called a Patient's Bill of Rights. During the 106th Congress, both the House and the Senate passed patient protection bills, but they couldn't agree on a single bill to send to the president for his signature. During the 107th Congress, this issue is being debated again. Many people believe that passage of a Patient's Bill of Rights would help ensure health care quality and access for all Americans. You can use the Internet to learn the current status of the Patient's Bill of Rights.

Just as you check your bill at a retail store or restaurant, you should also check the bills you receive from health care providers to make sure all the charges are correct. If you believe there are errors, you will want to alert the billing staff so they can make the proper corrections. If you are not satisfied with the medical services and attention you receive from your physician, you should first attempt to resolve the problem directly with the physician. Sometimes there is simply a misunderstanding that can be easily corrected. If the problem is not resolved to your satisfaction, however, you may want to change physicians. If you believe the problem is a danger to your health or the health of others, you can file a complaint with the local medical society or the Department of Health in your state.

BUILDING YOUR Wellness Plan

An important component of your wellness plan is becoming a wise consumer. You may want to search the Internet for more information about topics that you don't understand as well as you would like. You can also talk with your parents or other trusted adults for helpful hints about how to become a wise consumer. Are there any areas you want to improve? Make a note of these in your wellness plan. In this chapter, we discussed some of the important considerations necessary to be a wise consumer:

- Developing your shopping skills
- Becoming aware of advertising motives for profit
- Learning how credit cards work
- Understanding how health insurance works
- Reducing health care costs

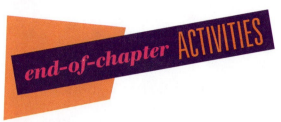

end-of-chapter ACTIVITIES

Weblinks

Managing Your Checking or Savings Account

eFunds, Inc.: **http://aboutchecking.com** (click on "Checkbook Basics" to get started)

Money Management

Institute of Consumer Financial Education: **http://www.financial-education-icfe.org** (take the "Young Spender's Profile Quiz" and the "Credit Risk Profile for Youth" located under "Children and Money")

Short-Answer Questions

1. Identify three types of products teens might buy to improve their personal appearance.
2. List five shopping skills of a wise consumer.
3. Identify three items that teens might buy with disposable income.
4. List five things to do in case your wallet or purse is stolen.
5. Identify five "red flags" for weight-loss advertisements.

Discussion Questions

1. Describe the differences among shoppers, buyers, and consumers.
2. Explain some of the key reasons why teenagers are a popular target market for advertisers.
3. Describe how credit cards work.
4. Describe how the health insurance system works.
5. Explain what insurance premiums and claims are.

Chapter Vocabulary

Using a separate sheet of paper, list and define the following terms:

claims	out-of-pocket expense
consumer	premiums
disposable income	target market
identity theft	third-party payment
insurance	uninsured

Application Activities

Language Arts Connection

1. Write a short story about two people who have been diagnosed with cancer. Both of the individuals are employed, but one of them has insurance and the other does not.
2. Construct a role-play scenario about the differences between a shopper and a buyer who are both searching for a weight-loss product.

Math Connection

1. A highly advertised brand of shampoo costs $5.99 for 18 ounces. A "look-alike" brand costs $2.99 for 12 ounces. How much money would you save (per ounce) by buying the look-alike brand?
2. You are responsible for purchasing healthy snacks for a team of 10 people. You have $12 to spend. The most expensive item you purchased costs three times as much as the least expensive item. You have purchased eight items. What is the price of each item?

Social Studies Connection

1. Research the characteristics of the teenage target market. Describe techniques that advertisers use to reach this target market.
2. Research resources for teens to become more financially literate. Compile a list of the resources available in your area.

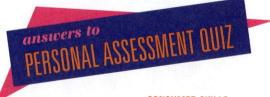

answers to PERSONAL ASSESSMENT QUIZ

personal assessment: CONSUMER SKILLS

Answers will vary. A higher proportion of Definitely True or Mostly True responses to odd-numbered questions indicates that you have already developed some skills associated with being a wise consumer. A higher proportion of Definitely True or Mostly True responses to even-numbered questions may suggest there is room for improvement in your consumer skills.

unit 8

Healthy Adulthood

Introduction

As you begin the last unit in this book, you should have a good understanding of the health risks you might face as a teen or young adult. You know what risk factors are and how they can be controlled by making good decisions and practicing healthy behaviors. Most likely you will have developed the health literacy skills that will help you create a personal wellness plan that can act as a road map on your wellness journey. Travel well!

This last unit will help enhance your wellness plan for adulthood. As an adult, you will encounter stressors specific to adulthood. You will have opportunities to contribute to the health of others. Should you become a parent, you will be responsible for the well-being of your family members. As a member of your community, you will have occasion to contribute to the health of your community. This unit will help you understand your role in the adult world and provide information for developing a wellness plan that will serve you well as an adult member of the community.

503

chapter 28

Stressors of Adulthood

Sarah is excited about the upcoming weekend. Her family is going to visit her mom's parents, Granddad and Grammy. Now that her grandfather is retired, her grandparents often spend special time with each grandchild. Last summer, for example, they took Sarah on a hiking trip to the mountains. This weekend they're going to plan a summer trip to take after school is out. Sarah hopes it includes an opportunity for her to see the ocean.

Sarah's thoughts wander to her dad's parents. Her dad's father died last year and her dad's mother, Granny, isn't in good health. She takes turns living with relatives because she can no longer take care of herself. Sarah overheard her mom and dad discussing the fact that Granny has financial problems and needs help paying bills. Sarah loves Granny, but she also feels sorry for her. She wonders what her own life will be like when she gets old. Will she be healthy and able to do fun things with her grandchildren, or will she be sick a lot and have to rely on other people to take care of her? She wonders if there is anything she can do now to make her life better when she gets older.

chapter OBJECTIVES

When you finish this chapter, you should be able to:

- Describe the process of maturation.
- Define a life event and give examples of different life events.
- Identify ways to investigate career options.
- Describe characteristics that contribute to marital longevity.
- Identify the six stages of the family life cycle.
- Identify typical stressors that occur during the various stages of life.
- Briefly explain the aging process.

key TERMS

ageism
empty nest
family life cycle
gerontologist
gerontology
life events
maturation
osteoporosis
similarity factors
social clock

Introduction

As a teen, you are probably looking forward to becoming an adult. You're eager to live independently and make all your own decisions. There are a lot of exciting things ahead of you! But in all the excitement about being in control of your own life as an adult, it's easy to forget that adulthood comes with its own set of stressors and challenges. This chapter discusses some of the stressors of adulthood. You will learn that rather than simply being one long stretch of time, adulthood can be divided into three stages: young adulthood, middle adulthood, and older adulthood. Each stage has its own set of stressors. If you begin as a teen to make preparations now to meet the challenges of adulthood and aging, you can save time, effort, money, and stress later in life.

personal assessment: BECOMING AN ADULT

Before reading this chapter, take this personal assessment to discover more about your thoughts and feelings about adulthood and aging. Read the questions below and answer them on a separate sheet of paper. Base your answers, using the following scale, on the way you feel most of the time: 1 = Definitely True; 2 = Mostly True; 3 = Mostly False; 4 = Definitely False. An interpretation of your results is located at the end of the chapter.

1. I will still like to do the same activities no matter how old I am.

2. The type of stressors that I experience will not change as I grow older.

3. There's really nothing I can do now to help me be happier when I am older.

4. Thinking about getting old is depressing to me.

5. There is no need to think about retirement until I am much older.

6. I believe I could be happy in more than one occupation.

7. Even when I am old, I expect to be healthy and active.

8. I believe you are only as old as you think you are.

9. Age has its privileges and benefits.

10. Parenting adolescents is probably a very difficult task.

ADOLESCENCE: PREPARING FOR ADULTHOOD

If you are like many teenagers, you have daydreamed about what life will be like when you become an adult. You can hardly wait until you are old enough to move out and have a place of your own. You may want to rush through these teen years and become an adult as soon as possible. You feel eager to start your "real life"—your life as an independent adult.

You may have fantasized about what kind of car you will buy, where you will live, what kind of job you will have, and if you will marry. It's normal to daydream about the future. The period of adolescence gives you an opportunity to think about your future, to set goals for your adult life, and to begin making plans to reach them. The choices and decisions you make as a teen help prepare you for assuming full responsibility for your adult life.

By now you are well aware that adolescence is a time of rapid change. Even though your body may have most of the physical characteristics of an adult, you probably still depend on your parents or other adults in a variety of ways. **Maturation** is the process of growing older and assuming more responsibility for your own life. Although the pace of change slows down when you are an adult, you will never stop (and shouldn't want to stop!) experiencing changes. Over the years, you are

maturation

the process of growing older and accepting increasing amounts of responsibility for your own life

take it on home

Show your parents or other adult family members Figure 28-1. Ask them how old they were when they experienced each of the events listed. Then ask them if there are other significant life events not mentioned on the list. Take notes and keep them in your Health Folio.

likely to continue changing physically, emotionally, mentally, socially, and spiritually. You will also face a variety of challenges. These changes and challenges are called **life events**. Some of the major life events that result from maturation are shown in Figure 28-1.

Teens often depend on their family members for help in meeting the challenges they face. When you find yourself in a difficult situation as a teen, your parents may step in to help you. They are not as likely to help when you are an adult. Adults have to make decisions for themselves and then accept the responsibility for the consequences of those decisions. Part of the maturation process is learning to make decisions and be responsible for yourself. You will be better able to make good decisions if you know what to expect during the various stages of your life.

YOUNG ADULTHOOD

Between the ages of 20 and 35, you will experience many external changes because this is a time when young adults must adapt to new roles and responsibilities. Young people entering adulthood typically experience more role changes during this period than during any other stage of life. Let's consider a young man named Mike. Mike graduated from college at 22 and got his first full-time job. Not too long after that, he broke up with his girlfriend, whom he had dated throughout college. When he was 24, he met Kate, and they fell in love. At 25, he was offered a new job in a neighboring state, so he and Kate married and moved to the new state. Mike had never lived so far away from his childhood home and found himself becoming more and more independent of his parents. When he was 28, he received a promotion at work. That same year he and Kate had their first child. The next year, at age 29, Mike and Kate bought their first house. Just two years later, Mike's father had a heart attack. Mike and Kate now have to decide if they should move their family to live closer to Mike's parents. In just a few short years, Mike experienced all of these life events: being a college student, becoming a full-time employee, breaking up with a girlfriend, dating, falling in love, getting a job promotion, marrying, moving far away from home, having children, and coping with the serious illness of a parent.

life events

physical, emotional, mental, social, and spiritual changes and challenges you will face throughout your life

- Leaving home
- Making educational choices
- Developing adult relationships
- Choosing an occupation
- Progressing at work
- Developing a financial plan
- Making decisions about marriage and a family
- Caring for aging parents
- Planning for retirement
- Confronting health issues
- Growing older
- Facing death

Figure 28-1
Major life events associated with maturation

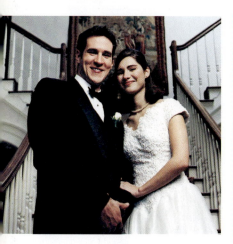

During their twenties and thirties, people undergo many life changes.

Developing good wellness skills as a teen will help you meet the challenges and role changes that young adulthood brings. As a young adult, you will continue developing your own set of personal values to guide your decision making. You will begin to set career and personal goals. At the same time, you must acquire the self-discipline needed to work and achieve those goals. As you become increasingly independent of your parents, you will take more and more responsibility for all aspects of your life.

Career Stressors

One of the biggest decisions you will ever make is choosing your career because this choice will affect many other aspects of your life. It may determine whether you need to attend college or professional school, how easily you will find employment, and how much money you will earn. If you work in a career you enjoy, your overall life is likely to be much more satisfying than if you choose a career you don't enjoy. To choose a career that is right for you, you need to consider your personality and interests as well as your job options. Here are several points to consider when choosing a career:

1. Choosing a career can be a way of expressing your personality. Many social scientists agree that personal traits such as aptitudes, abilities, and interests play a strong role in which career you are likely to choose.

2. You can be successful in more than one type of job. The U.S. Department of Labor produces a book called the *Dictionary of Occupational Titles.* There are more than 20,000 occupations listed in this book! Depending on your interests, you can probably find dozens of jobs that interest you and in which you can be successful.

3. Your level of education will affect your career options. Education past high school can help you achieve your goals and dreams. According to the U.S. Department of Labor, people who drop out of high school are 72% more likely to be unemployed than are those who finish high school. Education also plays a big role in how much money you earn. Dropouts who do have a job earn an average of 27% less than high school graduates. On average, people with a college degree earn more than twice what a high school dropout earns. So the more education you have, the more earning potential you are likely to have.

4. Career choices can be made throughout life. In the past, many people followed their parents in choosing their profession and worked their entire life in the same type job their parents had. Today, people usually choose occupations different from those of their parents. They are also more likely to switch jobs and even begin a whole new career area as they mature.

There are certain things you can do to increase the likelihood of choosing a career you find satisfying.

- ***Research job characteristics.*** Talk to people in occupations of interest to you, conduct research in the library, or go online to get more information. Find out which jobs interest you most. Learn about the working conditions, responsibilities, duties, and qualifications involved in the job. You should also consider the earning potential, opportunities for advancement, and personal satisfaction you can expect to obtain.

- ***See your guidance counselor to take an occupational interest inventory.*** An **occupational interest inventory** is a test that measures a person's interests as they are related to various jobs and careers. These tests can help you discover what types of careers might be the best fit for you.

- ***Set your goals early to obtain the job you choose.*** Determine how to best train for the job you want. If special courses or education are required, begin working to acquire those qualifications.

- ***Don't get stuck in a job you dislike.*** If you find that the first job you choose doesn't result in the job satisfaction you expected, find one that does. With more than 20,000 types of occupations available, surely you can find one that is right for you!

occupational interest inventory

a test that measures a person's interests as they are related to various jobs and careers

Financial Stressors

While you are living with your parents, they probably pay most of your expenses. As you get older, you will become more and more responsible for your own expenses. And when you become an independent young adult, your financial responsibilities will greatly increase.

Common Problems

Many people believe that if they just had more money, they would have fewer problems. But this is not necessarily true. Both the rich and the poor can have problems with money (as well as other kinds of problems). Have you heard the phrase "living from paycheck to paycheck"? Some people save little or nothing from what they earn. Perhaps they earn only enough to cover their bills, with little or no money left for personal spending or saving. Or they may spend a lot of money on things that aren't necessities. If unexpected emergencies arise, people who haven't saved can find themselves with serious financial problems.

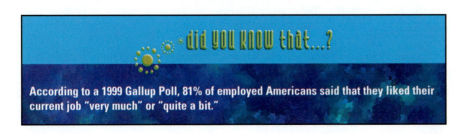

did you know that...?

According to a 1999 Gallup Poll, 81% of employed Americans said that they liked their current job "very much" or "quite a bit."

Another common problem is depending too heavily on borrowing. Buying a lot of things on credit can be an indication that people are living beyond their financial ability. You can begin learning good money management skills as a teen. Developing and practicing good money management skills now will help you manage your money well when you are an adult.

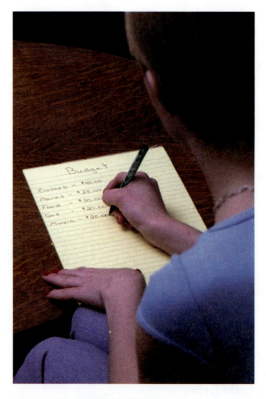

Money Management

Good money management requires balancing your expenses with your income. By acquiring the skills needed to make wise choices about spending and saving your money, you can begin to prepare for your future. Consider these strategies for practicing wise money management.

Determine Your Priorities. Your **priorities** are the things in life that are most important to you. These choices are based on your values and beliefs. They can be material things, such as a nice car, or nonmaterial things, such as good friends. Being clear about your priorities helps you decide where you want to invest your time, energy, and money.

Set Goals for Your Future. Once you have decided what is most important to you (your priorities), you can decide what you want to accomplish in the future (your goals). For instance, you may want to purchase a car, or you may want to travel with friends. Once you have set your goals, you can determine how much money you will need to achieve those goals.

priorities

items that are most important to you

Consider How and Where You Spend Your Money. Keep a record of all your purchases and expenses. You may discover that you spend a lot of your money on things that are not high priorities. If this is the case, you may need to reevaluate where you are spending your money in order to have enough money for those things that are most important to you.

Make a Commitment to Spend Money Wisely. Before making a purchase, ask yourself, "Will this purchase help me reach my financial goals and take care of my priorities? Is this purchase necessary? Can I wait to buy this?" If you decide to buy something, then comparison shop for the best bargain. Take your time to make sure you are getting the best deal.

Create a Budget. First list all your anticipated expenses. Next, write down how much money you expect to earn or receive. Do you have enough to cover your expenses? If you don't, look for expenses you can eliminate. Plan what to do with the money you have left, if any. You can spend it now, save it, or invest it. Learn to say no to purchases that don't fit your priorities and budget.

Use Credit Wisely. Credit cards often get people into trouble. On reaching age 18, many young adults apply for credit cards and begin purchasing items without a plan for paying off the debt. They don't think about what might happen if they get sick or lose their job. Many credit card companies charge a high interest rate, a percent of the balance added to what you owe each month. On cards with high interest rates, it is nearly impossible to pay off the debt by making only the minimum payment each month. If you use a credit card to make purchases, it is best to pay it off as soon as you can. Credit cards were discussed more fully in Chapter 27.

Relationship and Family Stressors

As they mature, young adults face many changes in their relationships. Friendships and romantic relationships from their teen years may end and new ones begin. Are you thinking of moving to another location after graduating from high school? If you move, you will be geographically distant from your family and the friends you grew up with. Some people find it difficult to leave their family. You'll have to cope with the changes and challenges of ending some relationships and beginning others.

Even when relationships are going well, young adults are often faced with important decisions. For example, consider Brad and Kerri, who have been dating for about four years. They just seemed to hit it off from the start. They love being together, but soon they will be graduating from college and looking for jobs. Brad is agonizing over whether to ask Kerri to marry him. "How do I know for sure this is really love?" he asks himself. "How do I know it will work out? Is there any test I can take to determine whether or not this is love?" He thinks about the things that he likes about Kerri. She has all the characteristics he wants in a partner: she's kind, trustworthy, loving, emotionally stable, dependable, ambitious, honest, and fun to be with. Brad examines their relationship. They have many things in common; they enjoy being together; and each of them cares about what happens to the other person. Still, Brad wonders how he can know for sure whether he and Kerri will be happy together for the rest of their lives.

Successful Relationships

There are no guarantees that two people will find a love and happiness that lasts forever. But there are some characteristics that help to determine compatibility (how well people get along) in relationships. In the United States, people tend to marry people who have a similar social standing. People also tend to marry individuals who have characteristics that are similar to their own. These characteristics are called **similarity factors**. The most important similarity factors that lead to successful long-term relationships in our culture include social class, geographic location, age, race, ethnic group, religion, and values.

similarity factors
the characteristics in which people are most alike

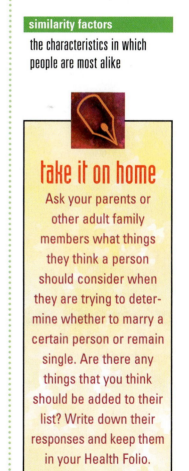

take it on home
Ask your parents or other adult family members what things they think a person should consider when they are trying to determine whether to marry a certain person or remain single. Are there any things that you think should be added to their list? Write down their responses and keep them in your Health Folio.

Relationships can cause stress, but not having relationships can cause stress, too. The lack of a romantic relationship is not necessarily a problem (unless the person wants to be in a relationship), but everyone needs friends and acquaintances with whom they feel comfortable. As you make the transition from adolescence to young adulthood, it's easy to become disconnected from the people who have been important in your life. You may have heard the old saying "Make new friends, but keep the old / one is silver, the other gold." As you become an adult, you will see that there is a great deal of value in both old and new friendships.

Entering the Family Life Cycle

Many young couples decide to start a family of their own. A child can bring great joy, but it can also bring many new stressors. Parents must adjust to a lifestyle that is totally different from the one they previously experienced as a couple. Social scientists have identified a **family life cycle** that describes the developmental stages of most families. There are six stages, and each stage has its own characteristics.

family life cycle

an orderly sequence of developmental stages that most families experience

1. *Between families.* This is the single young adult who has left his or her parents and has not married. Stressors during this stage can include learning to depend on peers for support and establishing new living, study, and work habits.

2. *Marriage–newly married couple.* The newly married couple tends to be very happy. But the husband and wife must each learn to live with another person, and new types of relationships must be formed with both sets of parents.

3. *Family with young children.* This can be one of the most stressful of the family life cycle stages. New parents must take on greater responsibility. Relationships with other family members change. What was once a couple is now a family. The couple's parents expand their roles, too, as they become grandparents.

4. *Family with adolescents.* Parents often rate this period as the most difficult time in childrearing. Even families who had little conflict earlier often experience family conflict during this time of transition. Families with adolescents begin to prepare their children to leave home. They must also deal with their own midlife issues and their aging parents.

empty nest

a family whose children have grown up and left home

5. *Beginning the empty nest.* An **empty nest** is a family whose children have grown up and left home. The original couple may need to learn to be a couple again. With children who are now adults, family relationships change. And when adult children marry, the family must accept outside members. The parents may also be dealing with the old age, disability, or death of the grandparents.

6. *Family in old age.* The original couple must face issues related to their advancing age. In some cases, these include serious health challenges. One spouse may die and leave the other widowed.

MIDDLE ADULTHOOD

Middle adulthood begins during the late thirties or early forties. When people enter middle adulthood, they may begin to ask themselves, "How am I doing for my age? Am I where I'm supposed to be?" Many people judge themselves by what is known as a **social clock**, a schedule of accomplishments they believe they must achieve by a certain age. When individuals don't accomplish one or more of the events or milestones of their social clock, they may become frustrated and disillusioned. This feeling is frequently referred to as a midlife crisis.

Middle adulthood is a transitional time. The excitement of young adulthood begins to diminish, and middle-aged adults are often faced with increased responsibilities for children and aging parents. At the same time, they are coping with the reality of their own aging and preparing for their retirement.

Career and Financial Stressors

In middle adulthood, individuals face many career and financial stressors. If one's chosen career has been successful and financially rewarding, these stressors may be minimal. When people are unhappy with their work, however, middle adulthood can be a time for career reevaluation. Individuals may decide to change jobs or return to school for additional training.

Financial stressors during this stage of life can be the result of trying to care for both children and aging parents as well as planning for one's own retirement. The retirement age in our culture varies from person to person but has steadily decreased. People are retiring at younger ages than ever before, with many leaving work between ages 60 and 65. They hope to have plenty of time to enjoy things they didn't have time to do when they were employed. If they are financially secure, the prospect of retirement can be something to look forward to. If retirement means a substantial decrease in financial security, however, it may be viewed with a great deal of anxiety.

Relationship and Family Stressors

It would be nice if everyone who married lived happily ever after, but this ideal is not always the case. When two people marry, they face many problems and challenges together. Sometimes these troubles become overwhelming to one or both of the spouses. Although marital challenges can occur early in a marriage, they often happen when the couple reaches middle adulthood.

Common Marital Challenges

Here are some of the most common marital challenges that may lead to divorce.

> **social clock**
>
> a schedule of accomplishments a person believes he or she can or should achieve by a certain age

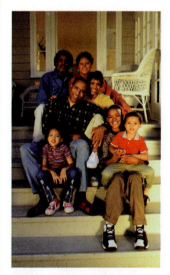

Middle adulthood is often a transitional time, with couples raising a family, dealing with their own aging, and often taking care of their parents, who may be facing health problems.

- *Unrealistic expectations.* When one of the partners has expectations of the other partner that are unrealistic, frustration and disappointment can occur. Unrealistic expectations can include role expectations. For instance, a husband may expect his wife to do all of the housework and cooking. She, on the other hand, may expect him to share those duties. Their conflicting expectations can result in a power struggle that leads to marital discontent.

- *Poor communication skills.* Poor communication is another common reason for divorce. To have a satisfying marriage, couples must recognize and resolve conflict in a positive manner in which both people feel like winners.

- *Work and career issues.* If one or both spouses are unhappy in their job, this unhappiness often shows up at home. Spouses may disagree about the amount of time that should be allocated to work or career and the amount of time that should be devoted to the needs of the family, particularly if there are children.

- *Financial difficulties.* Disagreement about how to spend money is one of the most common reasons for marital conflict. Couples who work together to make joint decisions about spending have fewer divorces than those who don't.

- *Problems with in-laws.* In-laws sometimes interfere in a marriage. Even if this interference is unintentional, it can create a lot of pressure for a couple. The spouse of the person whose parent is interfering may become resentful. The person whose parent is interfering may not know how to handle the situation without creating stress in his or her relationship with the parents.

- *Infidelity.* One or both partners' being unfaithful to the marriage commitment can create a great deal of emotional pain. This pain and the resulting lack of trust often cause marriages to dissolve.

Deciding to seek a divorce is usually very difficult for both spouses. In fact, it is common for the decision to divorce to be postponed repeatedly. It does not usually result from one incident but from a long chain of events. Adjusting to a divorce can be difficult for both spouses and for the children involved. It often causes frustration, conflict, pressure, and changes in the living situation. Most people who divorce eventually remarry. Unfortunately, divorce rates are even higher for second marriages than for first marriages. Some positive things about remarriages, however, are that partners often demonstrate better skills in conflict resolution and communication, and they share more of the housework and childrearing duties.

Childrearing

Childrearing can be a major family stressor during middle adulthood because this is often the time when the children are adolescents. As a teen, you probably realize how challenging it is for both you and your

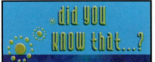

did you know that...?

According to National Center for Health Statistics data from 1990, the median age at first marriage was 24 for women and 25.9 for men. Both men and women are waiting longer to get married than in the past. The woman's median age for first birth has also risen, from 21.4 years in 1970 to almost 25 years in 2000. This trend is true in most of the developed countries of the world. In Switzerland, for example, the woman's median age for first birth in 2000 was 29 years old.

family as you are establishing your own separate independent identity. Shifting hormone levels during adolescence contribute to volatile emotions and mood swings. It can be difficult for parents to watch their teenage children deal with the challenges of adolescence.

Parents must prepare their adolescent emotionally and intellectually for life as an adult. They want their teens to be ready to live away from home, but, at the same time, they may still think of them as children. Some parents expect to help their children financially, so they can attend college or technical school. And parents today worry about their children growing up in a world threatened by violence in schools, bioterrorism, and the threat of nuclear weapons. In the midst of these concerns, parents may also be confronting their own personal challenges of middle adulthood and thinking about preparing for their upcoming retirement. The next time you say or think, "I'll never treat my kids like my parents treat me!" remember how much pressure there is on parents of teens today.

OLDER ADULTHOOD

The process of aging affects individuals physically, mentally, emotionally, and socially. Some people accept the effects of aging gracefully and learn to make the most of their later years. Others try to fight the aging process and end up depressed and frustrated.

The results of aging are more difficult for some people than for others. For example, serious health issues or financial difficulties can make older adulthood especially challenging. Learning now about the aging process and understanding upcoming life changes can influence your health and well-being as you become an older adult. The study of aging is called **gerontology**, and a scientist who studies aging is called a **gerontologist**. This is an important field of study because the elderly population is growing larger every year. In 2000, people over 65 represented about 13% of the total population in the United States. By 2050, about 20% of the population is expected to be over the age of 65.

In our culture, elderly people face many stressors. One of these stressors is ageism. **Ageism** is discrimination based on age and takes many forms. An example of ageism is the custom of requiring older Americans to retire at a certain age because of false beliefs about the competency of older people.

One of the best-known organizations formed by the elderly to fight ageism is the Gray Panthers, a political group. The Gray Panthers was formed in the 1970s and now has more than 15,000 members across the United States. Other organizations that fight ageism and do research on aging are the National Institute on Aging, the Administration on Aging, the National Council on Aging, and the American Association of Retired Persons.

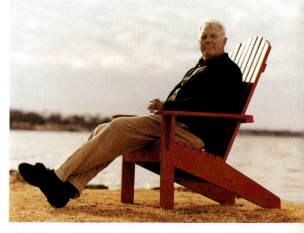

Older adults face many stressors, including ageism but organizations such as the Gray Panthers are working to fight ageism.

gerontology
the study of aging

gerontologist
a scientist who studies aging

ageism
discrimination based on age

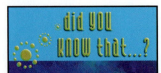

retiree

a person who is retired from an occupation

Career and Financial Stressors

Many older adults retire from their job at around age 65. If they planned ahead for their retirement, they are likely to adjust easily and enjoy their free time. A good retirement plan includes financial planning and goal setting.

Financial Planning

Financial planning means saving and investing regularly during the years you work in order to ensure a steady and reasonable income during the retirement years. Many companies have a retirement plan that allows workers to invest while they are employed. Government workers and state public employees, such as teachers, may be covered by a retirement plan. At certain ages, former employees can start drawing a living allowance from these various kinds of plans.

Goal Setting

Before people retire, they should decide what they want to accomplish during their retirement. These goals usually involve activities that keep the retiree occupied in a productive life. A **retiree** is a person who is retired from an occupation. People who retire without anything to do often end up bored and depressed.

Relationship and Family Stressors

As adults grow older, their children become grown adults and have families of their own. The parents now become grandparents and may eventually need extra help in performing their daily activities. When aging parents need extra help, the previous roles of the parents and children are reversed. The children become caregivers, and the older adults are the recipients of their care. These new roles can create stress for both the parents and the adult children. One or more of the adult children may have to assume a great deal of responsibility for their parents. In some cases, elderly parents move into the same house with their children. Some adult children decide to quit their job to care for their parents. For those adult children who work outside the home, elder adult day-care centers provide assistance. These centers are much like child day-care centers, providing a safe environment, activi-

What's News?

Scientists have discovered that a hormone called tumor necrosis factor (TNF) plays a role in aging. Healthy, active elderly people have a very low level of TNF, whereas people who are invalids have high levels of TNF. More research is needed to learn what causes the body to make this hormone.

real teens

Randy can't believe his neighbors! Why, they're more active than most of his friends! Every morning after breakfast, Mr. Saxon and his wife go for an hour-long walk together around the neighborhood. Mr. Saxon volunteers at the local library and is a handyman for "the little old people" at his church. In his free time, he builds furniture in his garage workshop. Three days a week, Mrs. Saxon cooks a large lunch. She divides it into small containers, and she and Mr. Saxon take the food to "the little old ladies at church." She's a whiz at working crossword puzzles and keeps up with her friends through e-mail. The Saxons' activities may not seem all that exceptional until you learn their ages. Mrs. Saxon is 81 years old and her husband is 83. Their children say they have to book appointments far in advance to spend time with their parents because they're so busy! Randy feels really lucky because Mr. Saxon is teaching him how to build bookshelves for his room. When they're finished with that project, Mr. Saxon says Randy will be able to build a computer desk (with a little help from him, of course). Randy hopes he'll be as active as Mr. and Mrs. Saxon when he's in his eighties!

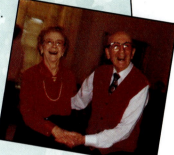

ties, and meals during the day. Adult children drop their elderly parents off at the centers in the morning on their way to work and pick them up in the afternoon on their way home.

Older couples who don't have children lack this potential support structure. They may have to rely on friends or other family members if they need assistance. One of the major challenges of the older adulthood years is accepting the fact that you are no longer able to be as independent as you once were.

Health Stressors

As people age, their body begins to change in many ways:

- *Changes in appearance.* Some older adults shrink in height. Their skin wrinkles and sags. They may begin balding, or their hair may turn gray.

- *Changes in taste, smell, hearing, and vision.* About a third of the elderly suffer hearing loss that requires corrective treatment. Vision often becomes weaker, and the senses of taste and smell diminish.

- *Diseases.* Older adults may begin to experience age-related diseases such as osteoporosis and arthritis. **Osteoporosis** is a thinning of the bones that results in their breaking easily. Arthritis is inflammation of the joints that causes painful swelling and stiffness.

osteoporosis

a thinning of the bones that results in their breaking easily

- *Changes in health status.* Organs of the body don't work as well as people age. Illnesses can affect older people more severely than younger people.

- *Cognitive changes.* Memory can decline as the aging process advances. The elderly may not remember things as easily as they did in the past. Learning and problem solving may become more difficult.

Although many of these changes occur naturally as part of the aging process, staying active both physically and mentally can help to slow the changes. Keeping active and practicing wellness behaviors throughout life have been shown to prevent many of the chronic diseases that affect older adults. It's never too early to start building the foundation for a healthy adulthood that extends into a happy old age.

Dealing with Death

One of the inevitable consequences of growing old is the fact that all human beings eventually die. Death is not a pleasant subject for most people, but it is something that has to be dealt with. Developing an understanding of death and the grieving process that goes with it is a healthy addition to any wellness plan.

Psychologists have studied death and dying for many years. The pioneering work on the dying process was done by Dr. Elisabeth Kubler-Ross. She studied people with terminal illnesses and found that there appeared to be five specific stages that most of them passed through as they were dying.

- *Denial.* The person doesn't accept the news that death is predicted by medical tests. Many people think that the diagnosis is wrong or theat the tests belong to someone else.

- *Anger.* The person lashes out because he or she does not want to face the inevitable. The anger may be directed toward hospital personnel, family members, or friends.

- *Bargaining.* The person may turn to prayer for help to find a cure for the condition. In essence, the person seeks a cure in exchange for promising to lead a better life.

- *Depression.* The person may withdraw to a very personal space and refuse visitors. During this time, they need the time to accept the reality that they will die.

- *Acceptance.* The person finally accepts the impending outcome and reaches a peaceful condition.

It is important to note that not every dying person passes through all these stages, and some people may float back and forth among the stages. Not every person acts the same, but all terminally ill people exhibit characteristics of some of these stages. Understanding the process can help you better respond to someone who needs help and understanding during a difficult time.

Grieving

Everyone responds to someone's death in their own way. Generally, we respond to death in a manner that reflects the values and personality of our family, and we may express our grief by participating in rituals and ceremonies defined by cultural and religious customs. These activities are designed to celebrate the deceased and help us overcome the loss.

Adults show grief much differently than do young children. Children generally do not understand the permanence of death until they become teenagers. A four-year-old, for example, may believe death is reversible and that the deceased person will return later. The grief response becomes deeper as a person gets older, largely due to the years of connection to the deceased and a mature understanding of the grieving process.

BUILDING YOUR Wellness Plan

As you age and mature, you will have stressors that correspond to the various stages of your life. Throughout your life, you will face career, financial, relationship, and family stressors. You may face health stressors as well, especially in later life. The stressors of adulthood are very different from the stressors of the teen years. Knowing what future stressors to expect and how to recognize them will help you lead a healthy, happy life. Here are some things to consider for your wellness plan.

- Consider which stressors you are most likely to face in each stage of adulthood.
- List some ways you might work through those stressors.
- Think about what you can do *now* as a teen to prepare for future stressors.
- List ways you can help your parents or grandparents either now or in the future.

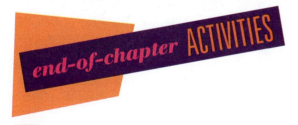

end-of-chapter ACTIVITIES

Weblinks

Aging

Administration on Aging: **http://www.aoa.gov**
Gray Panthers: **http://www.graypanthers.org**
National Council on the Aging: **http://www.ncoa.org**

Explore Your Future

icouldbe.org: **http://www.icouldbe.org** (click on "links for mentees")

How Education Improves Your Earning Potential

Bureau of Labor Statistics: **http://www.bls.gov**

Popular Jobs in the Future

U.S. Department of Labor: **http://www.dol.gov**

Retirement

American Association of Retired Persons:
  http://www.aarp.org

Short-Answer Questions

1. List five major life events.
2. Name the six stages of the family life cycle.
3. List four things to consider when choosing a career.
4. List six strategies for successfully managing your money.
5. Identify some of the physical changes associated with aging.

Discussion Questions

1. Describe how learning about aging contributes to the maturation process.
2. Explain how career counseling can help you choose a career.
3. Describe some of the major challenges of young adulthood.
4. Describe some of the major challenges of middle adulthood.
5. Explain why ageism is harmful to our society.

Chapter Vocabulary

Using a separate sheet of paper, list and define the following terms:

ageism	life events
empty nest	maturation
family life cycle	osteoporosis
gerontologist	similarity factors
gerontology	social clock

Application Activities

Language Arts Connection

1. Write an essay describing the characteristics of your ideal relationship.

2. Write an essay describing the characteristics of your ideal career.

Math Connection

1. Create a personal budget for a time when you will be living independently from your family. List the expenses you would expect to have for a month. Examples include rent, utility bills, food, entertainment, and insurance. Add these up. Ask the adult members of your family if your projected expenses seem reasonable. Calculate your current or expected income for a month. How much money will be left after all the bills and expenses have been paid? How much money could you expect to save or invest each month?

Social Studies Connection

1. Research and report on the social and economic status of the elderly in the United States as compared with their status in Japan, China, or another country of your choosing. What differences are there in the way the elderly are treated, how and where they live, and how much money they have?
2. Survey your community to find out what services are available for the elderly. Construct a sample resource list that could be distributed to the elderly at doctors' offices or in retirement communities.

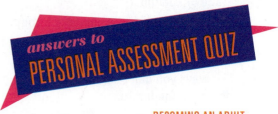

answers to PERSONAL ASSESSMENT QUIZ

personal assessment: BECOMING AN ADULT

Answers will vary. A higher proportion of Definitely True or Mostly True responses to the first five questions indicates that you have negative or unrealistic views of adulthood and aging. A higher proportion of Definitely True or Mostly True responses to the last five questions suggests that you have more positive or realistic views of adulthood and aging.

chapter 29

The Healthy Family

Ming is a pretty normal teen. She loves her family, but, at the same time, she is trying to create her own identity as a young adult. As with most teens, there are times when she disagrees with her parents. She gets especially frustrated when they don't have time to get together and discuss issues that are important to her. Ming decided to do some research on the Web to find information about improving family communication. She found a lot of good suggestions. One idea she really liked is to have designated mealtimes when the television is turned off and everyone in the family eats together. She also saw an idea for a family forum, a time when family members can discuss whatever is on their minds. Although Ming hasn't been able to convince her parents to practice these ideas on a regular basis, she has made a pledge to herself to try them when she has her own family. She also plans to continue learning ways to improve her communication skills.

chapter OBJECTIVES

When you finish this chapter, you should be able to:

- Explain when and how the concept of dating evolved.
- Discuss the importance of good communication to a romantic relationship.
- List and discuss factors that contribute to a successful marriage.
- List some of the important issues to consider when deciding whether to have children.
- Describe the stages of pregnancy and explain what takes place in the mother and fetus during each stage.
- Describe ways to raise healthy children.

key TERMS

cesarean section delivery
cohabitation
courtship
embryo
folate
morning sickness
placenta
prepared childbirth
trimester
umbilical cord

Introduction

The purpose of the family and the roles of family members are unique to every culture. The most universal family unit consists of two people who come together, have children, and raise them to be healthy, responsible, productive, and independent adults. All healthy families begin with healthy relationships. The wellness skills you learn as a teen, such as communication and decision making, will increase your own well-being now and the well-being of your own family, should you decide to create one of your own.

This chapter contains information to help you prepare for the important relationships that will define your life as an adult. You will learn about dating, marriage, childbirth, and parenting. As a teen, you can use this information to start thinking about your future and the important decisions you will someday be making. What you learn may encourage you to find out more about building the successful adult relationships that serve as the foundation of a healthy family. Unit 5 contains background information about relationships, so you may want to review the key points in that unit before reading this chapter.

personal assessment: MARRIAGE QUIZ

Let's see what you already know about marriage. Read each of the statements below and mark down on a separate sheet of paper whether you think each statement is true or false. The correct answers and comments appear at the end of the chapter.

1. The keys to a successful, long-term marriage are hard work, dedication, good communication, and commitment.

2. Marriage offers more benefits to men that it does to women.

3. People today are getting married at a younger age than they did 10 years ago.

4. The more education a woman has, the greater her chance of getting married.

5. Married couples tend to be happier after they have children.

6. Marriage puts a woman at greater risk for physical abuse than if she stays single.

DATING AND COURTSHIP

What does "dating" mean to you? In Chapter 19, we defined *dating* as "going out with another person in whom you have a romantic interest." But, as discussed, there can be many levels of romantic interest. For some people, including many teens, dating can mean casual outings with friends of the opposite sex. For others, dating is an activity that leads to marriage. In our culture, it is customary for people to spend time together to learn about each other and see how well they get along. If all goes well, the couple may decide to get married.

You may be surprised to learn that dating, something we take for granted today, is a relatively new idea. It is not something that people always did. In fact, dating is an American custom that started only about 100 years ago. Let's see how dating evolved.

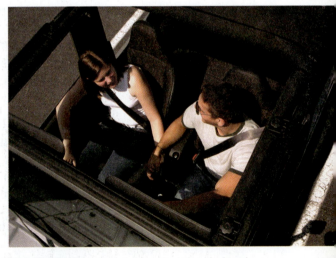

Dating as we have come to know it evolved in America.

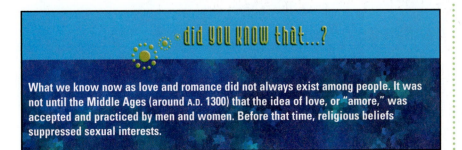

did you know that...?

What we know now as love and romance did not always exist among people. It was not until the Middle Ages (around A.D. 1300) that the idea of love, or "amore," was accepted and practiced by men and women. Before that time, religious beliefs suppressed sexual interests.

Romance in Colonial America

During colonial times, marriage was encouraged as a means of producing children who would grow up and contribute to building the new country. In fact, some towns didn't even allow bachelors to live in them. Others had a "bachelor's tax," and it was to escape this tax in Philadelphia that Benjamin Franklin married. Being single was viewed as a sign of laziness, whereas having a wife and family and the financial means to support them was viewed as socially desirable. In colonial times, marriage had a practical purpose. Love was something that developed *after* marriage, not before.

Marriages in Europe during this time were not any more romantic, being arranged by parents and based on what families could gain, such as power and wealth. If a young man did not marry according to his father's wishes, he might be disinherited. At least in America, young men were free to choose their marriage partner.

Courtship in the 1800s

Dating still didn't exist in the 1800s. A romantic relationship consisted of a young man "courting" a young lady. Courting meant visiting with a woman he found attractive and usually took place at the young lady's home, at church, or at community picnics and gatherings. When a man decided he wanted to get married, it was customary for him to ask the woman's father for permission to marry. It was during this time period that the engagement ring became a custom.

Dating in the Twentieth Century

Courtship customs at the beginning of the twentieth century began to change. By 1920, the practice of dating prospective marriage partners was firmly in place. Dating was an opportunity for couples to go off by themselves, away from the watchful eyes of parents and family. The most significant influence on the growth of dating customs was the invention of the automobile, which gave young people the freedom to meet and spend time together away from their homes. There were also social factors that contributed to the practice of dating. For example, young women broke away from parental control and socialized with men at gatherings outside their homes.

MARRIAGE

What do you think of when you hear the word *marriage*? Perhaps you picture a wedding ceremony. Or you may think about a couple you know who have been together for many years.

Marriage has been the cornerstone of the family unit for centuries. In the past, marriages joined two people legally and spiritually for the purpose of having children. Until fairly recently, marriages were

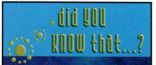

did you know that...?

In 1950, the median age of first marriage was at its lowest point in U.S. history: age 22 for men and age 20 for women.

"children centered," meaning that they took place to create a family. Children-centered marriages were characterized by:

- More than two children in the family
- One parent, almost always the mother, staying home with the children while the other parent worked
- The couple doing all they could to keep the marriage together, even if the relationship weakened, so the children could be raised in an intact family

After more than a century of social evolution, marriages today are very different. Current research shows that marriages are not primarily for the purpose of having children; rather, they are more "parent centered." Parent-centered marriages are characterized by:

- No more than two children, if any
- Both parents working outside the home and relying on other people to care for the children
- Parents sometimes choosing to divorce rather than "sticking it out for the sake of the kids"

Deciding to Marry

You may believe, as many people do, that marriage is about two people being in love, sharing a home, and living "happily ever after." This is certainly the ideal toward which couples strive, but good marriages don't just happen; they require planning, communication, and commitment. Marriage should be the natural outcome of a couple's caring for each other enough to want to spend a lifetime together. The truth is that most couples enter marriage without being well prepared for the reality of life together. In fact, most couples put more time and energy into planning the 20-minute wedding ceremony and party afterward than they put into preparing for a lifetime as a couple.

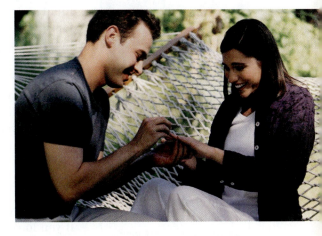

The decision to get married is a serious one, involving a lifetime commitment, and should be considered very carefully. An important first step to ensuring a successful marriage is for the couple to think about and discuss how

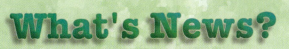

What's News?

New research indicates that men are less interested in marriage than they were years ago. Why? Because couples are more willing to live together, and men are comfortable with this living together and the sexual relationships that go with it without the legal entanglements.

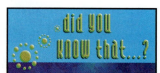

teen forum

Cost of Getting Married

Do you know how much a wedding ceremony and reception cost? You may want to do some research. What you find may surprise you. On a recent television show, a couple was in disagreement because the bride-to-be wanted a luxurious wedding that would put them $45,000 in debt.

• How do you feel about borrowing that much money for a wedding?

• How much do you think you would spend on a wedding?

ready each is to accept the responsibilities of marriage. They should spend enough time together to get to know each other very well. And there are some key issues that should be discussed and resolved *before* wedding plans are made:

• *Promise of commitment.* When two people marry, they commit themselves to each other for a lifetime. Commitment also means they support each other unconditionally.

• *Agreement about life goals.* The couple should share the same goals for the relationship. Does one of the partners want to attend school? Do both want to buy a house? Do both want children?

• *Agreement on roles.* Deciding in advance who will do what in the marriage will help the couple answer questions that range from "Who will pay the bills?" to "If one of us gets offered a job in another city, what will we do?"

• *Acceptance of lifestyle change.* When two people blend their lives, they create a new relationship. Sharing your life with another person is quite different from being single.

• *Financial considerations.* There is no set amount of money needed for a good marriage, but the couple should feel confident they have sufficient financial resources to get their marriage off to a good start. They should also feel they have the ability to plan their financial future and control their spending responsibly.

Couples who base their decision to marry on love and commitment and who prepare well for their life together have a greater chance for success than couples who do not. Some couples struggle because they get married for the wrong reason. Examples include financial gain, sex, or escape from an unhappy home situation. Some people marry the first person who finds them attractive because they don't believe anyone else ever will. They believe they better take what they can get. Other people marry despite being in a bad relationship, such as one in which they are already living with an abusive person and believe they have nowhere else to go.

Responsibilities in Marriage

Imagine yourself some years in the future thinking about marriage. If you look carefully at this special relationship, you see that it actually has three parts: you, your partner, and the relationship itself. Each partner has a responsibility to each part. Let's look more closely at each part:

• You have a responsibility for your own needs. You need to take care of yourself and develop the life skills needed to be an *independent* person in a *dependent* relationship. For example, you take time to get physical exercise and practice other wellness habits.

• You have a responsibility for your partner's needs. This doesn't mean that you do everything for that person, but rather, that you are

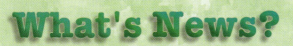

What's News?

The **Monitoring the Future Survey** reports that 64% of the female and 57% of the male teens surveyed believed that a good marriage and family life are "extremely important." Also reported was the fact that most males and females who planned to marry expected to stay married for life.

sensitive to his or her feelings, problems, and needs. Doing extra work around the house if your spouse has to study for a test is an example.

- You have a responsibility to the relationship. Each of the partners must act in support of the relationship. If one partner believes they need to save money and the other wants to make a major purchase, they should talk it out and find a solution that is best for the relationship, meaning for both partners, in the long run.

Living Together before Marriage

Living together before marriage, known as **cohabitation**, is a trend that started in the 1970s. Several factors contributed to the growth of this practice. First, the divorce rate in the United States was rising quickly at that time. Young people thought it made sense for couples to live together and "test" their compatibility for marriage. If all went well after living together for a while, then they would marry. A second reason was

cohabitation

two persons living together as if they were married

At a workshop, married couples were asked to name one thing that would strengthen a marriage. Here are some of the recommendations:

1. **Communicate. Communicate. Communicate.**

2. **Be best friends first. Keep the friendship alive each day.**

3. **Don't do anything to violate the trust and safe feeling of being together.**

4. **Always maintain an open mind and listen...keep practicing listening skills.**

5. **No matter what, somehow, someway, keep yourself from going to bed angry.**

6. **Share, say, or give something nice to your partner every day.**

7. **Don't ever forget anniversaries and birthdays.**

Keys to a successful marriage

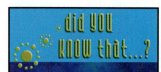

About 40 years ago, all across the United States, it was illegal for unmarried couples to live together.

the general rebellion among young people against many of the traditional rules and customs of society and their parents.

On the surface, cohabitation may seem like a good idea. It allows a couple to get to know one another and test their relationship in a setting like marriage before actually investing in marriage and its legal entanglements. If things go badly during cohabitation, they can leave the relationship and move on. Evidence shows, however, that this strategy does not ensure a successful marriage. In fact, people who live together before they marry or become pregnant before marriage are more likely to divorce than people who enter into marriage without these conditions. It may be that these marriages start out with weaker commitments.

Issues in Teen Marriages

The rate of teen marriages in the United States declined during the 1980s but then rebounded during the 1990s, increasing from 3.4% in 1990 to 5.4% in 2000. Although the percentage of teen marriages is still very low compared with marriages for the rest of the population, researchers were interested in explaining this upward trend. One explanation was the response to the "don't have sex until you are married" messages teens were receiving because of the AIDS epidemic.

Despite the trends, teen marriages are very risky. This is one reason why our culture encourages young people to delay marriage until they complete their education. For some individuals, this means high school graduation; for others, it may be earning a college degree. Completing an education increases the likelihood that couples have both the maturity and the financial means to support a successful marriage. Young people in the United States who marry as teenagers have a 60% chance of getting divorced within 5 years. Current research shows that 50% of the young women who marry before age 18 will be divorced within 10 years.

teen forum

What Is a Successful Marriage?

"A successful marriage requires falling in love many times, always with the same person" (Anonymous). There is no instruction book for a successful marriage. When two people feel right about each other and decide to commit to each other for a lifetime, they may forget that there *are* things each person can do and say to strengthen the relationship.

- Consider the quote above. What do you think it means?
- Do you agree with its message?
- Discuss it with your friends and see what they think about the words.

did you know that...?

Many of our current wedding customs and superstitions are very old. Have you heard about or seen any of these customs?

- Carrying the bride over the threshold—from 1549. The purpose is not clear, but it seems to be related to bringing good luck to the household and the relationship.
- Tossing of the garter—from 1648. Originally the garter went to the groomsmen only. The current custom is to toss it to all the unmarried males at the reception.
- Bride's left stocking thrown—from 1604. The members of the bridal party took turns throwing over their shoulder to try and hit the head of the bride or groom. Whoever was successful would be the next to marry. Now it is the bouquet and the garter.

Challenges to Marriage

Anyone who enters a marriage expecting the relationship to always be fun and free from conflicts and problems is likely to find that the reality is something quite different. Marriage, as does life in general, has rough spots along the way. The secret to a successful marriage is not finding the "perfect partner." It is *creating a partnership* in which two people communicate well, discuss their concerns, and work together to resolve their problems.

Research shows the following to be major challenges to a marital relationship:

- Poor communication
- Disagreements about finances
- Misuse of alcohol or drugs
- **Extramarital affairs**
- Differences in childrearing philosophies
- Poor sexual relations
- Problems with intimacy
- Problems with in-laws

Of all factors, the single most important factor associated with marital problems and divorce is poor communication.

extramarital affair

a sexual relationship outside the marriage

Warning Signs of a Bad Relationship

Certain behaviors can spell trouble for a relationship. If any of the following behaviors are present in a relationship, they should be addressed *before* marriage is considered.

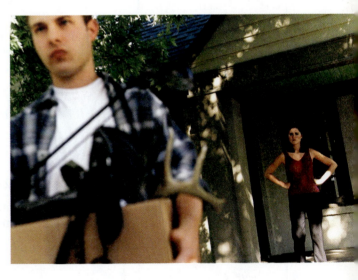

1. *Violence.* Using threats and physical abuse to resolve conflicts or satisfy needs is never appropriate. Remember, a person who truly loves someone does not hit him or her.

2. *Drug or Alcohol Abuse.* Abusing drugs or alcohol can lead to violence and instability in a relationship.

3. *Trouble with the Law.* Having problems with the rules of our society or trying to "beat the system" may very well be evidence of also having problems respecting the unwritten "rules" of relationships.

4. *Employment or Money Problems.* Discussing money matters before marriage is a must. Neither partner should take financial advantage of the other. Both partners in today's marriages are likely to work outside the home, an economic necessity in many areas.

real teens

Mira's parents said that Brady was no good, but their objections only made her angry and even more interested in him. She felt her parents misjudged him, and she was going to prove them wrong. Mira argued with her parents about how much she loved him, how ready she was for this relationship, and how she would continue seeing him no matter what they said. At first, her parents refused to give her permission, but after a while they got tired of fighting with her. They were having problems of their own, and when Mira went to court to get legal approval to marry Brady, her father told the judge, "If she wants to get married, let her." At the time, Mira was 16 and Brady was 18.

Mira felt certain that after they got married, Brady would settle down and become more responsible. But it wasn't long before Brady began to mistreat Mira, and eventually he physically abused her. Mira stuck with the marriage for a while after the abuse began because she loved him, but she finally left him and is now seeking a divorce from a marriage that lasted a little less than three years.

take it on home

It is extremely important to make the right decision about having children. You may have questions about how to make this decision and about what impact children have on parents' lives. Talk with the adults in your family to get their views about having children. Find out what it was that influenced their decisions to have, or not to have, children. Keep a record of your conversation in your Health Folio.

DECIDING TO HAVE CHILDREN

A couple's decision to have a child is the most significant decision the two of them will make. If they prepared well for their marriage, they will already have discussed children. Have you ever thought about how much children change the lives of parents? In fact, every aspect of marriage and life is different when there are children. And, although they bring great joy, children also bring many challenges. Mature partners who are considering becoming parents should ask the following questions of themselves and each other:

- Do I want to have a child?
- If I do want to have a child, why?
- What kind of parent will I be?
- What are my views on childrearing?
- How will a new baby affect the relationship with my spouse?
- If there are other children in the family, how will having another baby affect them?
- What would my life be like without children?

Pregnancy

In Chapter 7, you read about the male and female reproductive systems, the process of conception, and the development of the fetus. Now let's take a closer look at pregnancy and childbirth.

The First Trimester

Pregnancy is divided into three stages known as trimesters. The first trimester lasts for 14 weeks. This is probably the most important period of a pregnancy because this is when the vital structures are forming in the **embryo**. Good prenatal care, as discussed in Chapter 7, is extremely important early in the pregnancy to ensure both the health of the mother and the proper development of the child.

The Mother. During the first trimester, some women experience a condition known as **morning sickness**. This is the result of the significant changes taking place in the mother's body, particularly changes in her hormone levels. The symptoms of morning sickness can be reduced by eating four or five small meals a day instead of three large ones, eating a couple of crackers when first waking up in the morning, and avoiding spicy foods. If morning sickness is serious enough, the mother may require bed rest and will need extra help from her partner to take care of daily activities. By the time a woman reaches the second trimester, morning sickness usually has disappeared.

In addition to morning sickness, it is not uncommon for a woman to feel less romantic during the first trimester because of the discomfort of hormonal changes. She needs patience and understanding from her partner during this time.

The Baby. During the first trimester, the embryo develops all of its body organs and grows to a length of about 1½ inches. In addition to its organs, the embryo also develops an **umbilical cord**, which connects it to the placenta. The **placenta** is a structure in the mother's uterus that allows the passage of nutrients from the mother's blood into the fetus's blood and the passage of waste materials from the fetus's blood to the mother's blood. This exchange takes place throughout the pregnancy.

The Second Trimester

The second trimester lasts from week 14 through week 28. The baby is now referred to as a fetus because it has developed its organs.

The Mother. As a woman enters the second trimester, several changes are likely to take place: her morning sickness goes away; her appetite improves; and her energy level increases. She now has to be careful not to eat *too* much. Some women think they need to eat a lot because they are "eating for two." But this is not exactly the case. The mother needs to eat for herself and for a "very little person." Because of the growing fetus, she does have special nutritional needs: protein, calcium, iron, and **folate**. During this trimester, fetal growth causes the mother's abdomen to swell, so she now finds it more comfortable to wear loose clothing.

embryo

animal organism in the early stages of development; in humans, this stage begins with conception and lasts for 14 weeks

morning sickness

a feeling of nausea experienced by some women during the first trimester of pregnancy

umbilical cord

flexible structure that contains the arteries and veins that connect the embryo or fetus to the placenta

placenta

an organ that forms in the uterus during pregnancy to aid in the exchange of nutrients and waste products between mother and embryo or fetus

folate

a water-soluble B vitamin that occurs naturally in food

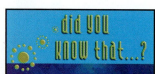

did you know that...?

Loud or persistent noise is more than a nuisance, it is an environmental hazard! Rock concerts, loud boom boxes or radios, street and airport jet traffic are all examples of environmental sources of noise. For pregnant mothers, it is very important to protect the developing fetus from environmental noise. Some studies have shown that pregnant women who are exposed to high levels of noise may deliver prematurely, have low-birthweight babies, and their babies may have a higher risk for some hearing loss.

prepared childbirth

a birthing technique that uses relaxation techniques and procedures to deliver the fetus without surgery

C-section delivery

birthing procedure in which the fetus is surgically removed from the uterus

The Baby. All the fetus's organs have formed by the time the second trimester begins, and its heartbeat can be heard. Early in the trimester, the heartbeat makes a swishing noise, but as the trimester progresses, the sound begins to resemble a regular heartbeat. Sometime around the middle of this trimester, the fetus begins to move around. This is an exciting time for the family because it is a clear sign that the fetus is doing well. By the time the second trimester is over, the fetus is about 14 or 15 inches long and weighs approximately 2 pounds.

The Third Trimester

The third trimester is the home stretch, the most exciting part of the pregnancy. The parents become anxious to deliver the baby and will decide, with input from the doctor, how the baby will be delivered. Approximately two-thirds of all deliveries in the United States are vaginal deliveries, and most of them use a **prepared childbirth** technique. Another method of delivery is a **C-section delivery** where the baby is removed through an incision in the uterus. Birthing classes are available to give couples information about labor and delivery. These classes usually teach the couple about prepared childbirth practices and explain the procedures used during a C-section. The classes give expectant fathers the opportunity to be actively involved with pregnancy and the birth process.

The Mother. Visits to the health care provider usually become more frequent as the physician monitors the last weeks of the pregnancy. The mother notices that the fetus is moving less as the trimester progresses because it has grown so large there isn't room for it to move freely. Near the end of the trimester, the mother feels somewhat uncomfortable as the baby continues to grow and starts to settle down in her pelvis in preparation for birth. At this time, it may be difficult for the mother to sleep comfortably because her abdomen is so large. The best sleeping position is on her side with a pillow between her legs.

The Baby. Although the fetus is completely formed by the beginning of the third trimester, there are significant events that take place at this time. The fetus gets a little fatter to make the transition from the comfortable warm place in the mother to the colder air outside. During the latter part of this trimester, the fetus turns upside down and gets positioned at the bottom of the uterus to prepare for birth.

Childbirth

The birthing process normally takes place around the fortieth week of pregnancy, though 10 days before or after is not unusual. Delivery usually begins when the fetus is completely ready to be born. Even though the mother is expecting the birth, the actual start may be a surprise, usually beginning with contractions of the uterus. The birthing process is broken down into three stages (see Figure 29-1).

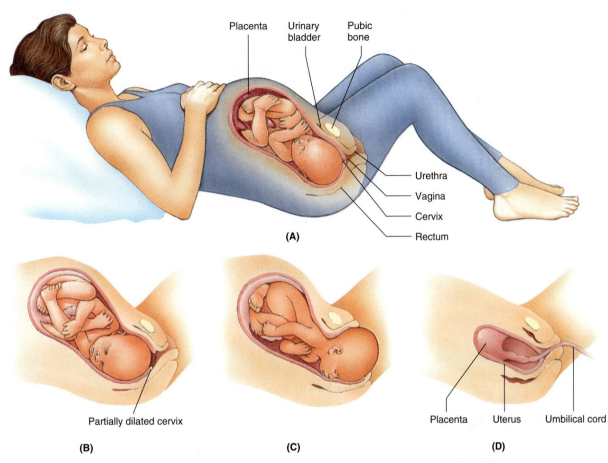

Placenta Urinary bladder Pubic bone

Urethra
Vagina
Cervix
Rectum

(A)

Partially dilated cervix

(B)

(C)

Placenta Uterus Umbilical cord

(D)

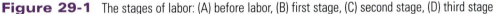

Figure 29-1 The stages of labor: (A) before labor, (B) first stage, (C) second stage, (D) third stage

- *Stage 1.* The uterus alternates episodes of contractions with periods of rest. During this time, the baby is moving downward from the uterus.
- *Stage 2.* The baby emerges from the uterus head first. The head is the largest part of the baby, so after the head has emerged, the rest of the baby slips out easily. The pressure of the birthing process on

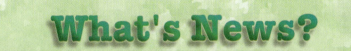

What's News?

Researchers in Norway reported in 2003 that pregnant and breast-feeding women who take cod liver oil may be increasing the intelligence levels of their children. Children of mothers who used cod liver oil supplement scored higher on intelligence and problem-solving tests than children whose mothers were not taking the oil. Cod liver oil is a type of omega-3 fatty acid that is crucial for the development of the central nervous system.

the baby's chest causes the heart and lungs to become fully functional for its first breaths.

- *Stage 3.* The placenta detaches from the uterus and leaves the uterus through the vagina.

MOTHERHOOD

Motherhood comes easily for many women because the instinct to care for a child comes naturally, and the bond that occurs with the baby is very special. It is believed that when children play with dolls they are developing and practicing nurturing behaviors.

The mother's role today is not the same as it was many years ago. Until the last half of the twentieth century, a wife and mother had the responsibility for all matters domestic such as childrearing, housekeeping, meal preparation, and so on. Large numbers of women now work outside the home, creating special child-care needs. And in many households, the mother is a single parent, making child care even more challenging.

FATHERHOOD

Fatherhood today is also much different than it was in the past when married couples had defined roles in the relationship. Dad did the outside chores and worked hard to earn enough to support the family. Mom was responsible for taking care of the children, cooking, cleaning the house, and doing the laundry. Today, the roles are much more blended. Sometimes Mom mows the lawn, and Dad occasionally cooks dinner. In some families, the couples have even agreed on role reversal. If the wife has a very good job, the husband may agree to stay home and care for the house and kids.

Fathers are very important to children. In fact, a recent study by the U.S. Department of Justice disclosed the most important factor that predicts whether a child will commit a violent crime. This factor is not education level, social class, or even substance abuse. It is the absence of the child's father. It is important to remember that it is not just the physical presence of the father that is important but also his active participation in helping his children grow.

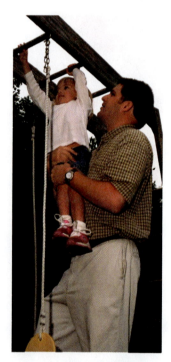

A father's active participation in his child's growth is important.

GOOD CHILDREARING PRACTICES

Raising children is not easy. Babies don't come home from the hospital with an instruction manual, and many parents raise their children using the same methods their parents used with them. These aren't always the best methods, and new parents may seek information to learn to be good parents.

When a couple decides to have a child, the *two of them* are committing to care for the child for a lifetime. The fundamental secret to successful parenting is to make sure a child knows that he or she is loved. It is important to show and tell children that they are loved and valued. There are many books available to help parents with childrearing. Some of the important and basic things to do include the following.

1. ***Be a parent to your children.*** This means doing things such as loving, protecting, encouraging, guiding, and disciplining. Be sure the children's behavioral boundaries are clear, and be consistent in enforcing rules. Some parents make the mistake of attempting to be friends with their children or wanting to keep the children happy at the expense of teaching them discipline and behavioral consequences.

2. ***From the very beginning, talk to your children.*** Research shows that children are far less likely to get into trouble if parents talk with them. Talk with your children about anything at all, even if the topics are childlike and seemingly unimportant. Be sure to be a good listener as well. The communication should not be one-sided. Establishing good lines of communication increases the chance that your kids will listen when you need to talk about really important things especially when they become adolescents.

3. ***Encourage self-reliance.*** Children need to have a sense of responsibility and empowerment. A parent's role is to prepare children to create a life for themselves away from home. Empowerment can come from a variety of activities, including not letting kids sleep in the same bed with parents (this practice creates a sense of dependence rather than independence), providing opportunities for the children to be successful, and praising successes and helping children learn from overcoming obstacles.

Support from Family Members

Couples will find a considerable amount of support for their childrearing and many other health-related issues from their siblings, parents, and grandparents. A healthy family unit extends beyond just the mother, father, and their child. A family reflects the blending of two family units to create a new unit. This means seeking and excepting the values of relatives outside the household. Other family members, especially the couple's parents, have many experiences and resources they can share with the couple and their baby. Couples can take advantage of the enthusiasm their parents and grandparents can bring to childrearing activities. Sometimes, a couple may have childrearing values that conflict with each other or with their parents' values. In these cases, it is a time for the couple to call on problem-solving and communication skills to create the healthiest conditions possible for their relationship and their child.

BUILDING YOUR Wellness Plan

There is no doubt that your decisions about marriage and family will be shaped by many factors, including what you learned from the family life you experience as a teen. The components of this section of your wellness plan are very personal. You will be responsible for the nature and quality of your adult relationships. Applying your wellness skills can help make these relationships happy and fulfilling. Good communication with your family and friends can help you build a good foundation for making wise decisions now and later. Your wellness plan should include:

- A set of values you develop to guide you through your romantic relationships. Clarify the characteristics you expect your romantic partner to possess. You might want to list these characteristics in order of importance. Identify your own expectations of romance and marriage.

- A self-inventory. Take a good look at yourself and write down the attributes you bring to a relationship. Is there anything you need to change, or are there skills you need to develop?

- A resource list. Go to the Web and visit sites that are related to the topics in this chapter, such as relationships, conception, pregnancy, and childbirth. Make a list of sites you find most informative.

- Good communication skills. Strive continually to develop and improve your communication skills. Be open with and understanding of those with whom you have relationships.

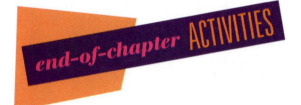

end-of-chapter ACTIVITIES

Weblinks

Information about Each Week of a Pregnancy

Parent's Place: **http://www.parentsplace.com**

Maintaining a Good Relationship

Dr. Phil McGraw: **http://www.drphil.com**

Nutritional Needs during Pregnancy

National Women's Health Information Center: **http://www.4woman.gov/faq/preg-nutr.htm**

Raising a Child

iVillage: **http://www.ivillage.com** (click on "parenting" or "babies")

☀ Short-Answer Questions

1. In what country did dating originate?
2. List the three characteristics of a "child-centered" family.
3. What is the chance that teens who marry end up divorcing within five years?
4. Name three important things a couple should consider before getting married.
5. List three suggestions for raising a healthy child.

☀ Discussion Questions

1. Explain the difference between courting and dating.
2. Discuss the trends and disadvantages of teen marriages.
3. Describe the condition of the mother and the baby during each trimester of pregnancy.
4. List and describe warning signs of a bad relationship.
5. Describe the difference between prepared childbirth and C-section.

☀ Chapter Vocabulary

Using a separate sheet of paper, list and define the following terms:

c-section delivery	morning sickness
cohabitation	placenta
courtship	prepared childbirth
embryo	trimester
folate	umbilical cord

☀ Application Activities

Language Arts Connection

Search the Web for quotations related to love, marriage, and family. Choose three quotations, one for each of the topics, that describe your views of the topics. For each quote, state its source and write a few paragraphs explaining why it is meaningful to you.

Social Studies Connection

Search the Web or your local library to learn more about wedding customs for various cultures, for example European, Chinese, African, and Hispanic. Choose one of these cultures and prepare a report comparing the customs from the chosen culture with a typical wedding in the United States.

Science Connection

Use your health literacy skills to find answers to the following questions. Prepare a one-page report for each of the topics and include your reports in your Health Folio.

- What kinds of food should a woman eat during pregnancy?
- Is it best to breast-feed a newborn?
- If a baby is crying, what do I do?
- What does it mean to "childproof" a home? How is it done?
- What is postpartum depression, and how is it treated?

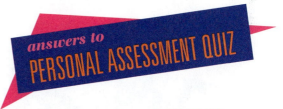

answers to
PERSONAL ASSESSMENT QUIZ

personal assessment: MARRIAGE QUIZ

Based on research conducted over many years:

1. **True.** Good marriages don't just happen; they develop over time with good communication and commitment.
2. **False.** Studies indicate that men and women benefit equally from being married.
3. **False.** The age at first marriage has risen to the middle twenties.
4. **True.** Currently, college-educated women are more likely to be married than are non-college-educated women even though they marry later than non-college-educated women do.
5. **False.** It appears that the first child in a marriage tends to bring stress into the marriage.
6. **False.** Reported research indicates that being *unmarried*—especially living with a man outside of marriage—increases her chances of being physically abused.

chapter 30

Contributing to a Healthy Community

Calvin and Eddie first started learning about the environment when they were in elementary school. The topic was interesting, but they didn't really understand the importance of their role in the human ecosystem. As older teens, they now realize there is a strong connection between the people in their community and the quality of their physical environment. They see how both the quality and the health of the community are influenced by what people do for each other and what actions they take to protect the environment. Calvin heard that the community center was running some community improvement projects, and he talked to Eddie about getting involved. They went to the community center wondering if they would be able to help and were put on a project right away. Not only did they feel good about what they did to help their community, they also made a new friend that day who was also a volunteer.

chapter OBJECTIVES

When you finish this chapter, you should be able to:

- Explain what a community is.
- Describe the characteristics of healthy communities.
- Explain what the health care system is.
- Discuss why it is important to get involved in community activities.
- Describe the roles and contributions of voluntary health agencies.

Introduction

When you were a child, you depended on your parents and your community to take care of most of your needs. As a teen, you are making more of your own decisions and learning to accept more responsibility. Your social skills are expanding, and you can recognize the needs of others. As a young adult, then, your social health extends beyond your own needs. You now have opportunities, as well as the ability, to help make your community a better place. The quality of life in your neighborhood, town, or city is a reflection of the positive actions people take, both individually and collectively. This chapter defines communities, explains what makes a healthy community, and tells how the actions of individuals, working together, contribute to community wellness.

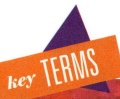

key TERMS

anti-drug coalition
economic development
voluntary health agency

personal assessment: ARE YOU A GOOD VOLUNTEER?

Strong, healthy communities have many people who volunteer to help make the community a better place for everyone. Read each of the questions below and choose the response that most closely describes you. Record your responses and the scores they represent on a separate sheet of paper. The answers are located at the end of the chapter. 1 = Definitely True; 2 = Mostly True; 3 = Mostly False; 4 = Definitely False

1. I enjoy talking with my neighbors.

2. If a friend asks a favor of me, I am willing to help.

3. I think it's important to keep my house and property clean.

4. I do things for other people.

5. I see other people doing volunteer work.

6. I appreciate the things my community has to offer.

WHAT IS A COMMUNITY?

What do you think of when you hear the word *community*? Perhaps you picture a town with houses, schools, businesses, and lots of people. Actually, there are many kinds of communities. They range in size from just a few people to entire countries. Each of us belongs to many communities, such as our nation, state, town, neighborhood, school, place of worship, and special-interest groups. The common element of communities is the relationship of the people in them—people who interact in some way and have a common bond with each other. This bond can range from a shared government to the same hobby.

Communities give individuals a sense of belonging by providing them with opportunities to form friendships, relationships, and networks. An important thing to understand about a geographic community, such as a town, is that it includes *everyone* who lives there.

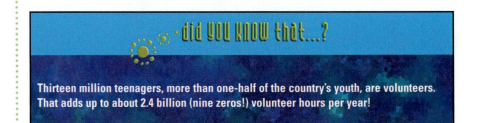

did you know that...?

Thirteen million teenagers, more than one-half of the country's youth, are volunteers. That adds up to about 2.4 billion (nine zeros!) volunteer hours per year!

Individuals often think about community in terms of "everyone else," a mass of people who are *separate* from them. Individuals who have this attitude of separation tend to believe they have little or no responsibility to the community as a whole. This belief contradicts the concept of community because if everyone thinks that someone else is responsible for the good of the group, nothing gets done. In a true community, every individual feels connected to the group. When people join together and participate, there is power to make positive changes that improve the quality of life for everyone.

WHAT MAKES A HEALTHY COMMUNITY?

All healthy communities share certain positive characteristics. These characteristics are related to the attitudes and actions of the members. It is important to understand that the health of a community is not solely determined by its wealth, size, or attractiveness. It is possible for a large, wealthy community to have unhealthy characteristics.

Sense of Community

"Sense of community" means that members feel connected to the community and are willing to be responsible for their part in it. This attitude creates an environment that enables the community to act in the best interest of its citizens, both individually and collectively. People and organizations recognize their obligations to the community and are willing to act.

Participation

A healthy community has members who actively participate in community affairs. No society can flourish if all the members of the community simply tend to their own business and think only about what others can do for them. You may remember from a history class that in colonial times, the colonists fought the British to secure independence with a *volunteer* army. All the Americans who fought at the Alamo were

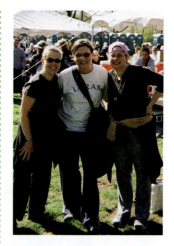

When people have a strong sense of community, they participate in community activities, such as this walk for breast cancer, to help make a difference.

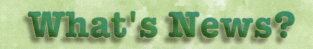

What's News?

AmeriCorps is a network of national service programs that engage more than 50,000 Americans each year in intensive service to meet critical needs in education, public safety, health, and the environment. This network received a congressional appropriation of approximately $300 million for 2004 programs and some unfunded programs from 2003.

volunteers. Following the terrorist incidents in New York City on September 11, 2001, thousands of volunteers, many of them from outside of New York, volunteered to help with recovery from the tragedy. Today, Americans continue to volunteer in many ways.

In reality, not everyone gets involved in community activities. In a typical community, 20%–30% of its members actively participate in some way, so that many people benefit from the actions of a few. How much good do you think could be accomplished if there were 50% participation?

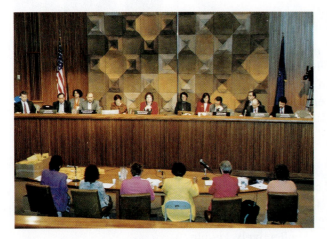

The democratic principles that guide the United States also encourage everyone to share their views and opinions with community and government leaders.

Communication

Good relationships are vital in a healthy community, and relationships depend on good communication. Information, opinions, and recommendations for improvement must be distributed among a community's members. In turn, people are encouraged to share their views and express their needs to community leaders. The United States was founded on democratic principles and respect for the views of the majority as well as protection of the minority. You may believe your opinion doesn't count, but this is not true because decisions are made by many *individuals* who are willing to listen to the opinions of others and engage in the exchange of ideas.

Acceptance

A healthy community accepts and welcomes the input of all its members regardless of their gender, race, religion, income, and level of education. Without diverse views and opinions, the community cannot move forward in *everyone's* best interests. Equal opportunities for employment, education, health care, housing, and civic leadership should be encouraged and accepted.

Vision of the Future

Healthy communities create a shared vision for their future. Members are clear about where they want to go and realize that much of what happens to them as communities is under their control. They understand, for example, the importance of economic development and environmental issues to their future well-being, and they set goals and take action to achieve them.

Resources

Community members have different health needs, and strong communities do their best to connect people with resources to help them. Large cities are likely to have a wide variety of resources, such as health centers, hospitals, and trained health care providers. Rural communities, on the other hand, may have few resources. For example, in some rural areas, people have to travel a hundred miles or more just to reach a hospital. But it is not how many resources there are that determines the quality of the community. Rather, it is the value the community puts on the welfare of all its members. Rural communities are challenged to use existing resources to develop new programs to help people.

Health Care in the Community

Health issues affect everyone and have an impact on everything we do. Unhealthy people lose time from their jobs. When they are not working, a business is not as productive, and the economy of the community can be negatively affected. Strong communities value wellness and recognize that good health means more than simply the absence of disease. This belief encourages communities to emphasize prevention and create the means necessary to support a high quality of life for their citizens.

When health is valued, a community will provide opportunities for wellness. It will create health-promoting features such as playgrounds and recreation centers, maintain healthy environmental conditions, and ensure access to health care facilities. Individuals in a community that shares a vision of good health recognize their own roles in contributing to the overall good of the community by practicing good personal wellness habits.

Health and the Economy

Communities tend to grow when they enjoy a good economy. Do you think the reverse is also true, that growth encourages a good economy? Because many communities think so, they create **economic development** plans. The purpose of these plans is to encourage business and industry to locate in the community. When businesses come, they provide jobs, and the money paid to the workers often ends up in the local economy. Businesses also pay property taxes to the community, and

economic development
a planned set of activities that encourages businesses and investors to become part of a community and contribute to its economic growth

What's News?

Recent research reported that two-thirds of the parents surveyed believed that the common cold is caused by bacteria that can be killed with antibiotics. Researchers also found that 25% of those surveyed thought they should take their children to the emergency room to be treated for a cold, whereas 60% reported they would take their kids to the doctor's office for a cold. People need to know that taking a child to an emergency room for a simple cold does not represent good use of the community's health care resources.

this money can be used to support community services such as police protection, fire departments, and hospitals.

Communities that have few financial resources, a small number of businesses, and high rates of unemployment lack the resources needed for the development of health care, transportation, and communication services. Communities with a high level of poverty have limited access to the health care system. As a result, these communities tend to receive low marks when the health status of its individual citizens is measured.

A weak economy even changes how people think about health care. Families that live in poverty for long periods of time tend to view good health as a luxury or as something beyond their control. Individuals in deep poverty don't even consider hospitalization or proper treatment through medication as options when they are ill. Instead, they may rely on less expensive, alternative medicines such as "home remedies." These remedies will be fine for mild illnesses such as the common cold. But problems may arise when home remedies are used to treat serious ailments, such as pneumonia, tuberculosis, or cancer.

Health and the Environment

What do you think about when you hear the words *our environment*? Many people immediately think about the problems of pollution because of what they hear in the media. The quality of our air and water may be important, but there are many other aspects of our physical and natural environment that affect health. The climate of the region in which you live is one example. Extreme temperatures encourage people to stay inside rather than engaging in exercise and outdoor activities. The natural vegetation in an area can either relieve or aggravate allergies. And the natural landscape can affect the flow of the wind, resulting in either a reduction or an increase in air pollution. Los Angeles, for example, is located in a basin that traps polluted air because the cool ocean air acts as a lid. And air quality is affected not only by artificial pollutants but also by natural phenomena such as radioactive radon gas, which can be found all over the United States. Sometimes the environment is in our favor. Did you know that a high level of natural salts in drinking water tends to prevent tooth decay by hardening the teeth? (This doesn't mean, however, that you can skip brushing and flossing!)

What we normally think of as our environment is actually a collection of many types of environments. There are social, political, and economic environments, and these all affect the health of the community, each in a different way. If your community has a good economy, for example, you are likely to have access to health services. The political and economic environment can affect our health in ways we may not even notice. If a city doesn't spend tax dollars building sidewalks and pedestrian overpasses, many people will get little physical exercise because they don't feel safe walking or jogging on busy streets.

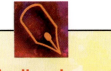

take it on home

Have a conversation with your family members about your community. Ask them how they feel about living there. Discuss the various environments that affect your lives. Does your family feel good about your living environments? Are there any things you think could be changed or improved? What do your family members do to contribute to a healthy community environment? Write a report of this conversation and keep it in your Health Folio.

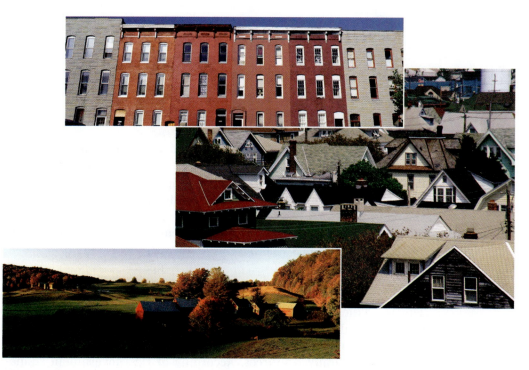

Where you live can have an effect on your health.

Community Health Challenges

All communities are faced with events and conditions that challenge the well-being of community members. The first step to improving the health of our communities is to assess what problems exist and what resources are available to address these problems. Conditions that have an impact on the health of the community include violence, substance abuse, natural disasters, and teen pregnancy.

Although some of these events are outside of human control, many are the result of negative human behaviors. Regardless of the causes, taking care of these conditions requires the attention of the community members. Even serious problems can be corrected if families, neighbors, civic groups, schools, businesses, and churches become involved in solving them.

Violence

Violent behavior continues to be a problem in many of our communities, becoming so prevalent in some places that teens accept it as a normal part of daily life. The 2001 Youth Risk Behavior Surveillance (YRBS) survey revealed that significant percentages of students engage in violent behavior. Here are some of the YRBS summaries from high school students:

- 33.2% had been in a physical fight one or more times during the 12 months preceding the survey.

- 6.4% had carried a weapon on school property on one or more of the 30 days preceding the survey.

- 12.5% had been in a physical fight on school property at least once during the 12 months preceding the survey.

- 9.5% had been hit, slapped, or physically hurt on purpose by their boyfriend or girlfriend at least once during the 12 months preceding the survey.

Communities address the problems of violence in many ways. Schools, for example, teach relationship and communication skills. Public and private agencies organize antigang programs and support the creation of women's shelters and children's safe homes (special shelters for abused children). Violence is a community concern that requires community efforts that can prevent violence and provide programs to help persons who have been abused.

Substance Abuse

The use of illegal drugs and abuse of alcohol are unhealthy, not only for the user but also for the community as a whole. Dealing with substance abuse and repairing the damage caused by drug users are expensive uses of community resources. According to U.S. government studies, the social cost of alcohol and drug abuse was approximately $246 billion in 1998:

- Health care for drug and alcohol abusers and the victims of drug-related crimes

- Loss of productivity in the work force caused by drug users' absenteeism and loss of employment, prison time, and early death

- Maintaining drug users and dealers in prison

- Repair of property damage

- Law enforcement

- Legal defense

These costs negatively affect the community in two ways. First, they deprive it of a full productive work force. Second, they drain it of financial resources that could otherwise be used to contribute to the life quality of its members.

Substance-abuse prevention has long been addressed by individual families, schools, and faith-based institutions. Many towns and cities are now fighting substance abuse at the community level by forming **antidrug coalitions**. These organizations bring the strength and resources of individuals and groups together to create a community-wide approach to prevent and reduce substance abuse. The success of these programs is related to how much time people are willing to donate to accomplish their objectives. Antidrug coalitions, according to government research studies, are achieving positive results. This is a good example of what can be accomplished when people come together to work on solving specific tough problems.

antidrug coalition

a large group of individuals and organizations that work cooperatively to prevent or reduce drug abuse in their community

Natural Disasters

Although many natural disasters take place with little or no warning, communities can prepare in advance to deal with them. In fact, communities that have emergency plans in place lose fewer lives and experience more rapid recovery from disasters than do communities that don't have plans in place. The reason is that communities with advance preparation can respond faster and in more organized and effective ways.

You should be aware of the types of emergencies your area is most likely to experience, based on its geographic location and weather patterns. You should know which local radio stations carry emergency information. As a contributing member of your community, you might want to volunteer to be part of your community's emergency-preparedness program.

Teen Pregnancy

Teen pregnancies are considered a challenge to the community because many teen parents are unable to support themselves and their children. Teen pregnancies cost taxpayers more than $7 billion a year. These costs include Medicaid and welfare expenditures, plus the loss of the teen mother's productivity in the workplace. Teen pregnancies tend to involve high risk because many teen mothers seek prenatal care late in their pregnancies, if at all. Although the rate of teenage pregnancies is declining, the United States still has the highest teen pregnancy rate, teen birth rate, and teen abortion rate in the Western industrialized world.

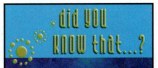

did you know that...?

The cost of teen pregnancy to taxpayers is more than $7 billion a year. The cost of STIs to taxpayers is almost $10 billion. These amounts could be reduced dramatically if teens practiced sexual abstinence until marriage. Abstinence is the only 100% effective method of preventing pregnancy and the transmission of STIs.

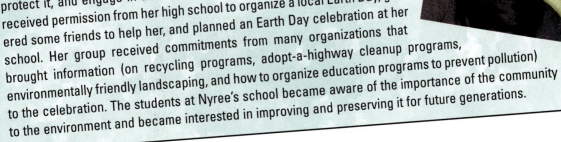

real teens

At one time Nyree wondered what she could do to help the environment. Although she had learned about the importance of the environment in her biology course, she was not sure how she could get involved in a program that would make a real difference in environmental quality. After thinking it over and talking with her friends, parents, and biology teacher, she decided that if something effective was going to get done, she would have to get it started herself. She heard about International Earth Day, which is typically celebrated on March 21 each year. Earth Day is a time when people are reminded of the importance of Planet Earth, learn about what they can do to protect it, and engage in activities that honor and support the earth. Nyree received permission from her high school to organize a local Earth Day, gathered some friends to help her, and planned an Earth Day celebration at her school. Her group received commitments from many organizations that brought information (on recycling programs, adopt-a-highway cleanup programs, environmentally friendly landscaping, and how to organize education programs to prevent pollution) to the celebration. The students at Nyree's school became aware of the importance of the community to the environment and became interested in improving and preserving it for future generations.

Opportunities for Community Involvement

We all have an obligation to contribute to making our communities healthy. Without our help, our towns and cities can't be expected to be comfortable places where we enjoy living. As a teen, you can make important contributions to your communities now, starting with very simple things such as keeping your property clean and disposing of trash appropriately. Other ways to help include:

- Participating in school activities
- Volunteering to help with special events, such as fun runs that raise money for the local library or family shelter
- Attending meetings, such as the school board, and sharing your views
- Joining a service organization such as Scouts, Lions Club, or Rotary
- Participating in activities at your place of worship
- Taking on responsibilities in youth organizations that provide teens with leadership opportunities

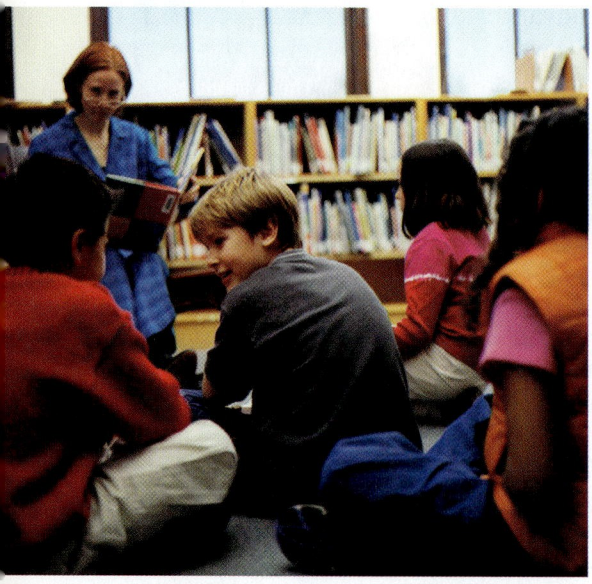

Public libraries often offer many free or low-cost programs, such as story hour. What other community programs are available where you live?

As an adult, you will be able to expand your service to the community. You will have more skills and additional experience to offer and there will be many ways you can contribute, including taking leadership positions. The following sections describe ways in which you might consider volunteering, both now and later as an adult.

Voluntary Health Agencies

voluntary health agency
organization dedicated to improving health through activities that depend on voluntary support from people in the community

Voluntary health agencies (VHAs) are organizations that work to improve health by providing patient and family services, community services, and health-related advocacy for millions of individuals who have chronic diseases or disabilities. The American Cancer Society,

teen forum

Volunteering

Communities depend on volunteers to provide many types of services. Many of the volunteers are adults who recognize the importance of helping people in need.

- How do you feel about teens serving as volunteers?
- Should volunteering be an adult responsibility, or should teens be expected to help out as well?

American Heart Association, and American Diabetes Association are examples of VHAs. These agencies depend on volunteers and charitable contributions to reach their objectives.

School

You may already be involved in school activities. As an adult, especially if you have children attending school, you may want to again volunteer your services. Many parents volunteer as teachers' assistants and chaperones for field trips and dances. Others help with sporting events and fund-raising activities. Many school districts also have parent–teacher councils that are always looking for people to help out.

House of Worship

Every community has places of worship that serve the variety of spiritual needs of its members. The congregations that make up religious organizations are referred to as faith-based communities. As does the larger community, faith-based communities both serve us and, at the same time, depend on our involvement. Individuals in faith-based communities often feel a special sense of belonging because they share the same values as the other members. Houses of worship offer many opportunities to serve others, such as working in a soup kitchen that feeds the needy, providing child care while parents attend services, and collecting donations for the poor.

Hospitals and Clinics

There are many volunteer opportunities in hospitals and clinics. Can you imagine how lonely it is to be a patient in a hospital and have no visitors? Visiting patients is one kind of volunteer activity. Others include reading to kids and helping hospital staff with their daily activities. When you are older, you may want to help the medical community by donating blood or being part of an emergency response team. You can contribute to the health of both your family and your community by learning to administer first aid.

Community Programs

Community programs are vital to the growth and well-being of a community. Many of these important programs depend on volunteers to remain in operation. Programs and projects arise from faith-based organizations, voluntary health organizations, and civic groups. Examples include Meals on Wheels, which delivers hot meals to elder adults; prenatal clinics; food pantries; the Salvation Army; and Goodwill. These programs provide free or low-cost products and services to the disabled, elderly, and low-income families in the community.

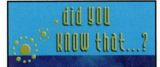

...did you know that...?

In his 2003 State of the Union Address, President Bush announced he was forming the President's Council on Service and Citizenship. The purpose of the council is to encourage more people to serve their communities and to honor those who contribute in outstanding ways.

BUILDING YOUR Wellness Plan

Developing your wellness plan for community wellness requires you to think outside of yourself and beyond your own needs. The key to community wellness is volunteerism, and volunteerism is based on having compassion for the people around you. Once you decide to become involved, there are many things you can do as a teen to improve your community. Here are some activities to consider for your wellness plan:

- Write a description of what your community means to you and what you believe you can do to make your community a better place.

- Take care of your environment by helping to keep it clean and safe for yourself and others.

- Volunteer for something related to your school. There are opportunities for everyone, and they usually don't require special skills or talents. Moreover, the work you do while you volunteer may teach you some new skill.

- Make a list of voluntary health agencies in your area. Contact them to see how you can help. Choose the one that matches your interests and the amount of time you have available to commit.

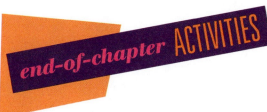

Weblinks

AmeriCorps*VISTA and Funding Part of a College Education

AmeriCorps*VISTA: **http://www.americorps.org**

Healthy Communities

American Hospital Association:
   http://www.hospitalconnect.com

Department of Health and Human Services, Healthy People 2010: **http://www.healthypeople.gov/ Publications/HealthyCommunities2001**

Teen Volunteer Ideas

Volunteer Center of Clark County, Ohio:
   http://www.volunteerservices.org (click on "Agencies with Opportunities for Teens" for ideas)

Short-Answer Questions

1. List five characteristics of a healthy community.
2. What percentage of the nation's teenagers get involved in volunteer activities?
3. List four major community health challenges.
4. What happens to communities when they have a good economy?
5. List some ways that people can help their communities.

Discussion Questions

1. Explain why volunteers are important to our communities.
2. List and describe the characteristics of a healthy community.
3. Discuss some of the major health issues facing today's communities.
4. Describe the nature of voluntary health organizations and what they do for the community.
5. List and discuss things people can do to get involved in their community.

Chapter Vocabulary

Using a separate sheet of paper, list and define the following terms:

   antidrug coalition

   economic development

   voluntary health agency

Application Activities

Math Connection

Survey 20 of your teen friends, neighbors, or classmates and ask if they (1) have volunteered in the community, (2) haven't volunteered but would like to if they had the chance, (3) have no interest in volunteering. Create a pie chart or bar graph to illustrate the results of your survey. Create a second pie chart showing a breakdown of where volunteers donated their time: school, hospital, church, voluntary health agency, scouting programs, and so on.

Social Studies Connection

Use the Web or the library to find information about voluntary health agencies. Choose one agency and prepare a report in which you describe the agency's mission, the types of programs it offers, the address of its office closest to you, and how the agency receives funding.

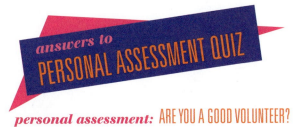

personal assessment: ARE YOU A GOOD VOLUNTEER?

If you scored between 6 and 12 points, you would be an excellent volunteer. If you scored more than 14 points, you may want to reflect on your role in the community.

Glossary

A

abusive relationship – relationship in which one of the partners uses power and control over the other in order to get what he or she wants

acquired immunodeficiency syndrome (AIDS) – a condition caused by HIV infection whereby a portion of the immune system is destroyed, making it easy for the infected person to get life-threatening diseases

acronym – a word that is formed from the first letter or letters of a series of words

actinic keratosis – a precancerous condition in which sores form on the skin as a result of sun exposure

active listening – paying attention and being completely engaged in the communication process

addictive relationship – relationship in which the object of your affection is the center around which your world revolves, or your "drug of choice"

adrenal glands – a set of glands on top of each kidney that produce two types of hormones that regulate the stress response and sexual development

adrenaline and noradrenaline – hormones produced in the adrenal medulla that regulate blood pressure and blood flow under conditions of stress

advertising – a form of communication that uses the mass media to sell a product or service to an intended audience

advocate – to speak or write in support of something or someone

aerobic activities – activities that require a continual supply of oxygen during the activity

aerobic capacity – the maximum amount of oxygen that can be delivered to and used by the cells of the body during vigorous workouts

ageism – discrimination based on age

agility – the ability to move easily, quickly, and lightly

alcohol dehydrogenase – an enzyme in the liver responsible for alcohol metabolism

alcohol poisoning – overdose of alcohol that can lead to death

alimentary canal – the tubular passage from mouth to rectum that functions in digestion, the absorption of food and water, and the elimination of waste

allied health care practitioners – health care workers with specialized technical skills who support and assist the physician in providing some types of patient care

alveoli – structures at the ends of the bronchioles that inflate with air when we breathe

amino acids – organic compounds that are the building blocks of protein

amphetamines – powerful stimulant medications that are sometimes abused to create an energetic euphoria (exaggerated feelings of well-being)

anabolic steroids – a class of synthetic drugs designed to build muscle

anaerobic activities – activities that require short bursts of energy that cannot be sustained for long periods of time because the body cannot supply enough oxygen quickly enough to keep up with the demand

androgens – male sex hormones produced in the adrenal cortex

angioplasty – medical procedure in which a small balloon is inserted into a clogged coronary artery and inflated to reduce an obstruction

anorexia nervosa – an eating disorder in which a person does not eat enough food for the body to function at a healthy level or maintain a healthy weight; it can result in death by starvation

antibiotics – a class of medications that kill bacteria and clear up infection

antidrug coalition – a large group of individuals and organizations that work cooperatively to prevent or reduce drug abuse in their community

553

antioxidant – compound that interferes with the damaging effects of certain compounds in the body; may help lower LDL in the blood and prevent certain cancers

asthma – a condition of the lungs characterized by periodic episodes of airway spasms, causing shortness of breath

atherosclerosis – a buildup of firm fatty deposits along the inner lining of the arteries, which causes the opening inside the artery to narrow and lose elasticity

attempted suicide – a deliberate, intentional, self-inflicted act that is intended to cause death but does not

auricle – the external part of the ear

autonomic nervous system – the division of the nervous system that controls basic body processes that are largely involuntary, such as breathing, heartbeat, blood pressure, and digestion

B

basal metabolism – the amount of energy needed to maintain body functions at rest

benign tumors – abnormal growth of cells that form a noncancerous tumor

binge drinking – drinking that consists of five or more alcoholic drinks in a row for males and four or more for females

binge-eating disorder – a condition in which a person eats large amounts of food frequently and repeatedly

biopsy – the removal of a tiny piece of a tumor for examination under a microscope

bioterrorism – a form of terrorism in which biological agents (pathogens) are used to infect large segments of a population

blastocyst – a mass of cells that implants in the uterus after fertilization of the ovum

blended family – a family created when one or both of the partners who remarry bring children from a previous marriage into the new family unit

blood alcohol concentration – the percent of ethyl alcohol present in the bloodstream after drinking alcoholic beverages

body composition – the relationship between fat-free mass (muscle, bone, and water) and fat tissue in the body

body image – the way you see yourself when you look in the mirror or when you picture yourself in your mind

body language – the nonverbal part of communication expressed through facial expressions, gestures, movements, postures, and appearance

body mass index – a commonly used measure of the relationship (or ratio) of weight to height expressed in a mathematical formula

botulism – a strong toxin that affects muscles in the body that can result in death if not treated quickly and properly; most often due to improperly canned foods

boundaries – imaginary lines that indicate a limit beyond which you will not go

brainstorming – generating a list of possible solutions to a problem through free and creative thought

brand-name drug – a drug whose manufacturer has an exclusive right to sell it

bronchiectasis – a condition in which the airways of the lungs become scarred, swollen, and filled with mucus

bronchiole – the very ends of the bronchial tree

bronchi – the branches of the airway that enter the lungs

bronchitis – inflammation of the bronchi (airways)

bulbourethral gland – small gland near the base of the urethra that produces a fluid that conditions the urethra for the movement of sperm

bulimia nervosa – an eating disorder in which a person eats a great deal of food and then vomits or uses other methods, such as laxatives or overexercising, to avoid gaining weight from the overeating

bullying – the use of threats or force by one person or group to intimidate another person or group

buyers – consumers who purchase a product or service without making comparisons

C

c-section delivery – birthing procedure in which the fetus is surgically removed from the uterus

calorie – a measure of the amount of energy needed to raise the temperature of 1 kilogram of water 1 degree centigrade; scientists burn foods to measure the number of calories they contain

cancer – the uncontrolled growth and spread of abnormal cells in the body

capillaries – the smallest of blood vessels, where oxygen and nutrients are exchanged for carbon dioxide and waste at the cell level

carbohydrates – food substances that provide energy for the body

carbon monoxide – a colorless, odorless poisonous gas

carcinogen – a substance that causes cancer

cardiomyopathy – damage to the heart muscle caused by long-term alcohol abuse

cardiorespiratory fitness – the ability of the respiratory and circulatory systems to provide enough oxygen to sustain moderate levels of activity for long periods of time

cardiovascular disease – a disease condition that affects the heart or circulatory system

carrier – an infected person who does not show symptoms of a disease but who can spread it to others

cartilage – a firm but elastic material that keeps the trachea open for the passage of air

cataracts – clouding of the lens of the eye, causing blurred vision

cervix – opening to the uterus

cholesterol – a soft, waxy type of fat that circulates in the bloodstream

chronic bronchitis – bronchitis that continues for a long time

chronic disease – a disease condition that continues for a long time

cilia – microscopic hairlike projections on certain cells that line the airways and sweep mucus and debris up the airway to the throat

circadian rhythms – daily rhythms, such as sleep, that are created by the body's internal clock

circumcision – surgical removal of the foreskin

claims – in reference to insurance, requests for payment that are made by health care providers to insurers

cochlea – spiral, fluid-filled structure that is the essential organ of hearing

coercion – the use of physical or psychological threat or force to get what you want

cohabitation – two persons living together as if they were married

collagen – firm, flexible connective tissue in the body, made of protein

commitment – the determination to continue in a relationship, often accompanied by an agreement or a pledge

communicator – a person who is transmitting information to another

complementary, or alternative, medicine – health care and medical practices that are not commonly part of conventional or Western medicine

complete protein – protein source that contains all nine essential amino acids

completed suicide – a term used to describe a suicide attempt that results in death

compromise – a conflict resolution in which both parties give up something

compulsion – a repetitive behavior that is performed in response to obsessive thoughts

cones – specialized cells in the eye that are sensitive to color

conflict – a struggle caused by incompatible or opposing interests, values, needs, or desires

conflict resolution – a structured problem-solving process that uses reflective awareness, communication skills, problem-solving skills, and decision-making skills to prevent, manage, and peacefully resolve conflicts

constructed – in reference to the media, pertains to the process of taking objective reality and interpreting it according to a particular viewpoint

consumer – a person who purchases a product or service

conventional, or Western, medicine – the type of health care and medical practices taught by most U.S. medical schools and offered in most U.S. hospitals

cornea – the transparent covering of the outer eye

coronary artery disease – atherosclerosis in the coronary arteries

credentials – titles, education, or training that verify a person's intellectual or professional ability

credible – believable; reliable

critical thinking – evaluating the worth, accuracy, or authenticity of issues and information, leading to a level of conclusion that can direct thoughts or actions

cross-promotions – the creation and advertising of products related to other products or forms of entertainment

cross-training – participating in two or more different physical activities to achieve cardiorespiratory fitness

D

Daily Reference Values (DRVs) – reference values of eight selected nutrients for a 2,000-calorie diet; the basis of nutrition labels

date rape or acquaintance rape – any forced sexual activity in which the victim is acquainted with or is dating the rapist

dating – going out with another person in whom you have a romantic interest

decibel – a measure of the intensity, or loudness, of a sound

decode – to interpret a word or behavior pattern

deductive reasoning – reasoning that begins with the general and ends with the specific. Arguments are based on laws, rules, and established principles. Conclusions are based on two or more premises

defense mechanisms – mental strategies and behaviors used to protect ourselves from situations that cause conflict or anxiety

dermis – the inner layer of the human skin

diabetes – disease in which the pancreas does not produce enough insulin, which is needed to properly use sugar for energy

diaphragm – a muscle just above the abdomen that causes breathing

diastolic pressure – pressure measured in the arteries as the heart relaxes to fill with blood

dieting – temporary patterns of eating that restrict calories for the purpose of losing weight

disordered eating patterns – conditions in which dieting, food restriction, fear of becoming overweight, and body image dissatisfaction interfere with normal daily life

disposable income – money that is left over after basic needs have been satisfied

distress – a negative form of stress that occurs in reaction to something we perceive as bad

dose related – referring to the effects of a substance that are related to how much of the substance is consumed over time

drug abuse – the use of chemical substances to achieve an abnormal mental state

drug dependence – a need for a drug that results in continuous use of the drug

ductus deferens – duct that transports sperm from the epididymis to the penis

duration – the number of minutes you engage in an activity at one time

dysfunctional family – a family in which family interactions negatively affect the physical, emotional, and social development and well-being of the individuals in the family

E

eating disorders – problems related to food, weight, and body image that are harmful to physical or psychological health

economic development – a planned set of activities that encourages businesses and investors to become part of a community and contribute to its economic growth

ecosystem – a complex collection of living things that share a specific environment

ejaculation – the process of ejecting semen from the penis

embryo – animal organism in the early stages of development; in humans, this stage begins with conception and lasts for 14 weeks

emotionally healthy – refers to a person who is in touch with his or her entire range of feelings and can express those feelings in an appropriate way

empathy – sensitivity to and understanding of another person's emotions

emphysema – a condition in which the alveoli tear because of overinflation

empty nest – a family whose children have grown up and left home

enamel – the hard outer covering of the tooth

encode – to develop a thought into a word or behavior pattern

endocrine system – a system of glands, tissues, and cells that produce hormones to help regulate bodily processes

endometrium – the innermost lining of the uterus, where a fertilized ovum becomes implanted

endotoxins – poisons that come from the cell wall of certain bacteria when they die

environmental tobacco smoke – smoke that people breathe when they are in a smoky environment; also called secondhand smoke

enzyme – a complex protein substance in the body that helps create chemical reactions

epidermis – the outermost layer of the human skin

epididymis – structure adjacent to the testes where sperm are stored

essential amino acids – the amino acids that humans must get in their diet and that cannot be manufactured by the body

essential body fat – the amount of fat necessary for use by the body to provide insulation, cushion body organs, and maintain normal bodily functions

essential fatty acids – fats needed by the body that must be consumed in the diet because the human body cannot manufacture them

estrogen – the female hormone produced by the ovaries to repair the uterine lining after menstruation and to enhance feminine characteristics

ethical – conforming to moral standards

eustachian tube – passageway connecting the middle ear to the back of the throat

eustress – a form of stress that occurs in reaction to something we perceive as good

exhaled mainstream smoke – smoke that is exhaled by the smoker

exotoxin – poison produced by and released from certain baccteria

extramarital affair – a sexual relationship outside the marriage

F

fact – something that has actually occurred or has been proved to be true

fad – something that is very popular for a short period of time

fad diets – eating regimens that overemphasize one particular food or type of food and contradict the guidelines of good nutrition

family household – a householder and persons who live in the same household who are related to the householder by birth, marriage, or adoption

family life cycle – an orderly sequence of developmental stages that most families experience

feedback – a way to check if you understand what someone has said. A common method is to restate in your own words what you heard and to ask the speaker if this is what he or she meant

fermentation – the process of converting sugars into ethyl alcohol and carbon dioxide

fetal alcohol syndrome – a characteristic set of birth defects that can occur among babies whose mother drank alcohol during her pregnancy

fiber – the indigestible material in food

fight-or-flight response – the response of the nervous and endocrine systems to supply the body with energy to fight back or escape from a stressor

flashback – an unexpected hallucinogenic ex-perience that occurs long after the effects of the drug have worn off

flexibility – the ability to move the joints of the body through a full range of motion

folate – a water-soluble B vitamin that occurs naturally in food

follicles – special structures in the skin where hair growth takes place

fomite – an inanimate object that transmits pathogenic organisms

frequency – in reference to fitness, the number of times each week that you engage in an activity

frequency – in reference to a social network, the amount of time you spend with members of your social network

frequency – in reference to sound, how often the material in a medium vibrates when a wave passes through the medium

functional alcoholic – a person who frequently consumes alcohol to the point of drunkenness but who is able to carry out responsibilities of daily life

G

general adaptation syndrome (GAS) – the body's physiological response to continuous stress; it includes three phases: alarm, resistance, and exhaustion

generic drug – a drug not protected by a trademark granting an exclusive right to market the product

genes – the small units of hereditary material found inside the nucleus of a cell

genitalia – the reproductive sex organs

gerontologist – a scientist who studies aging

gerontology – the study of aging

glans – the rounded head of the penis

glucagon – a hormone produced in the pancreas that regulates the level of blood sugar.

H

hardiness – resilience when confronted with stressors identified by the characteristics of challenge, control, and commitment

health fraud – claims by a manufacturer that a product is effective for treating a particular condition when it is not

health literacy – the ability to obtain, interpret, understand, and apply basic health information and services

health-related fitness – the level of fitness necessary to gain health benefits

healthy family – a family that consistently demonstrates positive qualities and skills that are characteristic of a strong, supportive family unit

heart attack – the death of heart muscle cells due to an inadequate supply of oxygen

Heimlich maneuver – the use of abdominal thrusts to dislodge items that are causing choking; it is named after the physician who invented the technique, Henry Heimlich

hemoglobin – an iron-rich compound in blood that carries oxygen

hepatitis C – a liver disease that is transmitted via the hepatitis C virus when blood products or injection instruments are shared

hertz (Hz) – unit used to measure the frequency of sound

high-density lipoprotein – fatty protein in the blood that helps carry cholesterol

homeostasis – the state of balance in which all the body's systems are working in harmony

homicide – the deliberate killing of one human being by another

hormones – chemical messengers produced by the endocrine system to help regulate bodily processes

household – a person or group of persons who occupy the same housing unit

human immunodeficiency virus (HIV) – a virus that can multiply and destroy a portion of the immune system

hydrogenation – the addition of hydrogen molecules to liquid fats to make them firm at room temperature

hypertension – increased pressure in the arteries against which the heart must pump the blood

hypothalmus – an area in the center of the brain that exerts nervous system control over the pituitary gland and the rest of the endocrine system

hypothermia – loss of body heat due to exposure to extreme cold

I

ideal body weight – the weight at which you feel strong and energetic and are able to lead a healthy life

identity – the recognition and expression of your uniqueness as a person, including your attitudes, beliefs, and behaviors

identity theft – another person's use of your personal information to create a new identity and use your financial resources

immunization – a process that enables the body to become immune to specific infectious diseases

in-patient – referring to treatment programs that take place while the patient stays in a hospital or other health care setting

incomplete protein – a protein source that does not contain all nine of the essential amino acids

inductive reasoning – reasoning that moves from the specific to the general; reasoning in which arguments are based on experience or observations rather than on laws or proven facts

infatuation – an idealizing, obsessive attraction to another person, characterized by a high degree of physiological arousal

infectious diseases – diseases that are caused by some form of pathogenic organism

insulin – a hormone produced in the pancreas that is used by the body to turn sugar into energy

insurance – a form of full or partial coverage for health services that is based on collecting a certain amount of money in advance from a consumer in return for payment for approved charges when they occur

intangible – not capable of being perceived by touch, for example, emotional aid or assistance

intensity – (exercise) how much effort you expend, or how hard you work, during a typical workout

intensity – (social network) the depth of interaction and intimacy you have with members of your social network

intentional injury – any harm, injury, or death that is caused deliberately

interest – the monthly amount that companies charge you for the privilege of purchasing on credit

interpersonal conflict – disagreement or argument between persons or groups

intimacy – a close personal knowledge of another person, characterized by feelings of warmth and closeness

intimate partners – current or former spouses and boyfriends or girlfriends

intrapersonal conflict – confusion or struggle within yourself

iris – the colored part of the eye that regulates the amount of light entering the eye

K

ketosis – buildup of ketone bodies, potentially poisonous by-products of protein metabolism

L

labia – folds of skin at the entrance to the vagina

leukoplakia – a precancerous sore that develops after prolonged exposure to tobacco

life events – physical, emotional, mental, social, and spiritual changes and challenges you will face throughout your life

life expectancy – a measure of how long a person has left to live based on data related to current causes of death

lipids – fatty compounds in foods that provide energy and transport certain vitamins

loneliness – an emotion that occurs when your current relationships don't match your expectations for ideal social relationships

longevity – the length of a person's life

love – a feeling of strong affection and devotion, characterized by unselfish and loyal concern for the well-being of another

M

mainstream smoke – smoke that comes directly to the smoker from the cigarette

malignant tumor – abnormal growth of cells forming a cancerous tumor

malleus, incus, and stapes – three very small bones in the middle ear that transmit sound from the eardrum to the inner ear

manic – referring to mania, excessive mental and physical energy often associated with mood disorders

Maslow's hierarchy of needs – a well-known representation of human needs progressing from most to least urgent; these needs include physical needs, safety and security, love and belonging, self-esteem, and self-actualization

mass media – channels for communication of messages that are produced by a few people and intended for consumption by many people

maturation – the process of growing older and accepting increasing amounts of responsibility for your own life

media – methods of mass communication such as radio, television, movies, magazines, and newspapers

media literacy – the ability to read, analyze, evaluate, and produce communication messages in a variety of media forms

media target audience – the group of people identified to receive a particular media message

mediation – a process in which two disputing parties work out their problems by talking through them with an outside person who facilitates the discussion

Medicaid – a joint federal-state program that provides medical insurance for people whose income falls below a certain level

Medicare – a federal program that provides medical insurance for citizens 65 years of age and older and those who are disabled

medications – drugs used to treat an illness or injury

medicine – a chemical substance used to treat an ailment or illness

medium – any method used to communicate; *medium* is the singular form of the word *media*

megadose – dosage that is much larger than what is recommended, approximately 5–10 times the RDI

meiosis – the process of reducing chromosome numbers in reproductive cells to one half the original number

melanin – substance in the skin that contributes to skin color

melatonin – a hormone produced by the pineal gland to help regulate sleep cycles

menstruation – a cyclical shedding of the uterine lining in response to changes in hormone levels

mentally healthy – refers to a person who has the ability to perceive reality in terms of facts and can respond appropriately to the challenges that life presents

metabolic rate – the rate at which your body uses food and oxygen to carry out various body processes

metabolism – the process of converting food substances into energy for the body

metastasis – the spread of cancer from one site to another location in the body

migraine – brain and nervous system disorder characterized by recurring attacks of severe headache

milligram – a unit of metric weight that is 1/1,000 of a gram; 100 milligrams is equal to 0.0035 of an ounce – about the same weight as a pinch of salt

mind mapping – a technique that enables you to organize and illustrate your thoughts using both sides of your brain

mindful eating – paying attention to the food you are eating and enjoying its tastes, smells, and textures

mirroring – repeating, copying, or paraphrasing the speaker's communication style

mitosis – the process of duplicating living cells

mode of transmission – a way for a pathogenic organism to enter the body

monounsaturated fat – types of oils containing fats that contribute very little to the development of heart disease

morbidity – pertaining to the amount of illness in a given number of people

morning sickness – a feeling of nausea experienced by some women during the first trimester of pregnancy

mortality – pertaining to the number of deaths in a given number of people

muscular endurance – the ability of a muscle to contract repeatedly without becoming fatigued

muscular strength – the amount of force a muscle is capable of exerting against a resistance with a single maximum effort

N

negotiation – a process in which two disputing parties work out their problems by talking through them without the assistance of an outside party

neuron – specialized body cell that is the basic unit of nerve tissue

neurotransmitter – chemical substance that enables transmission of information among neurons

nicotine – an addictive chemical substance in tobacco

nutrients – various substances that are needed for the body to function

O

obese – a term used to describe an excessively high amount of body fat in relation to height

obsession – an unwanted and distressing thought or impulse that occurs repeatedly

occupational interest inventory – a test that measures a person's interests as they are related to various jobs and careers

olfactory area – region of the nasal passage where odors are detected

opinion – a belief based on what seems to be true rather than on tested knowledge

opium – a narcotic drug derived from the sap of the opium poppy

opportunistic infections – specific infectious diseases that occur when part of the body's immune system is damaged

optimal health – the condition in which a person is the healthiest he or she can possibly be

osteoporosis – a condition in which the bones lose their density and strength

otitis media – infection of the middle ear

out-of-pocket expense – payment for health care made directly by the person receiving the care

out-patient – refers to treatment given to a patient during periodic visits to a health care facility or physician's office

oval window – a membrane that connects the middle ear to the inner ear

ovary – structure responsible for producing reproductive cells and female sex hormones

over-the-counter medications – medicines that do not require a doctor's prescription

overweight – a term to describe body weight that is too high in relation to height

ovulation – the release of an ovum from one of the ovaries

ovum – the female reproductive cell (the plural is ova)

ozone layer – layer of gas that protects the earth from harmful ultraviolet rays

P

paraphrase – to restate the speaker's message in your own words

parasite – an organism that relies on a host organism for survival; usually the host organism is harmed in some way

parasympathetic nervous system – the branch of the autonomic nervous system that slows down body processes and returns the body to homeostasis after a stressful situation has passed

parathyroid glands – four very small glands located on the thyroid gland that help regulate calcium

passion – a strong liking for, desire for, or romantic attraction to another person

pathogenic organism – also called a pathogen; a living organism that can cause disease by invading the body's tissues and multiplying; commonly referred to as germs

peer pressure – occurs when someone your own age tries to talk you into doing something you would not normally do

peers – people in your age group; those with whom you have something in common, such as level of education, musical interests, or religion

periodontal disease – loss of supporting structures around the tooth caused by bacterial plaque; if left untreated, it leads to tooth loss

periodontal tissue – supporting tissue around the tooth root

perpetrator – a person who commits an act of violence

personal identity – a unified sense of self, expressing attitudes, beliefs, and actions that are uniquely characteristic of you

phobia – overwhelming, illogical fear of an event or object

physical activity – any activity performed by the skeletal muscles (muscles concerned with body movement) that requires the body to use more energy than it does when it is at rest

pituitary gland – pea-sized gland in the center of the brain that regulates most of the endocrine glands in the body

placenta – an organ that forms in the uterus to control the movement and exchange of nutrients and wastes between the fetus and the mother

plaque – a mixture of bacteria and food residue that forms on the teeth

polyunsaturated fats – fats that come from plant sources that are better for heart health than saturated fats

post-traumatic stress disorder (PTSD) – a mental disturbance that results from experiencing or witnessing a traumatic event, which is replayed over and over in the mind after the event is over

power of accommodation – the ability of the eye to focus on objects at various distances because of changes in the shape of the lens

premiums – monthly payments made to an insurer in exchange for the insurer's commitment to pay any covered claims received

prenatal care – all the things done to safeguard the health of the mother and fetus throughout pregnancy

prepared childbirth – a birthing technique that uses relaxation techniques and procedures to deliver the fetus without surgery

prescription drug abuse – the use of a medical drug product for nonmedical reasons

prescription medicines – medicines that must be prescribed by a trained physician to ensure they fit the medical condition for which they are being taken

priorities – items that are most important to you

prioritize – rank items in order of importance

product placement – a form of advertising that takes place within entertainment, rather than as a separate commercial

progesterone – the female hormone responsible for developing the uterus during pregnancy

proof – the measure of the amount of alcohol in a liquor; a 90-proof liquor is 45% alcohol

prostate gland – accessory structure of the male reproductive system that supports movement of sperm

protein – nutrient used by the body to build and repair tissue and to manufacture enzymes

psychiatrist – a medical doctor who specializes in treating mental illnesses

psychoneuroimmunology (PNI) – the study of the interrelationships among the emotions, brain, nervous system, and immune system

psychotherapist – a mental health professional who is trained to treat mental disorders using psychological counseling techniques

psychotic – referring to a mental disorder in which the patient loses touch with reality by way of hallucinations, paranoid behavior, and fantasy thoughts

public health – sum of the federal, state, and local health agencies and organizations that work together to promote health and prevent disease for the community as a whole

purging – removing undesirable substances; in the case of bulimia nervosa, it refers to vomiting or using laxatives or exercise to remove excessive amounts of food consumed

Q

quackery – the practice of health fraud

R

receptor – nerve ending that receives stimuli, as from the sense organs

reciprocity – the "give-and-take" of a relationship; the evenness of exchange between the people involved

Reference Daily Intake (RDI) – the level of a vitamin or mineral recommended to be included in the diet each day

reflective awareness – the ability to identify to yourself what you are thinking or feeling at any given moment in time

refusal skills – strategies to help you avoid situations in which you don't want to be involved

relapse – a condition in which a person experiences an illness a second time before completely recovering from the first occurrence

reliability – the extent to which the information reported can be tested and confirmed by multiple trusted sources

resiliency – the ability to bounce back after experiencing distressing or traumatic events

retina – innermost area of the eye, where the image is received by the rods and cones

retiree – a person who is retired from an occupation

risk factors – identifiable conditions or behaviors that increase one's risk of getting ill or injured

risk reduction – activities and behaviors intended to reduce the threat of a disease or to minimize the possibility of accidental injury or death

rods – specialized cells in the eye that are sensitive to light

romantic love – a type of love that includes an attraction to another person based on affection and sexual interest

S

saliva – digestive fluid that is produced by the salivary glands to aid food digestion

salmonella – food poisoning caused by Salmonella bacteria that are found in food sources, especially chicken and other meat products

saturated fats – fats from animal sources that are firm at room temperature

scabies – infection caused by a small mite

schizophrenia – a brain disease that is perhaps the most severe of the mental illnesses

sebaceous glands – glands in the skin by each hair follicle that produce sebum

sebum – an oily substance that keeps the skin lubricated

second opinion – an opinion from a physician or other health care provider about diagnoses and treatment options in addition to the one made by the original treating physician

secondary infection – an infection that arises at a location other than the original site; usually involves a second pathogen or irritant

secondary sex characteristics – changes in the body that occur as someone passes through puberty

self-actualization – the highest level in Maslow's hierarchy of needs, representing an optimal level of mental and emotional function

self-care – managing a health-related situation on your own without direction from a health care professional

self-disclosure – revealing personal information

self-imposed quarantine – voluntarily staying away from other people when you are ill so as not to spread disease

semen – a milky fluid containing sperm and fluids from the seminal vesicles and prostate

semicircular canals – fluid-filled structures in the inner ear that are responsible for helping to maintain balance

seminal vesicles – structures that produce a component of semen that nourishes and protects sperm

serotonin – a hormone produced by the pineal gland to help regulate nerve impulses

sexual assault – a violent crime involving the use of force or threat of force to have sexual relations with someone without that person's voluntary consent

sexual harassment – any unwelcome sexual advances, requests for sexual favors, or other conduct that is sexual in nature and creates an intimidating atmosphere in an academic or work environment

shoppers – consumers who use their knowledge and skills to research and make comparisons to seek out the best product or service for the best price

side effects – unintended results of taking a medication

sidestream smoke – smoke that comes from the burning end of a cigarette

similarity factors – the characteristics in which people are most alike

size – in reference to a social network, the number of social relationships you have

skill-related fitness – the type of fitness required for participating in sports or other skill-related activities; includes such components as power, agility, coordination, speed, and balance

smokeless tobacco – tobacco that is not smoked but is used orally, such as snuff or chewing tobacco

social clock – a schedule of accomplishments a person believes he or she can or should achieve by a certain age

social network – a person-centered web of social relationships

social support – aid or assistance provided by people who care about you

social support network – a network of family, friends, and acquaintances who encourage, support, and provide positive feedback

specialist – a health care provider who focuses on one area of care, such as cardiology or gynecology

sperm – reproductive cells manufactured in the testes

sphygmomanometer – a device used to measure blood pressure

statutory rape – any sexual relations with an individual who is under the legal age of consent

stigma – something not considered normal; a mark of disgrace

storage fat – body fat that is a result of excess calories stored by the body

stress – the physical and emotional states experienced as a result of changes and challenges in our lives

stress response – the physiological reactions that occur in the body when a stressor is experienced

stressors – situations that trigger physical and emotional reactions in our bodies

stroke – an event in the brain that cuts off the blood supply to a section of brain tissue

suicide – a deliberate, intentional, self-inflicted act that results in one's own death

sun protection factor – ability of a sunscreen to protect the user from ultraviolet radiation; the higher the SPF value, the greater the amount of protection

Surgeon General – highest-ranking medical officer in the United States

sympathetic nervous system – the branch of the autonomic nervous system that responds to a stressor by accelerating body processes

symptoms – signals from the body, such as fever, cough, or chills, that you have a health problem

synesthesia – condition in which stimulation of one sense creates a response in both the stimulated sense and another sense

systolic pressure – pressure measured in the arteries as the heart is pumping blood into the arteries

T

tangible – concrete or physical; touchable

target heart rate range – the percentage of the predicted maximum heart rate that must be reached to obtain improvements in aerobic capacity

target market – the intended group of consumers for a particular product or service

tartar – a hard, scaly substance between the teeth and the gum line caused when plaque is not removed properly

tendon – dense connective tissue that attaches muscle to bone

testes – male sex glands that are located in the scrotum and are responsible for male sexual development and sperm production

testimony – a firsthand declaration of fact

testosterone – the male hormone that is produced in the testes

tetanus – a bacterial disease that affects the nervous system, commonly known as lockjaw; results in death about 10% of the time

third-party payment – a health insurance term meaning that approved charges are paid by the insurance provider rather than by the patient

thymus – endocrine gland that helps with the development of a child's immune system

thyroid gland – gland that produces hormones that influence growth and development by regulating metabolism

tolerance – (drug dependence) the physical adjustment to a drug that causes the user to require increased doses to feel the same effect

tolerance – (interpersonal) respect for people whose beliefs and practices differ from yours

"toxic" relationship – romantic involvement that results in negative consequences for one or both partners

trachea – the airway that extends from the throat to the lungs

traditional family – a family that consists of two parents and their biological or adopted children

trans fats – liquid fats that have been intentionally enhanced with hydrogen to make them firm at room temperature or more suitable for frying

tympanic membrane – the membrane that separates the outer from the middle ear; commonly known as the eardrum

type 2 diabetes – a condition in which the body cannot transport enough glucose (sugar) to the cells to be converted into energy

U

umami – a recently discovered taste sensation described as "beefy"

umbilical cord – flexible structure that contains the arteries and veins that connect the embryo or fetus to the placenta

uninsured – referring to people who do not have insurance

unintentional injuries – injuries that happen when no harm was intended to occur; formerly called accidents

unsaturated fats – fats that come from vegetable oil sources

urethra – passageway from the bladder to the outside of the body

uterine tube – passageway that transports the ovum from the ovary to the uterus

uterus – a pear-shaped, muscular structure that provides the proper environment where the fertilized ovum develops into a fetus

V

vagina – a muscular, flexible passageway between the labia and the uterus

validity – the accuracy of the information obtained

valid – based on evidence or supported by scientifically accurate data

vegetarianism – the practice of consuming foods only from plant sources, except eggs or dairy products in some instances

violence – the use of physical force with the intent to inflict harm, injury, or death

violent victimization statistics – statistics for rape, sexual assault, robbery, aggravated assault (assault with a weapon), and simple assault; statistics do not include murder

voluntary health agency – organization dedicated to improving health through activities that depend on voluntary support from people in the community

W

wellness – behaviors and habits that have a positive influence on health

wellness motives – the sum of knowledge, beliefs, and values that contribute to forming reasons that encourage wellness behaviors

withdrawal – feelings of discomfort that occur when the body is deprived of a drug to which it is addicted

Y

years of potential life lost – the difference in years between an individual's life expectancy and that individual's age at the time of death

Credits

PHOTOGRAPHS (AND PAGE NUMBERS)

© Digital Vision: 10, 11, 16, 207, 227, 299 (bottom), 350, 352, 372, 392, 508, 515, 525, 529

© Photodisc/Getty Images: cover, v, viii, ix, x, xi, xii, 2, 7, 14, 20, 28, 30, 31, 36, 44, 49, 50, 53, 65, 75, 80, 88, 110, 112, 123, 136, 151, 159, 163, 174, 184, 188 (bottom), 200, 216, 219, 224, 232, 240, 256, 259, 271, 275 (bottom), 279, 303, 304, 311, 316, 318, 320, 322, 333, 351, 262, 376, 381, 389, 398, 417, 445, 469, 474, 493, 498, 504, 517, 547, 548

© Thinkstock: 123

Photo courtesy of the Ellis Island Immigration Museum, U.S. Department of the Interior: 419

Photos courtesy of U.S. Centers for Disease Control and Prevention: 423, 437

FIGURES, PERSONAL ASSESSMENTS, AND TABLES

Page 5. Table 1-1 sources: *National Vital Statistics Report*, 50 (16), September 2002, and *Leading Causes of Death*, 1900–1998. Retrieved December 1, 2003, from http://www.cdc.gov/nchs/data/statab/lead1900_98.pdf.

Page 12. Figure 1-3 source: U.S. Centers for Disease Control and Prevention Behavioral Risk Factor Surveillance System

Page 13. Figure 1-4 source: National Center for Health Statistics. (2002). *Health, United States, 2002*.

Pages 42–43. Personal Assessment reproduced with permission from U.S. Centers for Disease Control and Prevention.

Page 45. Figures 3-1 and 3-2 source: U.S. Centers for Disease Control and Prevention (2000)

Page 87. Figure 5-2 source: Courtesy of Robert A. Silverman M.D., Pediatric Dermatology, Georgetown University

Page 369. Figure 20-2 reprinted by the permission of the American Cancer Society, Inc.

Page 370. Figure 20-3 reprinted by the permission of the American Cancer Society, Inc.

Page 407. Figure 22-2 source: Substance Abuse and Mental Health Services Administration. (2002). *Results from the 2001 National Household Survey on Drug Abuse: Volume I. Summary of National Findings* (Office of Applied Studies, NHSDA Series H-17, DHHS Publication No. SMA 02-3758). Rockville, MD. Retrieved December 1, 2003, from http://www.samhsa.gov/centers/clearinghouse/clearinghouses.html.

Page 421. Figure 23-1 courtesy of National Center for Infectious Diseases, U.S. Centers for Disease Control and Prevention. (2003). *2002–03 U.S. Influenza Season Summary*. Retrieved December 1, 2003, from http://www.cdc.gov/ncidod/diseases/flu/weeklyarchives2002-2003/02-03summary.htm

Page 425. Figure 23-3 courtesy of U.S. Centers for Disease Control and Prevention.

Page 431. Table 23-2 adapted from National Immunization Program of the Centers for Disease Control and Prevention.

Page 448. Table 24-1 adapted from the National Heart, Lung, and Blood Institute.

Index